Sirtuin Biology in Endocrinology and Metabolic Disease

Sirtuin Biology in Endocrinology and Metabolic Disease

Editor: Shay Welch

AMERICAN
MEDICAL PUBLISHERS
www.americanmedicalpublishers.com

AMERICAN
MEDICAL PUBLISHERS
www.americanmedicalpublishers.com

Cataloging-in-Publication Data

Sirtuin biology in endocrinology and metabolic disease / edited by Shay Welch.
p. cm.
Includes bibliographical references and index.
ISBN 979-8-88740-455-4
1. Sirtuins. 2. Proteins. 3. Molecular endocrinology. 4. Metabolism--Disorders.
5. Sirtuins--Metabolism. 6. Sirtuins--Health aspects. I. Welch, Shay.
QP551 .S57 2023
572.6--dc23

American Medical Publishers,
41 Flatbush Avenue,
1st Floor, New York,
NY 11217, USA

ISBN 979-8-88740-455-4 (Hardback)

Contents

Preface

Sirtuins refer to a class of signaling proteins involved in metabolic regulation. They are members of the class III family of NAD-dependent histone deacetylases (HDAC). They are involved in a variety of physiological processes ranging from metabolism and endocrine function control to immune coordination and cellular responses to stress. Sirtuin-1 (SIRT1) plays an important role in epigenetics, immunology, and endocrinology. SIRT1's diverse roles include energy sensing metabolic homeostasis regulation, and deacetylation of histone and non-histone proteins in numerous tissues. It also facilitates neuro-endocrine regulation through hypothalamus-pituitary axis stimulation, and synthesis and maintenance of reproductive hormones via steroidogenesis. Some of the other functions involve maintenance of innate and adaptive immune systems via T and B cell maturation regulation, chronic inflammation, and autoimmune diseases. This book provides significant information of sirtuin biology as well as its importance in endocrinology and metabolic disease. It will provide comprehensive knowledge to the readers.

After months of intensive research and writing, this book is the end result of all who devoted their time and efforts in the initiation and progress of this book. It will surely be a source of reference in enhancing the required knowledge of the new developments in the area. During the course of developing this book, certain measures such as accuracy, authenticity and research focused analytical studies were given preference in order to produce a comprehensive book in the area of study.

This book would not have been possible without the efforts of the authors and the publisher. I extend my sincere thanks to them. Secondly, I express my gratitude to my family and well-wishers. And most importantly, I thank my students for constantly expressing their willingness and curiosity in enhancing their knowledge in the field, which encourages me to take up further research projects for the advancement of the area.

Editor

1

17β-Estradiol Promotes Apoptosis in Airway Smooth Muscle Cells Through CD38/SIRT1/p53 Pathway

Yu Liu[1†], Yinfang Guo[2†], Weilu Huang[1], Ke-Yu Deng[1], Yisong Qian[1] and Hong-Bo Xin[1*]*

[1] Cardiovascular Research Center, Institute of Translational Medicine, Nanchang University, Nanchang, China, [2] Department of Medical Records, The First Affiliated Hospital of Nanchang University, Nanchang, China

***Correspondence:**
Yisong Qian
qianyisong@ncu.edu.cn
Hong-Bo Xin
xinhb@ncu.edu.cn

† These authors have contributed equally to this work

17β-Estradiol (E2) is the major estrogen secreted by the premenopausal ovary and shows dual effects on cell apoptosis under pathological conditions. E2 was previously shown to increase CD38 mRNA and protein expression in myometrial smooth muscle, but its function and mechanism remain largely unknown. Here we investigated the role of E2 in hypoxia-induced apoptosis in mouse airway smooth muscle cells (ASMCs) and explored the underlying mechanisms. Results showed that E2 significantly increased CD38 expression at both mRNA and protein levels, accompanied with decreased SIRT1 levels in ASMCs. By using primary ASMCs from the wild type (WT) and the smooth muscle-specific CD38 knockout (CD38 KO) mice, we found that the down-regulation of SIRT1 induced by E2 was abolished in CD38 KO AMSCs. E2 promoted the acetylation of p53 in WT cells, and this effect was also diminished in the absence of CD38. In addition, E2 further activated CD38/SIRT1/p53 signal pathway and promoted cell apoptosis during hypoxia. However, these effects were reversed in CD38 KO ASMCs and by the specific SIRT1 activator Resveratrol. We also found that E2 enhanced CD38 expression through estrogen receptor. The data suggested that CD38 is a direct target for E2 which promotes hypoxia-induced AMSC apoptosis through SIRT1/p53 signal pathway.

Keywords: 17β-estradiol, CD38, SIRT1, hypoxia, apoptosis

INTRODUCTION

Hypoxia is recognized as a critical contributor to pulmonary diseases including asthma, airway obstruction and pulmonary hypertension (1–3). Hypoxia stimulates airway inflammation and remodeling, and subsequently induces apoptosis in airway smooth muscle cells (ASMCs) during airway remodeling (4). There is emerging evidence for sex differences in the incidence and progression of lung diseases, and sex hormones play crucial roles in these pathological processes (5). Especially, estrogen regulates ASMCs in various manners. Estrogens reduce $[Ca^{2+}]i$ and promote human ASM relaxation via activation of cAMP and PKA, thereby facilitating bronchodilation (6). In addition, testosterone and E2 exhibit mitogenic effects in ASMCs, probably through estrogen receptors and the MAPK and PI3K signaling pathways, thus promote ASMC proliferation and airway remodeling (7). Estrogen signaling is also involved in allergic inflammation and contributes to sex differences in asthma and allergy (8). However, the effect of estrogen on ASMCs apoptosis during hypoxia remains largely unknown.

CD38 is a type II membrane-bound glycoprotein and functions as the major NADase responsible for the regulation of NAD-dependent deacetylase such as SIRT1 (9). In addition, CD38 is an NAADP synthase required for NAADP-mediated Ca^{2+} release from lysosomal stores (10). CD38/cyclic ADP-ribose (cADPR)-mediated calcium signaling plays critical roles in the regulation of intracellular calcium in a variety of smooth muscle cells, including that of the airway smooth muscle (11–13). Estrogens were shown to increase CD38 gene expression and leads to increased calcium mobilization and contractility of the myometrium (14, 15). It has also been recently reported that E2 downregulated SIRT1 expression in vascular smooth muscle cells, with increased apoptosis, reduced proliferation and migration, which were reversed by the SIRT1 activator Resveratrol (16). SIRT1 regulates p53-dependent apoptosis by deacetylating the Lys382 residue of p53, thus enhancing the transcriptional activity of p53 and inhibiting p53-induced apoptosis (17). However, whether E2 modulates the expression of CD38 and SIRT1 in ASMCs and the detailed mechanisms of E2 in the regulation of hypoxia-induced apoptosis have not been addressed.

In this study, we investigated the role of E2 in apoptosis during hypoxia by using primary ASMCs from the wild type (WT) and the smooth muscle-specific knockout of CD38 (CD38 KO) mice. CD38-mediated SIRT1/p53 signal pathway was also detected, with the purpose to elucidate the mechanism by which E2 promotes apoptosis in ASMCs.

MATERIALS AND METHODS

Materials

E2 and Resveratrol were purchased from Sigma-Aldrich (St. Louis, MO). ICI182,780 was from Abcam (Cambridge, MA). The anti-CD38 antibody was obtained from R&D Systems, Inc. (Minneapolis, MN); the anti-SIRT1 antibody was from EMD Millipore Corp. (Temecula, CA); the anti-p53, anti-Acetyl-p53 (K379), anti-Bax and anti-Bcl-2 antibodies were from Cell Signaling Technology, Inc., (Danvers, MA), and the anti-glyceraldehyde phosphate dehydrogenase (GAPDH) antibody was obtained from KangChen Bio-tech Inc., (Shanghai, China).

Preparation of Smooth Muscle-Specific CD38 Knockout Mice

Mice with LoxP flanking of exon 2 and exon 3 of the CD38 gene (CD38-fl/fl, produced by Cyagen Inc., Suzhou, China) were bred with mice expressing Cre recombinase under the control of a smooth muscle-specific promoter (SMA-Cre, from Collaborative Innovation Center of Model Animal, Wuhan University). The progeny with the genotype SMA-Cre-CD38-fl/fl is the homozygote used in the experiment.

Isolation, Culture, and Characterization of ASMCs

Primary mouse ASMCs were prepared as previously described (18), with some modifications. Male, 8–10 weeks old WT or CD38 KO mice were anesthetized and the tracheas were aseptically excised and placed in Ca^{2+}, Mg^{2+}-free Hanks' balanced salt solution (HBSS). The isolated tracheas were cleaned of connective tissues, cut longitudinally through the cartilage, and enzymatically dissociated with HBSS containing elastase type I (2 mg/ml) and BSA (2.5 mg/ml) for 1 h in a water bath at 37°C. Dissociated cells in suspension were centrifuged and resuspended in Dulbecco's modified Eagle's medium (DMEM) supplemented with 10% fetal bovine serum (FBS), 100 U/ml penicillin, 100 μg/ml streptomycin, and 2.5 μg/ml amphotericin β. Cells were plated on culture flasks and grew until confluence at 37°C in humidified air containing 5% CO_2. The confluent cells were passaged with 0.25% trypsin-0.02% EDTA solution. The cultures typically contained more than 98% ASMCs as assessed by immunocytochemical staining for the smooth muscle-specific marker α-actin. Cells at passages 3–5 were used for the experiments.

Cell Culture Treatment and Hypoxia Exposure

For the concentration response assay, ASMCs were pre-treated with various concentrations of E2 (0.1, 1, 10, and 100 nM) for 24 h. For the time course assay, 10 or 100 nM of E2 were added to the cultures for 24 or 48 h incubation. In the subsequent experiments, WT and CD38 KO ASMCs were pre-treated with 10 nM of E2 for 48 h respectively, followed by the exposure of sustained hypoxia. Cells were maintained in a hypoxia chamber (1% O_2, 5% CO_2; balance N_2 and water vapor) for 6 h to induce sustained hypoxia as described previously (19). A normoxic control experiment was performed in parallel by maintaining the cells under normoxia (21% O_2, 5% CO_2; 37°C). The specific SIRT1 activator Resveratrol (RSV, 10 μM) or the estrogen receptor antagonist ICI182,780 (ICI, 10 nM) was added to the cultures 2 h before E2 incubation.

Real-Time PCR

Total RNA was isolated from ASMCs using the TRIzol™ reagent (Life Technologies, CA, USA) according to the manufacturer's instructions. One microgram of total RNA was reverse-transcribed using a One Step PrimeScript™ RT-PCR Kit (Takara, Dalian, China) with a thermocycler. Real-time PCR was performed using the ABI ViiA™ 7 system with a reaction mixture that consisted of SYBR Green 2×PCR Master Mix (Applied Biosystems, CA, USA), cDNA template (0.5 μg), forward primer and reverse primer. Primer sequences were as follows: 5′-GAGCCTACCACGAAGCACTTTT-3′ and 5′-GGC CGGAGGATCTGAGTGTA-3′ (CD38), 5′-GCCAAACTTTGT TGTAACCCTGTA-3′ and 5′-TGGTGGCAACTCTGATAAATG AA-3′ (SIRT1), and 5′-ACATGGCCTCCAAGGAGTAAGAA-3′ and 5′-GGGATAGGGCCTCTCTTGCT-3′ (GAPDH). The PCR protocol consisted of 40 cycles of denaturation at 95°C for 15 s followed by 60°C for 1 min to allow extension and amplification of the target sequence. Data were analyzed using ABI 7500 sequence detection system software. The amount of mRNA was normalized to GAPDH using the $2^{-\Delta\Delta CT}$ method. The results were from three independent experiments performed in triplicate.

Western Blot

The cells were collected and lysed in RIPA lysis buffer. Equal amounts of protein per sample were loaded in each lane, separated by SDS-PAGE, and transferred to PVDF membranes.

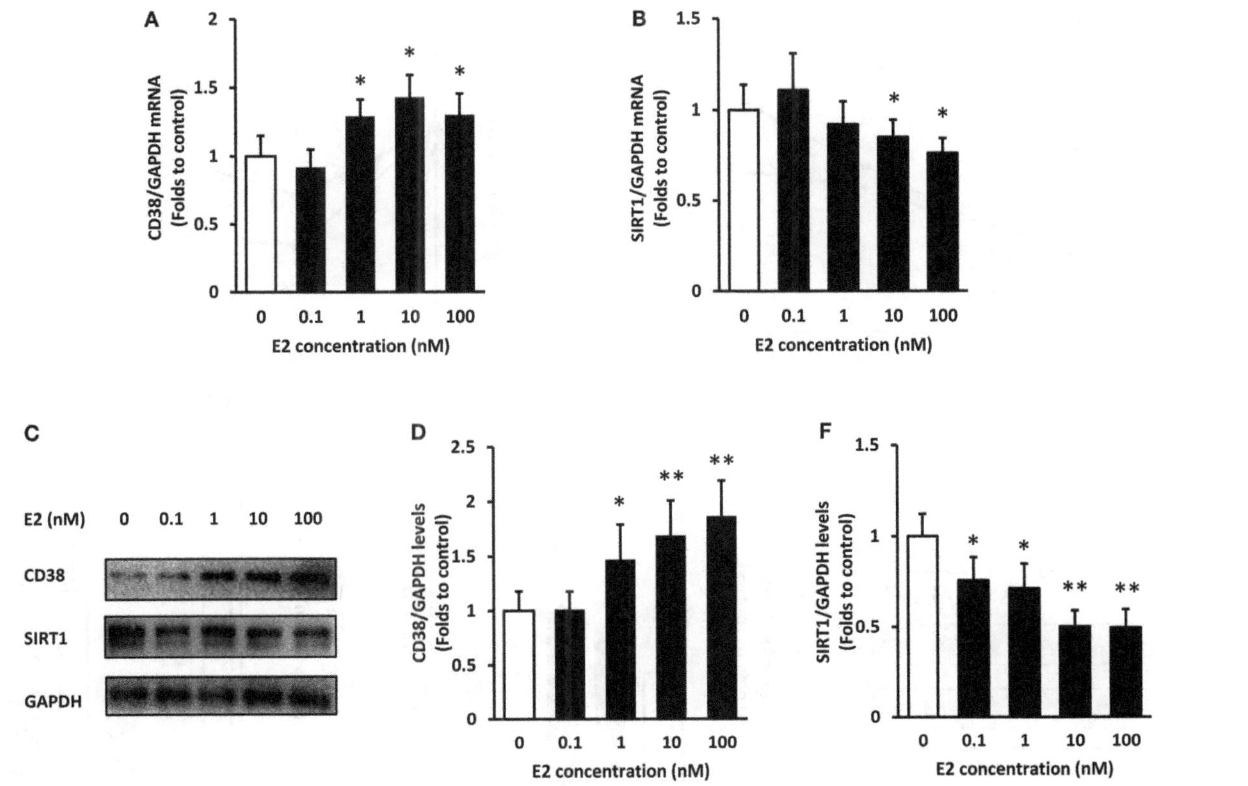

FIGURE 1 | Expression of CD38 and SIRT1 in ASMCs after E2 treatment. ASMCs were pre-treated with the indicated concentrations of E2 for 24 h. **(A)** CD38 and **(B)** SIRT1 mRNA levels were detected by real-time PCR. **(C)** CD38 and SIRT1 protein levels were determined by western blot and quantitative analysis of **(D)** CD38 and **(E)** SIRT1 levels was normalized to GAPDH levels. $^{*}P < 0.05$, $^{**}P < 0.01$ vs. the control group. $N = 3$.

The membranes were blocked with skimmed milk for 1 h, washed in Tris buffered saline containing 0.1% Tween-20 (TBST) and incubated overnight with the primary antibodies. After washing three times with TBST, the membranes were incubated for 1 h at room temperature with horseradish peroxidase-conjugated goat anti-rabbit or anti-mouse IgG and donkey anti-sheep IgG. Bands were visualized using the SuperSignalWest Pico Chemiluminescent Substrate Trial Kit (Pierce, Rockford, IL, USA). Images were taken using the ChemiDoc XRS system with Quantity One software (Bio-Rad, Richmond, CA, USA).

Hoechst 33258 Staining

Cell apoptosis was detected with DNA staining by Hoechst 33258. At the end of the treatment, cells were rinsed with phosphate-buffered saline (PBS, pH 7.4) and fixed with 4% paraformaldehyde for 30 min at room temperature, followed by incubation with Hoechst 33258 (5 μM, final concentration) at room temperature for 20 min. Fluorescence images were examined under the fluorescence microscope (Olympus IX71, Tokyo, Japan).

Caspase-3 Activity Assay

Caspase-3 activity was measured in lysates of AMSCs using the CaspACE^{TM} Assay System, Colorimetric (Promega, Madison, WI) following the instructions of the manufacturer. Briefly, cells were lysed by freeze-thaw, and then incubated on ice for 20 min to ensure complete cell lysis. Cell lysates were centrifuged at 12 000 rpm for 10 min at 4°C, and the supernatant fraction was collected for the determination. An aliquot of culture supernatant was incubated with 200 mM of DEVDpNA substrate at 37°C for 4 h. The absorbance was measured at 405 nm. The luminescence was measured in a microplate reader and the protein levels in the lysates were determined by the method of Bradford. Results were expressed as a percentage of the control cells.

Statistical Analysis

All values are expressed as the mean ± SD of at least three independent preparations. Differences among the groups were compared using one-way ANOVA analysis followed by a Tukey *post-hoc* test. A difference with $P < 0.05$ was considered statistically significant.

RESULTS

E2 Increases CD38 Expression and Decreases SIRT1 Levels in ASMCs

The expression of CD38 and SIRT1 at mRNA and protein levels were detected by real-time PCR and western blot, respectively. Non-normalized Ct values and non-cropped non contrasted western-blot images were provided in **Supplementary Material.**

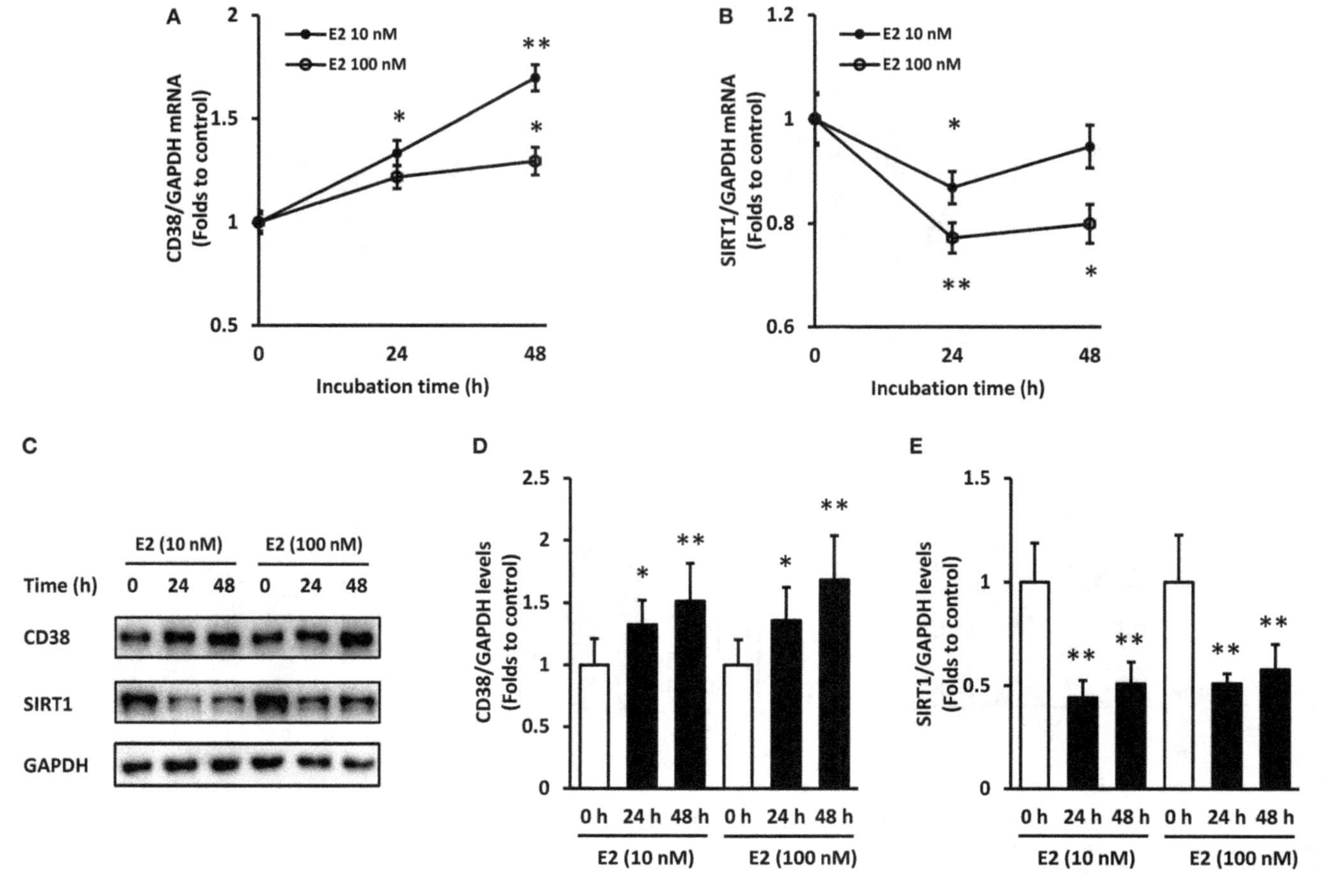

FIGURE 2 | Time course of CD38 and SIRT1 expression in ASMCs with E2 treatment. ASMCs were pre-treated with 10 or 100 nM of E2 for 24 h and 48 h respectively. **(A)** CD38 and **(B)** SIRT1 mRNA levels were detected by real-time PCR. **(C)** CD38 and SIRT1 protein levels were determined by western blot and quantitative analysis of **(D)** CD38 and **(E)** SIRT1 levels was normalized to GAPDH levels. $^{*}P < 0.05$, $^{**}P < 0.01$ vs. the control group. $N = 3$.

Firstly, ASMCs were pre-treated with various concentrations (0.1, 1, 10, and 100 nM) of E2 for 24 h. The mRNA levels of CD38 raised with the increase of E2 concentration, and the expression achieved maximum at 10 nM. There were no significant differences in CD38 expression between the 10 and 100 nM group (**Figure 1A**). By contrast, SIRT1 mRNA levels significantly decreased by the treatment of E2 at 10 and 100 nM (**Figure 1B**). In accordance with the PCR results, CD38 protein levels elevated whereas SIRT1 levels dropped in the presence of E2 in a concentration-dependent manner (**Figures 1C–E**).

In time course experiments, E2 at 10 and 100 nM were added to ASMCs for 24 and 48 h incubation, respectively. Results showed that CD38 mRNA continued to increase within 48 h and the effect was stronger in the 10 nM E2-treated group (**Figure 2A**). SIRT1 mRNA levels decreased at 24 h but partly restored at 48 h time point (**Figure 2B**). The protein levels of CD38 and SIRT1 showed a significant negative correction at 24 and 48 h, and there were no statistical differences between the 10 and 100 nM groups (**Figures 2C–E**). Therefore, pre-treatment with 10 nM of E2 for 48 h were selected for the subsequent experiments.

E2 Acts on SIRT1/p53 Signaling Through CD38 in ASMCs

We used the WT and CD38 KO ASMCs to confirm whether E2 affects SIRT1 expression through CD38. E2 promoted CD38 expression in WT ASMCs as expected (**Figures 3A,B**). The levels of SIRT1 were down-regulated by E2 in WT group compared with the vehicle treated cells. CD38 deficiency induced a marked increase in SIRT1 protein levels compared with the WT group, but this increase was not reversed by E2 treatment (**Figures 3A,C**).The acetylation of p53, one of the downstream targets of SIRT1, was assayed. In WT ASMCs, E2 increased the Ac-p53 levels, which were not changed in CD38 KO cells. The expression of p53 was not significantly altered (**Figures 3A,D**). These results indicated that E2 suppressed SIRT1/p53 signaling directly through CD38.

CD38 Deficiency Reverses the Effect of E2 on SIRT1/p53 Pathway During Hypoxia

We further investigated the role of E2 during hypoxia in WT and CD38 KO ASMCs. Hypoxia exposure induced an obvious down-regulation of CD38 mRNA, which was inhibited by E2

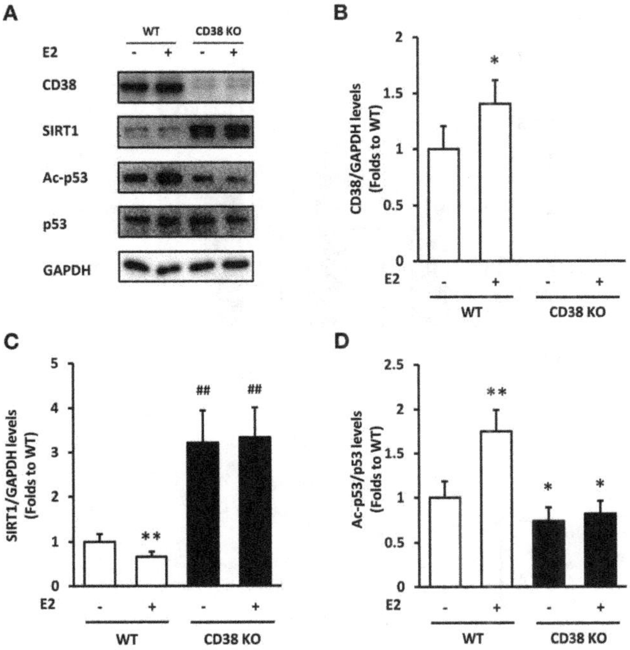

FIGURE 3 | The effects of E2 on SIRT1/p53 signal pathway in WT and CD38 KO ASMCs. **(A)** CD38, SIRT1, p53, and Ac-p53 levels were determined by western blot. Quantitative analysis of **(B)** CD38 and **(C)** SIRT1 levels was normalized to GAPDH levels, and **(D)** Ac-p53 levels were normalized to total p53 levels. $^*P < 0.05$, $^{**}P < 0.01$ vs. the WT control group. $^{\#\#}P < 0.01$ vs. the E2-treated WT group. $N = 3$.

treatment in WT cells (**Figure 4A**). SIRT1 mRNA reduced after hypoxia, and E2 further suppressed its expression in WT ASMCs. However, the effect of E2 on SIRT1 expression was abolished in the absence of CD38 (**Figure 4B**). At protein levels, hypoxia resulted in an increase in CD38 and a decrease in SIRT1. E2 further promoted CD38 expression and suppressed SIRT1 levels. By contrast, the effect of E2 on SIRT1 disappeared in CD38 KO cells (**Figures 4C–E**). Hypoxia induced the acetylation of p53, which was also aggravated by E2 treatment. Accordingly, this effect was diminished in CD38 KO ASMCs (**Figures 4C,F**).

CD38/SIRT1 Signaling Attenuates E2-Mediated ASMC Apoptosis After Hypoxia

We examined the apoptosis in ASMCs following hypoxia exposure. Hoechst 33258 staining was employed to evaluate the nuclear condensation and characteristic features of apoptotic cells. In WT ASMCs, control cells showed intact, light blue nuclei whereas cells exposed to hypoxia displayed typical nuclear apoptotic morphology, as indicated by bright, condensed and rounded nuclei. The apoptotic cells significantly increased after E2 treatment. In addition, E2 did not induce ASMC apoptosis under normoxia. However, CD38 deficiency showed an obvious protection against hypoxia exposure, with a marked reduction in apoptosis, and E2 did not further promote apoptosis in CD38 KO AMSCs (**Figure 5A**). The percentage of apoptotic cells was quantified in **Figure 5B**. Bax and Bcl-2 are the major members of Bcl-2 family which play a key role in promoting and inhibiting intrinsic apoptotic pathway. Bax promotes cell death while Bcl-2 prevents apoptosis by inhibiting the activity of Bax (20). The Bax/Bcl-2 ratio was significantly increased after hypoxia and E2 further aggravated the ratio. However, CD38 deficiency showed a lower Bax/Bcl-2 ratio compared with WT and the pro-apototic effect of E2 was antagonized in CD38 KO cells (**Figures 5C,D**). The effects of E2 on caspase-3 activation was further measured following hypoxia exposure. The activity of caspase-3 was comparable between the control and E2-treated cells under normoxia. Hypoxia induced a 2.05-fold increase in caspase-3 activity, and E2 further promoted caspase-3 activation in hypoxic WT AMSCs. However, in CD38 KO ASMCs, a lowed caspase-3 activity was observed after hypoxia exposure both in the absence and presence of E2 (**Figure 5E**).

The specific SIRT1 activator Resveratrol (RSV) was employed to verify whether SIRT1 is essential in E2-induced ASMC apoptosis. Single treatment with E2 or E2 combined with RSV did not affect apoptosis under normal conditions. However, E2 induced-Bax/Bcl-2 ratio change and caspase-3 activation were significantly reversed by RSV following hypoxia (**Figure 6**). The above data confirmed that E2 promoted ASMC apoptosis via CD38/SIRT1 signaling.

E2 Enhanced CD38 Expression Through Estrogen Receptor

To verify whether estrogen receptors (ER) mediate the action of E2 on CD38 expression, we used compound ICI 182,780, an estrogen receptor antagonist with no partial agonist activity (21).Treatment with ICI182,780 significantly decreased CD38 mRNA and protein levels, and E2-indcued CD38 expression was completely abolished in the presence of ICI182,780 (**Figure 7**). This result suggested that E2 promotes CD38 expression through ER.

DISCUSSION

Here, we demonstrated that pretreatment with E2 significantly up-regulated CD38 expression and suppressed SIRT1 activation, thus increasing the acetylation of p53 in mouse ASMCs. E2 further exaggerated hypoxia-induced AMSC apoptosis while this effect disappeared in CD38 KO cells and in the presence of SIRT1 activator. By using the ER antagonist we also found that E2 enhanced CD38 expression through ER. These results suggested that E2 promotes apoptosis through CD38/SIRT1/p53 signaling pathway.

There is increasing evidence that sex differences exist in a variety of lung diseases including asthma and COPD, and sex steroids have complex effects in modulating the processes. For example, in adult women, the cyclical variations in sex steroid levels with the menstrual cycle may influence asthma symptoms. Worsening of symptoms usually occurs when estrogen levels reduce, suggesting that estrogens may be protective for asthma (22). However, Use of estrogen by hormone replacement therapy increases asthma symptoms and the risk of asthma onset (23). The confounding effects request much more research in

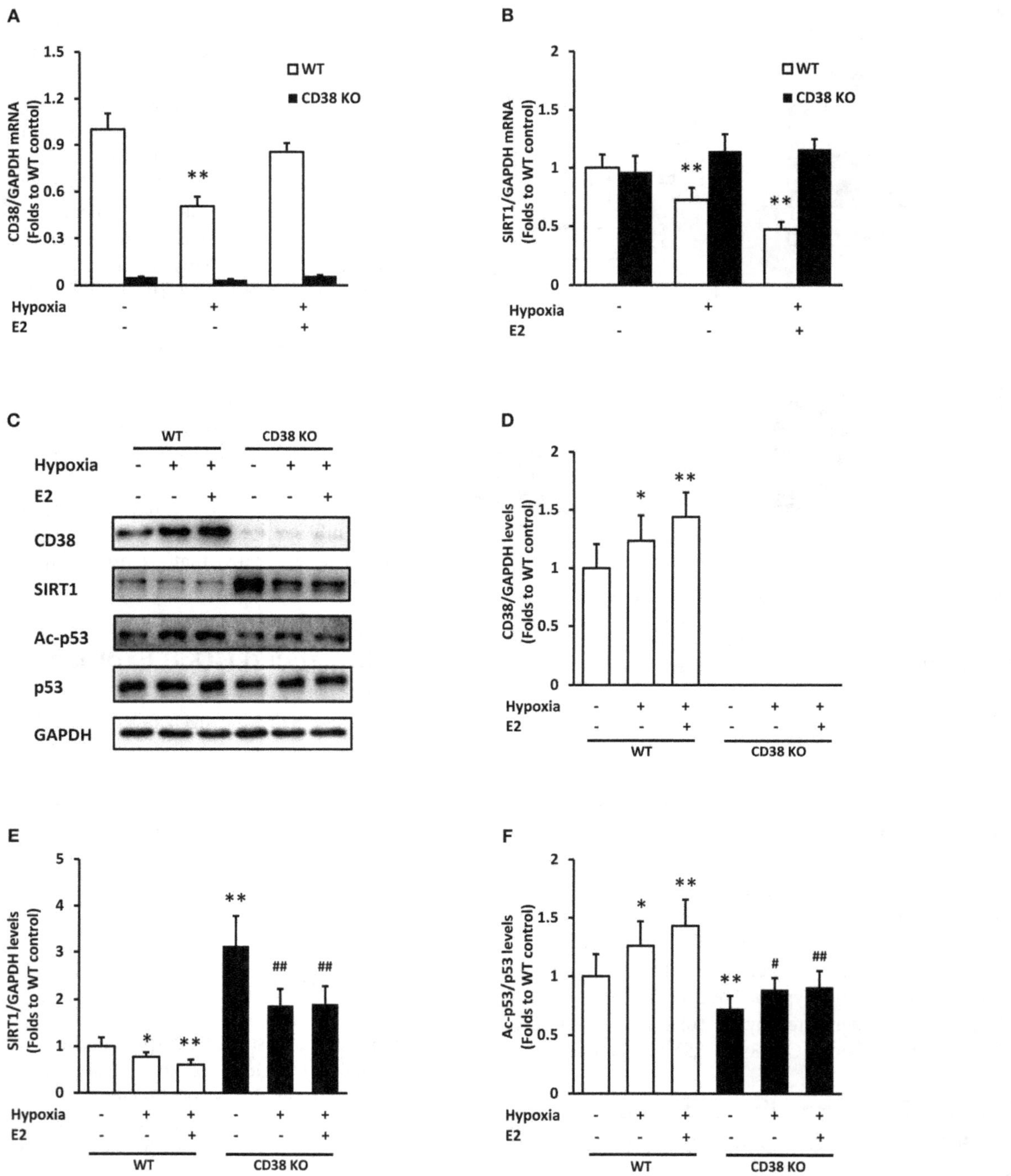

FIGURE 4 | The effects of E2 on SIRT1/p53 signal pathway in WT and CD38 KO ASMCs after hypoxia exposure. **(A)** CD38 and **(B)** SIRT1 mRNA levels were detected by real-time PCR. **(C)** CD38, SIRT1, p53, and Ac-p53 levels were determined by western blot. Quantitative analysis of **(D)** CD38 and **(E)** SIRT1 levels was normalized to GAPDH levels and **(F)** Ac-p53 levels were normalized to total p53 levels. $^*P < 0.05$, $^{**}P < 0.01$ vs. the WT control group; $^{\#}P < 0.05$, $^{\#\#}P < 0.01$ vs. the corresponding WT group. $N = 3$.

modulation of asthma and other lung diseases to elucidate the mechanisms underlying sex differences.

Sex steroids modulate airway smooth muscle contractility in a variety of manners. Estrogens potentiate bronchodilation through prostaglandin synthesis and cGMP modulation, and further influence Ca^{2+} influx channels (24). The mechanism by which estrogens decrease Ca^{2+} responses probably involve ERα (25), inhibition of L-type channels and store-operated calcium channels (26). CD38 is a critical regulator for intracellular Ca^{2+} homeostasis. CD38 is capable of cleaving nicotinamide adenine dinucleotide (NAD) to cyclic ADP ribose (cADPR) which is a trigger for intracellular Ca^{2+} release and hydrolyzing cADPR

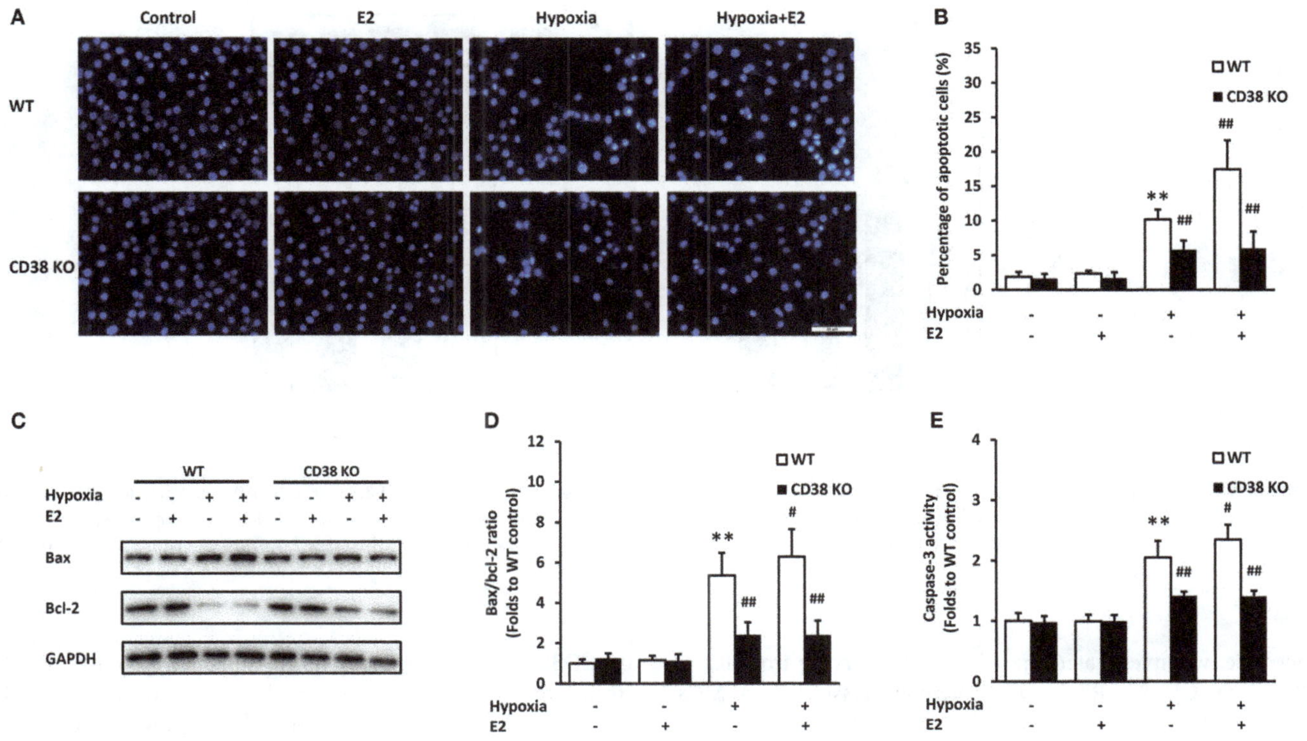

FIGURE 5 | The effects of E2 on apoptosis in WT and CD38 KO ASMCs after hypoxia exposure. **(A)** Representative images of Hoechst 33258 staining in ASMCs. Scale bar, 50 μm. **(B)** Quantitative analysis of apoptosis expressed as the percentage of total cell count. **(C)** Bax and Bcl-2 levels were determined by western blot and **(D)** the Bax/Bcl-2 ratio were quantitatively analyzed. **(E)** The activity of caspase-3 was measured by colorimetry. $^{**}P < 0.01$ vs. the WT control group; $^{\#}P < 0.05$, $^{\#\#}P < 0.01$ vs. the WT hypoxia group. $N = 3$.

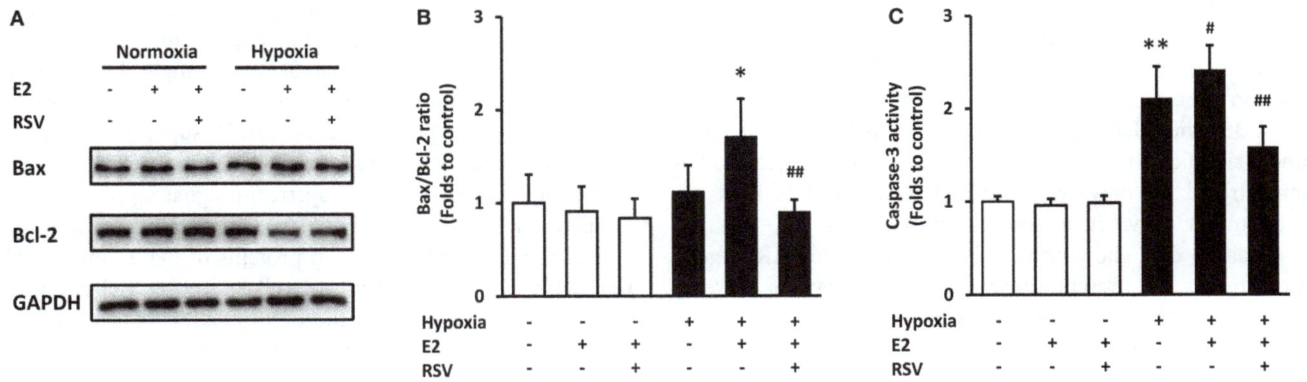

FIGURE 6 | The effects of combined treatment with E2 and SIRT1 activator Resveratrol (RSV) on apoptosis after hypoxia exposure. RSV (10 μM) was added to ASMCs for 2 h incubation followed by 24 h of E2 treatment. **(A)** Bax and Bcl-2 levels were determined by western blot and **(B)** the Bax/Bcl-2 ratio were quantitatively analyzed. **(C)** The activity of caspase-3 was measured by colorimetry. $^{*}P < 0.05$, $^{**}P < 0.01$ vs. the control group; $^{\#}P < 0.05$, $^{\#\#}P < 0.01$ vs. the E2-treated group under hypoxia. $N = 3$.

to ADPR (27). In addition, CD38 is an NAADP synthase required for NAADP-mediated Ca^{2+} release from lysosomal stores (10). CD38 KO mice exhibit very low cADPR levels in the lungs, attenuated $[Ca^{2+}]i$ responses to spasmogens, and decreased airway responsiveness (28). Cytokines such as IL-13 or TNF-α caused significantly lower inflammation and hyperresponsiveness in the CD38 KO mice compared to WT controls (29, 30), suggesting the crucial roles of CD38 in the contractility of airway smooth muscle and airway hyperresponsiveness. Studies showed that E2 increased CD38 mRNA and protein expression, resulting in increased cADPR synthesis, which may contribute to calcium regulation and myometrial contractility in rat myometrium (31). However, there has no data for CD38 expression in airway smooth muscle.

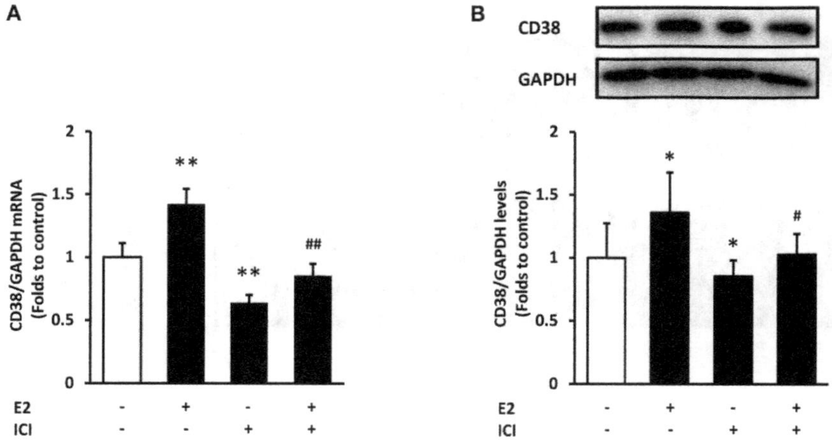

FIGURE 7 | The effects of estrogen receptor antagonist on CD38 expression. The estrogen receptor antagonist ICI182,780 (ICI, 10 nM) was added to ASMCs for 2 h incubation followed by 24 h of E2 treatment. **(A)** CD38 mRNA levels were detected by real-time PCR. **(B)** CD38 protein levels were determined by western blot and quantitative analysis of CD38 levels was normalized to GAPDH levels. *$P < 0.05$, **$P < 0.01$ vs. the control group; #$P < 0.05$, ##$P < 0.01$ vs. the E2-treated group. $N = 3$.

Therefore, we investigated the effect of E2 varying from 0.1 to 100 nM on CD38 mRNA and protein expression in ASMCs. In accordance with the result from myometrium, E2 showed a concentration-dependent increase in CD38 mRNA and protein levels. The time course assay revealed that CD38 mRNA and protein maintained a high level till 48 h with the treatment of physiological concentration of E2 (10 and 100 nM).

CD38 functions as the primary NAD^+ hydrolase that maintains low intracellular NAD^+ levels with a consequent low sirtuin activity (32) There is an increased NAD^+ levels as well as SIRT1 enzymatic activity in CD38 knockout mice, which is responsible for the deacetylation of the SIRT1 substrate p53 (9). This non-genomic regulation may explain our current results that CD38 gene deletion markedly increases SIRT1 protein levels without significant effect on its mRNA expression. Several studies demonstrated the down-regulation of SIRT1 protein levels by E2 treatment in vascular smooth muscle cells (16, 33), but there was no data showing that E2 had effects on SIRT1 gene expression. In the present study, E2 induced obvious decrease in SIRT1 mRNA and protein levels in WT ASMCs but not in CD38 KO cells, suggesting that other unknown mechanisms may exist in E2's actions associated with CD38 and warrants further investigation in our feature work. Taken together, these results suggested that CD38 is necessary for the modulation of SIRT1/p53 signaling pathway by E2. We for the first time demonstrated that E2 modulates the CD38/SIRT1/p53 signal pathway in mouse AMSCs.

The SIRT1/p53 pathway mediated cell apoptosis in many pathological processes. It has been reported that high concentration of glucose results in neuronal apoptosis through downregulation of SIRT1 and increased acetylation of p53, which likely contribute to the development of cognitive impairment in diabetes (34). In another study, rotenone treatment promotes p53 transcription and apoptosis through targeting SIRT1 and H3K9 SH-SY5Y cells, leading to nigrostriatal degeneration in Parkinson's disease (35). Here we investigated whether E2 acts on CD38/SIRT1/p53 signal pathway during hypoxia in ASMCs. Results showed that hypoxia caused a marked decrease in CD38 mRNA levels, which is consisted with the previous study (36). However, CD38 protein levels was up-regulated after hypoxia exposure. Although both *in vivo* and *in vitro* studies have confirmed that CD38 is activated during the process of hypoxia or ischemia, triggering CD38-mediated NADP(H) depletion with loss of eNOS-mediated NO generation and increased eNOS uncoupling (37, 38), no studies showed the changes of CD38 protein levels under hypoxia. We speculated that different time course changes may exist in mRNA and protein expression following hypoxia, or there might be a negative feedback regulation that inhibits CD38 mRNA expression. E2 exacerbated hypoxia-induced SIRT1 suppression and p53 acetylation, and these effects were abolished in CD38 KO cells, suggesting that CD38 is an upstream signaling molecule that regulates hypoxia-induced SIRT1/p53 activation.

Bcl-2 and Bax are two main proteins of Bcl-2 family, which is notable for the regulation of cell apoptosis. Bcl-2, an anti-apoptotic protein, inhibits the accumulation of cytochrome c in the cytosol, thereby preventing caspase-3 activation and blocking the apoptotic cascade, whereas Bax was identified as the proapoptotic member that triggers the release of caspases. Therefore, the Bax/Bcl-2 ratio is a determining factor in the regulation of apoptotic cell death (39). The ratio of Bax to Bcl-2 increased following hypoxia exposure in different models (40, 41). The expression of Bcl-2 and Bax is regulated by p53. The activation of p53 induces the expression of bcl-2 while simultaneously stimulates the expression of bax (42). By measuring the fluorescence of Hoechst 33258, the Bax/Bcl-2 ratio and the activity of caspase-3, we demonstrated that E2 aggravated cell apoptosis following hypoxia stimulation. The application of CD38 KO cells and the SIRT1 activator further confirmed the direct role of CD38/SIRT1 in E2-mediated AMSC apoptosis.

Finally, we explored the underlying mechanism by which E2 modulates CD38 expression. It has been widely considered that estrogens perform physiological function through receptor-mediated signaling pathways. The nuclear ERs exist in two main isoforms termed ERα and ERβ, and the classical mechanism of estrogen action involves ligand-induced dimerization of ER which interacts with estrogen responsive elements (EREs) in target gene promoters and results in transcriptional activation (43). Here we determined whether E2 mediated CD38 transcription through ER, by using ICI 182,780. ICI 182,780 is a selective estrogen antagonist that has been used for assessing ER-mediated actions of estrogens (21). Results showed that ICI 182,780 suppressed CD38 mRNA levels and counteracted the effect of E2, indicating the involvement of ER in the regulation of CD38. However, much more work is needed to elucidate the molecular mechanism, including the identification of the isoform (ERα or ERβ) which mediates the effect, and exploring possible ERE on CD38 promoters.

According to our results, the physiological concentration of E2 affects CD38 expression and promotes apoptosis, indicating that E2 have adverse effects on ASMCs. This may probably explain why women are more susceptible to respiratory diseases and the clinical application of estrogens should be more cautious. Further research into the effects of estrogen on the proliferation and inflammatory response in ASMCs are necessary, and the animal models of specific pulmonary diseases such as asthma and pulmonary hypertension in the smooth muscle-specific CD38 KO mice will also provide essential tools for elucidating the function of E2 on ASMCs. These studies are now ongoing in our laboratory.

In summary, the estrogen E2 acts on CD38/SIRT1/p53 signal pathway, resulting the acetylation of p53 and pro-apoptotic effects in mouse ASMCS following hypoxia. The findings may provide novel evidence for the prevention and treatment of respiratory disease through CD38 inhibition.

ETHICS STATEMENT

All experimental procedures involving animal and their care were carried out in accordance with the National Institutes of Health Guidelines. All experimental protocols were approved by Institutional Animal Care and use Committee of Nanchang University. All efforts were made to minimize animal suffering and reduce the number of animals used.

AUTHOR CONTRIBUTIONS

H-BX, K-YD, and YQ designed the experiments. The experimental procedures were performed by YL, YG, and WH. YQ and YL prepared the manuscript. H-BX revised the manuscript.

ACKNOWLEDGMENTS

We are grateful to Dr. Ling-Fang Wang, Dr. Xiao-Hui Guan, and Ms. Shui-Zhen Shi for their skilled technical assistance and good proposals.

REFERENCES

1. Jernigan NL, Resta TC, Gonzalez Bosc LV. Altered redox balance in the development of chronic hypoxia-induced pulmonary hypertension. *Adv Exp Med Biol.* (2017) 967:83–103. doi: 10.1007/978-3-319-63245-2_7
2. Keglowich L, Baraket M, Tamm M, Borger P. Hypoxia exerts dualistic effects on inflammatory and proliferative responses of healthy and asthmatic primary human bronchial smooth muscle cells. (2014) *PLoS ONE* 9:e89875. doi: 10.1371/journal.pone.0089875
3. Thompson M, Britt RDJr, Pabelick CM, Prakash YS. Hypoxia and local inflammation in pulmonary artery structure and function. *Adv Exp Med Biol.* (2017) 967:325–34. doi: 10.1007/978-3-319-63245-2_20
4. Wang J, Wang HS, Su ZB. MicroRNA-142 inhibits proliferation and promotes apoptosis in airway smooth muscle cells during airway remodeling in asthmatic rats via the inhibition of TGF-beta -dependent EGFR signaling pathway. *Cell Physiol Biochem.* (2018) 47:1682–95. doi: 10.1159/000490986
5. Townsend EA, Miller VM, Prakash YS. Sex differences and sex steroids in lung health and disease. *Endocr Rev.* (2012) 33:1–47. doi: 10.1210/er.2010-0031
6. Intapad S, Dimitropoulou C, Snead C, Piyachaturawat P, Catravas JD. Regulation of asthmatic airway relaxation by estrogen and heat shock protein 90. *J Cell Physiol.* (2012) 227:3036–43. doi: 10.1002/jcp.23045
7. Stamatiou R, Paraskeva E, Papagianni M, Molyvdas PA, Hatziefthimiou A. The mitogenic effect of testosterone and 17beta-estradiol on airway smooth muscle cells. *Steroids* (2011) 76:400–8. doi: 10.1016/j.steroids.2010.12.010
8. Keselman A, Heller N. Estrogen signaling modulates allergic inflammation and contributes to sex differences in asthma. *Front Immunol.* (2015) 6:568. doi: 10.3389/fimmu.2015.00568
9. Aksoy P, Escande C, White TA, Thompson M, Soares S, Benech JC, et al. Regulation of SIRT 1 mediated NAD dependent deacetylation: a novel role for the multifunctional enzyme CD38. *Biochem Biophys Res Commun.* (2006) 349:353–9. doi: 10.1016/j.bbrc.2006.08.066
10. Cosker F, Cheviron N, Yamasaki M, Menteyne A, Lund FE, Moutin MJ, et al. The ecto-enzyme CD38 is a nicotinic acid adenine dinucleotide phosphate (NAADP) synthase that couples receptor activation to Ca2+ mobilization from lysosomes in pancreatic acinar cells. *J Biol Chem.* (2010) 285:38251–9. doi: 10.1074/jbc.M110.125864
11. Deshpande DA, Walseth TF, Panettieri RA, Kannan MS. CD38/cyclic ADP-ribose-mediated Ca^{2+} signaling contributes to airway smooth muscle hyper-responsiveness. *FASEB J.* (2003) 17:452–4. doi: 10.1096/fj.02-0450fje
12. Barata H, Thompson M, Zielinska W, Han YS, Mantilla CB, Prakash YS, et al. The role of cyclic-ADP-ribose-signaling pathway in oxytocin-induced Ca^{2+} transients in human myometrium cells. *Endocrinology* (2004) 145:881–9. doi: 10.1210/en.2003-0774
13. Barone F, Genazzani AA, Conti A, Churchill GC, Palombi F, Ziparo E, et al. A pivotal role for cADPR-mediated Ca^{2+} signaling: regulation of endothelin-induced contraction in peritubular smooth muscle cells. *FASEB J.* (2002) 16:697–705. doi: 10.1096/fj.01-0749com

14. Chandran S, Cairns MT, O'Brien M, Smith TJ. Transcriptomic effects of estradiol treatment on cultured human uterine smooth muscle cells. *Mol Cell Endocrinol.* (2014) 393:16–23. doi: 10.1016/j.mce.2014.05.020
15. Dogan S, Deshpande DA, White TA, Walseth TF, Kannan MS. Regulation of CD 38 expression and function by steroid hormones in myometrium. *Mol Cell Endocrinol.* (2006) 246:101–6. doi: 10.1016/j.mce.2005.11.014
16. Lee CH, Su SC, Chiang CF, Chien CY, Hsu CC, Yu TY, et al. Estrogen modulates vascular smooth muscle cell function through downregulation of SIRT1. *Oncotarget* (2017) 8:110039–51. doi: 10.18632/oncotarget.22546
17. Solomon JM, Pasupuleti R, Xu L, McDonagh T, Curtis R, DiStefano PS, et al. Inhibition of SIRT1 catalytic activity increases p53 acetylation but does not alter cell survival following dna damage. *Mol Cell Biol.* (2005) 26:28–38. doi: 10.1128/MCB.26.1.28-38.2006
18. An SS, Laudadio RE, Lai J, Rogers RA, Fredberg JJ. Stiffness changes in cultured airway smooth muscle cells. *Am J Physiol Cell Physiol.* (2002) 283:C792–801. doi: 10.1152/ajpcell.00425.2001
19. Philippe C, Boussadia Y, Pruliere-Escabasse V, Papon JF, Clerici C, Isabey D, et al. Airway cell involvement in intermittent hypoxia-induced airway inflammation. *Sleep Breath.* (2015) 19:297–306. doi: 10.1007/s11325-014-1019-4
20. Mohan S, Abdelwahab SI, Kamalidehghan B, Syam S, May KS, Harmal NS, et al. Involvement of NF-kappaB and Bcl2/Bax signaling pathways in the apoptosis of MCF7 cells induced by a xanthone compound Pyranocycloartobiloxanthone A. *Phytomedicine* (2012) 19:1007–15. doi: 10.1016/j.phymed.2012.05.012
21. Rabaglino MB, Keller-Wood M, Wood CE. A transcriptomics model of estrogen action in the ovine fetal hypothalamus: evidence for estrogenic effects of ICI 182,780. *Physiol Rep.* (2018) 6:e13871. doi: 10.14814/phy2.13871
22. Farha S, Asosingh K, Laskowski D, Hammel J, Dweik RA, Wiedemann HP, et al. Effects of the menstrual cycle on lung function variables in women with asthma. *Am J Respir Crit Care Med.* (2009) 180:304–10. doi: 10.1164/rccm.200904-0497OC
23. Hepburn MJ, Dooley DP, Morris MJ. The effects of estrogen replacement therapy on airway function in postmenopausal, asthmatic women. *Arch Intern Med.* (2001) 161:2717–20. doi: 10.1001/archinte.161.22.2717
24. Pang JJ, Xu XB, Li HF, Zhang XY, Zheng TZ, Qu SY. Inhibition of beta-estradiol on trachea smooth muscle contraction *in vitro* and *in vivo*. *Acta Pharmacol Sin.* (2002) 23:273–7.
25. Townsend EA, Thompson MA, Pabelick CM, Prakash YS. Rapid effects of estrogen on intracellular Ca2+ regulation in human airway smooth muscle. *Am J Physiol Lung Cell Mol Physiol.* (2010) 298:L521–30. doi: 10.1152/ajplung.00287.2009
26. Ay B, Prakash YS, Pabelick CM, Sieck GC. Store-operated Ca^{2+} entry in porcine airway smooth muscle. *Am J Physiol Lung Cell Mol Physiol.* (2004) 286:L909–17. doi: 10.1152/ajplung.00317.2003
27. Lee HC. Enzymatic functions and structures of CD38 and homologs. *Chem Immunol.* (2000) 75, 39–59. doi: 10.1159/000058774
28. Deshpande DA, White TA, Dogan S, Walseth TF, Panettieri RA, Kannan MS. CD38/cyclic ADP-ribose signaling: role in the regulation of calcium homeostasis in airway smooth muscle. *Am J Physiol Lung Cell Mol Physiol.* (2005) 288:L773–88. doi: 10.1152/ajplung.00217.2004
29. Guedes AG, Paulin J, Rivero-Nava L, Kita H, Lund FE, Kannan MS. CD38-deficient mice have reduced airway hyperresponsiveness following IL-13 challenge. *Am J Physiol Lung Cell Mol Physiol.* (2006) 291:L1286–93. doi: 10.1152/ajplung.00187.2006
30. Guedes AG, Jude JA, Paulin J, Kita H, Lund FE, Kannan MS. Role of CD38 in TNF-alpha-induced airway hyperresponsiveness. *Am J Physiol Lung Cell Mol Physiol.* (2008) 294:L290–9. doi: 10.1152/ajplung.00367.2007
31. Dogan S, White TA, Deshpande DA, Murtaugh MP, Walseth TF, Kannan MS. Estrogen increases CD38 gene expression and leads to differentialregulation of adenosine diphosphate (ADP)-ribosyl cyclase and cyclic ADP-ribose hydrolase activities in rat myometrium. *Biol Reprod.* (2002) 66:596–602. doi: 10.1095/biolreprod66.3.596
32. Escande C, Nin V, Price NL, Capellini V, Gomes AP, Barbosa MT, et al. Flavonoid apigenin is an inhibitor of the NAD+ ase CD38: implications for cellular NAD+ metabolism, protein acetylation, and treatment of metabolic syndrome. *Diabetes*(2013) 62:1084–93. doi: 10.2337/db12-1139
33. Toniolo A, Warden EA, Nassi A, Cignarella A, Bolego C. Regulation of SIRT1 in vascular smooth muscle cells from streptozotocin-diabetic rats. *PLoS ONE* (2013) 8:e65666. doi: 10.1371/journal.pone.0065666
34. Shi X, Pi L, Zhou S, Li X, Min F, Wang S, et al. Activation of Sirtuin 1 attenuates high glucose-induced neuronal apoptosis by deacetylating p53. *Front Endocrinol.* (2018) 9:274. doi: 10.3389/fendo.2018.00274
35. Feng Y, Liu T, Dong SY, Guo YJ, Jankovic J, Xu H, et al. Rotenone affects p53 transcriptional activity and apoptosis via targeting SIRT1 and H3K9 acetylation in SH-SY5Y cells. *J Neurochem.* (2015) 134:668–76. doi: 10.1111/jnc.13172
36. Ota H, Tamaki S, Itaya-Hironaka A, Yamauchi A, Sakuramoto-Tsuchida S, Morioka T, et al. Attenuation of glucose-induced insulin secretion by intermittent hypoxia via down-regulation of CD38. *Life Sci.* (2012) 90:206–11. doi: 10.1016/j.lfs.2011.11.011
37. Boslett J, Hemann C, Christofi FL, Zweier JL. Characterization of CD38 in the major cell types of the heart: endothelial cells highly express CD38 with activation by hypoxia-reoxygenation triggering NAD(P)H depletion. *Am J Physiol Cell Physiol.* (2018) 314:C297–309. doi: 10.1152/ajpcell.00139.2017
38. Boslett J, Hemann C, Zhao YJ, Lee H-C, Zweier JL. Luteolinidin protects the postischemic heart through CD38 inhibition with preservation of NAD(P)(H). *J Pharmacol Exp Ther.* (2017) 361:99–108. doi: 10.1124/jpet.116.239459
39. Korsmeyer SJ. Regulators of cell death. *Trends Genet.* (1995) 11:101–5. doi: 10.1016/S0168-9525(00)89010-1
40. Kim SW, Kim IK, Ha JH, Yeo CD, Kang HH, Kim JW, et al. Normobaric hyperoxia inhibits the progression of lung cancer by inducing apoptosis. *Exp Biol Med.* (2018) 243:739–48. doi: 10.1177/1535370218774737
41. Joles JA, Abuyassin B, Badran M, Ayas NT, Laher I. Intermittent hypoxia causes histological kidney damage and increases growth factor expression in a mouse model of obstructive sleep apnea. *Plos ONE* (2018) 13:e0192084. doi: 10.1371/journal.pone.0192084
42. Miyashita T, Krajewski S, Krajewska M, Wang HG, Lin HK, Liebermann DA, et al. Tumor suppressor p53 is a regulator of bcl-2 and bax gene expression *in vitro* and *in vivo*. *Oncogene* (1994) 9:1799–805.
43. Nilsson S, Gustafsson JA. Biological role of estrogen and estrogen receptors. *Crit Rev Biochem Mol Biol.* (2002) 37:1–28. doi: 10.1080/10409230290771438

2

High Levels of SIRT1 Expression as a Protective Mechanism Against Disease-Related Conditions

Birsen Elibol[1] *and Ulkan Kilic*[2]*

[1] *Department of Medical Biology, Faculty of Medicine, Bezmialem Vakif University, Istanbul, Turkey,* [2] *Department of Medical Biology, Faculty of Medicine, University of Health Sciences, Istanbul, Turkey*

Correspondence:
Ulkan Kilic
uckilic@yahoo.com

SIRT1 protein, a member of Silent Information Regulator 2 (Sir2) protein family, have gained considerable attention as epigenetic regulators for a great area in the human physiology. Changes in sirtuin expression are critical in several diseases, including metabolic syndrome, cardiovascular diseases, cancer and neurodegeneration. Here, we provide an overview of the association of the increasing level of SIRT1 protein for regulating some disease related conditions such as obesity, cardiovascular diseases and neurodegeneration. This review also provides a detailed molecular understanding of the interaction of the some basic molecules with increasing SIRT1 levels rather than reduction of the SIRT1 expression. In this context, the current approaches to enhancing the expression of SIRT1 points the importance of epigenetics in several age-related diseases to provide a healthy aging by developing novel therapies which can prevent or damp the progression of some diseases.

Keywords: SIRT1 expression, oxidative stress, metabolic diseases, cardiovascular diseases, neurodegenerative diseases

INTRODUCTION

Sirtuin 1 (SIRT1) which is encoded by the *SIRT1* gene is the most conserved mammalian nicotinamide adenine dinucleotide (NAD+) dependent histone deacetylase (1). Besides its role being a target for histone and non-histone proteins, SIRT1 functions as a transcription factor for many different physiological processes (2). According to the previous experiments which were performed using yeast, worms and flies as model organisms, sirtuins were accepted as evolutionarily conserved epigenetic mediators of longevity (3–5). In addition to the key role on extending life by regulating the response to some conditions such as fasting, caloric restriction and exercise, SIRT1 regulates many endocrine functions, protects organism from oxidative stress-related cellular events, promotes DNA stability, and decreases various age-related disorders, such as neurodegenerative disease, metabolic abnormalities, and cancer (6–9).

SIRT1 protein is expressed in most of the body parts including brain, heart, kidney, liver, pancreas, spleen, skeletal muscle, endothelial tissue and white adipose tissue. By expression and activation of SIRT1, modulation of its downstream pathways occurs by targeting several cellular proteins, such as nuclear factor kappa-light-chain-enhancer of activated B cells (NF-κB), peroxisome proliferators-activated receptor-gamma (PPAR-γ) and its coactivator peroxisome proliferator-activated receptor gamma coactivator 1-alpha (PGC-1α), protein tyrosine phosphatase (PTP), forkhead transcriptional factors (the FoxO subgroup), adenosine monophosphate activated protein kinase (AMPK), CRE-binding protein regulated transcription coactivator 2 (CRTC2), endothelial nitric oxide synthase (eNOS), p53, myogenic differentiation (MyoD), liver X receptor (LXR), and transcription factor E2F1 (10, 11). Through its deacetylation activity, SIRT1 modulates functions of these critical molecules and shows its critical and multifaceted roles in cellular physiology (**Figure 1**).

Alterations of the level of SIRT1 expression were determined in several diseases including metabolic diseases, neurodegenerative diseases, cancer and aging. Whereas an increase in the expression of the SIRT1 protein was observed in cancer (12, 13), reductions in the SIRT1 level was more common in other diseases such as Alzheimer's Diseases (AD), Parkinson Disease (PD), obesity, diabetes, and cardiovascular diseases (14–18). Recent developments elucidated the relation between downregulation of SIRT1 levels and disease progression as an increase in the oxidative stress and inflammation (16, 17). For example, due to a significant decrease in SIRT1 levels which correlated with an increase in the oxidative stress parameters, accumulation of Tau proteins in AD, enhancement of acetylated p53 expression levels in coronary artery disease and increase in the fatty acid oxidation in obesity were observed in the patients (15, 17, 19, 20).

Previous studies showed that SIRT1 overexpression significantly increased cell viability, decreased cell apoptosis and reduced the release of pro-inflammatory cytokines (21–24). In addition, the regulation of metabolism and longevity by SIRT1 occurs through controlling the maturation of hypothalamic peptide hormones (25, 26). Specificity for SIRT1 increases in the relevant metabolic pathways in the hypothalamic circuitries which is also associated with altered downstream factors of SIRT1 such as FoxO transcription factors (27, 28). In the light of this information, we reviewed recent findings related to the association of the increasing level of SIRT1 protein rather than reduction of the SIRT1 expression and regulation of some disease related conditions such as obesity, cardiovascular diseases and neurodegeneration. The overarching aim of this paper is to provide a basis for hypothesizing that the level of SIRT1 are mechanistically increased to overcome the dysfunction of SIRT1 activity in the diseased conditions.

SIRT1 AND METABOLIC DISEASES

SIRT1 protein protects the functions of adipose tissue and liver in several aspects (29, 30) such as glucose homeostasis and fat metabolism against severe obesity (31, 32). It is also involved in energy balance and stress. Insulin sensitivity is increased in the pancreatic beta cells which have insulin resistance due to overexpression of SIRT1 (30, 33). The activity of PPARγ which have a role in the storage of glucose and fatty acid in adipose tissue is repressed by SIRT1 (34). During short term fasting, the CRTC2 is also depressed by SIRT1 and thus gluconeogenesis is declined in the liver tissue. During long term fasting, SIRT1 expression deacetylates and activates the PGC-1α to decrease adiposity and lipogenesis and to increase fatty acid oxidation (35–37). In addition, SIRT1 deacetlylates sterol regulatory element binding protein (SREBP), farnesoid X receptor (FXR), as well as liver X receptor (LXR) to increase bile acid production and to reverse cholesterol transport (30, 38). Thus, SIRT1 can be called as a "Master Metabolic Regulator" (30). Indeed, the dysregulation of energy sensing may cause inflammation and insulin resistance. Because of prevention of pro-inflammatory responses, SIRT1 behaves as a positive regulator of insulin in the adipose tissue (39). In one of the recent study, after feeding with high dietary fructose, the liver of rats were investigated in response to SIRT1 expression as a main energy sensing protein (40). However, they demonstrated a significant increase in the SIRT1 expression in the fructose-induced inflammation suggesting compensatory rise in the level of SIRT1 to decline the inflammation-related metabolic reactions (40). In addition, overexpression of SIRT1 in obesity which was formed by high-fat diet protects lipid-induced inflammation and hepatic steatosis while providing better glucose tolerance (41). These favorable effects of SIRT1 may be related with the activation of the antioxidant enzymes and stimulation of PGC1α to decrease the level of pro-inflammatory cytokines (41).

In some neurodegenerative diseases, a number of neuropeptide systems in the hypothalamus are affected from activity of SIRT1 which indicate an impact on metabolism. For example, SIRT1 upregulates the level of orexin receptor specifically in the lateral hypothalamic area and the ventromedial nucleus of the hypothalamus, whereas the expression of orexin and melanin-concentrating hormone is reduced in the hypothalamus due to inhibition of the active state of orexin neurons (25, 42, 43). In addition, SIRT1 also regulates the expression of BDNF in the brain. It was found that increased SIRT1 level diminished BDNF signaling which resulted in severe hyperphagia and obesity both in humans and animals (44, 45). These results showed that compensatory increase in the SIRT1 level to cope with the disease outcomes such as oxidative stress brings some additional metabolic dysfunctions in the body due to altered peptides in the endocrine system.

In addition to the obesity, SIRT1 has a role in the hepatic energy metabolism by modulating it nutritionally and hormonally. This modulation is mostly occurred through the deacetylation of metabolic regulators (46). Previous studies also showed that obese patients with non-alcoholic fatty-liver disease (NAFLD), which is the most common liver disease caused by elevated hepatic lipids, inflammation and oxidative stress, had high plasma levels of SIRT1 producing a potential against the physiological mechanisms related to NAFLD (47). In this type of disease, the action mechanism of SIRT1 acted through the modulation of PPARα activity and fatty acid oxidation (48).

On the other hand, it was found that increase in the SIRT1 activity upregulates genes-related metabolic functions, promotes insulin sensitivity and reduces inflammatory gene expressions in the adipose tissue of diet-induced obese animals (49). In addition, we found a polymorphism in the promoter region of *SIRT1* gene in obese children drawing attention to the association between altered SIRT1 activity and the risk of obesity (50). Previous reports also showed the protective role of SIRT1 on the development of osteoarthritis by upregulation of cartilage extracellular matrix genes and downregulation of matrix-degrading enzymes (51, 52). In addition, increase in the SIRT1 activity had a protective effect against osteoarthritis in

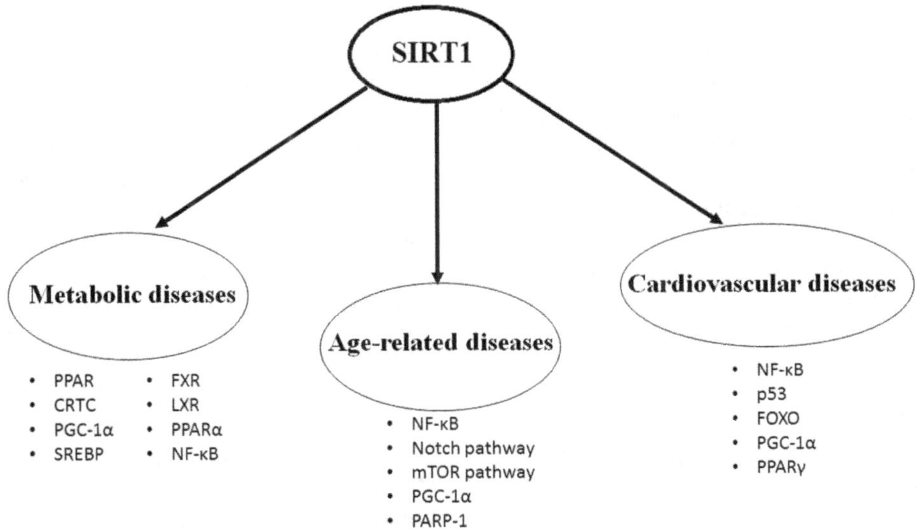

FIGURE 1 | The most studied targets of SIRT1 in the metabolic diseases, age-related diseases and cardiovascular diseases.

animal models (53, 54). Therefore, the investigators suggested that the increase both in the activity and expression of SIRT1 might be a protective strategy for progression of osteoarthritis via the modulation of the NF-κB pathway (55).

SIRT1 AND AGE-RELATED NEURODEGENERATIVE DISEASES

The relationships between SIRT1 and age were investigated in the previous studies related to interaction of lifespan elongation and calorie restriction which is thought as an enhancer for SIRT1 activity (56, 57). Most of these studies showed that calorie intake restriction innervates the extension of life by the inducement of defense of cells against to free radicals and toxins for attenuation of apoptosis or amelioration of cell repair which are desired factors in aging (58–60). That means, altered SIRT1 expression and activity is thought to be a potent way to keep the cells and organs properly functioning for longer times. The positive correlation between age and SIRT1 expression and/or activity may be a compensation against unexpected situations such as oxidative stress (61, 62). For example, in one of our previous study, it was noted higher level of SIRT1 protein in older people compared with the SIRT1 level in the younger people (62). It was thought that increased protein level of SIRT1 in older people may be a compensatory mechanism due to accumulation of oxidative stress-related products and elimination of antioxidant enzyme level in elderly (62). However, increase in the expression does not mean increase in the activity of protein. An oxidative stress-dependent decrease in the SIRT1 activity was noted in aged animals that had high levels of SIRT1 protein (63, 64). The decline in the activity of SIRT1 may not be related directly with SIRT1 protein but also its downstream or upstream molecules such as a decline in NAD+ levels with aging (65).

One of the main risk factor for several neurodegenerative diseases such as Alzheimer's disease (AD) and Parkinson's disease (PD) is age. The common underlying mechanisms of neurodegeneration are increase in the neuroinflammation, mitochondrial damages and oxidative stress (66, 67). In literature, it was shown that sirtuins' hyperactivity could reduce these negative outcomes both *in vivo* and *in vitro* due to its neuroprotective role (68–71). In the AD pathology, SIRT1 deacetylates substrates in favor of the non-amyloidogenic pathway or acts directly on the Aβ and Tau proteins (72). Molecular studies showed that SIRT1 activation prevents the accumulation of Aβ plaques and tau pathology through the NF-κB signaling pathway by upregulation of the *ADAM10* gene, induction of the Notch pathway, and inhibition of the mTOR pathway (20, 73, 74). As shown in previous studies, SIRT1 epigenetically reprograms inflammation taking about AD formation at the earlier stages by altering transcription factors (24, 75, 76). In addition, it was observed that brains of AD patients have consistently reduced NAD+ levels and SIRT1 transcription and/or protein levels involved in chronic inflammation that can also be altered by increased levels of the activated proinflammatory transcription factor NF-κB (77–79). In one of our studies, we found a significant increase in the SIRT1 level of dementia patients (80). Furthermore, in the patients with Huntington's disease (HD), Baldo and his colleagues found higher expression of SIRT1 protein level in the most affected brain regions, especially hypothalamic regions important for metabolic regulation, compared to brain regions which were less affected from the mutant huntingtin protein (28). In PD, SIRT1 inhibits α-synuclein aggregation by deacetylating proteins such as heat shock proteins and PGC-1α and, therefore, it protects dopaminergic neurons against cell death which occur due to the formation of insoluble fibrils called Lewy bodies (81, 82). In the *in vitro* PD model, it was observed that an overexpression of SIRT1 due to application of toxin (rotenone or MPTP) which causes neurodegeneration was rescued cells from oxidative stress (16, 83). The neuroprotection against to PD occurred by the mechanism of decreasing in the expression of NF-κB and cleaved PARP-1. In a postmortem study, the levels of SIRT1 showed a slight increase in the dementia patients with Lewy bodies (16, 83). However, as seen in the AD, the activity of the SIRT1 protein also decreased in the PD patients producing neurodegeneration in correlation with possible higher oxidative stress, synaptic and cell loss, and neuroinflammation (16).

We thought that the high levels of SIRT1 protein might have a role in alleviating the oxidative stress that is significantly increased in neurodegeneration because an induction of the SIRT1 expression occurs when the organism encounters a biological stress such as aging or an age-related disorder due to the role function of SIRT1 as an important stress sensor molecule.

Also, in literature, it was stated that high levels of SIRT1 may increase the expression of genes related to neuronal protection (84–86). On the other hand, SIRT1 behaves as a double edged sword in response to inflammation which is a cause of neurodegeneration. That means, low levels of SIRT1 cause early acute inflammation-related damages to tissues by increasing NF-kB, and high levels of SIRT1 during late inflammation cause immunosuppression and increased the rate of death (87). In a previous study, investigators observed that increase in the expression level of SIRT1 cannot protect the brain from neurodegeneration without increasing the activity level of SIRT1. For example, Ciriello and his colleagues observed a significant decrease in the level of phosphorylated SIRT1, the active form of SIRT1, in the patients with multiple sclerosis (88). Interestingly, a significant negative correlation between phosphorylated and non-phosphorylated forms of SIRT1 was observed explaining both the SIRT1 overexpression and inactivity of SIRT1 in diseased state. In addition, when a SIRT1-activating molecules were given to the organisms, profound therapeutic benefits and neuroprotective effects were recorded against age-dependent neurodegenerative diseases (89).

SIRT1 AND CARDIOVASCULAR DISEASE

Nowadays, the sirtuin protein family is thought as one of the important target for cardiovascular diseases (CVD). Therefore, the role of SIRT1 protein and its downstream molecules also gains importance in the experimental studies related with CVD development. In cardiomyocytes, during prenatal period, SIRT1 is found in the nucleus, however, it is mostly located in the cytoplasm of myocytes of adult heart of rodents (90). Previously, we found that the level of the SIRT1 expression was significantly higher in the CVD patients compared to the levels of SIRT1 in healthy subjects pointing the cross-talk between SIRT1 protein expression and reactive oxygen species (61). In this previous study, we also found a significant increase in the oxidative stress parameters which may be an inducer for SIRT1 expression. In cardiomyocytes, myoblast gains resistance against to oxidative stress by increasing expression of nuclear SIRT1 protein. To do produce this antioxidative activity, SIRT1 protein enhances the level of MnSOD expression through p53 deacetylation (90). In addition, activation of FoxO1-dependent oxidative pathway by overexpression of SIRT1 protein is another regulatory way of protection of cardiomyocytes from oxidative stress (91). By the help of this pathway, cardiac infarct volume is reduced to ameliorate and recover cardiac function after ischemia/reperfusion in mice (92). It is also thought that transcriptional activity of NF-κB protein, a preconditioner in cardiac ischemia, is inhibited by SIRT1 protein to promote cell protection (93, 94). In literature, it was reported that the activity of SIRT1 protein is directly or indirectly controlled via the JNK1-SIRT1 link by accumulated oxidative stress which is caused by an increase in the ROS level due to aging or age-related diseases enzyme (1). It was demonstrated that ROS inhibited JNK phosphatases which activated the JNK1 to phosphorylate SIRT1 (95, 96). Furthermore, this phosphorylation increased the activity of SIRT1 resulting its translocation into the nuclei (97). Alcendor et al. (91) noted that the rate of SIRT1 overexpression had two-sided action in the cardiovascular system. For example, 2.5- to 7.5-fold increase in the SIRT1 expression attenuated apoptosis, the symptoms of cardiac dysfunction, age-related cardiac hypertrophy and expression of senescence markers. On the other side, 12.5-fold increase in the expression of SIRT1 resulted in increased cardiac hypertrophy due to oxidative stress and apoptosis. This study explained clearly the relation between oxidative stress and overexpression of SIRT1 to the pathological levels in CVD patients. In one of our previous studies (61), we found a positive correlation between total antioxidant level and SIRT1 level in CVD patients. Therefore, we can conclude that the increase in the SIRT1 level may be a compensatory mechanism to increase the antioxidants against oxidative stress in CVD patients.

Contrary to some previous studies (98, 99), the SIRT1 level significantly decreased approaching to control values in the CVD patients receiving statin therapy (100). The decline in the SIRT1 level by statins can be explained by the statins' inducement effect on PPARγ activity to protect patients against the progression of atherosclerosis (101). On the other hand, PPARγ inhibits SIRT1 expression at the transcriptional level which interrupting compensatory action of increased SIRT1 expression (102).

CONCLUSION

Recent studies have shown that age-related diseases or endocrine system dysfunctions are associated with an increase in SIRT1 expression levels, but with a decrease in their activity. The oxidative stress produced during these processes may lead to compensatory or protective increase in the SIRT1 expression to deal with the decline of the SIRT1 activity.

AUTHOR CONTRIBUTIONS

BE wrote the draft of the manuscript and UK finalized the manuscript.

REFERENCES

1. Salminen A, Kaarniranta K, Kauppinen A. Crosstalk between oxidative stress and SIRT1: impact on the aging process. *Int J Mol Sci.* (2013) 14:3834–59. doi: 10.3390/ijms14023834
2. Yamamoto H, Schoonjans K, Auwerx J. Sirtuin functions in health and disease. *Mol Endocrinol.* (2007) 21:1745–55. doi: 10.1210/me.2007-0079
3. Rogina B, Helfand SL. Sir2 mediates longevity in the fly through a pathway related to calorie restriction. *Proc Natl Acad Sci USA.* (2004) 101:15998–6003. doi: 10.1073/pnas.0404184101
4. Tissenbaum HA, Guarente L. Increased dosage of a sir-2 gene extends lifespan in Caenorhabditis elegans. *Nature* (2001) 410:227–30. doi: 10.1038/35065638
5. Kaeberlein M, McVey M, Guarente L. The SIR2/3/4 complex and SIR2 alone promote longevity in Saccharomyces cerevisiae by two different mechanisms. *Genes Dev.* (1999) 13:2570–80. doi: 10.1101/gad.13.19.2570
6. Guarente L, Franklin H. Epstein lecture: sirtuins, aging, and medicine. *N Engl J Med.* (2011) 364:2235–44. doi: 10.1056/NEJMra1100831
7. Longo VD, Kennedy BK. Sirtuins in aging and age-related disease. *Cell* (2006) 126:257–68. doi: 10.1016/j.cell.2006.07.002
8. Koubova J, Guarente L. How does calorie restriction work? *Genes Dev.* (2003) 17:313–21. doi: 10.1101/gad.1052903
9. Jeśko H, Wencel P, Strosznajder RP, Strosznajder JB. Sirtuins and their roles in brain aging and neurodegenerative disorders. *Neurochem. Res.* (2017) 42:876–90. doi: 10.1007/s11064-016-2110-y
10. Valle I, Alvarez-Barrientos A, Arza E, Lamas S, Monsalve M. PGC1alpha regulates the mitochondrial antioxidant defense system in vascular endothelial cells. *Cardiovasc Res.* (2005) 66:562–73. doi: 10.1016/j.cardiores.2005.01.026
11. Olmos Y, Brosens JJ, Lam EW. Interplay between SIRT proteins and tumour suppressor transcription factors in chemotherapeutic resistance of cancer. *Drug Resist Update* (2011) 14:35–44. doi: 10.1016/j.drup.2010.12.001
12. Chen WY, Wang DH, Yen RC, Luo J, Gu W, Baylin SB. Tumor suppressor HIC1 directly regulates SIRT1 to modulate p53-dependent DNA-damage responses. *Cell* (2005) 123:437–48. doi: 10.1016/j.cell.2005.08.011
13. Wang C, Chen L, Hou X, Li Z, Kabra N, Ma Y, et al. Interactions between E2F1 and SirT1 regulate apoptotic response to DNA damage. *Nat Cell Biol.* (2006) 8:1025–31. doi: 10.1038/ncb1468
14. Lutz MI, Milenkovic I, Regelsberger G, Kovacs GG. Distinct patterns of sirtuin expression during progression of Alzheimer's disease. *Neuromol Med.* (2014) 16:405–14. doi: 10.1007/s12017-014-8288-8
15. Costa Cdos S, Hammes TO, Rohden F, Margis R, Bortolotto JW, Padoin AV, et al. SIRT1 transcription is decreased in visceral adipose tissue of morbidly obese patients with severe hepatic steatosis. *Obes Surg.* (2010) 20:633–9. doi: 10.1007/s11695-009-0052-z
16. Singh P, Hanson PS, Morris CM. SIRT1 ameliorates oxidative stress induced neural cell death and is down-regulated in Parkinson's disease. *BMC Neurosci.* (2017) 18:46. doi: 10.1186/s12868-017-0364-1
17. Chan SH, Hung CH, Shih JY, Chu PM, Cheng YH, Lin HC, et al. SIRT1 inhibition causes oxidative stress and inflammation in patients with coronary artery disease. *Redox Biol.* (2017) 13:301–9. doi: 10.1016/j.redox.2017.05.027
18. Aditya R, Kiran AR, Varma DS, Vemuri R, Gundamaraju R. A Review on SIRtuins in Diabetes. *Curr Pharm Des.* (2017) 23:2299–307. doi: 10.2174/1381612823666170125153334
19. Julien C, Tremblay C, Emond V, Lebbadi M, Salem N Jr, Bennett DA, et al. Sirtuin 1 reduction parallels the accumulation of tau in Alzheimer disease. *J Neuropathol Exp Neurol.* (2009) 68:48–58. doi: 10.1097/NEN.0b013e3181922348
20. Braidy N, Jayasena T, Poljak A, Sachdev PS. Sirtuins in cognitive ageing and Alzheimer's disease. *Curr Opin Psychiatry* (2012) 25:226–30. doi: 10.1097/YCO.0b013e32835112c1
21. Li K, Lv G, Pan L. Sirt1 alleviates LPS induced inflammation of periodontal ligament fibroblasts via downregulation of TLR4. *Int J Biol Macromol.* (2018) 119:249–54. doi: 10.1016/j.ijbiomac.2018.07.099
22. Yang SR, Wright J, Bauter M, Seweryniak K, Kode A, Rahman I. Sirtuin regulates cigarette smoke-induced proinflammatory mediator release via RelA/p65 NF-kappaB in macrophages *in vitro* and in rat lungs *in vivo*: implications for chronic inflammation and aging. *Am J Physiol Lung Cell Mol Physiol.* (2007) 292:L567–76. doi: 10.1152/ajplung.00308.2006
23. Rajendrasozhan S, Yang SR, Kinnula VL, Rahman I. SIRT1, an antiinflammatory and antiaging protein, is decreased in lungs of patients with chronic obstructive pulmonary disease. *Am J Respir Crit Care Med.* (2008) 177:861–70. doi: 10.1164/rccm.200708-1269OC
24. Yeung F, Hoberg JE, Ramsey CS, Keller MD, Jones DR, Frye RA, et al. Modulation of NF-kappaB-dependent transcription and cell survival by the SIRT1 deacetylase. *EMBO J.* (2004) 23:2369–80. doi: 10.1038/sj.emboj.7600244
25. Satoh A, Brace CS, Ben-Josef G, West T, Wozniak DF, Holtzman DM, et al. SIRT1 promotes the central adaptive response to diet restriction through activation of the dorsomedial and lateral nuclei of the hypothalamus. *J Neurosci.* (2010) 30:10220–32. doi: 10.1523/JNEUROSCI.1385-10.2010
26. Nillni EA. The metabolic sensor Sirt1 and the hypothalamus: interplay between peptide hormones and pro-hormone convertases. *Mol Cell Endocrinol.* (2016) 438:77–88 doi: 10.1016/j.mce.2016.09.002
27. Parker JA, Vazquez-Manrique RP, Tourette C, Farina F, Offner N, Mukhopadhyay A, et al. Integration of beta-catenin, sirtuin, and FOXO signaling protects from mutant huntingtin toxicity. *J Neurosci* (2012) 32:12630–40. doi: 10.1523/JNEUROSCI.0277-12.2012
28. Baldo B, Gabery S, Soylu-Kucharz R, Cheong RY, Henningsen JB, Englund E, et al. SIRT1 is increased in affected brain regions and hypothalamic metabolic pathways are altered in Huntington disease. *Neuropathol Appl Neurobiol.* (2018) doi: 10.1111/nan.12514. [Epub ahead of print].
29. Pedersen SB, Ølholm J, Paulsen SK, Bennetzen MF, Richelsen B. Low Sirt1 expression, which is upregulated by fasting, in human adipose tissue from obese women. *Int J Obes.* (2008) 32:1250–5. doi: 10.1038/ijo.2008.78
30. Schug TT, Li X. Sirtuin 1 in lipid metabolism and obesity. *Ann Med.* (2011) 43:198–211. doi: 10.3109/07853890.2010.547211
31. Li X. SIRT1 and energy metabolism. *Acta Biochim Biophys Sin (Shanghai)* (2013) 45:51–60. doi: 10.1093/abbs/gms108
32. Cakir I, Perello M, Lansari O, Messier NJ, Vaslet CA, Nillni EA. Hypothalamic Sirt1 regulates food intake in a rodent model system. *PLoS ONE* (2009) 4:e8322. doi: 10.1371/journal.pone.0008322
33. Banks AS, Kon N, Knight C, Matsumoto M, Gutiérrez-Juárez R, Rossetti L, et al. SirT1 gain of function increases energy efficiency and prevents diabetes in mice. *Cell Metab.* (2008) 8:333–41. doi: 10.1016/j.cmet.2008.08.014
34. Picard F, Kurtev M, Chung N, Topark-Ngarm A, Senawong T, Machado De Oliveira R, et al. Sirt1 promotes fat mobilization in white adipocytes by repressing PPAR-gamma. *Nature* (2004) 429:771–6. doi: 10.1038/nature02583
35. Nemoto S, Fergusson MM, Finkel T. SIRT1 functionally interacts with the metabolic regulator and transcriptional coactivator PGC-1α. *J Biol Chem.* (2005) 280:16456–60. doi: 10.1074/jbc.M501485200
36. Purushotham A, Schug TT, Xu Q, Surapureddi S, Guo X, Li X. Hepatocyte-specific deletion of SIRT1 alters fatty acid metabolism and results in hepatic steatosis and inflammation. *Cell Metab.* (2009) 9:327–38. doi: 10.1016/j.cmet.2009.02.006
37. Rodgers JT, Lerin C, Haas W. Nutrient control of glucose homeostasis through a complex of PGC-1alpha and SIRT1. *Nature* (2005) 434:113–8. doi: 10.1038/nature03354
38. Li X, Zhang S, Blander G. SIRT1 deacetylates and positively regulates the nuclear receptor LXR. *Mol Cell* (2007) 28:91–106. doi: 10.1016/j.molcel.2007.07.032
39. Alageel A, Tomasi J, Tersigni C, Brietzke E, Zuckerman H, Subramaniapillai M, et al. Evidence supporting a mechanistic role of sirtuins in mood and metabolic disorders. *Prog Neuropsychopharmacol Biol Psychiatry* (2018) 86:95–101. doi: 10.1016/j.pnpbp.2018.05.017
40. Veličković N, Teofilović A, Ilić D, Djordjevic A, Vojnović Milutinović D, Petrović S, et al. Modulation of hepatic inflammation and energy-sensing pathways in the rat liver by high-fructose diet and chronic stress. *Eur J Nutr.* (2018). doi: 10.1007/s00394-018-1730-1. [Epub ahead of print].
41. Pfluger PT, Herranz D, Velasco-Miguel S, Serrano M, Tschöp MH. Sirt1 protects against high-fat diet-induced metabolic damage. *Proc Natl Acad Sci USA.* (2008) 105:9793–8. doi: 10.1073/pnas.0802917105
42. Froy O, Sherman H, Bhargava G, Chapnik N, Cohen R, Gutman R, et al. Spontaneous caloric restriction associated with increased leptin levels

in obesity-resistant alphaMUPA mice. *Int J Obes (Lond)* (2011) 35:226–35. doi: 10.1038/ijo.2010.125

43. Hayakawa K, Hirosawa M, Tabei Y, Arai D, Tanaka S, Murakami N, et al. Epigenetic switching by the metabolism-sensing factors in the generation of orexin neurons from mouse embryonic stem cells. *J Biol Chem.* (2013) 288:17099–110. doi: 10.1074/jbc.M113.455899
44. Unger TJ, Calderon GA, Bradley LC, Sena-Esteves M, Rios M. Selective deletion of Bdnf in the ventromedial and dorsomedial hypothalamus of adult mice results in hyperphagic behavior and obesity. *J Neurosci.* (2007) 27:14265–74. doi: 10.1523/JNEUROSCI.3308-07.2007
45. Cordeira JW, Felsted JA, Teillon S, Daftary S, Panessiti M, Wirth J, et al. Hypothalamic dysfunction of the thrombospondin receptor alpha2delta-1 underlies the overeating and obesity triggered by brain-derived neurotrophic factor deficiency. *J Neurosci.* (2014) 34:554–65. doi: 10.1523/JNEUROSCI.1572-13.2014
46. Del Campo JA, Gallego-Durán R, Gallego P, Grande L. Genetic and epigenetic regulation in nonalcoholic fatty liver disease (NAFLD). *Int J Mol Sci.* (2018) 19:E911. doi: 10.3390/ijms19030911
47. Mariani S, Fiore D, Basciani S, Persichetti A, Contini S, Lubrano C, et al. Plasma levels of SIRT1 associate with non-alcoholic fatty liver disease in obese patients. *Endocrine* (2015) 49:711–6. doi: 10.1007/s12020-014-0465-x
48. Mukhopadhyay P, Horváth B, Rajesh M, Varga ZV, Gariani K, Ryu D, et al. PARP inhibition protects against alcoholic and non-alcoholic steatohepatitis. *J Hepatol.* (2017) 66:589–600. doi: 10.1016/j.jhep.2016.10.023
49. Nawaz A, Mehmood A, Kanatani Y, Kado T, Igarashi Y, Takikawa A, et al. Sirt1 activator induces proangiogenic genes in preadipocytes to rescue insulin resistance in diet-induced obese mice. *Sci Rep.* (2018) 8:11370. doi: 10.1038/s41598-018-29773-0
50. Kilic U, Gok O, Elibol-Can B, Ozgen IT, Erenberk U, Uysal O, et al. SIRT1 gene variants are related to risk of childhood obesity. *Eur J Pediatr.* (2015c) 174:473–9. doi: 10.1007/s00431-014-2424-1
51. Fujita N, Matsushita T, Ishida K, Topark-Ngarm A, Senawong T, Machado De Oliveira R, et al. Potential involvement of SIRT1 in the pathogenesis of osteoarthritis through the modulation of chondrocyte gene expressions. *J Orthop Res.* (2011) 29:511–5. doi: 10.1002/jor.21284
52. Matsuzaki T, Matsushita T, Takayama K, Matsumoto T, Nishida K, Kuroda R, et al. Disruption of Sirt1 in chondrocytes causes accelerated progression of osteoarthritis under mechanical stress and during ageing in mice. *Ann Rheum Dis.* (2014) 73:1397–404. doi: 10.1136/annrheumdis-2012-202620
53. Wang J, Gao JS, Chen JW Li F, Tian J. Effect of resveratrol on cartilage protection and apoptosis inhibition in experimental osteoarthritis of rabbit. *Rheumatol Int.* (2012) 32:1541–8. doi: 10.1007/s00296-010-1720-y
54. Li W, Cai L, Zhang Y, Cui L, Shen G. Intra-articular resveratrol injection prevents osteoarthritis progression in a mouse model by activating SIRT1 and thereby silencing HIF-2α. *J Orthop Res.* (2015) 33:1061–70. doi: 10.1002/jor.22859
55. Nishida K, Matsushita T, Takayama K, Tanaka T, Miyaji N, Ibaraki K, et al. Intraperitoneal injection of the SIRT1 activator SRT1720 attenuates the progression of experimental osteoarthritis in mice. *Bone Joint Res.* (2018) 7:252–62. doi: 10.1302/2046-3758.73.BJR-2017-0227.R1
56. Mercken EM, Hu J, Krzysik-Walker S, Wei M, Li Y, McBurney MW, et al. SIRT1 but not its increased expression is essential for lifespan extension in caloric-restricted mice. *Aging Cell* (2014) 13:193–6. doi: 10.1111/acel.12151
57. Satoh A, Brace CS, Rensing N, Cliften P, Wozniak DF, Herzog ED, et al. Sirt1 extends lifespan and delays aging in mice through the regulation of nk2 homeobox1 in the dmh and lh. *Cell Metab.* (2013) 18:416–30. doi: 10.1016/j.cmet.2013.07.013
58. Cantó C, Auwerx J. Caloric restriction, SIRT1 and longevity. *Trends Endocrinol Metab.* (2009) 20:325–31. doi: 10.1016/j.tem.2009.03.008
59. Cohen HY, Miller C, Bitterman KJ, Wall NR, Hekking B, Kessler B, et al. Calorie restriction promotes mammalian cell survival by inducing the SIRT1 deacetylase. *Science* (2004) 305:390–2. doi: 10.1126/science.1099196
60. Ungvari Z, Parrado-Fernandez C, Csiszar A, de Cabo R. Mechanisms underlying caloric restriction and lifespan regulation: implications for vascular aging. *Circ Res.* (2008) 102:519–28. doi: 10.1161/CIRCRESAHA.107.168369
61. Kilic U, Gok O, Bacaksiz A, Izmirli M, Elibol-Can B, Uysal O. SIRT1 gene polymorphisms affect the protein expression in cardiovascular diseases. *PLoS ONE* (2014) 9:e90428. doi: 10.1371/journal.pone.0090428
62. Kilic U, Gok O, Erenberk U, Dundaroz MR, Torun E, Kucukardali Y, et al. A remarkable age-related increase in SIRT1 protein expression against oxidative stress in elderly: SIRT1 gene variants and longevity in human. *PLoS ONE* (2015a) 10:e0117954. doi: 10.1371/journal.pone.0117954
63. Braidy N, Guillemin GJ, Mansour H, Chan-Ling T, Poljak A, Grant R. Age related changes in NAD+metabolism oxidative stress and Sirt1 activity in wistar rats. *PLoS ONE* (2011) 6:e19194. doi: 10.1371/journal.pone.0019194
64. Koltai E, Szabo Z, Atalay M, Bolodogh I, Naito H, Goto S, et al. Exercise alters SIRT1, SIRT6, NAD and NAMPT levels in skeletal muscle of aged rats. *Mech Ageing Dev.* (2010) 131:21–8. doi: 10.1016/j.mad.2009.11.002
65. Mills KF, Satoh A, Imai S. Age-associated loss of sirt1-mediated enhancement of glucose-stimulated insulin secretion in beta cell-specific sirt1-overexpressing (besto) mice. *Aging Cell* (2008) 7:78–88. doi: 10.1111/j.1474-9726.2007.00355.x
66. Cornelius C, Trovato Salinaro A, Scuto M, Fronte V, Cambria MT, Pennisi M, et al. Cellular stress response, sirtuins and UCP proteins in Alzheimer disease: role of vitagenes. *Immun Ageing* (2013) 10:41. doi: 10.1186/1742-4933-10-41
67. Herskovits AZ, Guarente L. Sirtuin deacetylases in neurodegenerative diseases of aging. *Cell Res.* (2013) 23:746–58. doi: 10.1038/cr.2013.70
68. Patel NV, Gordon MN, Connor KE, Good RA, Engelman RW, Mason J, et al. Caloric restriction attenuates A beta-deposition in Alzheimer transgenic models. *Neurobiol Aging* (2005) 26:995–1000. doi: 10.1016/j.neurobiolaging.2004.09.014
69. Guarente L. Mitochondria–a nexus for aging, calorie restriction, and sirtuins? *Cell* (2008) 132:171–6. doi: 10.1016/j.cell.2008.01.007
70. Bonda DJ, Lee HG, Camins A, Pallàs M, Casadesus G, Smith MA, et al. The sirtuin pathway in ageing and Alzheimer disease: mechanistic and therapeutic considerations. *Lancet Neurol.* (2011) 10:275–9. doi: 10.1016/S1474-4422(11)70013-8
71. Rizzi L, Roriz-Cruz M. Sirtuin 1 and Alzheimer's disease: an up-to-date review. *Neuropeptides* (2018) 71:54-60 doi: 10.1016/j.npep.2018.07.001
72. Wencel PL, Lukiw WJ, Strosznajder JB, Strosznajder RP. Inhibition of Poly(ADP-ribose) polymerase-1 enhances gene expression of selected sirtuins and app cleaving enzymes in amyloid beta cytotoxicity. *Mol Neurobiol.* (2018) 55:4612–23. doi: 10.1007/s12035-017-0646-8
73. Chen J, Zhou Y, Mueller-Steiner S, Chen LF, Kwon H, Yi S, et al. SIRT1 protects against microglia-dependent amyloid-beta toxicity through inhibiting NF-kappaB signaling. *J Biol Chem.* (2005) 280:40364–74. doi: 10.1074/jbc.M509329200
74. Song JH, Yu JT, Liu M, Yan CZ, Tan L. Genetic association between ADAM10 gene polymorphism and Alzheimer's disease in a Northern Han Chinese population. *Brain Res.* (2011) 1421:78–81. doi: 10.1016/j.brainres.2011.09.008
75. Xie J, Zhang X, Zhang L. Negative regulation of inflammation by SIRT1. *Pharmacol Res.* (2013) 67:60–7. doi: 10.1016/j.phrs.2012.10.010
76. Hardy J, Selkoe DJ. The amyloid hypothesis of Alzheimer's disease: progress and problems on the road to therapeutics. *Science* (2002) 297:353–6. doi: 10.1126/science.1072994
77. Qin W, Yang T, Ho L, Zhao Z, Wang J, Chen L, et al. Neuronal SIRT1 activation as a novel mechanism underlying the prevention of alzheimer disease amyloid neuropathology by calorie restriction. *J Biol Chem.* (2006) 281:21745–54. doi: 10.1074/jbc.M602909200
78. Serrano-Marco L, Chacón MR, Maymó-Masip E, Barroso E, Salvadó L, Wabitsch M, et al. TNF-α inhibits PPARβ/δ activity and SIRT1 expression through NF-kB in human adipocytes. *Biochim Biophys Acta* (2012) 1821:1177–85. doi: 10.1016/j.bbalip.2012.05.006
79. Vachharajani VT, Liu T, Wang X, Hoth JJ, Yoza BK, McCall CE. Sirtuins link inflammation and metabolism. *J Immunol Res.* (2016) 2016:8167273. doi: 10.1155/2016/8167273
80. Kilic U, Elibol B, Uysal O, Kilic E, Yulug B, Sakul AS, et al. Specific alterations in the circulating levels of the SIRT1, TLR4, and IL7 proteins in patients with dementia. *Exp Geront.* (2018) 111:203–9. doi: 10.1016/j.exger.2018.07.018.

81. Donmez G, Arun A, Chung CY, McLean PJ, Lindquist S, Guarente L. SIRT1 protects against alpha-synuclein aggregation by activating molecular chaperones. *J Neurosci Off J Soc Neurosci.* (2012) 32:124–32. doi: 10.1523/JNEUROSCI.3442-11.2012
82. Mudo G, Makela J, Di Liberto V, Tselykh TV, Olivieri M, Piepponen P, et al. Transgenic expression and activation of PGC-1alpha protect dopaminergic neurons in the MPTP mouse model of Parkinson's disease. *Cell Mol Life Sci.* (2012). 69:1153–65. doi: 10.1007/s00018-011-0850-z
83. Pallàs M, Pizarro JG, Gutierrez-Cuesta J, Crespo-Biel N, Alvira D, Tajes M, et al. Modulation of SIRT1 expression in different neurodegenerative models and human pathologies. *Neuroscience* (2008) 154:1388–97. doi: 10.1016/j.neuroscience.2008.04.065
84. Araki T, Sasaki Y, Milbrandt J. Increased nuclear NAD biosynthesis and SIRT1 activation prevent axonal degeneration. *Science* (2004) 305:1010–3. doi: 10.1126/science.1098014
85. Bedalov A, Simon JA. Neuroscience. *NAD* to the rescue. *Science* (2004) 305:954–55. doi: 10.1126/science.1102497
86. Huang PS, Son JH, Abbott LC, Winzer-Serhan UH. Regulated expression of neuronal SIRT1 and related genes by aging and neuronal β2-containing nicotinic cholinergic receptors. *Neuroscience* (2011) 196:189–202. doi: 10.1016/j.neuroscience.2011.09.007
87. Liu TF, Vachharajani VT, Yoza BK, McCall CE. NAD+-dependent sirtuin 1 and 6 proteins coordinate a switch from glucose to fatty acid oxidation during the acute inflammatory response. *J Biol Chem.* (2012) 287:25758–69. doi: 10.1074/jbc.M112.362343
88. Ciriello J, Tatomir A, Hewes D, Boodhoo D, Anselmo F, Rus V, et al. Phosphorylated SIRT1 as a biomarker of relapse and response to treatment with glatiramer acetate in multiple sclerosis. *Exp Mol Pathol.* (2018) 105:175–80. doi: 10.1016/j.yexmp.2018.07.008
89. Kim D, Nguyen MD, Dobbin MM, Fischer A, Sananbenesi F, Rodgers JT, et al. SIRT1 deacetylase protects against neurodegeneration in models for Alzheimer's disease and amyotrophic lateral sclerosis. *EMBO J.* (2007) 26:3169–79. doi: 10.1038/sj.emboj.7601758
90. Tanno M, Kuno A, Yano T, Miura T, Hisahara S, Ishikawa S, et al. Induction of manganese superoxide dismutase by nuclear translocation and activation of SIRT1 promotes cell survival in chronic heart failure. *J Biol Chem.* 285:8375–82. doi: 10.1074/jbc.M109.090266
91. Alcendor RR, Gao S, Zhai P, Zablocki D, Holle E, Yu X, et al. Sirt1 regulates aging and resistance to oxidative stress in the heart. *Circ Res.* (2007) 100:1512–21. doi: 10.1161/01.RES.0000267723.65696.4a
92. Hsu CP, Zhai P, Yamamoto T, Maejima Y, Matsushima S, Hariharan N, et al. Silent information regulator 1 protects the heart from ischemia/reperfusion. *Circulation* (2010) 122:2170–82. doi: 10.1161/CIRCULATIONAHA.110.958033
93. Teng FY, Tang BL. NF-kappaB signaling in neurite growth and neuronal survival. *Rev Neurosci.* (2010) 21:299–313. doi: 10.1515/REVNEURO.2010.21.4.299
94. Boyle EM Jr, Canty TG Jr, Morgan EN, Yun W, Pohlman TH, Verrier ED. Treating myocardial ischemia-reperfusion injury by targeting endothelial cell transcription. *Ann Thorac Surg.* (1999) 68:1949–53. doi: 10.1016/S0003-4975(99)01033-4
95. Kamata H, Honda S, Maeda S, Chang L, Hirata H, Karin M. Reactive oxygen species promote TNFalpha-induced death and sustained JNK activation by inhibiting MAP kinase phosphatases. *Cell* (2005) 120:649–61. doi: 10.1016/j.cell.2004.12.041
96. Matsukawa J, Matsuzawa A, Takeda K, Ichijo H. The ASK1-MAP kinase cascades in mammalian stress response. *J Biochem.* (2004) 136:261–5. doi: 10.1093/jb/mvh134
97. Nasrin N, Kaushik VK, Fortier E, Wall D, Pearson KJ, de Cabo R, et al. JNK1 phosphorylates SIRT1 and promotes its enzymatic activity. *PLoS ONE* (2009) 4:e8414. doi: 10.1371/journal.pone.0008414
98. Tabuchi T, Satoh M, Itoh T, Nakamura M. MicroRNA-34a regulates the longevity-associated protein SIRT1 in coronary artery disease: effect of statins on SIRT1 and microRNA-34a expression. *Clin Sci (Lond.)* (2012) 123:161–71. doi: 10.1042/CS20110563
99. Kok SH, Lin LD, Hou KL, Hong CY, Chang CC, Hsiao M, et al. Simvastatin inhibits cysteine-rich protein 61 expression in rheumatoid arthritis synovial fibroblasts through the regulation of sirtuin-1/FoxO3a signaling. *Arthr Rheum.* (2013) 65:639–49. doi: 10.1002/art.37807
100. Kilic U, Gok O, Elibol-Can B, Uysal O, Bacaksiz A. Efficacy of statins on sirtuin 1 and endothelial nitric oxide synthase expression: the role of sirtuin 1 gene variants in human coronary atherosclerosis. *Clin Exp Pharmacol Physiol.* (2015b) 42:321–30. doi: 10.1111/1440-1681.12362
101. Yano M, Matsumura T, Senokuchi T, Ishii N, Murata Y, Taketa K, et al. Statins activate peroxisome proliferator-activated receptor gamma through extracellular signal-regulated kinase 1/2 and p38 mitogen-activated protein kinase-dependent cyclooxygenase-2 expression in macrophages. *Circ Res.* (2007) 100:1442–51. doi: 10.1161/01.RES.0000268411.49545.9c
102. Han L, Zhou R, Niu J, McNutt MA, Wang P, Tong T. SIRT1 is regulated by a PPARγ-SIRT1 negative feedback loop associated with senescence. *Nucleic Acids Res.* (2010) 38:7458–71. doi: 10.1093/nar/gkq609

3

Long-Term L-Serine Administration Reduces Food Intake and Improves Oxidative Stress and Sirt1/NFκB Signaling in the Hypothalamus of Aging Mice

Xihong Zhou [1], Haiwen Zhang [2], Liuqin He [3], Xin Wu [1] and Yulong Yin [1,3]*

[1] Key Laboratory of Agro-Ecological Processes in Subtropical Region, Institute of Subtropical Agriculture, Chinese Academy of Sciences, Changsha, China, [2] Key Laboratory of Tropical Animal Breeding and Epidemic Disease Research of Hainan Province, Hainan University, Haikou, China, [3] Laboratory of Animal Nutrition and Human Health, College of Life Sciences, Hunan Normal University, Changsha, China

***Correspondence:**
Xin Wu
wuxin@isa.ac.cn

Serine has recently been shown to reduce oxidative stress and inflammation, which, when occurring in the hypothalamus, contribute to age-related obesity. To explore whether long-term serine administration reduces oxidative stress and body weight in aging mice, various concentrations of L-serine dissolved in water were administered to 18-month-old C57BL/6J mice for 6 months. The results showed that the administration of 0.5% (w/v) L-serine significantly reduced food intake and body weight gain during the experiment. Moreover, the administration of 0.5% L-serine decreased the concentrations of leptin, malondialdehyde, interleukin-1β, and interleukin-6, while it increased those of superoxide dismutase and glutathione, in both the serum and hypothalamus. Reactive oxygen species and the activity of nicotinamide adenine dinucleotide phosphate oxidase were reduced in the hypothalamus of aging mice treated with L-serine as compared with untreated control mice. Additionally, the expression of the leptin receptor increased while the levels of neuropeptide Y and agouti-related protein decreased in mice that had been treated with 0.5% L-serine. The expression of Sirt1 and phosphorylated signal transducers and activators of transcription 3 (pSTAT3) increased, while that of phosphorylated NFκB decreased in the mice treated with 0.5% L-serine. These results indicated that long-term L-serine administration reduces body weight by decreasing orexigenic peptide expression and reduces oxidative stress and inflammation during aging in mice, possibly by modulating the Sirt1/NFκB pathway. Thus, L-serine has the potential to be used in the prevention of age-related obesity.

Keywords: aging, inflammation, oxidative stress, serine, Sirt1

INTRODUCTION

The hypothalamus is a critical part of the central nervous system that modulates the stress response and senses nutrient-related inputs. However, in aging mice, increased levels of oxidative stress and inflammatory markers are observed in the hypothalamus (1–3). Low levels of antioxidant enzymes and high levels of lipid peroxidation make the hypothalamus vulnerable to reactive oxygen species

(ROS) (4–6). These elevations of oxidative damage and inflammatory responses in the central nervous system are believed to contribute to age-related diseases including obesity and various neurodegenerative disorders (7–9).

The nicotinamide adenine dinucleotide-dependent deacetylase sirtuin 1 (Sirt1) regulates the response to oxidative stress, which correlates with many diseases (10–12). Sirt1 activity in the hypothalamus decreases in association with aging, and its low expression contributes to a low level of antioxidants and increased oxidative damage (10). Importantly, Sirt1 is also a nutrient sensor and plays critical roles in the energy balance in the hypothalamus. Debate is ongoing as to whether hypothalamic Sirt1 has orexigenic or anorexigenic effects, although most of the evidence shows that inhibition of Sirt1 induces a negative energy balance by regulating the activity of forkhead transcription factor FKHR (FOXO1) (13–15) and the expression of agouti-related protein (AGRP) and neuropeptide Y (NPY) (16, 17). Additionally, the transcription factor nuclear factor-κB (NFκB) regulates numerous target genes to exert its biological functions. Importantly, NFκB functions as a central regulator of the immune response and controls the secretion of inflammatory cytokines in many tissues including the hypothalamus (18–20). Moreover, NFκB is also a central mediator of stress responses under conditions of oxidative stress and upon exposure to certain chemicals in the central nervous system (18).

L-Serine is traditionally considered a non-essential amino acid. Recently, dietary supplementation with L-serine has been shown to have antioxidant effects (21–24). L-Serine is a precursor of glycine and cysteine, which can be used for the synthesis of glutathione. In addition, L-serine exerts critical functions in the mammalian central nervous system. It serves as a precursor of the neuroactive substances L-serine and glycine, and mediates neuroprotective effects (25, 26). However, it remains unknown whether L-serine has any effects on age-related oxidative stress in the hypothalamus. Consequently, we conducted the present study to explore the effects of long-term L-serine supplementation on hypothalamic oxidative stress and Sirt1 expression in aging mice.

MATERIALS AND METHODS

Animals

Eighty 18-month-old C57BL/6J male mice were included in the study. The mice were obtained from SLAC Laboratory Animal Center (Changsha, China) and were housed in a temperature-controlled animal facility (lighting cycle: 12 h/d), with free access to food and water. All animals were randomly assigned into four groups: control mice, which were kept untreated, and mice administered with 0.1, 0.2, or 0.5% (w/v) L-serine dissolved in the drinking water. Eighteen-month-old adult mice were used as young controls. The experiment had the duration of 6 months. Food intake and body weight were recorded every week. Upon completion of the experiment, mice were euthanized with isoflurane and the blood was collected from the retro-orbital sinus. The hypothalamus was excised and collected according to the method described in a previous study (7). The hypothalamus samples were either immediately snap-frozen in liquid nitrogen or fixed in formaldehyde solution. This study was performed in accordance with the recommendations of the Guide for Care and Use of Laboratory Animals published by the Animal Welfare Committee of the Institute of Subtropical Agriculture, Chinese Academy of Sciences. The protocol was approved by the Animal Welfare Committee of the Institute of Subtropical Agriculture, Chinese Academy of Sciences.

Biochemical Assays

Superoxide dismutase (SOD), malondialdehyde (MDA), and glutathione (GSH) biochemical assays were performed with commercially available kits from Nanjing Jiancheng Bioengineering Institute (Nanjing, Jiangsu, China). Interleukin (IL)-1β, IL-6, and leptin biochemical assays were performed with kits from Cusabio Biotech (Wuhan, Hubei, China; https://www.cusabio.com/). Nicotinamide adenine dinucleotide phosphate (NADPH) oxidase activity was assayed as previously reported (27).

Determination of Reactive Oxygen Species

ROS content was determined as previously described (21). Hypothalamus samples were placed in optimum cutting temperature compound (Sakura Finetek, Tokyo, Japan) and flash-frozen in a methylbutane-chilled bath at $-81 \pm 2°C$, were sliced into 10-μm sections and stained with a solution of 1 μM dihydroethidium (Sigma-Aldrich, St. Louis, MO, USA), for 20 min, at 37°C in a humidified 5% CO_2 incubator. Results were observed and analyzed by fluorescence microscopy and Image Browser software (Leica, Wetzlar, Germany).

Immunohistochemistry Assay

Hypothalamus samples were cut into 4-μm sections and processed for immunohistochemical staining as previously described. Briefly, the samples were incubated with a primary antibody [leptin receptor (LepRb), NPY, or AGRP; Boster, Wuhan, China] overnight at 4°C and then with poly-horseradish peroxidase-conjugated IgG for 60 min at $22 \pm 4°C$. Subsequently, the avidin-biotin-peroxidase complex and the substrate 3,3′-diaminobenzidine were applied for 2 min and the samples were analyzed.

RT-qPCR Assay

Total hypothalamic RNA was isolated using the TRIzol® reagent and reverse-transcribed into cDNA with the PrimeScript™ RT reagent kit (TaKaRa Bio, Otsu, Japan). Quantitative PCR was performed as previously reported (28). Briefly, the reaction was performed with a total volume of 10 μL assay solution containing 5 μL SYBR® Green mix (TaKaRa Bio), 0.2 μL ROX internal reference dye, 1 μL cDNA template, 3 μL deionized H_2O, and 0.4 μL each of the forward and reverse primers. The comparative Ct method was applied to calculate the mRNA expression of the target genes relative to that of β-actin. The primer sequences are presented in **Supplementary Table 1**.

Western Blot Assay

Protein supernatants extracted from hypothalamus samples were run on 10% sodium dodecyl sulfate acrylamide gels and electro-blotted onto nitrocellulose membranes. The membranes were incubated with primary antibodies overnight

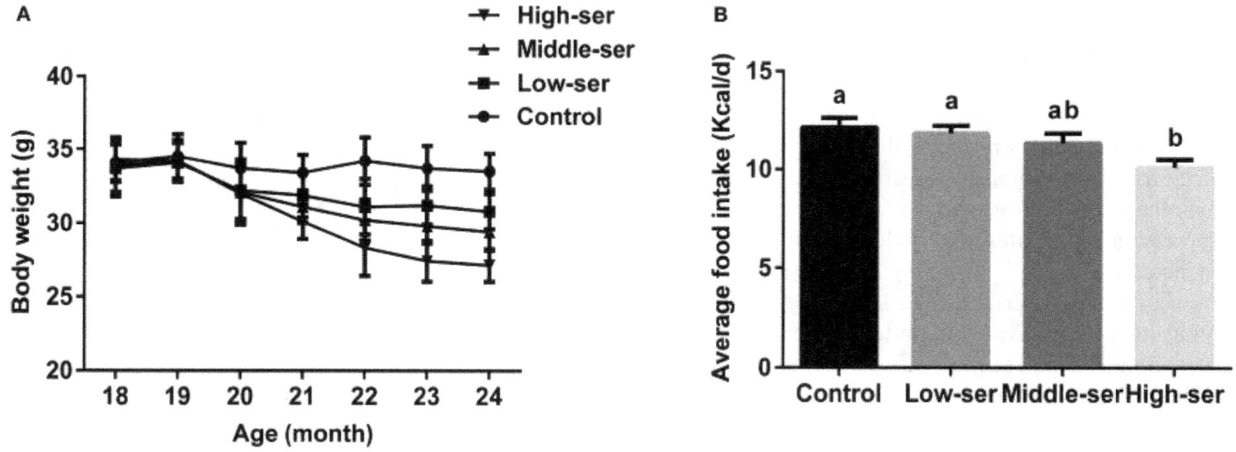

FIGURE 1 | Effects of long-term L-serine administration on body weight and food intake in aging mice. **(A)** Body weight; **(B)** average daily food intake. Control, untreated control mice; Low-ser, mice supplemented with 0.1% (wt/vol) L-serine dissolved in the drinking water; Middle-ser, mice supplemented with 0.2% (wt/vol) L-serine dissolved in the drinking water; High-ser, mice supplemented with 0.5% (wt/vol) L-serine dissolved in the drinking water. Values are expressed as mean ± standard error of the mean (SEM), $n = 20$; [a,b]Means of the bars with different letters were significantly different among groups ($P < 0.05$).

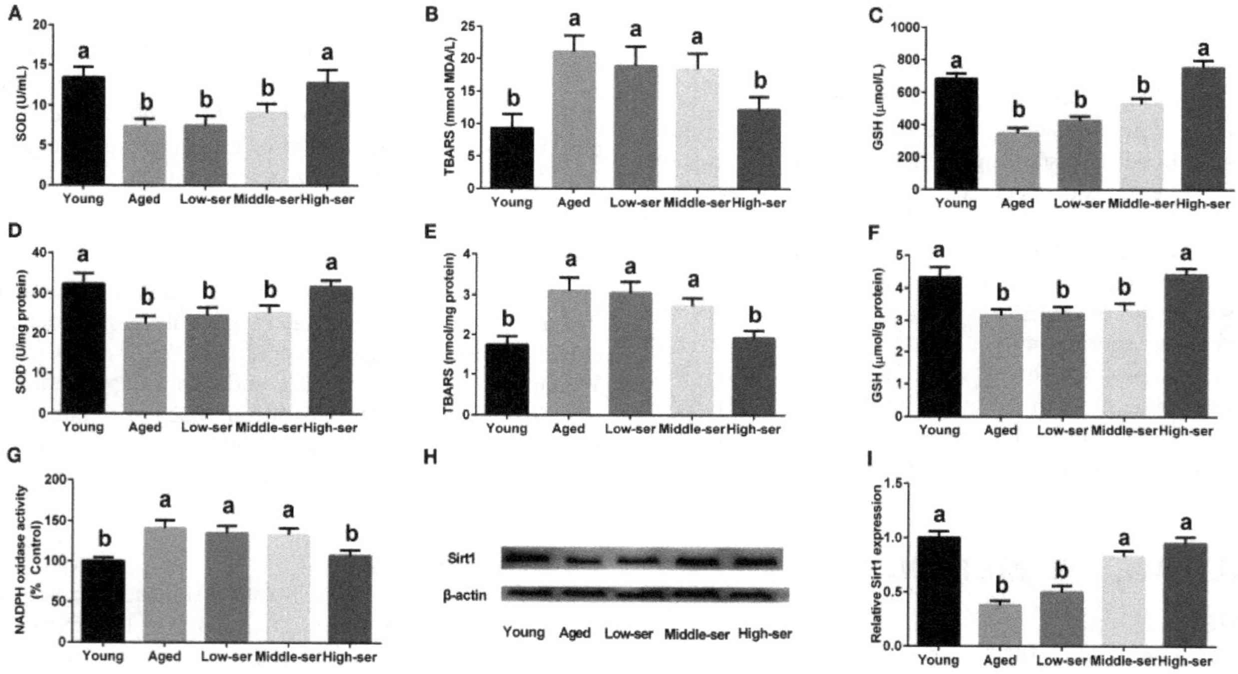

FIGURE 2 | Effects of long-term L-serine administration on oxidative stress in aging mice. **(A–C)** SOD, MDA, and GSH contents in serum; **(D–F)** SOD, MDA, and GSH contents in the hypothalamus; **(G)** NADPH oxidase activity; **(H,I)** Protein expression of Sirt1. Aged, untreated control mice; Low-ser, mice supplemented with 0.1% (wt/vol) L-serine dissolved in the drinking water; Middle-ser, mice supplemented with 0.2% (wt/vol) L-serine dissolved in the drinking water; High-ser, mice supplemented with 0.5% (wt/vol) L-serine dissolved in the drinking water. Young, adult male mice at the age of 18 months. SOD, superoxide dismutase; MDA, malondialdehyde; GSH, glutathione; NADPH, nicotinamide adenine dinucleotide phosphate. Values are expressed as mean ± SEM, $n = 3$ for the statistical analysis of western blotting data and $n = 8$ for the statistical analysis of other data; [a,b]Means of the bars with different letters were significantly different among groups ($P < 0.05$).

at 4°C, followed by a second incubation with anti-rabbit or anti-mouse IgG. Primary antibodies specific for Sirt1, STAT3, phospho-STAT3, and total NFκB (Cell Signaling Technology, Beverly, MA, USA) were used. Finally, the EZ-ECL chemiluminescence reagent (Biological Industries, Cromwell, CT, USA) was added onto the membrane and bands were obtained.

Statistical Analysis

All statistical analyses were performed with one-way analysis of variance, using the general linear model and the MIXED procedure (PROC MIXED) from SAS software version 9.2 (SAS Institute Inc., Cary, NC, USA). Data are presented as least squares means ± standard error of the mean. Mean values were considered significantly different when $P < 0.05$.

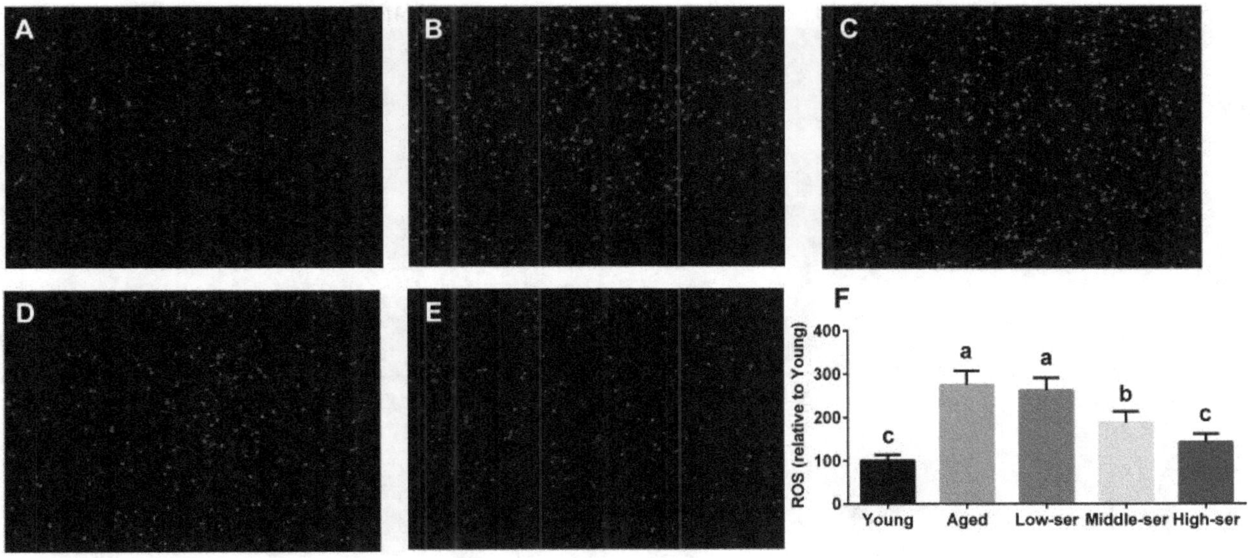

FIGURE 3 | Effects of long-term L-serine administration on the ROS content in aging mice. Representative images of ROS in mice from the Young **(A)**, Aged **(B)**, Low-ser **(C)**, Middle-ser **(D)**, and High-ser **(E)** groups; **(F)** Relative ROS content. Aged, untreated control mice; Low-ser, mice supplemented with 0.1% (wt/vol) L-serine dissolved in the drinking water; Middle-ser, mice supplemented with 0.2% (wt/vol) L-serine dissolved in the drinking water; High-ser, mice supplemented with 0.5% (wt/vol) L-serine dissolved in the drinking water. Young, adult male mice at the age of 18 months. ROS, reactive oxygen species. Values are expressed as mean ± SEM, $n = 4$. [a,b,c]Means of the bars with different letters were significantly different among groups ($P < 0.05$).

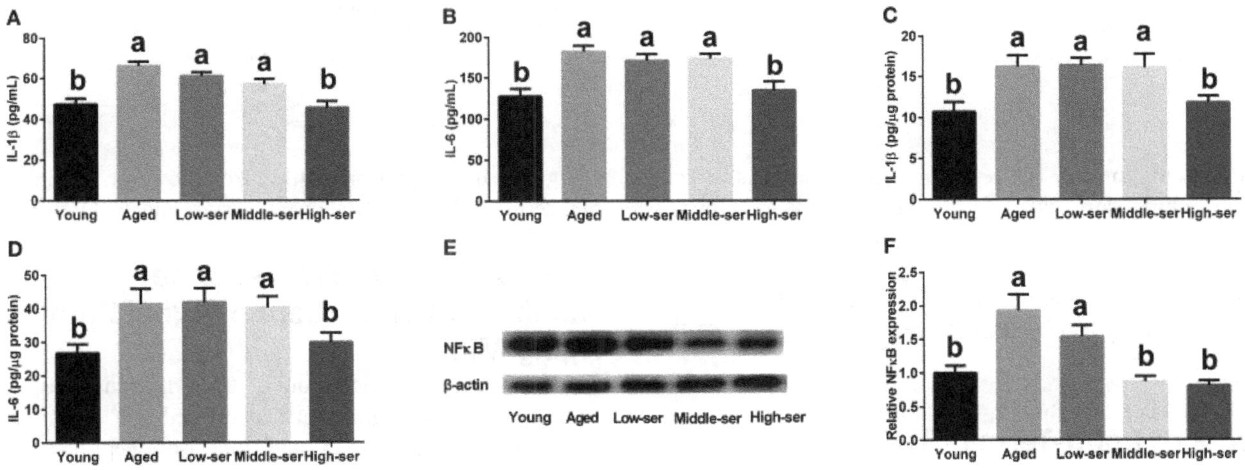

FIGURE 4 | Effects of long-term L-serine administration on the inflammatory response in aging mice. **(A,B)** Concentrations of IL-1β and IL-6 in serum; **(C,D)** Concentrations of IL-1β and IL-6 in the hypothalamus; **(E,F)** Relative NF-κB protein expression. Aged, untreated control mice; Low-ser, mice supplemented with 0.1% (wt/vol) L-serine dissolved in the drinking water; Middle-ser, mice supplemented with 0.2% (wt/vol) L-serine dissolved in the drinking water; High-ser, mice supplemented with 0.5% (wt/vol) L-serine dissolved in the drinking water. Young, adult male mice at the age of 18 months. Values are expressed as mean ± SEM, $n = 3$ for the statistical analysis of western blotting data and $n = 8$ for the statistical analysis of other data; [a,b]Means of the bars with different letters were significantly different among groups ($P < 0.05$).

RESULTS

Effects of Long-Term L-Serine Administration on Body Weight and Food Intake in Aging Mice

The long-term administration of 0.5% L-serine significantly decreased body weight and reduced food intake in aging mice when compared with controls (i.e., aging mice that did not receive L-serine), while the administration of 0.1 or 0.2% L-serine did not show such effects (**Figure 1**).

Effects of Long-Term L-Serine Administration on Oxidative Stress in Aging Mice

The long-term administration of 0.5% L-serine significantly increased the SOD and GSH levels while decreasing the

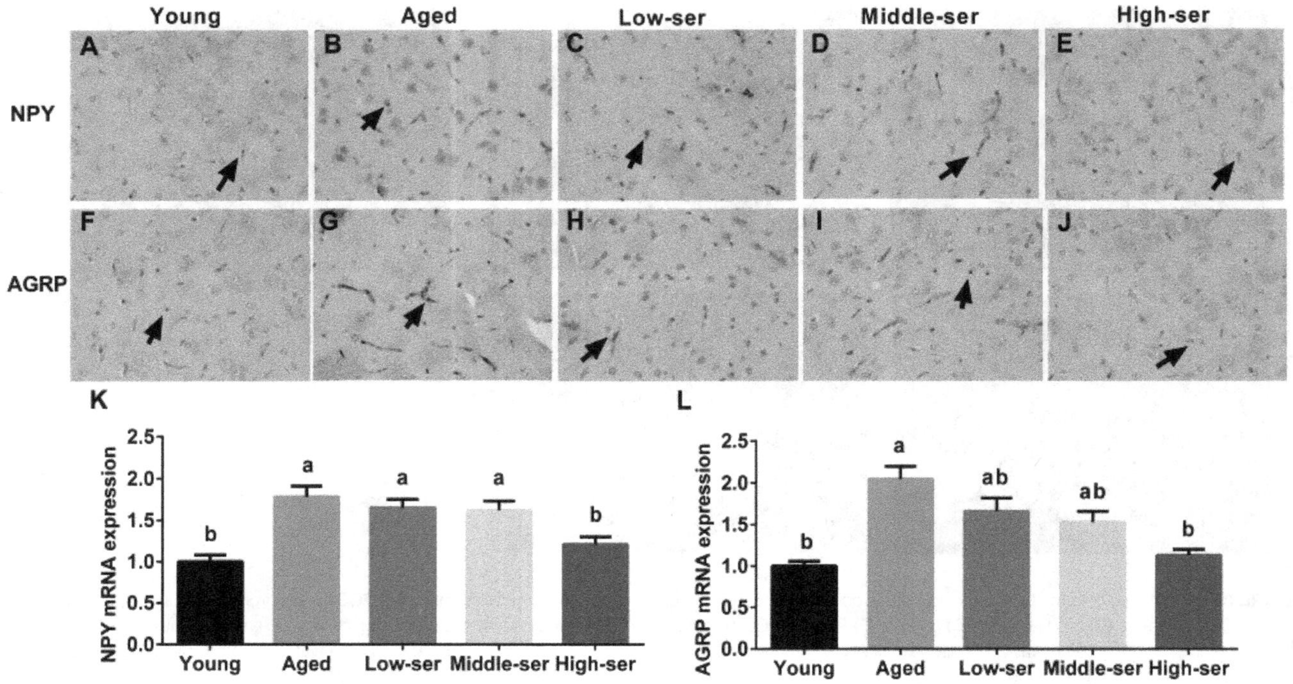

FIGURE 5 | Effects of long-term L-serine administration on orexigenic neuropeptide expression in aging mice. NPY **(A–E)** and AGRP **(F–J)** expression as determined by immunohistochemistry; relative NPY **(K)** and AGRP **(L)** mRNA expression. Aged, untreated control mice; Low-ser, mice supplemented with 0.1% (wt/vol) L-serine dissolved in the drinking water; Middle-ser, mice supplemented with 0.2% (wt/vol) L-serine dissolved in the drinking water; High-ser, mice supplemented with 0.5% (wt/vol) L-serine dissolved in the drinking water. Young, adult male mice at the age of 18 months. Arrow (yellow), expression of target proteins; NPY, neuropeptide Y; AGRP, agouti-related protein. Values are expressed as mean ± SEM, $n = 8$; [a,b]Means of the bars with different letters were significantly different among groups ($P < 0.05$).

MDA contents in both the serum and hypothalamus of aging mice in comparison with controls (**Figures 2A–F**). However, the administration of L-serine at 0.1 or 0.2% had no effect. Additionally, the administration of 0.5% L-serine significantly decreased NADPH oxidase activity (**Figure 2G**) and ROS content (**Figure 3**) while it increased Sirt1 expression (**Figures 2H,I**) in the hypothalamus.

Effects of Long-Term L-Serine Administration on the Inflammatory Response in Aging Mice

The long-term administration of 0.5% L-serine significantly decreased the concentrations of IL-1β and IL-6 in the serum and hypothalamus of aging mice when compared with the control animals. By contrast, L-serine at 0.1 or 0.2% had no effect (**Figures 4A–D**). In addition, the long-term administration of 0.5% L-serine significantly decreased NFκB expression in the hypothalamus (**Figures 4E,F**).

Effects of Long-Term L-Serine Administration on Orexigenic Neuropeptide Expression in Aging Mice

Long-term administration of 0.5% L-serine significantly decreased NPY and AGRP expression in the hypothalamus of aging mice in comparison with controls; however, administration of L-serine at 0.1 or 0.2% showed no such effects (**Figure 5**).

Effects of Long-Term L-Serine Administration on Leptin Signal Pathway in Aging Mice

The long-term administration of 0.5% L-serine, but not 0.1 or 0.2% L-serine, significantly decreased the leptin content (**Figure 6F**) in the serum and increased LepRb expression (**Figures 6A–E,G**) in the hypothalamus of aging mice when compared with controls. In addition, the long-term administration of 0.5% L-serine significantly increased the expression of phosphorylated STAT3 in the hypothalamus of aging mice (**Figures 6H,I**).

DISCUSSION

Our previous studies have shown that L-serine could alleviate oxidative stress in various tissues of different rodent models, including diquat- and long-term high-fat-induced oxidative stress in liver (21, 22) and lipopolysaccharides-induced oxidative damage in the small intestine (23). Based on these previous experiments, we chose the dose of 0.1, 0.2, and 0.5% (w/v) L-serine for the current 6-month study, respectively. Additionally, since patients who received the relatively high

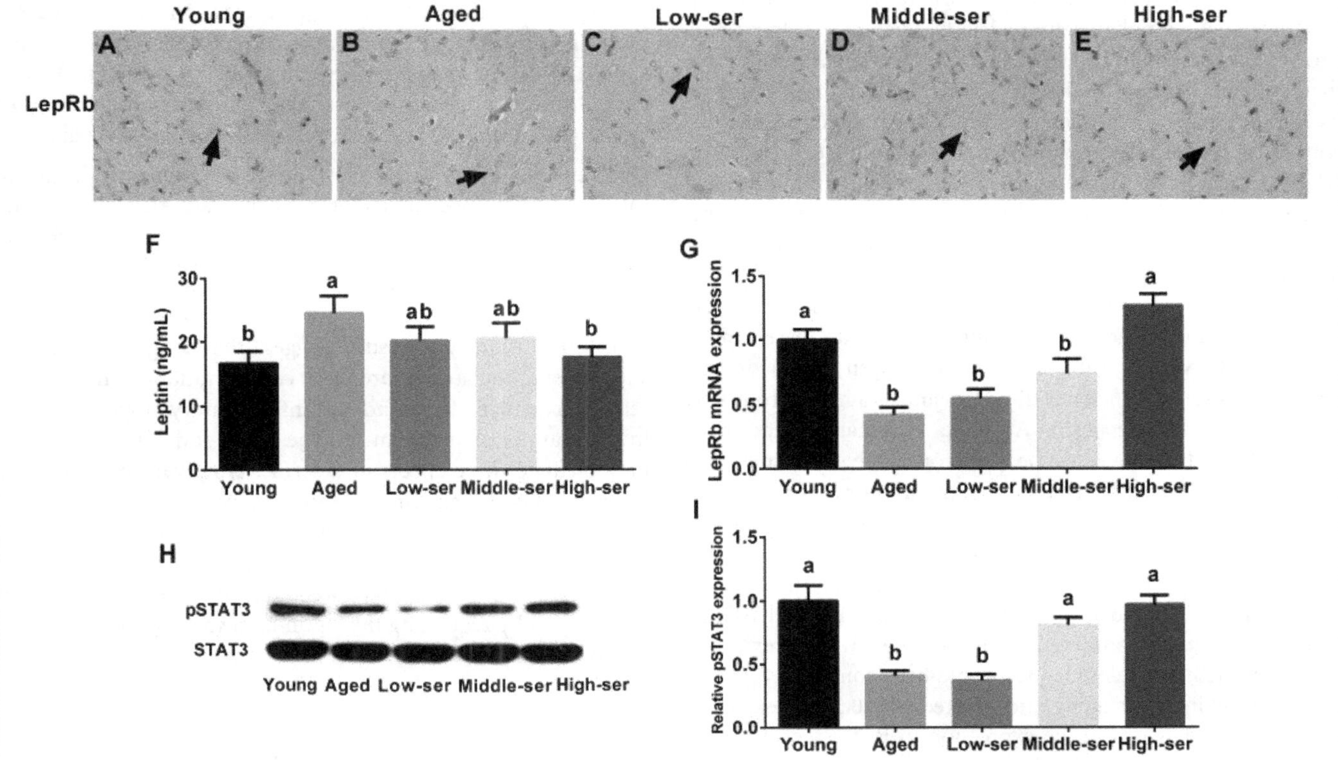

FIGURE 6 | Effects of long-term L-serine administration on the leptin signaling pathway in aging mice. **(A–E)** LepRb expression as determined by immunohistochemistry; **(F)** leptin content in the hypothalamus; **(G)** relative LepRb mRNA expression; **(H,I)** relative pSTAT3 protein expression. Aged, untreated control mice; Low-ser, mice fed with 0.1% (wt/vol) L-serine dissolved in the drinking water; Middle-ser, mice fed with 0.2% (wt/vol) L-serine dissolved in the drinking water; High-ser, mice fed with 0.5% (wt/vol) L-serine dissolved in the drinking water. Young, adult male mice at the age of 18 months. Arrow (yellow), expression of LepRb protein; LepRb, leptin receptor. Values are expressed as mean ± SEM, $n = 3$ for the statistical analysis of western blotting data and $n = 8$ for the statistical analysis of other data; [a,b]Means of the bars with different letters were significantly different among groups ($p < 0.05$).

amount of 30 g/day L-serine for 9 months in phase II clinical trials did not show any side effects and L-serine is generally regarded as safe by the United States Food and Drug Administration (25), we employed L-serine as a non-toxic agent. As expected, our results further supported that long-term L-serine supplementation may alleviate age-related oxidative damage, since it is shown herein that L-serine increased the levels of antioxidant enzymes while decreasing those of ROS in the hypothalamus.

The process of aging is associated with a redox imbalance and the accumulation of oxidative damage in many tissues, which is caused by an increase in ROS production and a decrease in antioxidant capacity (29). The hypothalamus is especially oxidatively challenged with increasing age and is vulnerable to oxidative stress (3). Since the hypothalamus plays a critical role in the central nervous system, age-related oxidative stress in this organ usually results in the loss of various physiological functions and the development of diseases such as age-related obesity and neurodegeneration. We found that long-term L-serine supplementation attenuated the decreases in the levels of antioxidants (GSH) and antioxidant enzymes (SOD) and the accumulation of ROS that are observed during aging. Based on these results, we believe that the functionality of the hypothalamus would be improved by long-term L-serine supplementation at an appropriate concentration in aging mice.

In age-related diseases, there is an antagonistic crosstalk between Sirt1 and NFκB. On the one hand, the inhibition of Sirt1 stimulates NFκB-induced inflammation directly through regulating the p65 subunit of the NFκB complex. On the other hand, NFκB inhibits Sirt1 activity mainly by affecting the production of factors such as ROS (30). Sirt1 plays a major role in the regulation of oxidative stress during aging. A reduction in Sirt1 expression with the progression of aging contributes to the upregulation of oxidative damage (31). Consequently, Sirt1-activating dietary supplements such as resveratrol, eicosapentaenoic acid, docosahexaenoic acid, and acetylshikonin show anti-aging effects (32, 33). Moreover, Sirt1 also plays a protective role against neuroinflammation in brain disease (33). Here, we found that L-serine supplementation at the concentration of 0.5% (w/v) restored the expression of Sirt1 after its age-related decrease. Thus, we suggest that the Sirt1 pathway may mediate the antioxidative and anti-inflammatory effects of L-serine in the hypothalamus of aging mice. Additionally, the activity of NFκB signaling was reported to increase in the hypothalamus with aging (34), suggesting that NFκB signaling is a promising target for preventing age-related inflammation.

The inhibition of this pathway by caloric restriction and dietary nutrients such as polyunsaturated fatty acids delays aging and extends the lifespan of rodents (33, 35). Our results also indicate that L-serine attenuated the inflammatory response, which is usually associated with oxidative stress during aging, since the concentrations of inflammatory cytokines and the expression of NFκB decreased in the hypothalamus. These results indicated that NFκB pathway also plays an important role in mediating the preventive effects of L-serine against the increased inflammation in aged mice.

Unexpectedly, we found that long-term L-serine supplementation affected food intake and decreased age-related body weight gain. L-Serine has been used for the treatment of serine deficiency disorders and as a neuroprotective substance for decades (36). A phase I human clinical trial indicated that L-serine could be a generally safe supplement for patients with amyotrophic lateral sclerosis/motor neuron disease (37). However, we noticed that, in these reports, two patients showed a slightly decreased food intake. Supplementation with a high dose of L-serine for a long period might have some effects on food intake. The decreased expression of NPY and AGRP, which are highly conserved neuropeptides with orexigenic actions in the hypothalamus (38), could have contributed to the reduced food intake in aging mice treated with 0.5% L-serine. In addition, the increases in the expression of leptin receptor and the phosphorylation of STAT3, which is involved in the leptin signaling pathway in the hypothalamus, induced by serine would also affect food intake because of the anorectic effects of leptin. However, a high leptin level was found in aged mice; therefore, we suggest that leptin resistance may occur in these aged animals. The preventive effects of long-term L-serine supplementation on age-induced oxidative stress and age-related obesity observed herein suggest that L-serine supplementation might have the same effects as lifelong caloric restriction. Furthermore, L-serine supplementation in aging mice activated *Sirt1*, which is defined as a "longevity gene," suggesting a life-extending effect of serine. Interestingly, researchers found that in the village of Ogimi, which is known as the "Village of Longevity" in Japan, the traditional food items of residents are rich in L-serine (25). Further studies are required to provide more convincing evidence of the life-extending effect of L-serine.

In conclusion, our results suggest that long-term L-serine supplementation at an appropriate concentration attenuates age-related oxidative stress and the inflammatory response in the hypothalamus of aging mice. The Sirt1 and NFκB pathways may mediate these effects of L-serine. However, the molecular mechanisms through which L-serine decreases the expression of NFκB while rescuing that of Sirt1 need to be further elucidated. Additionally, we unexpectedly found that L-serine reduced food intake and age-related body weight gain. L-Serine may exert these effects by regulating the leptin pathway and the orexigenic neuropeptides NPY and AGRP.

AUTHOR CONTRIBUTIONS

XZ, LH, and HZ conducted the experiment. XZ and LH collected and analyzed the data. XW and YY helped with the discussion. XZ and XW designed the experiment and wrote the manuscript. XW and YY revised the manuscript.

REFERENCES

1. MohanKumar SM, Kasturi BS, Shin AC, Balasubramanian P, Gilbreath ET, Subramanian M, et al. Chronic estradiol exposure induces oxidative stress in the hypothalamus to decrease hypothalamic dopamine and cause hyperprolactinemia. *Am J Physiol Regul Integr Comp Physiol.* (2011) 300:R693–9. doi: 10.1152/ajpregu.00481.2010
2. Manjula KR, Subramanyam MV, Asha Devi S. Protection against oxidative stress caused by intermittent cold exposure by combined supplementation with vitamin E and C in the aging rat hypothalamus. *Neurochem Res.* (2013) 38:876–85. doi: 10.1007/s11064-013-0993-4
3. Whidden MA, Kirichenko N, Halici Z, Erdos B, Foster TC, Tumer N. Lifelong caloric restriction prevents age-induced oxidative stress in the sympathoadrenal system of Fischer 344 x Brown Norway rats. *Biochem Biophys Res Commun.* (2011) 408:454–8. doi: 10.1016/j.bbrc.2011.04.051
4. Siqueira IR, Fochesatto C, de Andrade A, Santos M, Hagen M, Bello-Klein A, et al. Total antioxidant capacity is impaired in different structures from aged rat brain. *Int J Dev Neurosci.* (2005) 23:663–71. doi: 10.1016/j.ijdevneu.2005.03.001
5. Floyd RA, Hensley K. Oxidative stress in brain aging. Implications for therapeutics of neurodegenerative diseases. *Neurobiol Aging* (2002) 23:795–807. doi: 10.1016/S0197-4580(02)00019-2
6. Gilgun-Sherki Y, Melamed E, Offen D. Oxidative stress induced-neurodegenerative diseases: the need for antioxidants that penetrate the blood brain barrier. *Neuropharmacology* (2001) 40:959–75. doi: 10.1016/S0028-3908(01)00019-3
7. Toklu HZ, Scarpace PJ, Sakarya Y, Kirichenko N, Matheny M, Bruce EB, et al. Intracerebroventricular tempol administration in older rats reduces oxidative stress in the hypothalamus but does not change STAT3 signalling or SIRT1/AMPK pathway. *Appl Physiol Nutr Metab.* (2017) 42:59–67. doi: 10.1139/apnm-2016-0067
8. Sharma S, Singh R, Kaur M, Kaur G. Late-onset dietary restriction compensates for age-related increase in oxidative stress and alterations of HSP 70 and synapsin 1 protein levels in male Wistar rats. *Biogerontology* (2010) 11:197–209. doi: 10.1007/s10522-009-9240-4
9. Lv J, Jiang S, Yang Z, Hu W, Wang Z, Li T, et al. PGC-1alpha sparks the fire of neuroprotection against neurodegenerative disorders. *Ageing Res Rev.* (2018) 44:8–21. doi: 10.1016/j.arr.2018.03.004

10. Russomanno G, Corbi G, Manzo V, Ferrara N, Rengo G, Puca AA, et al. The anti-ageing molecule sirt1 mediates beneficial effects of cardiac rehabilitation. *Immun Aging* (2017) 14:7. doi: 10.1186/s12979-017-0088-1
11. Ma Z, Yang Y, Di S, Feng X, Liu D, Jiang S, et al. Pterostilbene exerts anticancer activity on non-small-cell lung cancer via activating endoplasmic reticulum stress. *Sci Rep.* (2017) 7:8091. doi: 10.1038/s41598-017-08547-0
12. Jiang S, Yang Z, Di S, Hu W, Ma Z, Chen F, et al. Novel role of forkhead box O 4 transcription factor in cancer: bringing out the good or the bad. *Semin Cancer Biol.* (2018) 50:1–12. doi: 10.1016/j.semcancer.2018.04.007
13. Jiang S, Li T, Yang Z, Hu W, Yang Y. Deciphering the roles of FOXO1 in human neoplasms. *Int J Cancer* (2018). doi: 10.1002/ijc.31338
14. Xin Z, Ma Z, Hu W, Jiang S, Yang Z, Li T, et al. FOXO1/3: potential suppressors of fibrosis. *Ageing Res Rev.* (2018) 41:42–52. doi: 10.1016/j.arr.2017.11.002
15. Ma Z, Xin Z, Hu W, Jiang S, Yang Z, Yan X, et al. Forkhead box O proteins: crucial regulators of cancer EMT. *Semin Cancer Biol.* (2018) 50:21–31. doi: 10.1016/j.semcancer.2018.02.004
16. Toorie AM, Nillni EA. Minireview: central sirt1 regulates energy balance via the melanocortin system and alternate pathways. *Mol Endocrinol.* (2014) 28:1423–34. doi: 10.1210/me.2014-1115
17. Nillni EA. The metabolic sensor Sirt1 and the hypothalamus: interplay between peptide hormones and pro-hormone convertases. *Mol Cell Endocrinol.* (2016) 438:77–88. doi: 10.1016/j.mce.2016.09.002
18. Li X, Stark GR. NFkappaB-dependent signaling pathways. *Exp Hematol.* (2002) 30:285–96. doi: 10.1016/S0301-472X(02)00777-4
19. Cai D. NFkappaB-mediated metabolic inflammation in peripheral tissues versus central nervous system. *Cell Cycle* (2009) 8:2542–8. doi: 10.4161/cc.8.16.9386
20. Kaltschmidt B, Kaltschmidt C. NF-kappaB in the nervous system. *Cold Spring Harb Perspect Biol.* (2009) 1:a001271. doi: 10.1101/cshperspect.a001271
21. Zhou X, He L, Zuo S, Zhang Y, Wan D, Long C, et al. Serine prevented high-fat diet-induced oxidative stress by activating AMPK and epigenetically modulating the expression of glutathione synthesis-related genes. *Biochim Biophys Acta* (2018) 1864:488–98. doi: 10.1016/j.bbadis.2017.11.009
22. Zhou X, He L, Wu C, Zhang Y, Wu X, Yin Y. Serine alleviates oxidative stress via supporting glutathione synthesis and methionine cycle in mice. *Mol Nutr Food Res.* (2017) 61:1700262 . doi: 10.1002/mnfr.201700262
23. Zhou XH, Zhang YM, He LQ, Wan D, Liu G, Wu X, et al. Serine prevents LPS-induced intestinal inflammation and barrier damage via p53-dependent glutathione synthesis and AMPK activation. *J Funct Foods* (2017) 39:225–32. doi: 10.1016/j.jff.2017.10.026
24. Cao G, Tao F, Xin L, Li Z, Zhou X. Effects of maternal serine supplementation on high-fat diet-induced oxidative stress and epigenetic changes in promoters of glutathione synthesis-related genes in offspring. *J Funct Foods* (2018) 47:316–24. doi: 10.1016/j.jff.2018.05.067
25. Metcalf JS, Dunlop RA, Powell JT, Banack SA, Cox PA. L-Serine: a naturally-occurring amino acid with therapeutic potential. *Neurotox Res.* (2018) 33:213–21. doi: 10.1007/s12640-017-9814-x
26. Dunlop RA, Powell JT, Metcalf JS, Guillemin GJ, Cox PA. L-serine-mediated neuroprotection includes the upregulation of the ER stress chaperone protein disulfide isomerase (PDI). *Neurotox Res.* (2018) 33:113–22. doi: 10.1007/s12640-017-9817-7
27. Jang JY, Min JH, Wang SB, Chae YH, Baek JY, Kim M, et al. Resveratrol inhibits collagen-induced platelet stimulation through suppressing NADPH oxidase and oxidative inactivation of SH2 domain-containing protein tyrosine phosphatase-2. *Free Radic Biol Med.* (2015) 89:842–51. doi: 10.1016/j.freeradbiomed.2015.10.413
28. Jin XL, Wang K, Li QQ, Tian WL, Xue XF, Wu LM, et al. Antioxidant and anti-inflammatory effects of Chinese propolis during palmitic acid-induced lipotoxicity in cultured hepatocytes. *J Funct Foods* (2017) 34:216–23. doi: 10.1016/j.jff.2017.04.039
29. Bokov A, Chaudhuri A, Richardson A. The role of oxidative damage and stress in aging. *Mech Ageing Dev.* (2004) 125:811–26. doi: 10.1016/j.mad.2004.07.009
30. Kauppinen A, Suuronen T, Ojala J, Kaarniranta K, Salminen A. Antagonistic crosstalk between NF-kappaB and SIRT1 in the regulation of inflammation and metabolic disorders. *Cell Signal.* (2013) 25:1939–48. doi: 10.1016/j.cellsig.2013.06.007
31. Lu TM, Tsai JY, Chen YC, Huang CY, Hsu HL, Weng CF, et al. Downregulation of Sirt1 as aging change in advanced heart failure. *J Biomed Sci.* (2014) 21:57. doi: 10.1186/1423-0127-21-57
32. Li Q, Zeng J, Su M, He Y, Zhu B. Acetylshikonin from Zicao attenuates cognitive impairment and hippocampus senescence in d-galactose-induced aging mouse model via upregulating the expression of SIRT1. *Brain Res Bull.* (2018) 137:311–8. doi: 10.1016/j.brainresbull.2018.01.007
33. Freitas HR, Ferreira GDC, Trevenzoli IH, Oliveira KJ, de Melo Reis RA. Fatty acids, antioxidants and physical activity in brain aging. *Nutrients* (2017) 9:E1263. doi: 10.3390/nu9111263
34. Zhang G, Li J, Purkayastha S, Tang Y, Zhang H, Yin Y, et al. Hypothalamic programming of systemic ageing involving IKK-beta, NF-kappaB and GnRH. *Nature* (2013) 497:211–6. doi: 10.1038/nature12143
35. Horrillo D, Sierra J, Arribas C, Garcia-San Frutos M, Carrascosa JM, Lauzurica N, et al. Age-associated development of inflammation in Wistar rats: effects of caloric restriction. *Arch Physiol Biochem.* (2011) 117:140–50. doi: 10.3109/13813455.2011.577435
36. de Koning TJ, Snell K, Duran M, Berger R, Poll-The BT, Surtees R. L-serine in disease and development. *Biochem J.* (2003) 371:653–61. doi: 10.1042/bj20021785
37. Levine TD, Miller RG, Bradley WG, Moore DH, Saperstein DS, Flynn LE, et al. Phase I clinical trial of safety of L-serine for ALS patients. *Amyotroph Lateral Scler Frontotemporal Degener.* (2017) 18:107–11. doi: 10.1080/21678421.2016.1221971
38. Mercer RE, Chee MJ, Colmers WF. The role of NPY in hypothalamic mediated food intake. *Front Neuroendocrinol.* (2011) 32:398–415. doi: 10.1016/j.yfrne.2011.06.001

4

Distinctive Roles of Sirtuins on Diabetes, Protective or Detrimental?

Jie Song [1,2], Bing Yang [1,3], Xiaobin Jia [1], Mingyu Li [3], Wei Tan [2], Shitang Ma [4], Xinhong Shi [1] and Liang Feng [1]*

[1] School of Traditional Chinese Pharmacy, China Pharmaceutical University, Nanjing, China, [2] Affiliated Hospital on Integration of Chinese and Western Medicine, Nanjing University of Chinese Medicine, Nanjing, China, [3] Nanjing University of Chinese Medicine, Nanjing, China, [4] Life and Health college, Anhui Science and Technology University, Fengyang, China

***Correspondence:**
Liang Feng
wenmoxiushi@163.com

Dysregulation of metabolic pathways leads to type 2 diabetes, characteristic of high glucose concentration caused by insulin resistance. The histone deacetylases sirtuins exhibit remarkable enzymatic activities. Accumulating evidence indicates that sirtuins can be pharmacologically activated to ameliorate diabetes. Here, we evaluated different roles of sirtuins (SIRT1-SIRT7) in diabetes progression and described their involvement in metabolic pathways of skeletal muscle, adipose tissue and liver. The nuclear sirtuins, SIRT1, SIRT6, and SIRT7, regulate the activity of key transcription factors and cofactors in almost all tissues with the cellular responses to energy demands. The mitochondrial sirtuins, SIRT3, SIRT4, and SIRT5, regulate the activity of mitochondrial enzymes in response to fasting and calorie restriction. Moreover, genetic polymorphisms of SIRT1 and SIRT2 have been reported to associate with diabetes development. It's worth noting that SIRT1, SIRT2, SIRT3, and SIRT6 are positive regulators of insulin resistance in most cases. In the opposite, SIRT4 and SIRT7 inhibit insulin secretion and fatty acid oxidation. Identification of SIRT1 activators for diabetes has gained wide attention, such as metformin, resveratrol, and resveratrol derivatives. Randomized, prospective, and large-scale clinical trials are warrant to uncover the responsibilities of SIRTs modulators on diabetes progress.

Keywords: SIRTs, diabetes, insulin resistance, glucose uptake, fatty acid oxidation

INTRODUCTION

Sirtuins belong to class III histone deacylases, and in each deacylation cycle one molecule NAD^+ is consumed (1). SIRTs isoforms have been defined in mammals, such as SIRT1–7. Although they are equipped with a highly conserved structure of about 275 amino acids, just like the silent information regulator 2 in yeast (2), the C-and N-terminal extensions are distinctive, which are the predominant factor of sirtuins subcellular localization (3). SIRT1, SIRT6, and SIRT7 are principally found in the nucleus. SIRT2 is mainly located in the cytoplasm, and SIRT3-5 are located in the mitochondria (**Figure 1**). The catalytic core is made up of a small zinc-binding domain, a large Rossmann-fold domain, and a few flexible loops which bind these domains together. The large domain of most sirtuins resembles each other, characteristic of a β-sheet encircled by six α-helices, excluding SIRT2, which has seven α-helices (4). In the small domain, diversities are observed in the principal sequence. Firstly, the helix bundle is only absent in SIRT7 and SIRT6. Next, SIRT5 and SIRT4 have a loop and a short helix, yielding an insertion in the small domain. This feature might be essential for the mitochondrial localization (5). Lastly, SIRT1 has a 5-residue loop in this domain, neighboring to the zinc-binding cysteine. Those dissimilarities in the catalytic core might closely relate with their key properties.

SIRT1-3 and SIRT6 exhibit remarkable demyristoylase activity (6, 7). Except for functioning as an ADP-ribosyltransferase (8, 9), SIRT4 also possesses a lipoamidase effect (10). By targeting carbamoyl phosphate synthetase (CPS1), SIRT5 can remove malonyl or succinyl groups in a manner very similar to deacetylation (11, 12). SIRT6 deacetylates histone H3K9 & H3K56, and mono-ADP-ribosyltransferate long-chain acyl and acetyl groups (13). SIRT7 is distributed in all organs and tissues (14) and activates RNA polymerase I transcription. Although several of its molecular substrate have been identified, including WSTF–ISWI chromatin remodeling complex (WICH), rDNA transcription factor UBF (the nucleolar upstream-binding factor) and RNA polI (15), SIRT7's catalytic activity remains elusive.

Diabetes is a global epidemic problem growing exponentially, posing a serious threat. Type 2 diabetes mellitus (T2DM) is a multifactorial metabolic and endocrine disorder for human beings, characteristic of abnormal glucose level in blood. T2DM individuals are estimated to be 642 million by 2,040 globally (16). T2DM is predominately attributed to insulin resistance and pancreatic β-cell dysfunction (17, 18). Insulin resistance, primarily in liver, muscle and adipose tissue as well, spoils glucose disposal, leading to β-cell insulin increase and hyperinsulinemia in a compensatory manner.

Blunted sirtuin activity has been reported to induce diabetes and metabolic syndrome, and aggravate high-fat diet (HFD) effects in mice. Exceptionally, SIRT4 prevents insulin secretion and stimulates T2DM. SIRT4 also negatively regulates fatty acid oxidation (FAO) in muscle and liver cells. A mutation in human SIRT1 caused a familial form of autoimmune diabetes (19–21). SIRT1 can interact with transcription factors and co-activators (RelA/p65, FOXO, and p53). T2DM group has lower SIRT1 mRNA levels compared with healthy group. There is a negative connection between fasting plasma glucose and SIRT1, as shown in the correlation analysis. The expression of SIRT1 in monocytes and granulocytes of T2DM might associate with glucose/lipid metabolism status (22). In both of the kidney and liver of diabetic rats, SIRT1 and SIRT2 gene expressions reduced considerably than blank control group (23). HFD triggers SIRT1 decrement in mice probably via proteolysis (19). SIRT1 expression is also reduced in obese humans (24, 25), and meanwhile diabetes is alleviated in SIRT1-overexpressed mice (26–28). SIRT6 is important for sustaining pancreatic β-cell function in mice. SIRT6 knockout leads to severe hypoglycemia in mice. SIRT6 deficiency results in liver steatosis and accelerates insulin resistance and obesity induced by diet. Overnutrition and aging decreased SIRT6 level as well as irregular lipid and glucose metabolism (29). SIRT7 deficiency in mice induces multi-systemic mitochondrial dysfunction. To fully understand the part SIRTs play in diabetes and to reveal regulatory mechanisms regarding SIRTs is the principal purpose in the current review.

SIRTs IN INSULIN RESISTANCE

Pancreatic β cells secret insulin after nutrient stimulation. In the fed state, glycolysis, glucose uptake, and glycogen formation will be promoted by insulin. The glucose homeostasis in adipose tissue and skeletal muscle can also be regulated by insulin (30). Insulin resistance will give rise to hyperuricemia, visceral adiposity, dyslipidemia, hypertension, and hyperglycemia. About 70% of glucose is disposed in muscle. Free fatty acids accumulation and inflammation in muscle triggeres abundant lipid deposition. Imbalanced muscle uptake promotes extra glucose to returns to the liver, which yields intense circulation of free fatty acids, finally leading to fat accumulation and insulin resistance.

As a major inhibitor of the insulin receptor, protein tyrosine phosphatase 1b (PTP1B) can be inhibited by SIRT1, thus increasing insulin sensitivity (31–33). In insulin-resistant obese mice, PTP1B level was raised, associated with decreased SIRT1 expression in skeletal muscle. SIRT1 overexpression brought PTP1B expression to the baseline and abrogated the insulin-stimulated signaling in skeletal muscle (**Figure 2** and **Table 1**). In β-cells, SIRT1 overexpression boosted insulin secretion and improved glucose tolerance, contributing to glucose homeostasis (34). Uncoupling protein 2 (UCP2) disturbs the electrochemical proton gradient, leading to shrink in ATP production and insulin secretion impairment afterwards (35). SIRT1 overexpression suppressed UCP2, finally enlarging ATP levels and insulin secretion (34, 36). UCP2 expression in MIN6 β-cells was reduced by SIRT1, as demonstrated in microarray assays. SIRT1 RNAi decreased the secretion capability of β-cells, which was renovated by UCP2 RNAi (36). On the other side, oxidative stress-induced hyperglycemia and cytokine toxicity was repressed by SIRT1 via deacetylating forkhead box O1 (FOXO1) and the NF-κB subunit p65 on β-cells, respectively (37, 38). Multiple feedback loops are involved in SIRT signaling network. Via binding to SIRT1 promoter, p53 successfully inhibited SIRT1 transcription activity (39). FOXO3a can block the effect of p53, in consequence SIRT1 promoter will be relieved (39). Peroxisome Proliferator Activated Receptor Gamma (PPARγ) is negatively associated with SIRT1 activity (40, 41), whereas PPARα and PPARβ function in the opposite way (42, 43). MiR-199a, MiR-34a, posttranslational modification, such as phosphorylation, also affect SIRT1 activity or transcription (44–47). Taken together, SIRT1 positively regulated insulin sensitivity.

Recently, SIRT2 has been implicated in sustaining insulin sensitivity and glucose homeostasis (48). In insulin-resistant livers and hepatocytes, SIRT2 expression was lowered, accompanied with mitochondrial dysfunction, extracellular signal-regulated kinase (ERK) activation, and amplified production of reactive oxygen species (ROS). On the contrary, insulin sensitivity and mitochondrial dysfunction was improved, and ROS generation was lessened in SIRT2-overexpressed insulin-resistant hepatocytes (49). In human peripheral blood mononuclear cells (PBMCs), insulin resistance and obesity negatively related with SIRT2 (50). As Protein Kinase B (Akt) substrates, FOXO transcription factors are deacetylated by SIRT2 (51–54). However, the function of SIRT2 in insulin

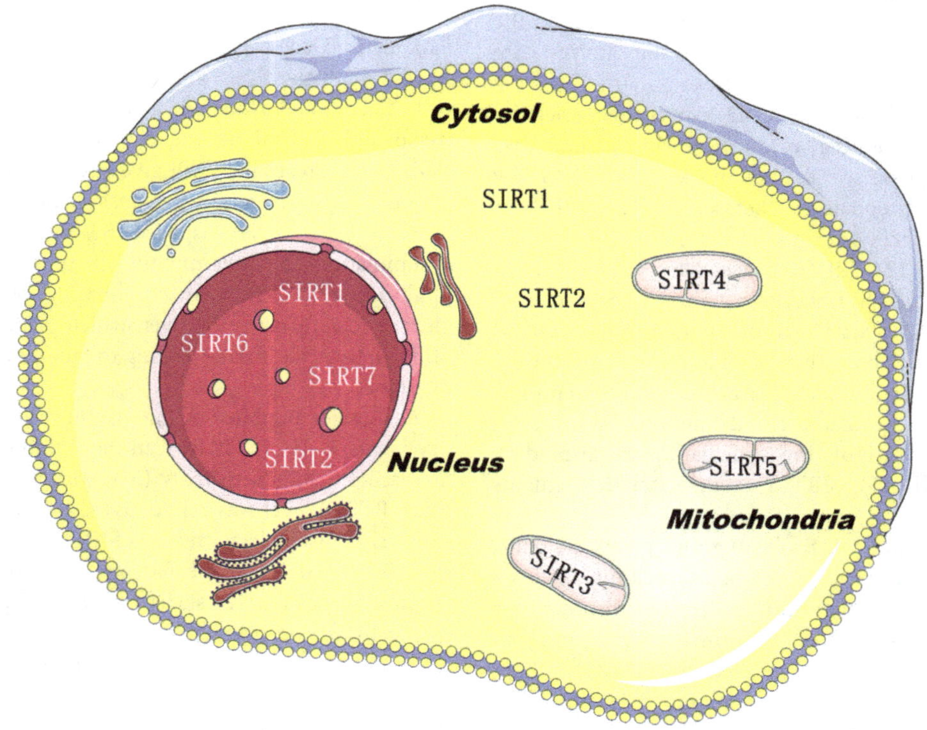

FIGURE 1 | The localization of SIRTs family in the cells.

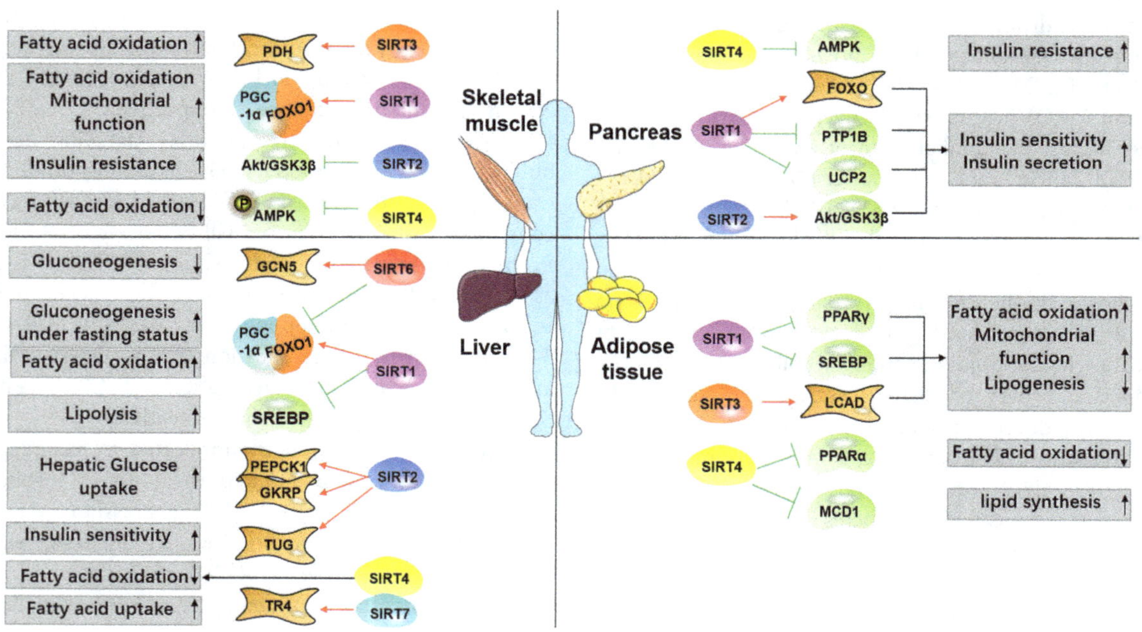

FIGURE 2 | Overview of SIRTs targets involved in diabetes. Major metabolic tissues, including liver, pancreas, adipose, and skeletal muscle are depicted to demonstrate SIRTs functions in the metabolic process modulating insulin resistance, glucose uptake, and lipid synthesis. Red arrows indicate promoting effect, and green arrows indicate inhibiting effect.

TABLE 1 | Summary of sirtuin functions in diabetes development.

Sirtuins	Subcellular localization	Enzyme actions	Substrates	Functions
SIRT1	Nuclear Cytoplasm	Deacetylase	PTP1B, UCP2, PPARα, PPARγ, PPARγ2, p53, FOXO1, PGC-1α, NF-κB, CRTC2, SREBP	Adipogenesis↓ Lipogenesis↓ Lipolysis↑ FAO↑ Glucose uptake↑ Mitochondrial biogenesis↑ Insulin secretion↑ in the fed state Hepatic gluconeogenesis↑ in fasted state Preserve glucose homeostasis under fasted and fed conditions
SIRT2	Cytoplasm (nuclear during interphase and mitosis)	Deacetylase ADP-ribosyltransferase Demyristoylase	ERK1/2, GSK3β, p70S6 Akt, FOXO, TUG, GKRP, PEPCK1, PGC-1α	Adipogenesis↓ Lipolysis↑ FAO↑ HGU↑ Regulation of adipocyte differentiation Insulin sensitivity↑ in insulin-resistant hepatocytes, mitochondrial dysfunction↓ Insulin sensitivity↓ in skeletal muscle cells Skeletal muscle glucose uptake↓
SIRT3	Mitochondrial	Deacetylase Decrotonylase	PGC-1α, AMPK, CREB, PDH, LCAD	FAO↑ Insulin resistance↓ in skeletal muscle Regulate mitochondrial antioxidant defense enzymes, ROS↓ Urea cycle and ketogenesis in liver↑
SIRT4	Mitochondrial	ADP-ribosyltransferase Deacetylase Lipoamidase	PGC-1α, AMPK, Adenine translocator, IDE, Glutamate dehydrogenase, MCD1	Lipogenesis↑ FAO↓ Hepatic lipid accumulation↑ Insulin secretion↓ Mitochondrial biogenesis↓
SIRT5	Mitochondrial	Deacetylase Desuccinylase Deglutarylase Demalonylase	IDH2, G6P, CPS1	Ammonia detoxification↑ Regulates glucose oxidation, FAO, ROS Cellular antioxidant defense↑
SIRT6	Nuclear, associated to chromatin	Deacetylase ADP-ribosyltransferase Demyristoylase	HIF-1α, Akt, FOXO1, GCN5, IGF-1, NF-κB, GLUT1, LDH, PGK1, PFK-1	Insulin resistance↓ Gluconeogenesis↓ Mimics the effect of calorie restriction Maintains glucose homeostasis and repress mitochondrial respiration by acting as an HIF-1α corepressor
SIRT7	Nucleolar	Deacetylase	TR4/TAK1, Cd36, PPARγ,	Adipogenesis↑ Fatty acid uptake↑ Hepatic lipid accumulation↑ Triglyceride synthesis/storage↑ Controversy of fatty liver development in SIRT7 knockout mice

Green shade infers detrimental effect, while red shade infers protective effect. The symbol ↑means increment, and ↓means decrement.

signaling is still controversial. Under standard nutrient conditions, it has been suggested that Akt activation in insulin-responsive cells is mainly attributed to SIRT2, other than SIRT1 (55, 56). However, SIRT2 overexpression strengthened insulin-induced Akt/GSK3β/p70S6 signaling in HeLa cells and 3T3-L1 preadipocytes (56). It's elusive whether the phenomenon was caused by alteration of Akt acetylation status. Further investigations are needed to explore whether Akt deacetylation mediated by SIRT2 disturbs both protein binding and downstream pathway. TUG (tether, containing a UBX domain, for GLUT4) plays a role in the exocytosis of glucose transporter type 4 (GLUT4) (57), and binds with SIRT2. SIRT2 regulated the acetylation of TUG *in vitro* and *in vivo* (58). Enhanced TUG acetylation was observed in the liver of SIRT2 knockout mice, alone with greater glucose uptake and more GLUT4 storage vesicles in response to insulin (58). Altogether, SIRT2 may exert distinctive and even opposing effect in response to insulin in different tissues.

However, SIRT4 has been reported to inhibit insulin secretion (9, 59, 60). SIRT4 overexpression promotes lipogenesis and dyslipidimeia, and meanwhile diminishes FAO. All these will lead to insulin resistance (21). SIRT4 mono-ADPribosylates insulin degrading enzyme and ATP/ADP translocases in β cells, leading to downregulation of insulin secretion induced by glucose (61). SIRT4 deletion declines ATP level and low ATP level will activate 5′adenosine monophosphate-activated protein kinase (AMPK), PGC-1α and its target genes, both of which are involved in mitochondrial biogenesis and FAO. Dysregulation of AMPK signaling leads to autophagy deactivation, oxidative stress, and inflammation which are implicated in pathogenesis of insulin resistance (62).

SIRT6 plays an essential role pancreatic β-cell function and survival in mice (63). SIRT6 protected against insulin resistance and obesity induced by HFD (64). Akt phosphorylation at Ser 473 and Thr 308 were negatively regulate by SIRT6 through interfering with insulin receptors, insulin receptor substrate and various upstream molecules (65). In SIRT6 deficiency mice, increased Akt phosphorylation and activated insulin signaling is observed, yielding more glucose uptake and even hypoglycemia. Additionally, glucose induced more cell apoptosis and impaired insulin secretion severely in MIN6 β-cells in SIRT6 ablation mice. Contrariwise, SIRT6 overexpression rescued β-cell apoptosis and dysfunction (66, 67).

Hence activating SIRT1, SIRT3, and SIRT6 would be a right option to struggle with T2DM due to the repression on PTP1B and UCP2 and final increment in insulin secretion. But SIRT4 functions in a negative way in diabetes development.

SIRTs IN GLUCOSE METABOLISM AND HOMEOSTASIS

During energy restriction status, glucose will be provided by the liver to sustain normoglycemia, initially in the glycogenolysis manner and then changing to gluconeogenesis (68). In the fed condition, insulin is secreted to suppress gluconeogenic enzymes transcription including phosphoenolpyruvate carboxykinase (PEPCK1), fructose-1,6-bisphosphatase, and glucose-6-phosphatase (G6P). PGC-1α and FOXO1 can upsurge gluconeogenic enzyme genes transcription (69, 70).

SIRT1 motivates hepatic gluconeogenesis in fasting status. In contrast, SIRT1 sensitizes insulin and lowers glucose under insulin-resistant condition (71). SIRT1 also deacetylates PGC-1α, and subsequently improves gluconeogenic genes expression in the liver (71, 72), finally encouraging hepatic glucose output during fasting. SIRT2 deacetylates and stabilizes PEPCK1 under glucose deprivation conditions (73). Compromised hepatic glucose uptake (HGU) is the cause of postprandial hyperglycemia in T2DM patients (74). In diabetic mice fed with HFD, SIRT2 overexpression in liver rises HGU and alleviates glucose tolerance. In liver-specific SIRT2 knockdown mice, HGU was diminished and glucose tolerance was imbalanced. It has been reported that SIRT2 stimulates HGU probably via deacetylating K126 of glucokinase regulatory protein (GKRP) (74).

SIRT5 manipulates protein substrates which are involved in ROS management, FAO, ammonia detoxification, ketone body formation, and glucose oxidation by glutarylation, malonylation, and succinylation (75).

SIRT6 interferes with FOXO1, thus reducing gluconeogenic genes such as G6P and PEPCK (76). Hepatic gluconeogenesis was meaningfully upregulated in SIRT6 knockout mice, suggesting a compensatory reaction to hypoglycemia (77). General control non-repressed protein 5 (GCN5) acetylated PGC-1α and diminished the transcriptional activity of PGC-1α (72). SIRT6 could activate GCN5 (77). A hypoxia-inducible factor 1α (HIF-1α) inhibitor would rescue the hypoglycemia phenotype in SIRT6 deficiency mice. Mice with SIRT6 knockout in brains exhibited lower levels of insulin-like growth factor 1 (IGF-1) and growth hormone than control mice, similar to the effect achieved in whole-body SIRT6 knockout mice (78), suggesting that the central nervous system is critical in glucose metabolism.

SIRTs IN CALORIE RESTRICTION AND EXERCISE

Calorie restriction (CR) has been reported to postpone the onset of diabetes. During the initial phase of CR, liver gluconeogenesis is activated by pancreatic α cells-secreted glucagon, during which the cyclic AMP response-element-binding protein (CREB) and CREB-regulated transcription coactivator 2 (CRTC2) are involved. CR and exercise is beneficial for health and longevity, and genetic ablation of SIRT1, SIRT3, and SIRT6 would block the benefits provided by CR and exercise (79–83).

SIRT1 encourages FOXO1-tirggered gluconeogenesis in fasting (84). SIRT1 activators exert similar effects like CR (85, 86). However, this effect is reversed by CRTC2 deacetylation mediated by SIRT1 (84). SIRT1 then deacetylates and activates PGC-1α to facilitate gluconeogenesis (71). CRTC2 supports gluconeogenesis in the initial stage of fasting. Hepatic SIRT1 reduced CRTC2 level via deacetylation and ubiquitination, at 18 h fasting. FOXO1 accounted for gluconeogenesis after 18 h of fasting (84). Mice exposed to long-term CR (18 months) displayed SIRT2 increment in kidney and white adipose tissue (WAT) but not in brain or liver (51). Likewise, short-term fasting (24 h) also enhances protein and mRNA expression of SIRT2 in WAT (53). SIRT6 also accounted for CR function. SIRT6 knockout eliminated CR-induced life extension. SIRT6 Overexpression mimics the effects of exercise and CR in mice, and extends lifespan and health span, including reduced glucose, insulin, adipokines, cholesterol, and body weight (64, 87, 88). In addition, CR-stimulated SIRT6 repressed NF-κB pathway (89). SIRT1 also transcriptionally activated SIRT6, therefore sirtuins might work in a coordinated way to modulate each phase of calorie restriction (29).

SIRTs IN MITOCHONDRIAL GLYCOLYSIS AND BIOGENESIS

ATP is generated in animal cells by two principal processes, glycolysis and mitochondrial oxidative phosphorylation. T2DM, obesity, and many other aging-related disorders are characteristic of amplified oxidative damage. ROS is generally produced in mitochondria, as superoxide (O_2^-) is a byproduct during electron transport system metabolism. In response to excess glucose, SIRTs will orchestrate the ratio of respiration and glycolysis, consuming energy through proton leak (90).

SIRT1 deacetylates PGC-1α, which is critical for mitochondrial function and gluconeogenesis. SIRT1 directly deacetylates and activates PGC-1α while SIRT3 enhances PGC-1α protein expression indirectly(91), through activating CREB and AMPK which accordingly increases downstream mitochondrial biogenesis targets (92–94). Significant mortality, defective thermogenesis, decreased hypoglycemia, and reduced FAO are obvious in SIRT3 knockout models (95). SIRT3 also deacetylates key genes in oxidative stress and mitochondrial antioxidant defense enzymes. The beneficial effects of SIRT3 on CR can chiefly be ascribed to inhibiting ROS (83). Actually, the alleviation in cellular oxidative stress that generates during CR is absent in SIRT3 knockout mice (82).

In contrast to SIRT3, SIRT4 inhibits mitochondrial biogenesis by suppressing PGC-1α expression. AMPK and SIRT4 interplay to retrograde PGC-1α signaling, suggesting that SIRT4 negatively manipulates mitochondrial biogenesis (96). SIRT5 has been reported to promote antioxidant defense and sustain NADPH homeostasis in cells by increasing G6P deglutarylation and isocitrate dehydrogenase 2 (IDH2) desuccinylation (97). Interestingly, SIRT6 interacts with HIF-1α to co-repress mitochondrial respiration (98). SIRT6 deficiency promoted HIF-1α activity and glycolysis by enhancing phosphofructokinase 1 (PGK1), glucose-6-phosphate isomerase, phosphoglycerate kinase (PFK-1), lactate dehydrogenase (LDH), and GLUT1 (98, 99).

SIRTs IN THE METABOLIC HOMEOSTASIS OF SKELETAL MUSCLE

Skeletal muscle is a critical tissue to maintain energy homeostasis. Storage of lipid metabolites and fatty acids in muscle prevents glucose uptake, finally leading to T2DM (100, 101). Induction of fatty acid β-oxidation has emerged as a hopeful method to attenuate muscle insulin resistance in muscle.

In skeletal muscle, SIRT1 expression is triggered by fasting. SIRT1 in turn deacetylates both FOXO1 and PGC-1α and facilitates fatty acid β-oxidation (91). Likewise, FAO and mitochondrial biogenesis genes are upregulated owning to SIRT1 activators SRT1720 treatment via deacetylating PGC-1α (27, 102). Moreover, SIRT1 plays a role in mitochondrial biogenesis induced by adiponectin in skeletal muscle (103).

SIRT2 negatively regulates insulin resistance and glucose uptake in C2C12 muscle cells. Akt/GSK3β signaling and glucose uptake which are driven by insulin was enlarged by inhibition of SIRT2 under insulin-resistance conditions (104). SIRT2 knockdown under insulin-resistant status enhanced insulin sensitivity in skeletal muscle cells. Nevertheless, blunt of SIRT3 and SIRT1 in C2C12 cells impairs insulin pathway and stimulates insulin resistance. Despite the fact that SIRTs possess a conserved catalytic domain, they exert a differential regulating effect on insulin resistance. SIRT3 Knockdown in muscle cells impairs insulin action and metabolic flexibility (105, 106), and muscle ability to adjust to fuel oxidation (107). SIRT3 deletion amplified acetylation of pyruvate hydrogenase (PDH), yielding declining PDH activity, and subsequent less glucose oxidation. All these gave rise to a switch to FAO, even with glucose available (106, 108).

SIRT4 negatively regulates mitochondrial biogenesis and FAO in muscles. SIRT4 regulates insulin secretion by modulating glutamate dehydrogenase. As expected, fat acid oxidative capability and mitochondrial metabolism enzymes in muscle and hepatocytes was upregulated in response to SIRT4 knockdown. In primary SIRT4 knockdown myotubes, phosphorylation of AMPK was activated, accompanied with intense cellular respiration and FAO. Moreover, protein and mRNA levels of SIRT1 were enhanced both *in vitro* and *in vivo*, largely attributed to the reduced SIRT4 levels (109).

SIRTs IN FATTY ACID OXIDATION

The development of T2DM and its complications is associated with lipid metabolism disorder. Inadequate FAO gives rise to the initiation of insulin resistance and lipid accumulation (110, 111).

SIRT1 fosters fat metabolism in liver cells, as demonstrated by the formation of fatty livers in mice with SIRT1 deletion in the liver (112, 113). SIRT1 knockout mice hardly suppressed lipogenic genes or increased FAO genes in the background of fasting (112). In normal hepatocytes, SIRT1 interacts with the PPARα response element where it deacetylates PGC-1α and increases PPARα expression, thus stimulating FAO (113, 114). Furthermore, once the fat anabolism-inducing factor PPARγ was deacetylated by SIRT1, the sterol regulatory element binding proteins (SREBPs) will be deactivated and become more susceptible to degradation (115), achieving more lipolysis. Deacetylation of PGC-1α and expression of β-oxidation genes was accordingly diminished due to SIRT2 function impairment (116).

SIRT3 plays an essential role in FAO in the mitochondria. Upon CR or fasting, SIRT3 is activated in mitochondria to stimulate FAO through inducing the deacetylation of long-chain-specific acyl coenzyme A dehydrogenase (LCAD) (95, 117). SIRT3 stimulates ketogenesis and urea cycle as well (118, 119). A chronic HFD reduced SIRT3 levels in mice, associated with LCAD function impairment and mitochondrial hyperacetylation (120).

SIRT4's effect is remarkably different from SIRT3 and SIRT1. Ablation of SIRT4 avoids steatosis during HFD (109). In addition, SIRT4 suppresses PPARα to prevent FAO, in the meantime SIRT4 inhibits malonyl CoA decarboxylase 1 (MCD1) to facilitate the synthesis of lipid (29). SIRT4 interferes with SIRT1-PPARα complex, therefore the activation effect of SIRT1 on PPARα and the inhibiting effect on FAO was abrogated.

Analogous to SIRT4, SIRT7 knockout in liver resulted in blunted triglyceride accumulation. Hepatic SIRT7 facilitated triglyceride storage/synthesis and fatty acid uptake by activating TR4/TAK1, a nuclear receptor participating in lipid metabolism. Moreover, the ubiquitin-proteasome pathway is also involved in the regulating effect of hepatic SIRT7 on lipid metabolism (121). SIRT7 also hinders TR4 degradation. TR4 involves in lipid balance by modulating monoacylglycerol O-acyltransferase 1, *Cidec*, cell death-inducing DFFA-like effector a (*Cidea*), and Cd36. SIRT7 has been reported to upsurge hepatic lipid accumulation owning to increasing Cd36 expression (121, 122). Yoshizawa et al. (121) observed that HFD failed to stimulate glucose intolerance, obesity, or fatty liver in SIRT7 knockout mice. The conclusion is controversial to the result that SIRT7 knockout promoted fatty liver development (123, 124). Compared with SIRT1, SIRT7 displays distinctive effect on maintaining liver lipid homeostasisa. Lipid storage is raised by SIRT7 by suppressing PPARα, like SIRT4 (125).

SIRTs IN THE METABOLIC HOMEOSTASIS OF ADIPOCYTE

Regarded as a storage compartment for fatty lipids, adipose tissue also serves as an important modulator for energy homeostasis, vascular remodeling endocrine functions, insulin sensitivity, and innate immune response (126). Adipokines, such as leptin and adiponectin, are systemically regulated by white adipose tissue (WAT). There is convincing evidence supporting that adiponectin derived from adipocyte plays an essential part in insulin resistance (127, 128). Moreover, adiponectin sustains glucose homeostasis and protects against diabetes and obesity.

Numerous SIRT1 benefits take place in WAT (129). SIRT1 inhibits lipogenesis and stimulates fat mobilization in adipocytes from WAT, via suppressing PPARγ. Eventually, peripheral utilization of the fat storages is raised (113). White fat can be switched to metabolically active brown fat due to SIRT1 deacetylation on PPARγ (130). Conversely, SIRT1 can be cleaved in WAT by caspase I and inflammasome which is activated by HFD (19).

SIRT1 knockdown reduced WAT mass in rats. The mRNA contents of PPARγ2 and PPARγ, both of which were adipogenic genes, are abridged in adipose, driving adipocyte differentiation and adipose loss. Adipocytes-specific SIRT1 knockdown led to lower plasma concentrations of adiponectin and leptin. In adipose of obese individuals, mRNA levels of SIRT1 were lower in than those of control group. In the opposite, obese patients have higher SIRT7 expressions in adipose. SIRT7 and SIRT1 promoters' methylation status are not closely associated with the upregulation or downregulation of their mRNA levels induced by obesity. In visceral adipose tissue (VAT) of obese patients, the content of miR-181a-3p and miR-34a-5p negatively associated with SIRT1 levels. In contrary, the expression of miR-125b-5p and miR-125a-5p negatively correlated with SIRT7 in VAT of slim subjects (131). Furthermore, MiR-93 impedes the metabolic target SIRT7 (132).

SIRT7 has been identified as a chief driver of adipogenesis by inducing differentiation and maturation of early adipocyte precursors. PPARγ is adipogenic and its expression is reduced in the WAT of mice with SIRT7 deletion (132), designating that SIRT7 stimulates adipogenesis. SIRT7 can remove long-chain fatty acyl groups more efficiently than removing acetyl groups (133, 134).

Inhibited SIRT2 expression and amplified HIF-1α expression are observed in VAT from obese individuals. HIF-1α hinders adipocyte-mediated fatty acid catabolism by blocking SIRT2-PGC-1α pathway, thereby favoring the progression of obesity (116). Diet-induced obesity was strengthened in SIRT6 knockout mice, principally attributed to hypertrophy of adipocyte other than differentiation of abnormal adipocyte (135).

SIRTs IN NEURONS UNDER DIABETIC CONDITIONS

In the anorexigenic proopiomelanocortin (POMC) neurons, SIRT1 is critical in preserving normal energy expenditure. POMC neurons-specific SIRT1 knockout mice are vulnerable to diet-induced obesity (136). SIRT1 is also defensive against diabetes and obesity in the steroidogenic factor 1 neurons (137). Additionally, the peptide release of orexigenic agouti is suppressed by SIRT1 via interacting with FOXO1 (138, 139). Nevertheless, SIRT1 ablation in neurons was related with insulin secretion in hypothalamic neurons (140).

SIRT2, PGC-1α, and P-AMPK declined dramatically in diabetic cortex. AMPK/SIRT/PGC-1α pathway, which mediates antioxidant abilities and mitochondrial biogenesis, is involved in cortex neurodegeneration progression under diabetic conditions (141). SIRT6 and SIRT2 expression were meaningfully reduced in the neural stem or embryo cells from pre-gestational maternal diabetes. Superoxide dismutase 1 (SOD1) mimetic and overexpression rescued the decrement of SIRT6 and SIRT2 in the diabetic embryopathy mouse model. Histone acetylation caused by Sirtuin decrement might participates in neural tube defects induced by diabetes.

SIRTs POLYMORPHISMS IN DIABETES

While abundant data point to the essential role of SIRTs activities, there are genetic polymorphisms of SIRT1 and SIRT2 concerning diabetes. rs10509291 and rs7896005 in SIRT1 genes are associated with T2DM development as well as reduced acute insulin response (142). In a report about Japanese patients with T2DM, four single nucleotide polymorphisms (SNPs) in SIRT1 that were positively correlated with diabetic nephropathy, and a haplotype containing the SNPs within SIRT1 locus had a stronger association (143). Moreover, SIRT1 mutation has been reported to link with autoimmune diabetes. Type 1 diabetes mellitus (T1DM) is an autoimmune disease characteristic of autoimmune-mediated β cell destruction. Lately, exome, and direct sequencing recognized a T-to-C exchange in exon 1 of *SIRT1* in a patient diagnosed with T1DM, corresponding to a leucine-to-proline mutation at residue 107. It is speculated that the SIRT1 L107P mutation, located within the N-terminal protein-binding domain, could also disturb the oligomerization and activity (20). Furthermore, the prenatally famine-exposed kids, who have minor alleles of SIRT1 gene (GA and AA of rs1467568 and AG and GG of rs7895833), have a lower risk for T2DM in adult life (144). DNA sequence variants (DSVs), including g.38900237G > A, g.38900359C > T, g.38900561C > T, and g.38900912G > T, might upsurge SIRT2 gene promoter activity and SIRT2 levels, contributing to T2DM as a risk factor (50).

CLINICAL TRIALS OF SIRTs ACTIVATORS IN DIABETES: CURRENT EVIDENCE

As mentioned above, SIRTs activators exert positive effects in neurodegenerative, and metabolism diseases. Identification of SIRT1 activators for T2DM treatment has become immediate areas of research focus, such as metformin, resveratrol, resveratrol derivatives (Resveratrol aliphatic acids, acetylated derivatives, 3,3′,4,4′,5,5′-hexahydroxystilbene) and polyphenols (quercetin, piceatannol, fisetin, pinosylvin, and butein) (145). Metformin is the recommended first-line oral glucose-lowering drug initiated to control hyperglycemia in T2DM, a synthetic dimethyl biguanid (146). SIRT1 level rises after metformin treatment. SIRT1 is obviously entangled into the mechanism of metformin action (147). In the largest Randomized Controlled Trial inspecting metformin for diabetes prevention (148, 149), 1073 subjects from 27 USA medical centers took metformin (850 mg twice every day) or placebo ($n = 1082$). As compared with placebo, diabetes occurrence was considerably decreased by 31% (95% $CI = 17\%, 43\%$) in the metformin group after almost 3 years follow-up.

When it comes to another potent SIRT activator resveratrol, SIRTris Pharmaceuticals had launched an oral resveratrol formulation (SRT501), which has entered Phase III clinical trials for T2DM therapy (150). Effects of trans-resveratrol extract from Polygonum in patients with type 2 diabetes has completed Phase I clinical trials, with trial number NCT01677611 (151). In a dose-escalation Phase I trial, resveratrol clearance (5 g in a single dose) was rapid, and urine excretion reached 77% within 4 h, signifying that derivatives structure optimization with longer half-life is in great need (152). Moreover, derivatives SRT-2183, SRT-1720, and SRT-1460 are also discovered. But SRT-1720 was terminated owing to limited effect. SRT-2104 was more potent and the Phase II clinical trials has completed successfully (153). The pharmacokinetics and safety study of SRT2379 evaluated in healthy male volunteers has finished the Phase I clinical trials (154).

CONCLUSION

SIRTs play a noticeable role in modulating insulin resistance and glucose uptake in adipose tissue, liver, and muscle. SIRT1, SIRT2, SIRT3, and SIRT6 has been implicated to positively sustain insulin sensitivity and glucose homeostasis, rendering them attractive potential drug targets. While SIRT4 and SIRT7 negatively regulate insulin secretion and FAO.

Specifically, SIRT1 enhances fat catabolism in adipose tissue, skeletal muscle and liver by modifying the activity of PPARα, PPARγ, and PGC-1α. Apart from inducing fat catabolism, SIRT1 also promotes FAO, mitochondrial oxidative capacity and energy expenditure in fat tissue and skeletal muscle, not only through direct activation of PPARα, but also through secondary activation of AMPK and PPARα by SIRT1-mediated adiponectin synthesis. SIRT1 prevents lipogenesis and motivates free fatty acid release by inhibiting SREBP and PPARγ. SIRT1 exhibits conflicting effects on maintaining glucose homeostasis under fed and fasted conditions. In fed condition, SIRT1 reinforces pancreatic insulin secretion. In fasted status, SIRT1 promotes hepatic gluconeogenesis by deacetylating FOXO1 and PGC-1α. SIRT1 exerts insulin-sensitizing effect by inhibiting PTP1B and UCP2 expression and regulating adiponectin synthesis. SIRT2 increases insulin sensitivity in insulin-resistant hepatocytes, while decreases insulin sensitivity in skeletal muscle cells. Nevertheless, there is very limited literature on SIRT5 enzyme activity until the recent finding as it can remove succinyl or malonyl groups, and this action resembles deacetylation. SIRT5 is broadly expressed, but SIRT5-deficient mice are healthy, fertile, and without major clinical phenotype (155), inferring that SIRT5 is not indispensable for metabolic homeostasis at least under basal conditions. SIRT6 supports pancreatic β-cell function and sustains glucose homeostasis by acting as a HIF-1α corepressor. Conversely, SIRT4 and SIRT7 exhibited negative effect on diabetes therapy, such as aggravating lipogenesis, and inhibiting insulin secretion.

The majority of sirtuins isoforms are protective on diabetes and a minority appears to be detrimental, but the antagonism effect on the whole body remains elusive. Although several metabolic pathways and targets have been proposed to mediate SIRTs function on T2DM, some outstanding questions need to be resolved. Moreover, do these SIRTs act independently or synergistically on diabetes? How do they communicate for cooperative actions in cells? SIRTs are regulated by protein-protein interactions and microRNAs at the level of translation and transcription (156), however, little is known about the epigenetic mechanisms modifying sirtuins. In some cases, sirtuins isoforms regulate certain essential enzymes in an opposite direction. For instance, PDH can be activated through deacetylation by SIRT3 (106), while both delipoamidating by SIRT4 or desuccinylating by SIRT5 inhibited PDH activity (157, 158), and the question that which effect will win out is quite a puzzle. Furthermore, when SIRTs display both ADP-ribosyltransferase and deacetylase activity, the circumstances that decide the predominant activity need to be determined.

A plenty of clinical trials has been carried out, including resveratrol, metformin, and other SIRT activators. It is possible that in the foreseeable future one or more SIRT activators will be approved for diabetes therapy. As a well-known pharmaceutical preparation, the widespread usage of metformin facilitates the recruit of a large randomized controlled trial. Metformin has been regarded as the most promising candidate. But it's a little harder to explore the natural compounds in a large scale, such as curcumin, berberine, and genistein. It is attributed to the complexity in reducing batches variability of supplements and the difficulty in evaluating dietary intake in observational studies (159–161). Long-term, outcomes-based placebo-controlled rigorous clinical trials would be crucial to confirm the function of SIRT activators on diabetes.

AUTHOR CONTRIBUTIONS

JS and LF drafted the manuscript. All authors contributed in the discussion section, and approved it for publication.

ACKNOWLEDGMENTS

We acknowledge the financial support from the National Natural Science Foundation Committee of China (No. 81603336, 81703775, 81873055), Jiangsu province high-level health personnel Six-One Project (LGY2017085), Jiangsu Province Youth Medical Key Talent Project (QNRC2016634), Innovative Research Team of Health Development Project with Science and

Education in Jiangsu Province (CXTDB2017003), Program for Innovative Research Team of Six Talent Peaks Project in Jiangsu Province (SWYY-CXTD-004). The Public Welfare Technology Application Research Linkage Project of Anhui Province (grant No. 1704f0704062). TCM for Public Interest Research from Ministry of Finance of China (No. 201507004).

REFERENCES

1. Imai S, Armstrong CM, Kaeberlein M, Guarente L. Transcriptional silencing and longevity protein Sir2 is an NAD-dependent histone deacetylase. *Nature* (2000) 403:795–800. doi: 10.1038/35001622
2. Chang HC, Guarente L. SIRT1 and other sirtuins in metabolism. *Trends Endocrinol Metab.* (2014) 25:138–45. doi: 10.1016/j.tem.2013.12.001
3. Haigis MC, Sinclair DA. Mammalian sirtuins: biological insights and disease relevance. *Annu Rev Pathol.* (2010) 5:253–95. doi: 10.1146/annurev.pathol.4.110807.092250
4. Parenti MD, Bruzzone S, Nencioni A, Del Rio A. Selectivity hot-spots of sirtuin catalytic cores. *Mol Biosyst.* (2015) 11:2263–72. doi: 10.1039/c5mb00205b
5. Schuetz A, Min J, Antoshenko T, Wang CL, Allali-Hassani A, Dong A, et al. Structural basis of inhibition of the human NAD+-dependent deacetylase SIRT5 by suramin. *Structure* (2007) 15:377–89. doi: 10.1016/j.str.2007.02.002
6. Houtkooper RH, Pirinen E, Auwerx J. Sirtuins as regulators of metabolism and healthspan. *Nat Rev Mol Cell Biol.* (2012) 13:225–238. doi: 10.1038/nrm3293
7. Rauh D, Fischer F, Gertz M, Lakshminarasimhan M, Bergbrede T, Aladini F, et al. An acetylome peptide microarray reveals specificities and deacetylation substrates for all human sirtuin isoforms. *Nat Commun.* (2013) 4:2327. doi: 10.1038/ncomms3327
8. Teng YB, Jing H, Aramsangtienchai P, He B, Khan S, Hu J, et al. Efficient demyristoylase activity of SIRT2 revealed by kinetic and structural studies. *Sci Rep.* (2015) 5:8529. doi: 10.1038/srep08529
9. Haigis MC, Mostoslavsky R, Haigis KM, Fahie K, Christodoulou DC, Murphy AJ, et al. SIRT4 inhibits glutamate dehydrogenase and opposes the effects of calorie restriction in pancreatic beta cells. *Cell* (2006) 126:941–54. doi: 10.1016/j.cell.2006.06.057
10. Osborne B, Bentley NL, Montgomery MK, Turner N. The role of mitochondrial sirtuins in health and disease. *Free Radic Biol Med.* (2016) 100:164–174. doi: 10.1016/j.freeradbiomed.2016.04.197
11. Du J, Zhou Y, Su X, Yu JJ, Khan S, Jiang H, et al. Sirt5 is a NAD-dependent protein lysine demalonylase and desuccinylase. *Science* (2011) 334:806–9. doi: 10.1126/science.1207861
12. Nakagawa T, Lomb DJ, Haigis MC, Guarente L. SIRT5 deacetylates carbamoyl phosphate synthetase 1 and regulates the urea cycle. *Cell* (2009) 137:560–70. doi: 10.1016/j.cell.2009.02.026
13. Kuang J, Chen L, Tang Q, Zhang J, Li Y, He J. The role of Sirt6 in obesity and diabetes. *Front Physiol.* (2018) 9:135. doi: 10.3389/fphys.2018.00135
14. Ford E, Voit R, Liszt G, Magin C, Grummt I, Guarente L. Mammalian Sir2 homolog SIRT7 is an activator of RNA polymerase I transcription. *Genes Dev.* (2006) 20:1075–80. doi: 10.1101/gad.1399706
15. Tsai YC, Greco TM, Boonmee A, Miteva Y, Cristea IM. Functional proteomics establishes the interaction of SIRT7 with chromatin remodeling complexes and expands its role in regulation of RNA polymerase I transcription. *Mol Cell Proteomics* (2012) 11:60–76. doi: 10.1074/mcp.A111.015156
16. Zhou Z, Sun B, Li X, Zhu C. DNA methylation landscapes in the pathogenesis of type 2 diabetes mellitus. *Nutr Metab.* (2018) 15:47. doi: 10.1186/s12986-018-0283-x
17. Freeman AM, Pennings N. Insulin resistance. In: *Treasure Island.* Lumberton, NC: StatPearls (2018), p. 34.
18. Kahn SE, Cooper ME, Del Prato S. Pathophysiology and treatment of type 2 diabetes: perspectives on the past, present, and future. *Lancet* (2014) 383:1068–83. doi: 10.1016/S0140-6736(13)62154-6
19. Chalkiadaki A, Guarente L. High-fat diet triggers inflammation-induced cleavage of SIRT1 in adipose tissue to promote metabolic dysfunction. *Cell Metab.* (2012) 16:180–8. doi: 10.1016/j.cmet.2012.07.003
20. Biason-Lauber A, Boni-Schnetzler M, Hubbard BP, Bouzakri K, Brunner A, Cavelti-Weder C, et al. Identification of a SIRT1 mutation in a family with type 1 diabetes. *Cell Metab.* (2013) 17:448–455. doi: 10.1016/j.cmet.2013.02.001
21. Choubey SK, Prabhu D, Nachiappan M, Biswal J, Jeyakanthan J. Molecular modeling, dynamics studies and density functional theory approaches to identify potential inhibitors of SIRT4 protein from Homo sapiens: a novel target for the treatment of type 2 diabetes. *J Biomol Struct Dyn.* (2017) 35:3316–3329. doi: 10.1080/07391102.2016.1254117
22. Song R, Xu W, Chen Y, Li Z, Zeng Y, Fu Y. The expression of Sirtuins 1 and 4 in peripheral blood leukocytes from patients with type 2 diabetes. *Eur J Histochem.* (2011) 55:e10. doi: 10.4081/ejh.2011.e10
23. Arab Sadeghabadi Z, Ziamajidi N, Abbasalipourkabir R, Mohseni R. Garlic (*Allium sativum*) increases SIRT1 and SIRT2 gene expressions in the kidney and liver tissues of STZ- and STZ+niacinamide-induced diabetic rats. *J Basic Clin Physiol Pharmacol.* (2018) 29:463–7. doi: 10.1515/jbcpp-2017-0079
24. Pedersen SB, Olholm J, Paulsen SK, Bennetzen MF, Richelsen B. Low Sirt1 expression, which is upregulated by fasting, in human adipose tissue from obese women. *Int J Obes.* (2008) 32:1250–5. doi: 10.1038/ijo.2008.78
25. Costa Cdos S, Hammes TO, Rohden F, Margis R, Bortolotto JW, Padoin AV, et al. SIRT1 transcription is decreased in visceral adipose tissue of morbidly obese patients with severe hepatic steatosis. *Obes Surg.* (2010) 20:633–9. doi: 10.1007/s11695-009-0052-z
26. Baur JA, Pearson KJ, Price NL, Jamieson HA, Lerin C, Kalra A, et al. Resveratrol improves health and survival of mice on a high-calorie diet. *Nature* (2006) 444:337–42. doi: 10.1038/nature05354
27. Lagouge M, Argmann C, Gerhart-Hines Z, Meziane H, Lerin C, Daussin F, et al. Resveratrol improves mitochondrial function and protects against metabolic disease by activating SIRT1 and PGC-1alpha. *Cell* (2006) 127:1109–22. doi: 10.1016/j.cell.2006.11.013
28. Bordone L, Cohen D, Robinson A, Motta MC, van Veen E, Czopik A, et al. SIRT1 transgenic mice show phenotypes resembling calorie restriction. *Aging Cell* (2007) 6:759–67. doi: 10.1111/j.1474-9726.2007.00335.x
29. Kim HS, Xiao C, Wang RH, Lahusen T, Xu X, Vassilopoulos A, et al. Hepatic-specific disruption of SIRT6 in mice results in fatty liver formation due to enhanced glycolysis and triglyceride synthesis. *Cell Metab.* (2010) 12:224–36. doi: 10.1016/j.cmet.2010.06.009
30. Saltiel AR, Kahn CR. Insulin signalling and the regulation of glucose and lipid metabolism. *Nature* (2001) 414:799–806. doi: 10.1038/414799a
31. Jukarainen S, Heinonen S, Ramo JT, Rinnankoski-Tuikka R, Rappou E, Tummers M, et al. Obesity is associated with low NAD(+)/SIRT pathway expression in adipose tissue of BMI-discordant monozygotic twins. *J Clin Endocrinol Metab.* (2016) 101:275–83. doi: 10.1210/jc.2015-3095
32. Sun C, Zhang F, Ge X, Yan T, Chen X, Shi X, et al. SIRT1 improves insulin sensitivity under insulin-resistant conditions by repressing PTP1B. *Cell Metab.* (2007) 6:307–19. doi: 10.1016/j.cmet.2007.08.014
33. Elchebly M, Payette P, Michaliszyn E, Cromlish W, Collins S, Loy AL, et al. Increased insulin sensitivity and obesity resistance in mice lacking the protein tyrosine phosphatase-1B gene. *Science* (1999) 283:1544–8.
34. Moynihan KA, Grimm AA, Plueger MM, Bernal-Mizrachi E, Ford E, Cras-Meneur C, et al. Increased dosage of mammalian Sir2 in pancreatic beta cells enhances glucose-stimulated insulin secretion in mice. *Cell Metab.* (2005) 2:105–17. doi: 10.1016/j.cmet.2005.07.001
35. Zhang CY, Baffy G, Perret P, Krauss S, Peroni O, Grujic D, et al. Uncoupling protein-2 negatively regulates insulin secretion and is a major link between obesity, beta cell dysfunction, and type 2 diabetes. *Cell* (2001) 105:745–55. doi: 10.1016/S0092-8674(01)00378-6
36. Bordone L, Motta MC, Picard F, Robinson A, Jhala US, Apfeld J, et al. Sirt1 regulates insulin secretion by repressing UCP2 in pancreatic beta cells. *PLoS Biol.* (2006) 4:e31. doi: 10.1371/journal.pbio.0040031

37. Kitamura YI, Kitamura T, Kruse JP, Raum JC, Stein R, Gu W, et al. FoxO1 protects against pancreatic beta cell failure through NeuroD and MafA induction. *Cell Metab.* (2005) 2:153–63. doi: 10.1016/j.cmet.2005.08.004
38. Lee JH, Song MY, Song EK, Kim EK, Moon WS, Han MK, et al. Overexpression of SIRT1 protects pancreatic beta-cells against cytokine toxicity by suppressing the nuclear factor-kappaB signaling pathway. *Diabetes* (2009) 58:344–51. doi: 10.2337/db07-1795
39. Nemoto S, Fergusson MM, Finkel T. Nutrient availability regulates SIRT1 through a forkhead-dependent pathway. *Science* (2004) 306:2105–8. doi: 10.1126/science.1101731
40. Bai P, Canto C, Brunyanszki A, Huber A, Szanto M, Cen Y, et al. PARP-2 regulates SIRT1 expression and whole-body energy expenditure. *Cell Metab.* (2011) 13:450–460. doi: 10.1016/j.cmet.2011.03.013
41. Han L, Zhou R, Niu J, McNutt MA, Wang P, Tong T. SIRT1 is regulated by a PPAR{gamma}-SIRT1 negative feedback loop associated with senescence. *Nucleic Acids Res.* (2010) 38:7458–71. doi: 10.1093/nar/gkq609
42. Hayashida S, Arimoto A, Kuramoto Y, Kozako T, Honda S, Shimeno H, et al. Fasting promotes the expression of SIRT1, an NAD+ -dependent protein deacetylase, via activation of PPARalpha in mice. *Mol Cell Biochem.* (2010) 339:285–92. doi: 10.1007/s11010-010-0391-z
43. Okazaki M, Iwasaki Y, Nishiyama M, Taguchi T, Tsugita M, Nakayama S, et al. PPARβ/δ regulates the human SIRT1 gene transcription via Sp1. *Endocr J.* (2010) 57:403–13. doi: 10.1507/endocrj.K10E-004
44. Yamakuchi M, Ferlito M, Lowenstein CJ. miR-34a repression of SIRT1 regulates apoptosis. *Proc Natl Acad Sci USA.* (2008) 105:13421–6. doi: 10.1073/pnas.0801613105
45. Rane S, He M, Sayed D, Vashistha H, Malhotra A, Sadoshima J, et al. Downregulation of miR-199a derepresses hypoxia-inducible factor-1alpha and Sirtuin 1 and recapitulates hypoxia preconditioning in cardiac myocytes. *Circ Res.* (2009) 104:879–86. doi: 10.1161/CIRCRESAHA.108.193102
46. Sasaki T, Maier B, Koclega KD, Chruszcz M, Gluba W, Stukenberg PT, et al. Phosphorylation regulates SIRT1 function. *PLoS ONE* (2008) 3:e4020. doi: 10.1371/journal.pone.0004020
47. Conrad E, Polonio-Vallon T, Meister M, Matt S, Bitomsky N, Herbel C, et al. HIPK2 restricts SIRT1 activity upon severe DNA damage by a phosphorylation-controlled mechanism. *Cell Death Differ.* (2016) 23:110–22. doi: 10.1038/cdd.2015.75
48. Gomes P, Fleming Outeiro T, Cavadas C. Emerging role of sirtuin 2 in the regulation of mammalian metabolism. *Trends Pharmacol Sci.* (2015) 36:756–68. doi: 10.1016/j.tips.2015.08.001
49. Lemos V, de Oliveira RM, Naia L, Szego E, Ramos E, Pinho S, et al. The NAD+-dependent deacetylase SIRT2 attenuates oxidative stress and mitochondrial dysfunction and improves insulin sensitivity in hepatocytes. *Hum Mol Genet.* (2017) 26:4105–17. doi: 10.1093/hmg/ddx298
50. Liu T, Yang W, Pang S, Yu S, Yan B. Functional genetic variants within the SIRT2 gene promoter in type 2 diabetes mellitus. *Diabetes Res Clin Pract.* (2018) 137:200–07. doi: 10.1016/j.diabres.2018.01.012
51. Wang F, Nguyen M, Qin FX, Tong Q. SIRT2 deacetylates FOXO3a in response to oxidative stress and caloric restriction. *Aging Cell* (2007) 6:505–14. doi: 10.1111/j.1474-9726.2007.00304.x
52. Jing E, Gesta S, Kahn CR. SIRT2 regulates adipocyte differentiation through FoxO1 acetylation/deacetylation. *Cell Metab.* (2007) 6:105–14. doi: 10.1016/j.cmet.2007.07.003
53. Wang F, Tong Q. SIRT2 suppresses adipocyte differentiation by deacetylating FOXO1 and enhancing FOXO1's repressive interaction with PPARgamma. *Mol Biol Cell* (2009) 20:801–8. doi: 10.1091/mbc.E08-06-0647
54. Motta MC, Divecha N, Lemieux M, Kamel C, Chen D, Gu W, et al. Mammalian SIRT1 represses forkhead transcription factors. *Cell* (2004) 116:551–63. doi: 10.1016/S0092-8674(04)00126-6
55. Chen J, Chan AW, To KF, Chen W, Zhang Z, Ren J, et al. SIRT2 overexpression in hepatocellular carcinoma mediates epithelial to mesenchymal transition by protein kinase B/glycogen synthase kinase-3beta/beta-catenin signaling. *Hepatology* (2013) 57:2287–98. doi: 10.1002/hep.26278
56. Ramakrishnan G, Davaakhuu G, Kaplun L, Chung WC, Rana A, Atfi A, et al. Sirt2 deacetylase is a novel AKT binding partner critical for AKT activation by insulin. *J Biol Chem.* (2014) 289:6054–66. doi: 10.1074/jbc.M113.537266
57. Bogan JS, Hendon N, McKee AE, Tsao TS, Lodish HF. Functional cloning of TUG as a regulator of GLUT4 glucose transporter trafficking. *Nature* (2003) 425:727–33. doi: 10.1038/nature01989
58. Belman JP, Bian RR, Habtemichael EN, Li DT, Jurczak MJ, Alcazar-Roman A, et al. Acetylation of TUG protein promotes the accumulation of GLUT4 glucose transporters in an insulin-responsive intracellular compartment. *J Biol Chem.* (2015) 290:4447–63. doi: 10.1074/jbc.M114.603977
59. Hutton JC, Sener A, Malaisse WJ. Interaction of branched chain amino acids and keto acids upon pancreatic islet metabolism and insulin secretion. *J Biol Chem.* (1980) 255:7340–6.
60. Huynh FK, Hu X, Lin Z, Johnson JD, Hirschey MD. Loss of sirtuin 4 leads to elevated glucose- and leucine-stimulated insulin levels and accelerated age-induced insulin resistance in multiple murine genetic backgrounds. *J Inherit Metab Dis.* (2018) 41:59–72. doi: 10.1007/s10545-017-0069-8
61. Ahuja N, Schwer B, Carobbio S, Waltregny D, North BJ, Castronovo V, et al. Regulation of insulin secretion by SIRT4, a mitochondrial ADP-ribosyltransferase. *J Biol Chem.* (2007) 282:33583–92. doi: 10.1074/jbc.M705488200
62. Li SZheng W. Mammalian sirtuins SIRT4 and SIRT7. *Prog Mol Biol Transl Sci.* (2018) 154:147–68. doi: 10.1016/bs.pmbts.2017.11.001
63. Qin K, Zhang N, Zhang Z, Nipper M, Zhu Z, Leighton J, et al. SIRT6-mediated transcriptional suppression of Txnip is critical for pancreatic beta cell function and survival in mice. *Diabetologia* (2018) 61:906–18. doi: 10.1007/s00125-017-4542-6
64. Kanfi Y, Peshti V, Gil R, Naiman S, Nahum L, Levin E, et al. SIRT6 protects against pathological damage caused by diet-induced obesity. *Aging Cell* (2010) 9:162–73. doi: 10.1111/j.1474-9726.2009.00544.x
65. Xiao C, Kim HS, Lahusen T, Wang RH, Xu X, Gavrilova O, et al. SIRT6 deficiency results in severe hypoglycemia by enhancing both basal and insulin-stimulated glucose uptake in mice. *J Biol Chem.* (2010) 285:36776–84. doi: 10.1074/jbc.M110.168039
66. Song MY, Wang J, Ka SO, Bae EJ, Park BH. Insulin secretion impairment in Sirt6 knockout pancreatic beta cells is mediated by suppression of the FoxO1-Pdx1-Glut2 pathway. *Sci Rep.* (2016) 6:30321. doi: 10.1038/srep30321
67. Xiong X, Sun X, Wang Q, Qian X, Zhang Y, Pan X, et al. SIRT6 protects against palmitate-induced pancreatic beta-cell dysfunction and apoptosis. *J Endocrinol.* (2016) 231:159–65. doi: 10.1530/JOE-16-0317
68. Bouche C, Serdy S, Kahn CR, Goldfine AB. The cellular fate of glucose and its relevance in type 2 diabetes. *Endocr Rev.* (2004) 25:807–30. doi: 10.1210/er.2003-0026
69. Koo SH, Flechner L, Qi L, Zhang X, Screaton RA, Jeffries S, et al. The CREB coactivator TORC2 is a key regulator of fasting glucose metabolism. *Nature* (2005) 437:1109–11. doi: 10.1038/nature03967
70. Puigserver P, Rhee J, Donovan J, Walkey CJ, Yoon JC, Oriente F, et al. Insulin-regulated hepatic gluconeogenesis through FOXO1-PGC-1alpha interaction. *Nature* (2003) 423:550–5. doi: 10.1038/nature01667
71. Rodgers JT, Lerin C, Haas W, Gygi SP, Spiegelman BM, Puigserver P. Nutrient control of glucose homeostasis through a complex of PGC-1alpha and SIRT1. *Nature* (2005) 434:113–8. doi: 10.1038/nature03354
72. Lerin C, Rodgers JT, Kalume DE, Kim SH, Pandey A, Puigserver P. GCN5 acetyltransferase complex controls glucose metabolism through transcriptional repression of PGC-1alpha. *Cell Metab.* (2006) 3:429–38. doi: 10.1016/j.cmet.2006.04.013
73. Jiang W, Wang S, Xiao M, Lin Y, Zhou L, Lei Q, et al. Acetylation regulates gluconeogenesis by promoting PEPCK1 degradation via recruiting the UBR5 ubiquitin ligase. *Mol Cell* (2011) 43:33–44. doi: 10.1016/j.molcel.2011.04.028
74. Watanabe H, Inaba Y, Kimura K, Matsumoto M, Kaneko S, Kasuga M, et al. Sirt2 facilitates hepatic glucose uptake by deacetylating glucokinase regulatory protein. *Nat Commun.* (2018) 9:30. doi: 10.1038/s41467-017-02537-6
75. Kumar S, Lombard DB. Generation and purification of catalytically active recombinant sirtuin5 (SIRT5) protein. *Methods Mol Biol.* (2016) 1436:241–57. doi: 10.1007/978-1-4939-3667-0_16
76. Zhang P, Tu B, Wang H, Cao Z, Tang M, Zhang C, et al. Tumor suppressor p53 cooperates with SIRT6 to regulate gluconeogenesis by promoting FoxO1 nuclear exclusion. *Proc Natl Acad Sci USA.* (2014) 111:10684–9. doi: 10.1073/pnas.1411026111

77. Dominy JE Jr, Lee Y, Jedrychowski MP, Chim H, Jurczak MJ, Camporez JP, et al. The deacetylase Sirt6 activates the acetyltransferase GCN5 and suppresses hepatic gluconeogenesis. *Mol Cell* (2012) 48:900–13. doi: 10.1016/j.molcel.2012.09.030
78. Schwer B, Schumacher B, Lombard DB, Xiao C, Kurtev MV, Gao J, et al. Neural sirtuin 6 (Sirt6) ablation attenuates somatic growth and causes obesity. *Proc Natl Acad Sci USA.* (2010) 107:21790–4. doi: 10.1073/pnas.1016306107
79. Boily G, Seifert EL, Bevilacqua L, He XH, Sabourin G, Estey C, et al. SirT1 regulates energy metabolism and response to caloric restriction in mice. *PLoS ONE* (2008) 3:e1759. doi: 10.1371/journal.pone.0001759
80. Chen D, Steele AD, Lindquist S, Guarente L. Increase in activity during calorie restriction requires Sirt1. *Science* (2005) 310:1641. doi: 10.1126/science.1118357
81. Hebert AS, Dittenhafer-Reed KE, Yu W, Bailey DJ, Selen ES, Boersma MD, et al. Calorie restriction and SIRT3 trigger global reprogramming of the mitochondrial protein acetylome. *Mol Cell* (2013) 49:186–99. doi: 10.1016/j.molcel.2012.10.024
82. Qiu X, Brown K, Hirschey MD, Verdin E, Chen D. Calorie restriction reduces oxidative stress by SIRT3-mediated SOD2 activation. *Cell Metab.* (2010) 12:662–7. doi: 10.1016/j.cmet.2010.11.015
83. Someya S, Yu W, Hallows WC, Xu J, Vann JM, Leeuwenburgh C, et al. Sirt3 mediates reduction of oxidative damage and prevention of age-related hearing loss under caloric restriction. *Cell* (2010) 143:802–12. doi: 10.1016/j.cell.2010.10.002
84. Liu Y, Dentin R, Chen D, Hedrick S, Ravnskjaer K, Schenk S, et al. A fasting inducible switch modulates gluconeogenesis via activator/coactivator exchange. *Nature* (2008) 456:269–73. doi: 10.1038/nature07349
85. Milne JC, Lambert PD, Schenk S, Carney DP, Smith JJ, Gagne DJ, et al. Small molecule activators of SIRT1 as therapeutics for the treatment of type 2 diabetes. *Nature* (2007) 450:712–6. doi: 10.1038/nature06261
86. Barger JL, Kayo T, Vann JM, Arias EB, Wang J, Hacker TA, et al. A low dose of dietary resveratrol partially mimics caloric restriction and retards aging parameters in mice. *PLoS ONE* (2008) 3:e2264. doi: 10.1371/journal.pone.0002264
87. Kanfi Y, Naiman S, Amir G, Peshti V, Zinman G, Nahum L, et al. The sirtuin SIRT6 regulates lifespan in male mice. *Nature* (2012) 483:218–21. doi: 10.1038/nature10815
88. Satoh A, Brace CS, Ben-Josef G, West T, Wozniak DF, Holtzman DM, et al. SIRT1 promotes the central adaptive response to diet restriction through activation of the dorsomedial and lateral nuclei of the hypothalamus. *J Neurosci.* (2010) 30:10220–32. doi: 10.1523/JNEUROSCI.1385-10.2010
89. Zhang HJ, Zhang XF, Ma ZM, Pan LL, Chen Z, Han HW, et al. Irisin is inversely associated with intrahepatic triglyceride contents in obese adults. *J Hepatol.* (2013) 59:557–62. doi: 10.1016/j.jhep.2013.04.030
90. de Moura MB, Uppala R, Zhang Y, Van Houten B, Goetzman ES. Overexpression of mitochondrial sirtuins alters glycolysis and mitochondrial function in HEK293 cells. *PLoS ONE* (2014) 9:e106028. doi: 10.1371/journal.pone.0106028
91. Gerhart-Hines Z, Rodgers JT, Bare O, Lerin C, Kim SH, Mostoslavsky R, et al. Metabolic control of muscle mitochondrial function and fatty acid oxidation through SIRT1/PGC-1alpha. *EMBO J.* (2007) 26:1913–23. doi: 10.1038/sj.emboj.7601633
92. Giralt A, Hondares E, Villena JA, Ribas F, Diaz-Delfin J, Giralt M, et al. Peroxisome proliferator-activated receptor-gamma coactivator-1alpha controls transcription of the Sirt3 gene, an essential component of the thermogenic brown adipocyte phenotype. *J Biol Chem.* (2011) 286:16958–66. doi: 10.1074/jbc.M110.202390
93. Kong X, Wang R, Xue Y, Liu X, Zhang H, Chen Y, et al. Sirtuin 3, a new target of PGC-1alpha, plays an important role in the suppression of ROS and mitochondrial biogenesis. *PLoS ONE* (2010) 5:e11707. doi: 10.1371/journal.pone.0011707
94. Shi T, Wang F, Stieren E, Tong Q. SIRT3, a mitochondrial sirtuin deacetylase, regulates mitochondrial function and thermogenesis in brown adipocytes. *J Biol Chem.* (2005) 280:13560–7. doi: 10.1074/jbc.M414670200
95. Hirschey MD, Shimazu T, Goetzman E, Jing E, Schwer B, Lombard DB, et al. SIRT3 regulates mitochondrial fatty-acid oxidation by reversible enzyme deacetylation. *Nature* (2010) 464:121–5. doi: 10.1038/nature08778
96. Ho L, Titus AS, Banerjee KK, George S, Lin W, Deota S, et al. SIRT4 regulates ATP homeostasis and mediates a retrograde signaling via AMPK. *Aging* (2013) 5:835–49. doi: 10.18632/aging.100616
97. Zhou L, Wang F, Sun R, Chen X, Zhang M, Xu Q, et al. SIRT5 promotes IDH2 desuccinylation and G6PD deglutarylation to enhance cellular antioxidant defense. *EMBO Rep.* (2016) 17:811–22. doi: 10.15252/embr.201541643
98. Zhong L, D'Urso A, Toiber D, Sebastian C, Henry RE, Vadysirisack DD, et al. The histone deacetylase Sirt6 regulates glucose homeostasis via Hif1alpha. *Cell* (2010) 140:280–93. doi: 10.1016/j.cell.2009.12.041
99. Hu CJ, Iyer S, Sataur A, Covello KL, Chodosh LA, Simon MC. Differential regulation of the transcriptional activities of hypoxia-inducible factor 1 alpha (HIF-1α) and HIF-2α in stem cells. *Mol Cell Biol.* (2006) 26:3514–26. doi: 10.1128/MCB.26.9.3514-3526.2006
100. Randle PJ, Garland PB, Hales CN, Newsholme EA. The glucose fatty-acid cycle. Its role in insulin sensitivity and the metabolic disturbances of diabetes mellitus. *Lancet* (1963) 1:785–9.
101. Furler SM, Poynten AM, Kriketos AD, Lowy AJ, Ellis BA, Maclean EL, et al. Independent influences of central fat and skeletal muscle lipids on insulin sensitivity. *Obes Res.* (2001) 9:535–43. doi: 10.1038/oby.2001.70
102. Feige JN, Lagouge M, Canto C, Strehle A, Houten SM, Milne JC, et al. Specific SIRT1 activation mimics low energy levels and protects against diet-induced metabolic disorders by enhancing fat oxidation. *Cell Metab.* (2008) 8:347–58. doi: 10.1016/j.cmet.2008.08.017
103. Iwabu M, Yamauchi T, Okada-Iwabu M, Sato K, Nakagawa T, Funata M, et al. Adiponectin and AdipoR1 regulate PGC-1α and mitochondria by Ca(2+) and AMPK/SIRT1. *Nature* (2010) 464:1313–9. doi: 10.1038/nature08991
104. Arora A, Dey CS. SIRT2 negatively regulates insulin resistance in C2C12 skeletal muscle cells. *Biochim Biophys Acta* (2014) 1842:1372–8. doi: 10.1016/j.bbadis.2014.04.027
105. Jing E, Emanuelli B, Hirschey MD, Boucher J, Lee KY, Lombard D, et al. Sirtuin-3 (Sirt3) regulates skeletal muscle metabolism and insulin signaling via altered mitochondrial oxidation and reactive oxygen species production. *Proc Natl Acad Sci USA.* (2011) 108:14608–13. doi: 10.1073/pnas.1111308108
106. Jing E, O'Neill BT, Rardin MJ, Kleinridders A, Ilkeyeva OR, Ussar S, et al. Sirt3 regulates metabolic flexibility of skeletal muscle through reversible enzymatic deacetylation. *Diabetes* (2013) 62:3404–17. doi: 10.2337/db12-1650
107. Muoio DM, Neufer PD. Lipid-induced mitochondrial stress and insulin action in muscle. *Cell Metab.* (2012) 15:595–605. doi: 10.1016/j.cmet.2012.04.010
108. Lantier L, Williams AS, Williams IM, Yang KK, Bracy DP, Goelzer M, et al. SIRT3 is crucial for maintaining skeletal muscle insulin action and protects against severe insulin resistance in high-fat-fed mice. *Diabetes* (2015) 64:3081–92. doi: 10.2337/db14-1810
109. Nasrin N, Wu X, Fortier E, Feng Y, Bare OC, Chen S, et al. SIRT4 regulates fatty acid oxidation and mitochondrial gene expression in liver and muscle cells. *J Biol Chem.* (2010) 285:31995–2002. doi: 10.1074/jbc.M110.124164
110. Kelley DE, Goodpaster B, Wing RR, Simoneau JA. Skeletal muscle fatty acid metabolism in association with insulin resistance, obesity, and weight loss. *Am J Physiol.* (1999) 277:E1130–41.
111. Kelley DE, He J, Menshikova EV, Ritov VB. Dysfunction of mitochondria in human skeletal muscle in type 2 diabetes. *Diabetes* (2002) 51:2944–50. doi: 10.2337/diabetes.51.10.2944
112. Rodgers JT, Puigserver P. Fasting-dependent glucose and lipid metabolic response through hepatic sirtuin 1. *Proc Natl Acad Sci USA.* (2007) 104:12861–6. doi: 10.1073/pnas.0702509104
113. Purushotham A, Schug TT, Xu Q, Surapureddi S, Guo X, Li X. Hepatocyte-specific deletion of SIRT1 alters fatty acid metabolism and results in hepatic steatosis and inflammation. *Cell Metab.* (2009) 9:327–38. doi: 10.1016/j.cmet.2009.02.006
114. Sugden MC, Caton PW, Holness MJ. PPAR control: it's SIRTainly as easy as PGC. *J Endocrinol.* (2010) 204:93–104. doi: 10.1677/JOE-09-0359
115. Ponugoti B, Kim DH, Xiao Z, Smith Z, Miao J, Zang M, et al. SIRT1 deacetylates and inhibits SREBP-1C activity in regulation of hepatic lipid metabolism. *J Biol Chem.* (2010) 285:33959–70. doi: 10.1074/jbc.M110.122978
116. Krishnan J, Danzer C, Simka T, Ukropec J, Walter KM, Kumpf S, et al. Dietary obesity-associated Hif1alpha activation in adipocytes restricts fatty

acid oxidation and energy expenditure via suppression of the Sirt2-NAD+ system. *Genes Dev.* (2012) 26:259–70. doi: 10.1101/gad.180406.111

117. Lombard DB, Alt FW, Cheng HL, Bunkenborg J, Streeper RS, Mostoslavsky R, et al. Mammalian Sir2 homolog SIRT3 regulates global mitochondrial lysine acetylation. *Mol Cell Biol.* (2007) 27:8807–14. doi: 10.1128/MCB.01636-07
118. Hallows WC, Yu W, Smith BC, Devries MK, Ellinger JJ, Someya S, et al. Sirt3 promotes the urea cycle and fatty acid oxidation during dietary restriction. *Mol Cell* (2011) 41:139–49. doi: 10.1016/j.molcel.2011.01.002
119. Shimazu T, Hirschey MD, Hua L, Dittenhafer-Reed KE, Schwer B, Lombard DB, et al. SIRT3 deacetylates mitochondrial 3-hydroxy-3-methylglutaryl CoA synthase 2 and regulates ketone body production. *Cell Metab.* (2010) 12:654–61. doi: 10.1016/j.cmet.2010.11.003
120. Hirschey MD, Shimazu T, Jing E, Grueter CA, Collins AM, Aouizerat B, et al. SIRT3 deficiency and mitochondrial protein hyperacetylation accelerate the development of the metabolic syndrome. *Mol Cell* (2011) 44:177–90. doi: 10.1016/j.molcel.2011.07.019
121. Yoshizawa T, Karim MF, Sato Y, Senokuchi T, Miyata K, Fukuda T, et al. SIRT7 controls hepatic lipid metabolism by regulating the ubiquitin-proteasome pathway. *Cell Metab.* (2014) 19:712–21. doi: 10.1016/j.cmet.2014.03.006
122. Karim MF, Yoshizawa T, Sobuz SU, Sato Y, Yamagata K. Sirtuin 7-dependent deacetylation of DDB1 regulates the expression of nuclear receptor TR4. *Biochem Biophys Res Commun.* (2017) 490:423–428. doi: 10.1016/j.bbrc.2017.06.057
123. Ryu D, Jo YS, Lo Sasso G, Stein S, Zhang H, Perino A, et al. A SIRT7-dependent acetylation switch of GABPbeta1 controls mitochondrial function. *Cell Metab.* (2014) 20:856–69. doi: 10.1016/j.cmet.2014.08.001
124. Shin J, He M, Liu Y, Paredes S, Villanova L, Brown K, et al. SIRT7 represses Myc activity to suppress ER stress and prevent fatty liver disease. *Cell Rep.* (2013) 5:654–65. doi: 10.1016/j.celrep.2013.10.007
125. Laurent G, de Boer VC, Finley LW, Sweeney M, Lu H, Schug TT, et al. SIRT4 represses peroxisome proliferator-activated receptor alpha activity to suppress hepatic fat oxidation. *Mol Cell Biol.* (2013) 33:4552–61. doi: 10.1128/MCB.00087-13
126. Rajala MW, Scherer PE. Minireview: the adipocyte–at the crossroads of energy homeostasis, inflammation, and atherosclerosis. *Endocrinology* (2003) 144:3765–73. doi: 10.1210/en.2003-0580
127. Berg AH, Scherer PE. Adipose tissue, inflammation, and cardiovascular disease. *Circ Res.* (2005) 96:939–49. doi: 10.1161/01.RES.0000163635.62927.34
128. Kadowaki T, Yamauchi T. Adiponectin and adiponectin receptors. *Endocr Rev.* (2005) 26:439–51. doi: 10.1210/er.2005-0005
129. Picard F, Kurtev M, Chung N, Topark-Ngarm A, Senawong T, Machado De Oliveira R, et al. Sirt1 promotes fat mobilization in white adipocytes by repressing PPAR-gamma. *Nature* (2004) 429:771–6. doi: 10.1038/nature02583
130. Qiang L, Wang L, Kon N, Zhao W, Lee S, Zhang Y, et al. Brown remodeling of white adipose tissue by SirT1-dependent deacetylation of Ppargamma. *Cell* (2012) 150:620–32. doi: 10.1016/j.cell.2012.06.027
131. Kurylowicz A, Owczarz M, Polosak J, Jonas MI, Lisik W, Jonas M, et al. SIRT1 and SIRT7 expression in adipose tissues of obese and normal-weight individuals is regulated by microRNAs but not by methylation status. *Int J Obes.* (2016) 40:1635–42. doi: 10.1038/ijo.2016.131
132. Cioffi M, Vallespinos-Serrano M, Trabulo SM, Fernandez-Marcos PJ, Firment AN, Vazquez BN, et al. MiR-93 controls adiposity via inhibition of Sirt7 and Tbx3. *Cell Rep.* (2015) 12:1594–605. doi: 10.1016/j.celrep.2015.08.006
133. Tong Z, Wang Y, Zhang X, Kim DD, Sadhukhan S, Hao Q, et al. SIRT7 Is activated by DNA and deacetylates histone H3 in the chromatin context. *ACS Chem Biol.* (2016) 11:742–7. doi: 10.1021/acschembio.5b01084
134. Tong Z, Wang M, Wang Y, Kim DD, Grenier JK, Cao J, et al. SIRT7 is an RNA-activated protein lysine deacylase. *ACS Chem Biol.* (2017) 12:300–10. doi: 10.1021/acschembio.6b00954
135. Kuang J, Zhang Y, Liu Q, Shen J, Pu S, Cheng S, et al. Fat-specific Sirt6 ablation sensitizes mice to high-fat diet-induced obesity and insulin resistance by inhibiting lipolysis. *Diabetes* (2017) 66:1159–71. doi: 10.2337/db16-1225
136. Ramadori G, Fujikawa T, Fukuda M, Anderson J, Morgan DA, Mostoslavsky R, et al. SIRT1 deacetylase in POMC neurons is required for homeostatic defenses against diet-induced obesity. *Cell Metab.* (2010) 12:78–87. doi: 10.1016/j.cmet.2010.05.010
137. Ramadori G, Fujikawa T, Anderson J, Berglund ED, Frazao R, Michan S, et al. SIRT1 deacetylase in SF1 neurons protects against metabolic imbalance. *Cell Metab.* (2011) 14:301–12. doi: 10.1016/j.cmet.2011.06.014
138. Sasaki T, Kim HJ, Kobayashi M, Kitamura YI, Yokota-Hashimoto H, Shiuchi T, et al. Induction of hypothalamic Sirt1 leads to cessation of feeding via agouti-related peptide. *Endocrinology* (2010) 151:2556–66. doi: 10.1210/en.2009-1319
139. Velasquez DA, Martinez G, Romero A, Vazquez MJ, Boit KD, Dopeso-Reyes IG, et al. The central Sirtuin 1/p53 pathway is essential for the orexigenic action of ghrelin. *Diabetes* (2011) 60:1177–85. doi: 10.2337/db10-0802
140. Lu M, Sarruf DA, Li P, Osborn O, Sanchez-Alavez M, Talukdar S, et al. Neuronal Sirt1 deficiency increases insulin sensitivity in both brain and peripheral tissues. *J Biol Chem.* (2013) 288:10722–35. doi: 10.1074/jbc.M112.443606
141. Roy Chowdhury S, Djordjevic J, Thomson E, Smith DR, Albensi BC, Fernyhough P. Depressed mitochondrial function and electron transport complex II-mediated H2O2 production in the cortex of type 1 diabetic rodents. *Mol Cell Neurosci.* (2018) 90:49–59. doi: 10.1016/j.mcn.2018.05.006
142. Dong Y, Guo T, Traurig M, Mason CC, Kobes S, Perez J, et al. SIRT1 is associated with a decrease in acute insulin secretion and a sex specific increase in risk for type 2 diabetes in Pima Indians. *Mol Genet Metab.* (2011) 104:661–5. doi: 10.1016/j.ymgme.2011.08.001
143. Maeda S, Koya D, Araki SI, Babazono T, Umezono T, Toyoda M, et al. Association between single nucleotide polymorphisms within genes encoding sirtuin families and diabetic nephropathy in Japanese subjects with type 2 diabetes. *Clin Exp Nephrol.* (2011) 15:381–90. doi: 10.1007/s10157-011-0418-0
144. Botden IP, Zillikens MC, de Rooij SR, Langendonk JG, Danser AH, Sijbrands EJ, et al. Variants in the SIRT1 gene may affect diabetes risk in interaction with prenatal exposure to famine. *Diabetes Care* (2012) 35:424–6. doi: 10.2337/dc11-1203
145. Sosnowska B, Mazidi M, Penson P, Gluba-Brzozka A, Rysz J, Banach M. The sirtuin family members SIRT1, SIRT3 and SIRT6: their role in vascular biology and atherogenesis. *Atherosclerosis* (2017) 265:275–82. doi: 10.1016/j.atherosclerosis.2017.08.027
146. Tan MH, Alquraini H, Mizokami-Stout K, MacEachern M. Metformin: from research to clinical practice. *Endocrinol Metab Clin North Am.* (2016) 45:819–43. doi: 10.1016/j.ecl.2016.06.008
147. Sliwinska A, Drzewoski J. Molecular action of metformin in hepatocytes: an updated insight. *Curr Diabetes Rev.* (2015) 11:175–81. doi: 10.2174/1573399811666150325233108
148. Knowler WC, Barrett-Connor E, Fowler SE, Hamman RF, Lachin JM, Walker EA, et al. Reduction in the incidence of type 2 diabetes with lifestyle intervention or metformin. *N Engl J Med.* (2002) 346:393–403. doi: 10.1056/NEJMoa012512
149. Moin T, Schmittdiel JA, Flory JH, Yeh J, Karter AJ, Kruge LE, et al. Review of metformin use for type 2 diabetes prevention. *Am J Prev Med.* (2018) 55:565–74. doi: 10.1016/j.amepre.2018.04.038
150. Kaleida Health. *Effect of Resveratrol on Insulin Resistance and Inflammatory Mediators in Obese and Type 2 Diabetic Subjects, 2010.* ClinicalTrials.gov. Identifier: NCT01158417 Available online at: http://clinicaltrials.gov/ct2/show/NCT01158417?term=NCT01158417.&rank$=$1
151. Mellini P, Valente S, Mai A. Sirtuin modulators: an updated patent review (2012–2014). *Expert Opin Ther Pat.* (2015) 25:5–15. doi: 10.1517/13543776.2014.982532
152. Boocock DJ, Faust GE, Patel KR, Schinas AM, Brown VA, Ducharme MP, et al. Phase I dose escalation pharmacokinetic study in healthy volunteers of resveratrol, a potential cancer chemopreventive agent. *Cancer Epidemiol Biomarkers Prev.* (2007) 16:1246–52. doi: 10.1158/1055-9965.EPI-07-0022
153. GlaxoSmithKline. *A Clinical Study to Assess the Safety, Tolerability, and Activity of Oral SRT2104 Capsules Administered for 28 Days to Subjects With Type 2 Diabetes Mellitus. 2011.* ClinicalTrials.gov. Identifier: NCT01018017 Available online at: http://clinicaltrials.gov/ct2/show/study/NCT01018017?term=NCT01018017.&rank=1

154. GlaxoSmithKline. *A Phase I Randomized, Placebo-Controlled, Single-Blind, Multiple-Dose, Dose-Escalation Clinical Study to Assess the Safety and Pharmacokinetics of SRT2379 in Normal Healthy Male Volunteers, 2011.* ClinicalTrials.gov.Identifier: NCT01018628 Available online at: http://clinicaltrials.gov/ct2/show/NCT01018628?term=NCT01018628&rank=1
155. Rardin MJ, He W, Nishida Y, Newman JC, Carrico C, Danielson SR, et al. SIRT5 regulates the mitochondrial lysine succinylome and metabolic networks. *Cell Metab.* (2013) 18:920–33. doi: 10.1016/j.cmet.2013.11.013
156. Cohen HY, Miller C, Bitterman KJ, Wall NR, Hekking B, Kessler B, et al. Calorie restriction promotes mammalian cell survival by inducing the SIRT1 deacetylase. *Science* (2004) 305:390–2. doi: 10.1126/science.1099196
157. Mathias RA, Greco TM, Oberstein A, Budayeva HG, Chakrabarti R, Rowland EA, et al. Sirtuin 4 is a lipoamidase regulating pyruvate dehydrogenase complex activity. *Cell* (2014) 159:1615–25. doi: 10.1016/j.cell.2014.11.046
158. Park J, Chen Y, Tishkoff DX, Peng C, Tan M, Dai L, et al. SIRT5-mediated lysine desuccinylation impacts diverse metabolic pathways. *Mol Cell* (2013) 50:919–30. doi: 10.1016/j.molcel.2013.06.001
159. Burns J, Yokota T, Ashihara H, Lean ME, Crozier A. Plant foods and herbal sources of resveratrol. *J Agric Food Chem.* (2002) 50:3337–40. doi: 10.1021/jf0112973
160. Hung CH, Chan SH, Chu PM, Tsai KL. Quercetin is a potent anti-atherosclerotic compound by activation of SIRT1 signaling under oxLDL stimulation. *Mol Nutr Food Res.* (2015) 59:1905–17. doi: 10.1002/mnfr.201500144
161. Affuso F, Mercurio V, Fazio V, Fazio S. Cardiovascular and metabolic effects of Berberine. *World J Cardiol.* (2010) 2:71–7. doi: 10.4330/wjc.v2.i4.71

5

SIRT1 in Secretory Organ Cancer

Raffaele Frazzi*

Laboratory of Translational Research, Azienda Unità Sanitaria Locale - IRCCS di Reggio Emilia, Reggio Emilia, Italy

***Correspondence:**
Raffaele Frazzi
raffaele.frazzi@ausl.re.it

Mammalian silent information regulator 1 (SIRT1) is reported to play a role in cancers of the secretory organs, including thyroid, pancreatic endocrine, and ovarian tumors (1–4). A recent meta-analysis conducted on 37 selected studies of human cancers analyzed the correlations of overall survival (OS), disease-free survival (DFS) and relapse-free survival (RFS) with SIRT1 expression (5). This study reported that SIRT1 overexpression was associated with a worse OS in liver and lung cancers, while it was not correlated with OS in breast cancer, colorectal cancer, or gastric carcinoma. Collectively, the meta-analysis revealed that an unfavorable OS was associated with SIRT1 expression for solid malignancies. Given the growing importance of this class of lysine/histone deacetylases in human endocrine malignancies, a rational and focused literature assessment is desirable in light of future clinical translations.

Keywords: SIRT1, cancer, secretory organs, acetylation, epigenetic modulation

INTRODUCTION

The epigenetic regulation of chromatin structure and gene expression represents a major field of study and intervention for researchers focused on cancer. The class III lysine/histone deacetylases are known as Sirtuins and are represented, in humans, by 7 members (6, 7). Silent information regulator 1 (SIRT1) is the most studied and well characterized among the class III deacetylases and its targets include p53, Ku70, peroxisome proliferator-activated receptor gamma (PPARγ), peroxisome proliferator-activated receptor gamma coactivator 1-alpha (PGC1α), Beclin 1 and β-catenin, among others (8–13). A relevant group of SIRT1 targets is the Forkhead box O (FOXO) family of transcription factors. FOXO3a hyperacetylation mediated by SIRT1 accompanies apoptosis while FOXO4 deacetylation activates this target enhancing its transcriptional and biological activity in the nucleus. FOXO4 activation enhances the cellular defenses against oxidative stress and leads to apoptosis resistance (8, 14, 15). Fibrosis is another aging-related disease involving FOXO1/3, well known modulators of aging and longevity playing a clear inhibitory effects on fibrogenic effector cells and extracellular matrix production (16).

Furthermore, the epigenetic regulation and dysregulation of the hypermethylated in cancer1 (HIC1)/SIRT1/p53 axis is relevant for the development of malignancies (17). SIRT1 is also a target for several miRNAs, small non-coding RNA molecules known to be deregulated in various cancers, whose expression is involved in tumorigenesis (18).

SIRT1, due to its NAD^{+} dependency, is also a metabolic sensor and its deacetylating activity toward regulatory target proteins affects cell metabolism (19).

The focus of this review is the role and involvement of SIRT1 in secretory organ cancers since the information recently gathered on this topic should bear new translational benefits. Correlations between SIRT1 and nuclear receptors, transcription factors, master regulators of gene expression, miRNAs and lncRNAs have been reported. The main glands in the body and the most recent literature are taken into consideration.

OVARIAN CANCER

Ovarian cancer is the fifth leading cause of female cancer mortality in the United States (20). This type of cancer is currently treated with a platinum and taxane-based chemotherapy after surgical cytoreduction. However, the rates of progression free survival (PFS) and OS for these patients remain dismal and no benefits seem to arise by the introduction of additional cytotoxic agents (21). Ovarian cancer is usually regarded as a single entity and current treatment protocols for the disease are not subtype specific. Actually, ovarian cancer is a heterogeneous disease that is classified by histopathological examination, including serous, clear cell, endometrioid, and mucinous subtypes. These subtypes develop differently and respond differently to chemotherapy (22).

SIRT1 overexpression is reported by many authors as associated with poor outcome and chemoresistance in ovarian cancer of epithelial origin (23–25). Ovarian cells (both normal and tumoral) express two kinds of estrogen receptors (ER), ERα and ERβ which play different roles in cell proliferation and aggressiveness (4). Specifically, ERα is associated to a poor outcome, while ERβ expression corresponds, on the contrary, to a favorable outcome. ERα levels are closely associated with estrogen-dependent growth and the increased metastatic potential of ovarian epithelial carcinoma (OEC) through the promotion of the epithelial to mesenchymal transition (EMT) (26). ERβ, in contrast, inhibits EMT in presence of 17β-estradiol (E2), thus mediating the opposite effect to ERα (26). SIRT1 is inversely correlated to ERβ mRNA and protein levels, and the specific ERβ activator KB9520 strongly inhibits SIRT1 mRNA expression. These data collectively support the role of SIRT1 as a tumor promoter in OEC (4).

Recently, another association between OEC and SIRT1 was reported (27). These observations are relevant, because OEC patients often acquire resistance to paclitaxel or cisplatin, and the increased expression in *SIRT1* and *TWIST1* (two genes associated with drug resistance) is observed in OVCAR-5 cells that show increased cisplatin resistance, migration and invasion potential (27).

SIRT1 is a downstream target of hypoxia inducible factor 1α (HIF1α) (28). Hypoxia is a condition associated with several types of tumors and, specifically, increased HIF1α expression predicts the poor prognosis of ovarian cancer. Notably it has been demonstrated that SIRT1 expression is induced by hypoxia and that HIF1α silencing indirectly hampers SIRT1 expression. Finally, the NF-κB signaling pathway is involved in hypoxia-induced SIRT1 up-regulation, strengthening the link between this class III lysine deacetylase and ovarian cancer (28).

THYROID CANCER

The incidence of thyroid cancer has increased over the past few decades worldwide. This increase is mainly driven by new cases of papillary thyroid cancer (29). SIRT1 is reported to be oncogenic in thyroid and prostate murine carcinomas initiated by PTEN deficiency (2). The mechanism unveiled by mRNA transcriptional analysis revealed that SIRT1 drives oncogenesis through c-MYC regulation (**Figure 1**). Two pathways upregulated via SIRT1 overexpression are related to translation and ribosomal biogenesis, which are both controlled by c-MYC. The protein product of the c-MYC oncogene lies at the intersection of a transcriptional network regulating cellular proliferation, replicative potential, cell–cell competition, cell size, differentiation, metabolism, and apoptosis (30).

c-MYC increases in response to mitogenic stimuli, and this is accompanied by SIRT1 upregulation. c-MYC activates SIRT1 by promoting NAMPT transcription and then the NAD-salvage pathway. Furthermore, c-MYC can bind directly to DBC1 (that is a SIRT1 inhibitor) thus preventing SIRT1 blockade (31, 32). On the other hand, SIRT1 activation leads to p53 deacetylation and consequent inactivation, decreasing the levels of PUMA and p21 and eventually counteracting the pro-apoptotic effects of p53. Finally, SIRT1 stabilizes c-MYC via lysine-specific deacetylation and increases its transcriptional activity. Altogether, these data demonstrate a positive feedback loop between c-MYC and SIRT1 (31).

The translational significance of these findings is highlighted by the consistent overexpression of SIRT1 in follicular and papillary thyroid carcinomas, positively correlates with c-MYC protein levels and stabilizes c-MYC (2).

The natural phytochemical resveratrol (RSV) is known to affect mammalian cell metabolism and aging by modulating SIRT1 (33, 34). Furthermore, SIRT1 is also a reported molecular target of RSV in cancer cells of both lymphoid and epithelial origin (35). RSV regulates thyroid stimulating hormone (TSH) secretion via SIRT1 activation. RSV also arrests follicular thyroid and papillary thyroid carcinoma growth by activating the mitogen-activated protein kinase (MAPK) signal transduction pathway and p53 phosphorylation (36, 37).

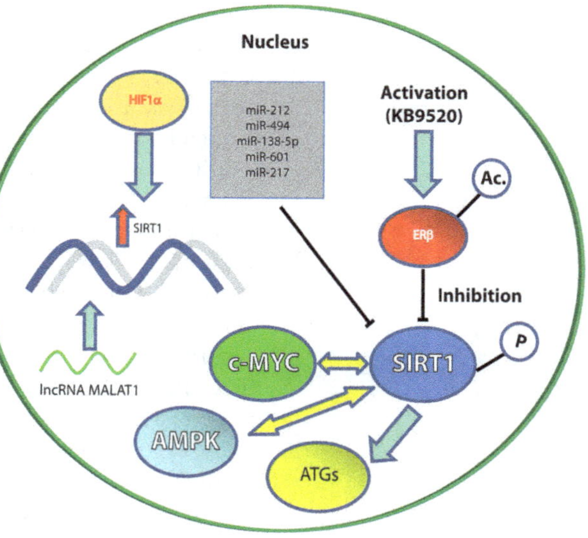

FIGURE 1 | The main SIRT1 molecular interactors (inhibitory or activatory) cited in the text. Solid blue arrows represent an activation; yellow arrows represent an interplay; blunt ended black lines represent an inhibition; red arrow represents upregulation of gene expression.

Among the few studies available, regarding the role of SIRT1 in the thyroid neoplasias, most report involvement as a direct target for miRNAs. miR-212 is a tumor suppressor miRNA that inhibits the proliferation, migration, and invasiveness of thyroid cancer cells. SIRT1 is a direct target of miR-212 and is inversely correlated to miR-212 expression in thyroid cancer tissues (42 samples of human thyroid cancer) (38).

PANCREATIC CANCER

Pancreatic cancer (PC) is one of the most deadly tumors in western countries and the 10th most common cancer in the United States. Pancreatic ductal adenocarcinoma is the most common subtype and is recognized as "incurable" due to its aggressive clinical course and resistance to available therapies (39, 40). miR-494 is specifically involved in PC proliferation (41). The overexpression of miR-494 inhibits PC cell proliferation *in vitro* and *in vivo* in addition to inhibiting invasion. The c-MYC/SIRT1 axis is a direct target of miR-494 and there is an inverse correlation between the two. The simultaneous interference of c-MYC and SIRT1 synergistically reduces the expression of these two targets and inhibits PC proliferation, eventually stimulating miR-494 expression (41). The interplay between c-MYC and SIRT1, therefore, plays a relevant role during PC tumorigenesis and should be taken into account when designing strategies aimed at combating this cancer.

Recent studies on the miRNA-mediated regulation of autophagy in PC have been published (42). Since it is known that hypoxia induces autophagy, PC cells were cultured under normoxic and hypoxic conditions. miR-138-5p emerged among the most down-regulated miRNAs in the hypoxia-grown cells. Targets can analysis further revealed that the *SIRT1* gene contains a classical and conserved domain that binds miR-138-5p. Notably, miR-138-5p specifically binds to the 3′-UTR of *SIRT1* and its overexpression leads to SIRT1 protein downregulation (42). Finally, the authors demonstrated that miR-138-5p also counteracts the hypoxia induction in cancer cells through SIRT1 inhibition in tumor xenografts.

Another player that emerged recently is miR-601, which suppresses PC proliferation and migration (43). The target of this miRNA's activity was identified, once more, as SIRT1. This Sirtuin is downregulated by miR-601 and its overexpression reverses the effect of miR-601 on PC cells (43).

miR-217 also directly targets SIRT1, it is inversely correlated to SIRT1 expression and is down-regulated in chronic pancreatitis and PC (44).

The Ex-527 synthetic inhibitor, which inhibits pancreatic cell proliferation *in vitro* and in combination with the first-line drug for this pathology, gemcitabine, is considered one of the most specific SIRT1 inhibitors currently available (45). The same inhibitor was shown to promote PC xenograft tumors in SCID mice and did not synergize with gemcitabine. Therefore, caution should be used when dealing with Ex-527 inhibitor to target SIRT1 *in vivo*.

The role of histone deacetylases (HDACs) is poorly understood in pancreatic neuroendocrine tumors (pNETs). A comprehensive expression pattern of all the five classes (I, IIa, IIb, III, and IV) of HDACs was recently described (3). The gene expression profiles of a total of $n = 57$ patients revealed a significant upregulation of all the HDAC classes in pNETs over controls with increased levels ranging from 1.5- to 7-fold. The expression of several HDACs, including SIRT1, correlates to the G3 stage and, thus, to pNETs tumor grading (3).

GASTRIC CANCER

Gastric cancer (GC) is among the most prevalent malignancies of the upper gastrointestinal tract. It is a solid aggressive carcinoma where new therapeutic options are warranted (46). Autophagy in GC may have the dual role of promoting the activity of irradiation and anticancer drugs or, on the contrary, may function as a protective mechanism for cancer cells (47–49).

SIRT1 plays a confirmed role in autophagy (50, 51). In GC, it has been demonstrated that SIRT1 deacetylates autophagy-related gene products (ATGs) and a series of histonic and non-histonic targets, eventually interfering with the autophagic process (**Figure 1**) (52).

GC is among the few human tumors where SIRT1 is downregulated, and in one study, the prognosis of low-SIRT1 expressing GC patients was good (52, 53). However, other authors reported a meta-analysis of SIRT1 expression in gastrointestinal cancer in which the results were heterogeneous (54). The overall results from 15 studies showed an association between worse OS and high SIRT1 expression in gastrointestinal cancer. The subgroup analysis revealed that this association was particularly strong in non-colorectal gastrointestinal cancers, especially GC and hepatocellular carcinoma (54). Therefore, SIRT1 is a promising prognostic factor in GC but not in colorectal tumors.

In contrast with the abovementioned results, a study of the clinicopathological parameters in GC patients was analyzed using the Kaplan-Meier plotter (55). Here, the data concerning the seven human Sirtuins were extrapolated from NCBI GEO databases containing mRNA profiles and the corresponding clinical data of a large number of GC patient samples. The Kaplan-Meier plotter was used to investigate the predictive value of mRNA expression of the Sirtuins for the OS of GC patients. Among a total of 631 available cases for SIRT1 expression, the survival curves suggested that a high expression of SIRT1 mRNA was favorable for OS and that different Sirtuins had diverse correlations with OS. Furthermore, the first progression (FP) was positively correlated with SIRT1 expression: in other words, a longer FP time was associated with a higher SIRT1 level (55).

Opposite evidence was reported from the immunohistochemical (IHC) staining of primary GC tissues. High SIRT1 expression, by IHC, was associated with lymphatic invasion ($p = 0.028$), vessel invasion ($p = 0.016$) and lymph node metastasis ($p = 0.014$) and tended to be associated with more advanced disease stages (56).

Clearly, no consistent data on the exact role of SIRT1 in GC are available at present. The evidence available thus far points to a dual role for SIRT1 (that is to say it may act as a tumor promoter as well as a tumor suppressor), possibly depending on its sub-cellular localization, p53 status, and microenvironmental conditions (57, 58).

ADRENAL GLANDS

The function of SIRT1 in the adrenal glands has been investigated the least. One study reports the researches performed on human adrenal NCI-H295R cells (59) and, in this setting, Sirtuins (including SIRT1) did not seem to be involved in the RSV-mediated lowering of androgen production.

Moreover, steroidogenesis in H295R cells was not affected by Sirtuins, even when SIRT1/3/5 are overexpressed through transgenesis, strengthening the fact that RSV-dependent effects in this setting are SIRT-independent (59).

HEPATIC CANCER

Hepatocellular carcinoma (HCC) is a highly malignant tumor with a higher frequency in East Asia than in Europe and North America (60). HCC is the predominant malignancy in the liver and recent evidence shows a role for SIRT1/PGC-1alpha/mitochondrial biosynthesis pathway in protecting the liver against lipid accumulation and mitochondrial dysfunction (61, 62). Senescence induction is a recently proposed strategy with the aim of counteracting HCC (63). Metformin, for instance, induce senescence via the activation of AMP-activated protein kinase (AMPK) when used at low doses. This effect is accompanied by the phosphorylation of SIRT1 as well as p53-acetylation (**Figure 1**). The prolonged exposure to low doses of metformin leads to human HCC senescence in murine xenografts via modulation of the AMPK-SIRT1 axis (63).

The long non-coding RNA (lncRNA) metastasis associated lung adenocarcinoma transcript 1 (MALAT1) was recently discovered to interfere with SIRT1 activity in hepatocellular cancer (64). MALAT1 is frequently upregulated in several types of cancers and contributes functionally to the development and malignancy of tumor cells (65). MALAT1 is, among lncRNAs, a stable and highly transcribed molecule localized in the nucleus, and it has been reported that, in breast cancer cells expressing ERα, 17β-estradiol treatment negatively regulates MALAT1 transcription, thus inhibiting proliferation, migration and invasion (66). MALAT1 is also regulated during endothelial differentiation in that hypoxia induces its transcription leading to the proliferation of the vasculature (67). In HCC specifically this lncRNA promotes aggressiveness in that releases SIRT1 by sponging miR-204 (64). SIRT1 is a direct downstream target of miR-204 and results inhibited by this interaction. MALAT1 can release the suppression on SIRT1 by base-pairing with miR-204 and leading to its post-transcriptional downregulation (64).

CONCLUSIONS

SIRT1 should be regarded as a multi-faceted enzyme and, as already suggested by several authors, studied in a context-dependent fashion. Secretory organs are no exception to this. **Table 1** summarizes the secretory organ tumors in which SIRT1 has been investigated, with the relevant experimental models. The most recent publications are taken into account.

TABLE 1 | Cancer models of the secretory organs in which SIRT1 has been studied.

	Experimental models and specimens	References
Ovarian cancer of epithelial origin	Normal ovaries, endometriosis with/without carcinoma, OvCa (endometrioid; clear cell; mucinous; serous). OvCa cell lines. Serous EOC.	(4, 23–28)
Thyroid carcinoma	Murine thyroid cancers. Thyroid cell lines. Nude mice models. Human normal and tumor thyroid specimens	(2, 37, 38)
Pancreatic cancer	Confirmed human PC and non-tumor pancreatic specimens. PC cell lines. Normal human pancreatic ductal epithelium. PC xenografts. Human chronic pancreatitis specimens	(41–45)
Pancreatic neuroendocrine tumors	Formalin fixed paraffin-embedded human samples	(3)
Gastric cancer	Human primary GC specimens. GC cell lines. Clinical trials concerning gastrointestinal cancers, overall survival and SIRT1. NCBI GEO databases of mRNA profiles. Formalin fixed paraffin-embedded human samples	(52–56)
Hepatic cancer	Primary liver cancer organoids (hepatocellular carcinoma; cholangiocarcinoma; combined HCC/CC; healthy liver). HCC mouse xenografts. HCC cell lines and primary human tissues	(61, 63, 64)

SIRT1 plays a confirmed role in ovarian, thyroid, and pancreatic cancers, while its role in GC is yet to be definitely established. The evidence available in thyroid cancer confirms that c-MYC and SIRT1 are valuable therapeutic targets, encouraging translational researches aimed at the related pathways. The recent meta-analysis spanning 37 selected studies on human solid cancers demonstrates a correlation between higher SIRT1 expression and worse OS in liver and lung cancers (5). These clinical data are consistent with the experimental ones reported for HCC where SIRT1 activation correlates to malignancy through MALAT1, a lncRNA highly expressed in various cancers including HCC (64, 68).

Furthermore, colorectal and GC do not show the correlation between OS and SIRT1 expression (5). SIRT1 overexpression has been reported either positively associated to FP or negatively associated to OS. Contradictory results also concern SIRT1 IHC and mRNA expression and prognosis of GC, suggesting that this class of lysine-deacetylases is not a reliable biomarker for GC.

In contrast, little evidence is available in the literature concerning the role (if any) of SIRT1 in the pituitary gland. In the testis, the role of SIRT1 is reported to be associated with spermatogenesis, fertility, and differentiation, but not testicular cancer (7).

In light of the literature presented here, further basic research is warranted in order to establish possible therapeutic strategies for ovarian, thyroid and pancreatic cancer, where a pro-tumorigenic role for SIRT1 has been established. Particular attention should be paid to the role of miRNAs in regulating SIRT1 levels (miR-212 in thyroid cancer; miR-494, miR-138-5p, miR-601, and miR-217 in PC; miR-204 in HCC). Furthermore, given the growing importance of lncRNAs in cancer pathology, the involvement of MALAT1 should be exploited. For instance, by measuring its levels in HCC biopsies and, possibly, by monitoring its expression during therapy administration or disease progression.

AUTHOR CONTRIBUTIONS

RF has been studied SIRT1 in cancer and is currently assessing a possible epigenetic regulation for this enzyme. RF conceived, wrote, and formatted the manuscript.

REFERENCES

1. Wu W, Zhang L, Lin J, Huang H, Shi B, Lin X, et al. Hypermethylation of the HIC1 promoter and aberrant expression of HIC1/SIRT1 contribute to the development of thyroid papillary carcinoma. *Oncotarget* (2016) 7:84416–27. doi: 10.18632/oncotarget.12936
2. Herranz D, Maraver A, Canamero M, Gomez-Lopez G, Inglada-Perez L, Robledo M, et al. SIRT1 promotes thyroid carcinogenesis driven by PTEN deficiency. *Oncogene* (2013) 32:4052–6. doi: 10.1038/onc.2012.407
3. Klieser E, Urbas R, Stattner S, Primavesi F, Jager T, Dinnewitzer A, et al. Comprehensive immunohistochemical analysis of histone deacetylases in pancreatic neuroendocrine tumors: HDAC5 as a predictor of poor clinical outcome. *Hum Pathol.* (2017) 65:41–52. doi: 10.1016/j.humpath.2017.02.009
4. Pinton G, Nilsson S, Moro L. Targeting estrogen receptor beta (ERbeta) for treatment of ovarian cancer: importance of KDM6B and SIRT1 for ERbeta expression and functionality. *Oncogenesis* (2018) 7:15. doi: 10.1038/s41389-018-0027-9
5. Wang C, Yang W, Dong F, Guo Y, Tan J, Ruan S, et al. The prognostic role of Sirt1 expression in solid malignancies: a meta-analysis. *Oncotarget* (2017) 8:66343–51. doi: 10.18632/oncotarget.18494
6. Das A, Huang GX, Bonkowski MS, Longchamp A, Li C, Schultz MB, et al. Impairment of an Endothelial NAD(+)-H2S signaling network is a reversible cause of vascular aging. *Cell* (2018) 173:74–89 e20. doi: 10.1016/j.cell.2018.02.008
7. Tatone, C. Di Emidio G, Barbonetti A, Carta G, Luciano AM, Falone S, et al. Sirtuins in gamete biology and reproductive physiology: emerging roles and therapeutic potential in female and male infertility. *Hum Reprod Update* (2018) 24:267–89. doi: 10.1093/humupd/dmy003
8. Frazzi R, Valli R, Tamagnini I, Casali B, Latruffe N, Merli F. Resveratrol-mediated apoptosis of hodgkin lymphoma cells involves SIRT1 inhibition and FOXO3a hyperacetylation. *Int J Cancer* (2013) 132:1013–21. doi: 10.1002/ijc.27748
9. Ma CH, Chiua YC, Wu CH, Jou IM, Tu YK, Hung CH, et al. Homocysteine causes dysfunction of chondrocytes and oxidative stress through repression of SIRT1/AMPK pathway: A possible link between hyperhomocysteinemia and osteoarthritis. *Redox Biol.* (2018) 15:504–12. doi: 10.1016/j.redox.2018.01.010
10. Sun T, Jiao L, Wang Y, Yu Y, Ming L. SIRT1 induces epithelial-mesenchymal transition by promoting autophagic degradation of E-cadherin in melanoma cells. *Cell Death Dis.* (2018) 9:136. doi: 10.1038/s41419-017-0167-4
11. Yu EJ, Kim SH, Kim HJ, Heo K, Ou CY, Stallcup MR, et al. Positive regulation of beta-catenin-PROX1 signaling axis by DBC1 in colon cancer progression. *Oncogene* (2016) 35:3410–8. doi: 10.1038/onc.2015.401
12. Choupani, J. Mansoori Derakhshan S, Bayat S, Alivand MR. Shekari Khaniani, M. Narrower insight to SIRT1 role in cancer: A potential therapeutic target to control epithelial-mesenchymal transition in cancer cells. *J Cell Physiol.* (2018) 233:4443–57. doi: 10.1002/jcp.26302
13. Lv J, Jiang S, Yang Z, Hu W, Wang Z, Li T, et al. PGC-1alpha sparks the fire of neuroprotection against neurodegenerative disorders. *Ageing Res Rev.* (2018) 44:8–21. doi: 10.1016/j.arr.2018.03.004
14. Jiang S, Yang Z, Di S, Hu W, Ma Z, Chen F, et al. Novel role of forkhead box O 4 transcription factor in cancer: Bringing out the good or the bad. *Semin Cancer Biol.* (2018) 50:1–12. doi: 10.1016/j.semcancer.2018.04.007
15. Jiang S, Li T, Yang Z, Hu W, Yang, Y. Deciphering the roles of FOXO1 in human neoplasms. *Int J Cancer* (2018). doi: 10.1002/ijc.31338
16. Xin Z, Ma Z, Hu W, Jiang S, Yang Z, Li T, et al. FOXO1/3: Potential suppressors of fibrosis. *Ageing Res Rev.* (2018) 41:42–52. doi: 10.1016/j.arr.2017.11.002
17. Tseng RC, Lee CC, Hsu HS, Tzao C, Wang YC. Distinct HIC1-SIRT1-p53 loop deregulation in lung squamous carcinoma and adenocarcinoma patients. *Neoplasia* (2009) 11:763–70. doi: 10.1593/neo.09470
18. Calin GA, Croce CM. MicroRNA signatures in human cancers. *Nat Rev Cancer* (2006) 6:857–66. doi: 10.1038/nrc1997
19. Knight JR, Milner J. SIRT1, metabolism and cancer. *Curr Opin Oncol.* (2012) 24:68–75. doi: 10.1097/CCO.0b013e32834d813b
20. Henderson JT, Webber EM, Sawaya GF. Screening for ovarian cancer: updated evidence report and systematic review for the us preventive services task force. *JAMA* (2018) 319:595–606. doi: 10.1001/jama.2017.21421
21. Oliver KE, McGuire WP. Ovarian cancer and antiangiogenic therapy: caveat emptor. *J Clin Oncol.* (2014) 32:3353–6. doi: 10.1200/JCO.2014.57.4574
22. Kobel M, Kalloger SE, Boyd N, McKinney S, Mehl E, Palmer C, et al. Ovarian carcinoma subtypes are different diseases: implications for biomarker studies. *PLoS Med.* (2008) 5:e232. doi: 10.1371/journal.pmed.0050232
23. Mvunta DH, Miyamoto T, Asaka R, Yamada Y, Ando H, Higuchi S, et al. Overexpression of SIRT1 is associated with poor outcomes in patients with ovarian carcinoma. *Appl Immunohistochem Mol Morphol.* (2017) 25:415–21. doi: 10.1097/PAI.0000000000000316
24. Mvunta DH, Miyamoto T, Asaka R, Yamada Y, Ando H, Higuchi S, et al. SIRT1 Regulates the chemoresistance and invasiveness of ovarian carcinoma cells. *Transl Oncol.* (2017) 10:621–31. doi: 10.1016/j.tranon.2017.05.005
25. Shuang T, Wang M, Zhou Y, Shi C. Over-expression of Sirt1 contributes to chemoresistance and indicates poor prognosis in serous epithelial ovarian cancer (EOC). *Med Oncol.* (2015) 32:260. doi: 10.1007/s12032-015-0706-8
26. Park SH, Cheung LW, Wong AS, Leung PC. Estrogen regulates Snail and Slug in the down-regulation of E-cadherin and induces metastatic potential of ovarian cancer cells through estrogen receptor alpha. *Mol Endocrinol.* (2008) 22:2085–98. doi: 10.1210/me.2007-0512
27. Akhter MZ, Sharawat SK, Kumar V, Kochat V, Equbal Z, Ramakrishnan M, et al. Aggressive serous epithelial ovarian cancer is potentially propagated by EpCAM(+)CD45(+) phenotype. *Oncogene* (2018) 37:2089–103. doi: 10.1038/s41388-017-0106-y
28. Qin J, Liu Y, Lu Y, Liu M, Li M, Li J, et al. Hypoxia-inducible factor 1 alpha promotes cancer stem cells-like properties in human ovarian cancer cells by upregulating SIRT1 expression. *Sci Rep.* (2017) 7:10592. doi: 10.1038/s41598-017-09244-8

29. Kitahara CM, Sosa JA. The changing incidence of thyroid cancer. *Nat Rev Endocrinol* (2016) 12:646–653. doi: 10.1038/nrendo.2016.110
30. Dang CV, O'Donnell KA, Zeller KI, Nguyen T, Osthus RC, Li F. The c-Myc target gene network. *Semin Cancer Biol.* (2006) 16:253–64. doi: 10.1016/j.semcancer.2006.07.014
31. Menssen A, Hydbring P, Kapelle K, Vervoorts J, Diebold J, Luscher B, et al. The c-MYC oncoprotein, the NAMPT enzyme, the SIRT1-inhibitor DBC1, and the SIRT1 deacetylase form a positive feedback loop. *Proc Natl Acad Sci USA.* (2012) 109:E187–96. doi: 10.1073/pnas.1105304109
32. Yuan J, Minter-Dykhouse K, Lou Z. A c-Myc-SIRT1 feedback loop regulates cell growth and transformation. *J Cell Biol.* (2009) 185:203–11. doi: 10.1083/jcb.200809167
33. Han HS, Choi BH, Kim JS, Kang G, Koo SH. Hepatic Crtc2 controls whole body energy metabolism via a miR-34a-Fgf21 axis. *Nat Commun/* (2017) 8:1878. doi: 10.1038/s41467-017-01878-6
34. Qiang L, Sample A, Liu H, Wu X, He YY. Epidermal SIRT1 regulates inflammation, cell migration, and wound healing. *Sci Rep.* (2017) 7:14110. doi: 10.1038/s41598-017-14371-3
35. Frazzi R, Tigano, M. The multiple mechanisms of cell death triggered by resveratrol in lymphoma and leukemia. *Int J Mol Sci.* (2014) 15:4977–93. doi: 10.3390/ijms15034977
36. Duntas, L. H. Resveratrol and its impact on aging and thyroid function. *J Endocrinol Invest.* (2011) 34:788–92.
37. Shih A, Davis FB, Lin HY, Davis PJ. Resveratrol induces apoptosis in thyroid cancer cell lines via a MAPK- and p53-dependent mechanism. *J Clin Endocrinol Metab.* (2002) 87:1223–32. doi: 10.1210/jcem.87.3.8345
38. Li D, Bai L, Wang T, Xie Q, Chen M, Fu Y, Wen Q. Function of miR-212 as a tumor suppressor in thyroid cancer by targeting SIRT1. *Oncol Rep.* (2018) 39:695–702. doi: 10.1007/s12094-017-1772-5
39. Notta F, Hahn SA, Real FX. A genetic roadmap of pancreatic cancer: still evolving. *Gut* (2017) 66:2170–78. doi: 10.1136/gutjnl-2016-313317
40. Gurusamy KS, Riviere D, C.van Laarhoven JH, Besselink M, Abu-Hilal M, Davidson BR, et al. Cost-effectiveness of laparoscopic versus open distal pancreatectomy for pancreatic cancer. *PLoS ONE* (2017) 12:e0189631. doi: 10.1371/journal.pone.0189631
41. Liu Y, Li X, Zhu S, Zhang JG, Yang M, Qin Q, et al. Ectopic expression of miR-494 inhibited the proliferation, invasion and chemoresistance of pancreatic cancer by regulating SIRT1 and c-Myc. *Gene Ther.* (2015) 22:729–38. doi: 10.1038/gt.2015.39
42. Tian S, Guo X, Yu C, Sun C, Jiang J. miR-138-5p suppresses autophagy in pancreatic cancer by targeting SIRT1. *Oncotarget* (2017) 8:11071–82. doi: 10.18632/oncotarget.14360
43. Cao W, Jin H, Zhang L, Chen X, Qian H. Identification of miR-601 as a novel regulator in the development of pancreatic cancer. *Biochem Biophys Res Commun.* (2017) 483:638–44. doi: 10.1016/j.bbrc.2016.12.090
44. Deng S, Zhu S, Wang B, Li X, Liu Y, Qin Q, et al. Chronic pancreatitis and pancreatic cancer demonstrate active epithelial-mesenchymal transition profile, regulated by miR-217-SIRT1 pathway. *Cancer Lett.* (2014) 355:184–91. doi: 10.1016/j.canlet.2014.08.007
45. Oon CE, Strell C, Yeong KY, Ostman A, Prakash J. SIRT1 inhibition in pancreatic cancer models: contrasting effects *in vitro* and *in vivo*. *Eur J Pharmacol.* (2015) 757:59–67. doi: 10.1016/j.ejphar.2015.03.064
46. Bolm L, Kasmann L, Paysen A, Karapetis C, Rades D, Wellner UF, et al. Multimodal Anti-tumor approaches combined with immunotherapy to overcome tumor resistance in esophageal and gastric cancer. *Anticancer Res.* (2018) 38:3231–42. doi: 10.21873/anticanres.12588
47. Wang K, Liu R, Li J, Mao J, Lei Y, Wu J, et al. Quercetin induces protective autophagy in gastric cancer cells: involvement of Akt-mTOR- and hypoxia-induced factor 1alpha-mediated signaling. *Autophagy* (2011) 7:966–78. doi: 10.4161/auto.7.9.15863
48. Humbert M, Medova M, Aebersold DM, Blaukat A, Bladt F, Fey MF, et al. Protective autophagy is involved in resistance towards MET inhibitors in human gastric adenocarcinoma cells. *Biochem Biophys Res Commun.* (2013) 431:264–9. doi: 10.1016/j.bbrc.2012.12.120
49. Hu X, Sui X, Li L, Huang X, Rong R, Su X, et al. Protocadherin 17 acts as a tumour suppressor inducing tumour cell apoptosis and autophagy, and is frequently methylated in gastric and colorectal cancers. *J Pathol.* (2013) 229:62–73. doi: 10.1002/path.4093
50. Lee IH, Cao L, Mostoslavsky R, Lombard DB, Liu J, Bruns NE, et al. A role for the NAD-dependent deacetylase Sirt1 in the regulation of autophagy. *Proc Natl Acad Sci USA.* (2008) 105:3374–9. doi: 10.1073/pnas.0712145105
51. Fullgrabe J, Klionsky DJ, Joseph, B. Histone post-translational modifications regulate autophagy flux and outcome. *Autophagy* (2013) 9:1621–3. doi: 10.4161/auto.25803
52. Qiu G, Li X, Che X, Wei C, He S, Lu J, et al. SIRT1 is a regulator of autophagy: Implications in gastric cancer progression and treatment. *FEBS Lett.* (2015) 589:2034–42. doi: 10.1016/j.febslet.2015.05.042
53. Yang Q, Wang B, Gao W, Huang S, Liu Z, Li W, et al. SIRT1 is downregulated in gastric cancer and leads to G1-phase arrest via NF-kappaB/Cyclin D1 signaling. *Mol Cancer Res.* (2013) 11:1497–507. doi: 10.1158/1541-7786.MCR-13-0214
54. Wu S, Jiang J, Liu J, Wang X, Gan Y, Tang Y. Meta-analysis of SIRT1 expression as a prognostic marker for overall survival in gastrointestinal cancer. *Oncotarget* (2017) 8:62589–99. doi: 10.18632/oncotarget.19880
55. Shen X, Li P, Xu Y, Chen X, Sun H, Zhao Y, et al. Association of sirtuins with clinicopathological parameters and overall survival in gastric cancer. *Oncotarget* (2017) 8:74359–70. doi: 10.18632/oncotarget.20799
56. Noguchi A, Kikuchi K, Zheng H, Takahashi H, Miyagi Y, Aoki I, et al. SIRT1 expression is associated with a poor prognosis, whereas DBC1 is associated with favorable outcomes in gastric cancer. *Cancer Med.* (2014) 3:1553–61. doi: 10.1002/cam4.310
57. Brooks CL, Gu W. How does SIRT1 affect metabolism, senescence and cancer?. *Nat Rev Cancer* (2009) 9:123–8. doi: 10.1038/nrc2562
58. Song NY, Surh YJ. Janus-faced role of SIRT1 in tumorigenesis. *Ann N Y Acad Sci.* (2012) 1271:10–9. doi: 10.1111/j.1749-6632.2012.06762.x
59. Marti N, Bouchoucha N, Sauter KS, Fluck CE. Resveratrol inhibits androgen production of human adrenocortical H295R cells by lowering CYP17 and CYP21 expression and activities. *PLoS ONE* (2017) 12:e0174224. doi: 10.1371/journal.pone.0174224
60. Shibata T, Arai Y, Totoki Y. Molecular genomic landscapes of hepatobiliary cancer. *Cancer Sci.* (2018) 109:1282–91. doi: 10.1111/cas.13582
61. Broutier L, Mastrogiovanni G, Verstegen MM, Francies HE, Gavarro LM, Bradshaw CR, et al. Human primary liver cancer-derived organoid cultures for disease modeling and drug screening. *Nat Med.* (2017) 23:1424–35. doi: 10.1038/nm.4438
62. Wang S, Wan T, Ye M, Qiu Y, Pei L, Jiang R, et al. Nicotinamide riboside attenuates alcohol induced liver injuries via activation of SirT1/PGC-1alpha/mitochondrial biosynthesis pathway. *Redox Biol.* (2018) 17:89–98. doi: 10.1016/j.redox.2018.04.006
63. Zhou X, Chen J, Chen L, Feng X, Liu Z, Zeng ZH, et al. Negative regulation of Sirtuin 1 by AMP-activated protein kinase promotes metformin-induced senescence in hepatocellular carcinoma xenografts. *Cancer Lett.* (2017) 411:1–11. doi: 10.1016/j.canlet.2017.09.027
64. Hou Z, Xu X, Zhou L, Fu X, Tao S, Zhou J, et al. The long non-coding RNA MALAT1 promotes the migration and invasion of hepatocellular carcinoma by sponging miR-204 and releasing SIRT1. *Tumour Biol.* (2017) 39:1010428317718135. doi: 10.1177/1010428317718135
65. Yoshimoto R, Mayeda A, Yoshida M, Nakagawa S. MALAT1 long non-coding RNA in cancer. *Biochim Biophys Acta* (2016) 1859:192–9. doi: 10.1016/j.bbagrm.2015.09.012
66. Fang D, Yang H, Lin J, Teng Y, Jiang Y, Chen J, et al. 17beta-estradiol regulates cell proliferation, colony formation, migration, invasion and promotes apoptosis by upregulating miR-9 and thus degrades

MALAT-1 in osteosarcoma cell MG-63 in an estrogen receptor-independent manner. *Biochem Biophys Res Commun.* (2015) 457:500–6. doi: 10.1016/j.bbrc.2014.12.114
67. Michalik KM, You X, Manavski Y, Doddaballapur A, Zornig M, et al. Long noncoding RNA MALAT1 regulates endothelial cell function and vessel growth. *Circ Res.* (2014) 114:1389–97. doi: 10.1161/CIRCRESAHA.114.303265
68. Lin R, Maeda S, Liu C, Karin M, Edgington TS. A large noncoding RNA is a marker for murine hepatocellular carcinomas and a spectrum of human carcinomas. *Oncogene* (2007) 26:851–8. doi: 10.1038/sj.onc.1209846

6

Advances in Cellular Characterization of the Sirtuin Isoform, SIRT7

Di Wu [1,2†], *Yinglu Li* [3†], *Kathy S. Zhu* [4], *Haiying Wang* [1,5*] *and Wei-Guo Zhu* [3*]

[1] Key Laboratory of Carcinogenesis and Translational Research (Ministry of Education), Beijing Key Laboratory of Protein Posttranslational Modifications and Cell Function, Peking University Health Science Center, School of Basic Medical Sciences, Beijing, China, [2] School of Basic Medical Sciences, Institute of Systems Biomedicine, Peking University Health Science Center, Beijing, China, [3] Department of Biochemistry and Molecular Biology, Shenzhen University Health Science Center, Shenzhen, China, [4] Peking University Health Science Center, School of Public Health, Beijing, China, [5] Department of Biochemistry and Molecular Biology, Peking University Health Science Center, School of Basic Medical Sciences, Beijing, China

***Correspondence:**
Wei-Guo Zhu
zhuweiguo@bjmu.edu.cn;
zhuweiguo@szu.edu.cn
Haiying Wang
wendy@bjmu.edu.cn

† These authors have contributed equally to this work

SIRT7 is one of seven mammalian sirtuins that functions as an NAD^+-dependent histone/protein deacetylase. SIRT7 is the least well-known member of the sirtuin family, but recent efforts have identified its involvement in various cellular processes, such as ribosome biogenesis, gene expression, cellular metabolism and cancer. Here we provide an update on the functions and mechanisms of SIRT7 in cellular regulation and disease.

Keywords: SIRT7, rDNA transcription, ribosome biogenesis, cellular stress, metabolism, aging, genome stability, cancer

INTRODUCTION

In the year 2000, researchers identified that silent information regulator 2 (Sir2)—a nicotinamide adenine dinucleotide (NAD)-dependent histone deacetylase—extends the lifespan of yeast (1, 2). Since then, the Sir2 homologs in mammals, known as sirtuins, have received increasing attention. There are seven sirtuin homologs in mammals (SIRT1 to SIRT7) that share a conserved NAD^+ binding domain, but their cellular localization, activities and functions differ (**Figure 1**). SIRT1, SIRT6, and SIRT7 predominantly localize to the nucleus (SIRT7 primarily resides in nucleolus), SIRT2 localizes to the cytoplasm and SIRT3, SIRT4, and SIRT5 localize to the mitochondria (3). Sirtuins mediate various cellular functions that regulate a wide range of physiological processes, including the cell cycle, proliferation, apoptosis, aging, genomic stability, stress resistance and metabolism (4). SIRT7 is the least well-studied of the sirtuins, but recent breakthroughs have shown that it is also involved in numerous cellular processes and its biological function is gradually becoming clear. In this review, we outline the current data regarding SIRT7 function and highlight the areas where SIRT7 may have a possible therapeutic role in disease.

SIRT7 ENZYMATIC ACTIVITY

SIRT7 encodes a 400 amino acid protein that functions as a class III histone deacetylase in *Homo sapiens.* (5) Compared to other nuclear-localized Sirtuins (SIRT1 and SIRT6), SIRT7 exhibits weak deacetylase activity (3). Within the SIRT7 catalytic domain, serine residue 111 (S111) and histidine residue 187 (H187) are responsible for the deacetylation activity (6, 7), but to date, only a few SIRT7 substrates have been identified. In 2012, Barber et al. (6) reported that SIRT7 is a highly selective histone H3 lysine 18 (H3K18) deacetylase, and that H3K18Ac deacetylation is associated with high-grade tumors and poor patient prognosis. Non-histone substrates have also been identified, including p53, PAF53, U3-55k, GABPβ1, NPM1, PGK1, CDK9, DDB1, FKBP51, FOXO3, SMAD4, and DDX21 (**Table 1**). We discuss the data for each of these substrates in turn below.

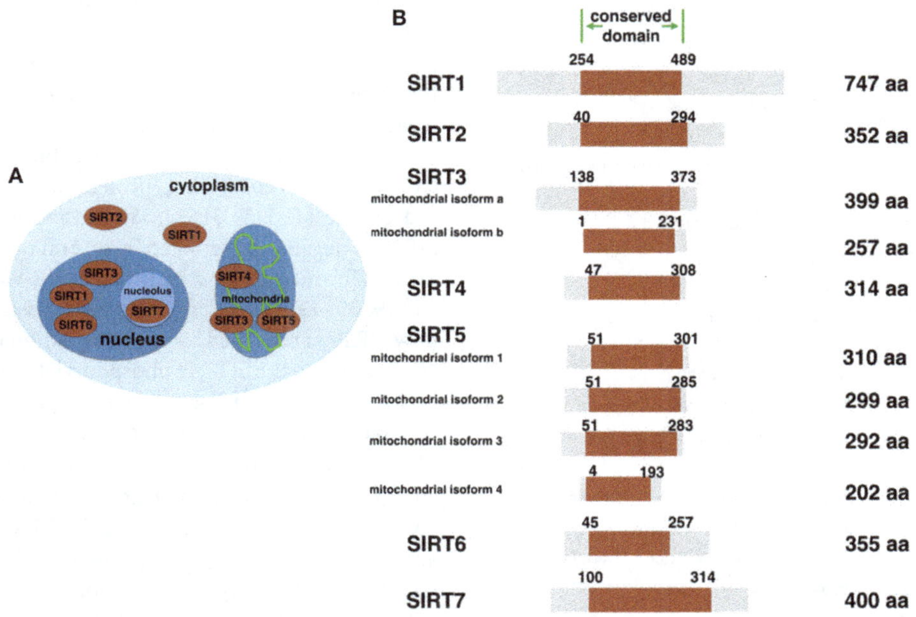

FIGURE 1 | Sirtuin family. **(A)** Sirtuins' intracellular location. **(B)** Human sirtuin proteins and their protein structures. The sequences are based on NCBI Protein database.

Vakhrusheva et al. found that p53 peptides were deacetylated *in vitro* by SIRT7 as efficiently as SIRT1, and mutant SIRT7 nearly abolished p53 decetylation (8). Conversely, Barber et al. did not detect SIRT7 deacetylase activity toward p53 both *in vivo* and *in vitro*, which questioned the ability of SIRT7 to deacetylate p53 (6). Kim et al. found an inverse correlation between p53 acetylation levels and SIRT7 expression in Hep3B cells (9). Finally, Nahalkova et al. identified an interaction between SIRT7 and p53, but did not assess SIRT7 deacetylase activity (10). p53 is debatable to be a SIRT7 substrate, for SIRT7 is found only effective toward p53 peptide, but not p53 protein both *in vivo* and *in vitro*. More studies are required, therefore, to resolve whether p53 is truly a SIRT7 substrate.

The wide variety of non-histone SIRT7 substrates suggests that SIRT7 participates in a diverse range of cellular processes. For example, SIRT7 can deacetylate nucleolar organizer polymerase-associated factor 53 (PAF53) and U3-specific protein U3-55k to regulate the synthesis and ripening of precursor ribose RNA (11, 12). By bioinformatic analysis, Ryu et al. found that GA-binding protein β1 (GABPβ1) is another substrate of SIRT7 (13). Here, SIRT7 interacts with and deacetylates GABPβ1 to regulate mitochondrion function (13). Lee et al. reported that SIRT7 deacetylates nucleophosmin (NPM1), which is involved in regulating aging processes (14), while Hu et al. found that SIRT7 deacetylates phosphoglycerate kinase 1 (PGK1) and participates in glycolysis regulation (15). Yu et al. showed that SIRT7 specifically interacts with and deacetylates FK506-binding protein 51 (FKBP51) at lysine residues 28 and 155 (K28 and K155), which enhances FKBP51–Akt–PHLPP complex formation, resulting in AKT inactivation and enhanced chemo-sensitivity in breast cancer cells (16). Blank et al. showed that SIRT7-dependent deacetylation of Cyclin-dependent kinase 9 (CDK9) activates its kinase activity; CDK9 subsequently phosphorylates the Pol II C-terminal domain (CTD) and facilitates transcription elongation (17). Li et al. observed that SIRT1/SIRT7 deacetylate FOXO3 *in vitro* and *in vivo* to prevent its phosphorylation and block apoptosis in response to lipopolysaccharide stimulation (18). Mo et al. found that SIRT7 is a major deacetylase of DNA damage-binding protein 1 (DDB1): DDB1 acetylation negatively regulates the DDB1–CUL4 interaction and CRL4 activity (19, 20). Tang et al. found that SIRT7 inhibits breast cancer lung metastasis by deacetylating and promoting SMAD4 degradation (21). Finally, Song et al. showed that deacetylation of the nucleolar DEAD-box helicase DDX21 by SIRT7 increases R-loop-unwinding activity and safeguards genome stability (22).

To widen the range of SIRT7 targets, our laboratory conducted the first proteomic screen of SIRT7 substrates. Using stable isotope labeling with amino acids in cell culture coupled with quantitative mass spectrometry, we produced a comprehensive list of candidates that are involved in a variety of functions, ranging from chromatin architecture homeostasis to gene silencing and metabolism. Some selected candidates, such as SIRT2, histone-lysine N-methyltransferase (EZH2), mitogen-activated protein kinase 2 (MAPK2) and glycogen synthase kinase-3 beta (GSK3β) have been validated by *in vitro* co-immunoprecipitation and deacetylation experiments. By combining this approach with predictive tools, we have started to greatly expand the list of SIRT7 candidate substrates. Such studies have enhanced our understanding of the physiological role of SIRT7 and raised awareness as to the global impact of sirtuins in cell homeostasis (23).

SIRT7 exhibits other enzymatic activities in addition to NAD^+-dependent deacetylation. In 2016, Li et al. found

TABLE 1 | SIRT7 catalytic substrates.

Substrate	Modification	Function
H3K18	Deacetylation	Tumorigenesis
p53	Deacetylation	Apoptosis
PAF53 and U3-55k	Deacetylation	Synthesis and ripening of precursor ribose RNA
GABPβ1	Deacetylation	Mitochondrial function
NPM1	Deacetylation	Aging
PGK1	Deacetylation	Glycolysis
FKBP51	Deacetylation	AKT inactivation and chemo-sensitivity in breast cancer cells
CDK9	Deacetylation	Transcription elongation
FOXO3	Deacetylation	Blocks apoptosis in response to LPS
DDB1	Deacetylation	Regulates DDB1-CUL4 interaction and CRL4 activity
SMAD4	Deacetylation	Inhibits breast cancer lung metastasis
DDX21	Deacetylation	Genome stability
H3K122	Desuccinylation	Chromatin remodeling during DNA repair
H3K36/K37	Deacetylation/ debutyrylation	Unknown

that SIRT7 is an NAD^+-dependent histone desuccinylase, and desuccinylates H3K122 to regulate chromatin remodeling during DNA repair (24). However, no non-histone substrates for SIRT7 desuccinylase have been identified. SIRT7 also interacts with some proteins without deacetylating them, such as mTOR, Myc, and TFIIIC2 (25); it is possible that SIRT7 regulates these proteins via its desuccinylase activity. Future investigations should investigate the spectrum of non-histone desuccinylation-mediated regulation by SIRT7. A recent report also showed that SIRT7 has robust deacetylase or debutyrylase activity on acetylated or butyrylated nucleosomes, mainly toward H3K36/K37 (26).

SIRT7 deacetylase activity is markedly enhanced by chromatin compositional DNA and RNA. SIRT7 also exhibits defatty-acylase activity, which can be effectively activated by RNA (27, 28). Conversely, Myb-binding protein 1a (Mybbp1a), a component of the chromatin remodeling complex B-WICH, inhibits SIRT7 deacetylation activity and increases H3K18 levels in cells (29), although the mechanistic details remain to be understood.

SIRT7 EXPRESSION AND REGULATION

SIRT7 is widely expressed in different organs and tissues of the human body: the highest expression is found in hyperplastic tissues, such as the spleen, liver and testis, and the lowest expression is found in the skeletal muscle, heart and brain (30). SIRT7 expression levels are associated with cellular proliferation, differentiation and the stress response, acting as a positive or negative regulator in different organs and tissues (31). Recent findings from the TCGA database suggest that SIRT7 expression is tightly correlated with the development of various types of cancer (32–34). The diverse roles of SIRT7 suggest it is tightly regulated by multiple mechanisms, as evidenced by SIRT1 (35, 36).

Previous reports have indicated that SIRT7 is regulated at the transcriptional, post-transcriptional and translational levels (**Figure 2**). At the transcriptional level, SIRT7 is regulated by upstream molecules, such as X-box binding protein 1 (XBP1), CCAAT-enhancer-binding protein α (C/EBPα), and histone deacetylase 3 (HDAC3) (37, 38). At the post-transcriptional level, SIRT7 is negatively regulated by several microRNAs, such as hsa-miR-125b, miR-125a-5p, miR-125b, miR-93, miR-3666, and miR-340 (9, 39–42). There are only few reports, however, describing how SIRT7 is regulated by post-translational modifications. Grob et al. found that SIRT7 is phosphorylated during mitosis by the cyclin-dependent kinase 1 (CDK1)-cyclin B pathway, although the phosphorylation sites and function have not been defined (43). Sun et al. found that SIRT7 is phosphorylated during cellular energy stress by 5′ AMP-activated protein kinase (AMPK), which has a crucial role in determining SIRT7 subcellular distribution and degradation (44). The researchers also showed that SIRT7 is modified by polyubiquitination (44), which is consistent with our study that showed that SIRT7 is modified by Lys-63-linked polyubiquitination (45). We also found that SIRT7 enzymatic activity is negatively regulated by ubiquitin-specific-processing protease 7 (USP7)-mediated deubiquitination, which helps control gluconeogenesis by regulating *G6PC* expression (45). Post-translational modifications have a crucial role in regulating protein stability, activity, structure and function; thus, further studies into SIRT7 post-translational modifications are warranted.

SIRT7 BIOLOGICAL FUNCTIONS

Ribosome Biogenesis and Protein Translation

Global proteomic studies have identified numerous SIRT7-associated proteins, with most of them having important roles in transcription, ribosome biogenesis and translation (7, 14, 25). Subsequent functional studies have confirmed that SIRT7 is involved in multiple pathways regulating ribosome biogenesis and protein translation. First, SIRT7 can regulate rDNA transcription. Ford et al. found that SIRT7 forms part of the RNA Polymerase I (RNA Pol I) complex, and activation of the RNA Pol I transcription *in vivo* is dependent on its enzymatic activity (30). Specifically, the researchers showed that SIRT7 over-expression increased Pol I-mediated transcription, whereas SIRT7 knockdown or catalytic inhibition decreased Pol I transcription (30). Grob et al. also found that SIRT7 activates Pol I transcription by interacting with upstream binding factor (UBF), which is a component of the RNA polymerase complex (43). Tsai et al. extended the mechanisms of SIRT7-mediated rDNA transcriptional regulation by showing that SIRT7 associates with the B-WICH complex, a chromatin remodeling complex involved in rDNA transcriptional regulation and chromatin structure changes. In addition, the researchers found that down-regulated SIRT7 reduced levels of RNA Pol I protein by decreasing the expression levels of RPA194, the

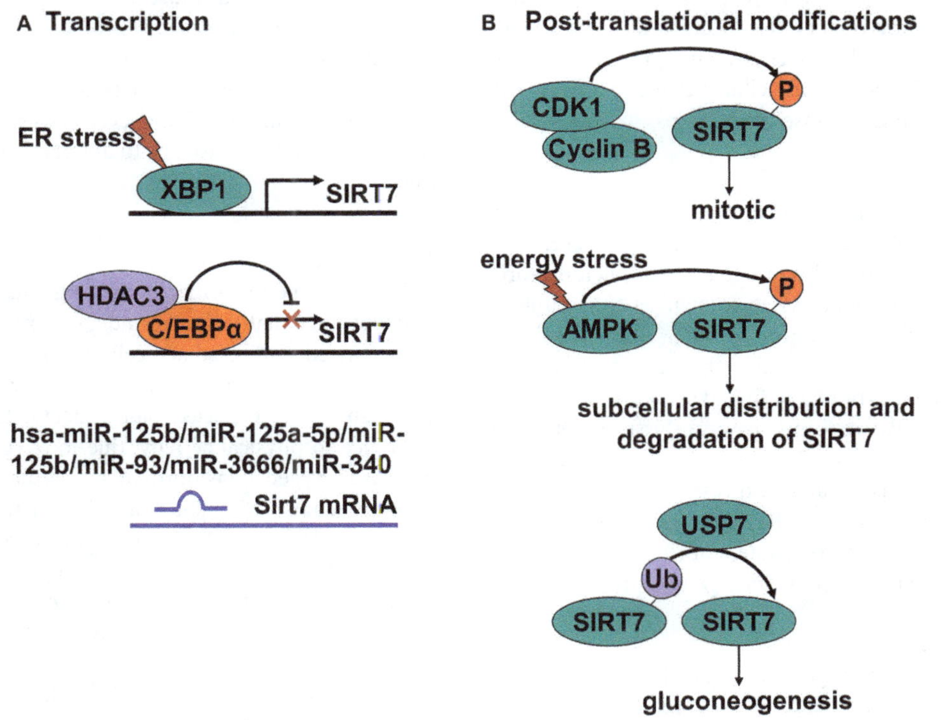

FIGURE 2 | Summary of regulation of SIRT7. **(A)** Various transcription factors regulate SIRT7 expression. The X-box binding protein 1 (XBP1) enhances SIRT7 expression, whereas Histone Deacetylase 3 (HDAC3) and CCAAT/enhancer-binding protein alpha (C/EBP alpha) repress SIRT7 expression. In addition, SIRT7 expression is also repressed by the microRNAs, such as hsa-miR-125b, miR-125a-5p, miR-125b, miR-93, miR-3666, and miR-340. **(B)** Some post-translational modifications affect SIRT7 activity. The cyclin-dependent kinase 1 (CDK1)–cyclin B pathway phosphorylates SIRT7 during mitosis. Under energy stress, SIRT7 can be phosphorylated by Adenosine 5′-monophosphate (AMP)-activated protein kinase (AMPK), thereby determining the subcellular distribution and degradation of SIRT7. Moreover, Ubiquitin-specific protease 7 (USP7) negatively regulates the enzymatic activity of SIRT7 through deubiquitination to control gluconeogenesis.

largest RNA polymerase I subunit (7). Others have shown that SIRT7 regulates Pol I transcription by deacetylating PAF53, another component of RNA polymerase I complex: PAF53 hypo-acetylation correlates with increased Pol I occupancy on rDNA and transcriptional activation (12).

SIRT7 also regulates the conversion between rDNA transcriptional activation and inhibition during the cell cycle. Here, SIRT7 is phosphorylated by the CDK1–cyclin B pathway during mitosis, rendering SIRT7 inactive such that rDNA transcription is inhibited. Upon exiting mitosis, SIRT7 is dephosphorylated by a phosphatase sensitive to okadaic acid such that rDNA transcription can resume (43).

SIRT7 is also involved in pre-rRNA processing and rRNA maturation. SIRT7 can deacetylate U3-55k, a component of the U3 small nucleolar RNP (snRNP) complex, which increases the association between U3-55k and U3 snRNP. This association is essential for processing pre-rRNA. Under stress conditions however, SIRT7 is released from the nucleoli, resulting in U3-55k hyper-acetylation and reduced pre-rRNA processing (11).

A role for SIRT7 in protein synthesis has also been suggested, as supported by Tsai et al. who found that SIRT7 knockdown suppresses both RNA and protein synthesis (25). They showed that SIRT7 associates with mTOR and TFIIIC2 to modulate Pol III-dependent tRNA transcription, and co-localizes with Pol III target genes. Supporting these observations, SIRT7 knockdown decreased tRNA levels and amino acid incorporation rates; however, SIRT7 over-expression did not increase the rate of protein synthesis, indicating that the observed reduction in protein synthesis may be an indirect effect of SIRT7 knockdown. In addition, the reduced amino acid incorporation rates in SIRT7 knockdown cells were due to reduced abundance of tRNAs for different amino acids (25).

Shin et al. found that Myc depletion significantly reduces SIRT7 occupancy at the promoters of ribosomal proteins. SIRT7 is targeted to the promoters of ribosomal proteins by interacting with Myc and repressing Myc-dependent expression (38).

Finally, SIRT7 may have a role in Pol II activation, as data indicate that SIRT7 associates with Pol II and regulates transcription of snoRNAs and other Pol II genes (17). Here, SIRT7 promotes the release of the elongation factor P-TEFb from the inactive 7SK snRNP complex and deacetylates CDK9, a component of the P-TEFb complex. CDK9 deacetylation promotes Pol II C-terminal domain (CTD) phosphorylation and transcription elongation (17).

Regulator of Cellular Stress

SIRT7 is resistant to various cellular stressors, such as endoplasmic reticulum (ER) stress, oxidative stress, mitochondrial protein folding stress, nutrition stress and genotoxic stress (8, 12, 38, 46). As such, it can be inferred that SIRT7 has an important role in regulating cell survival. The function of SIRT7 in regulating rRNA and protein synthesis also supports a role for SIRT7 in cellular stress, because both processes are reduced under stressed conditions.

ER Stress

The ER is an important intracellular organelle where protein synthesis, folding, modification and trafficking occur. The accumulation of unfolded proteins or depletion of calcium stores triggers the ER stress response (also known as the unfolded protein response, UPR), to restore protein homeostasis by increasing the expression of molecular chaperones, decreasing protein translation and degrading unfolded proteins (47).

SIRT7 can relieve ER stress in two ways. First, under stress conditions, XBP1 induces SIRT7 expression, which in turn reduces ER stress response protein expression, such as CHOP, XBP1s, and GRP78 (38). Second, SIRT7 can interact with Myc to facilitate its recruitment to the promoters of ribosomal proteins, such as RPS20 and RPS14 to repress their gene expression (38).

Mitochondrial Stress

The mitochondrion is an important organelle for regulating cellular energy homeostasis, and is thus sensitive to many stresses. Cellular stress leads to an accumulation of unfolded mitochondrial proteins resulting in mitochondrial protein folding stress (PFS^{mt}) and the unfolded protein response in mitochondria (UPR^{mt}) (48). Mohrin et al. found that SIRT7 alleviates PFS^{mt} by repressing NRF1 activity and reducing the expression of the mitochondrial translation machinery (46). NRF1 is a master regulator of mitochondria, and by interacting with SIRT7, targets it to the promoters of mitochondrial ribosomal proteins (mRPs) and mitochondrial translation factors (mTFs) to repress their expression. This mechanism helps alleviate PFS^{mt} and improve cellular survival under conditions of nutrient deprivation (46).

Oxidative Stress

Many diseases and disorders have been linked with a cellular oxidant–antioxidant imbalance. Data suggest that sirtuins are important in the homeostasis of cellular oxidation–reduction systems. Hypoxia-inducible factors HIF-1 and HIF-2 are essential transcription factors that mediate adaptation to hypoxia (49). Hubbi et al. found that SIRT7 interacts with HIF-1α and HIF-2α proteins and negatively regulates their expression (50). Over-expression of SIRT7 reduced the levels of HIF proteins as well as their transcriptional targets, independent of SIRT7 deacetylase activity and hydroxylation-mediated ubiquitinylation and the proteasomal and lysosomal-mediated degradation pathways. Vakhrusheva et al. found that SIRT7-deficient primary cardiomyocytes exhibit a drastic increase in basal apoptosis compared to wild-type primary cardiomyocytes upon exposure to hydrogen peroxide, suggesting a critical role for SIRT7 in regulating the oxidative stress response and cell death in the heart (8). The researchers speculated that this susceptibility of SIRT7 mutant cells to apoptosis may be due to hyperactive p53, as SIRT7 deacetylates p53 (8). Lewinska et al. also reported that vascular smooth muscle cells exposed to curcumin to induce oxidative damage, exhibited down-regulated SIRT7 and p53 stability (51). SIRT7 down-regulation also decreased Pol I mediated transcription, and the stabilized p53 activated its target protein p21, resulting in cell-cycle arrest. Thus, SIRT7 has a potential role in the resistance to different conditions of oxidative stress.

Cardiac Injury

SIRT7 has a role in cardiac homeostasis as illustrated by SIRT7 knockout mice that suffer from degenerative heart hypertrophy, as evidenced by cardiac cell fibrosis and inflammation, resulting in inflammatory cardiomyopathy (8). SIRT7 knockout mice also show increased blood lactate levels and decreased endurance to physical activity, due to oxygen insufficiency and decreased oxygen consumption by cardiac muscles stemming from mitochondrial respiratory dysfunction (13). A possible pathway by which SIRT7 maintains cardiac health may be through GABP. SIRT7 promotes GABP complex formation and activation by deacetylating GABPβ1 to enhance the expression of mitochondrial genes and promote mitochondrial respiration (13).

Araki et al. described another SIRT7 pathway that may regulate cardiac health (52). The researchers noted that SIRT7 expression increases at active wound healing sites upon acute cardiovascular injury and thus speculated that SIRT7 may be involved in tissue repair. Consistently, SIRT7 depletion led to reduced collagen production and insufficient angiogenic and inflammatory responses, resulting in impaired wound healing (52). TGF-β is essential to wound healing as it regulates fibroblast chemotaxis, differentiation and the epithelial-to-mesenchymal transition (EMT). TGF-β receptor protein 1 (TβR1) is an important component of the TGF-β signaling pathway (53). Researchers showed that SIRT7 depletion decreases TβR1 levels and reduces downstream signaling. The effect on TβR1, however, was indirect as SIRT7 did not interact with TβR1, but the mediator PICK1 (protein interacting with protein kinase C, alpha), which interacts with TβR1 and SIRT7 together. This study also showed that loss of SIRT7 activates autophagy and PICK1, again affecting TβRI status. Thus, the researchers concluded that SIRT7 maintains TβRI protein levels by modulating autophagy and PICK1 to regulate the TGF-β signaling pathway. In this way, SIRT7 can participate in scar formation, angiogenesis, inflammation and wound healing in response to acute cardiovascular injury (52). Based on these data, SIRT7 may be considered as a good predictor or therapeutic target for cardiac diseases.

Genome Stability

Sirtuins, including SIRT7, maintain genomic stability under stress conditions through a variety of mechanisms (24, 31, 54, 55). SIRT7 protects the genome largely by influencing chromatin structure, cell-cycle progression and DNA damage signaling and repair (**Figure 3**). SIRT7 knockout mice show an aging-like phenotype, associated with an increased sensitivity to oxidative

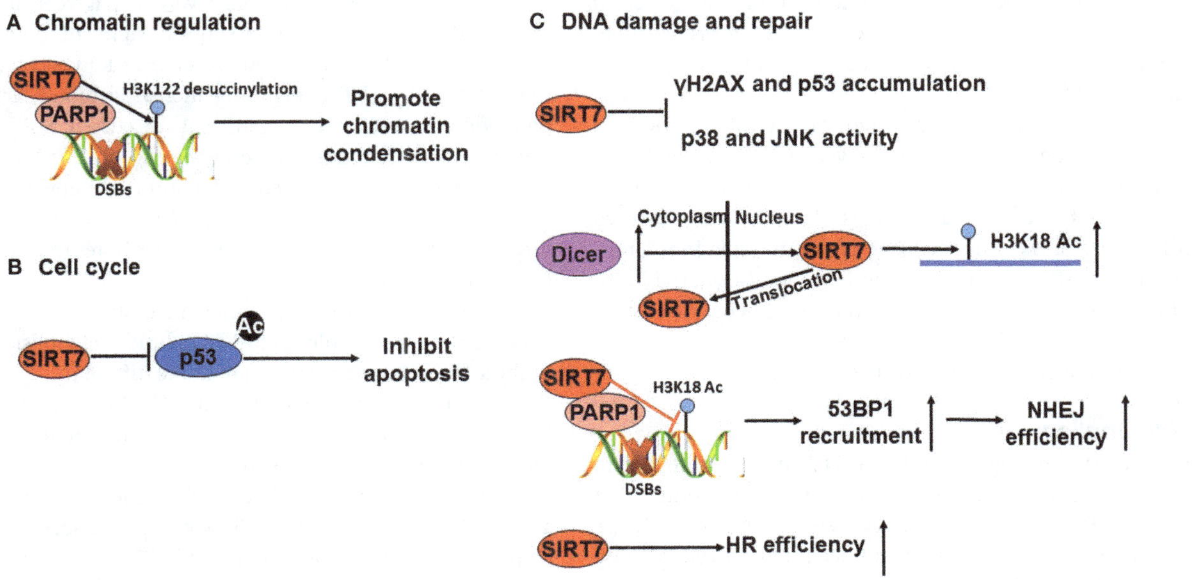

FIGURE 3 | SIRT7 maintains genome stability through multiple pathways. Under stress conditions, SIRT7 participates in the maintenance of genome stability via multiple mechanisms. **(A)** SIRT7 is recruited to DSBs in a PARP1-dependent manner to catalyze desuccinylation of H3K122 at DSBs to promote chromatin condensation. **(B)** SIRT7 can deacetylate p53 to inhibit apoptosis. **(C)** SIRT7 exerts a protective role during genomic insults by attenuating the DNA damage response (preventing γH2AX and p53 accumulation) and the stress-activated MAPK pathway (p38 and JNK activity inhibition). The upregulation of Dicer in cytoplasm promotes SIRT7 translocation from the nucleus to the cytoplasm, thereby causing a decrease in chromatin-associated SIRT7 and elevated H3K18Ac levels. Besides, SIRT7 overexpression increases the efficiency of non-homologous end joining (NHEJ) and homologous recombination (HR). The recruitment of SIRT7 to sites of DNA damage by a PARP1-dependent manner also modulates H3K18Ac levels, thereby influencing 53BP1 recruitment to DNA double-strand breaks (DSBs) to increase the efficiency of NHEJ.

and genotoxic stress, suggesting a link between SIRT7 and genomic protection (8).

SIRT7 can maintain genomic stability by regulating p53 or DNA damage repair. With regards to p53, Vakhrusheva et al. found that SIRT7 knockout mouse embryonic fibroblasts (MEFs) undergo higher levels of apoptosis than control MEFs upon adriamycin treatment. This process is as a result of p53 hyperacetylation in the absence of SIRT7 (8). Kiran et al. found that SIRT7 exerts a protective role during genomic insults by attenuating the DNA damage response (preventing γH2AX and p53 accumulation) and the stress-activated MAPK pathway (p38 and JNK activity inhibition) (31). Moreover, they found that SIRT7 transfers from the nucleolus to the nuclear matrix after doxorubicin chemotherapy (31). Similarly, Zhang et al. found that SIRT7 translocates from the nucleus to the cytoplasm in response to DNA damage. This translocation occurs through an interaction with Dicer, causing a decrease in chromatin-associated SIRT7 and elevated H3K18Ac levels (56).

Regarding DNA damage repair, Mao et al. found that SIRT7 overexpression increases the efficiency of non-homologous end joining (NHEJ) by 1.5-fold and homologous recombination (HR) by 2.8-fold in paraquat toxin-treated human fibroblast cells (57). A more recent study by Vazquez et al. elucidated a mechanism by which SIRT7 contributes to NHEJ. They demonstrated that SIRT7 is recruited to sites of DNA damage in a PARP1-dependent manner, where it modulates H3K18Ac levels, thereby influencing 53BP1 recruitment to DNA double-strand breaks (DSBs) to increase the efficiency of NHEJ (55). These data provide direct evidence for a role of SIRT7-mediated H3K18 deacetylation in maintaining genome integrity by DSB repair. At the same time, Li et al. also found that SIRT7 is recruited to DSBs in a PARP1-dependent manner, but showed that it catalyzes desuccinylation of H3K122 at DSBs to promote chromatin condensation and efficient DSB repair (24). These latest findings extend our understanding as to how SIRT7 helps maintain genome stability.

Metabolic Regulation

Glucose Metabolism

The enzymatic activity of SIRT7 depends on its metabolic co-substrate NAD^+, thus connecting its role to cellular metabolic status. SIRT7 is a low glucose stress sensor that, as discussed, modulates rDNA transcription to preserve energy and resist nutritional stress. Chen et al. identified that SIRT7 redistributes from the nucleoli to the nucleoplasm upon glucose deprivation or treatment with AICAR (a low energy mimic) (12). At the mechanistic level, PAF53 interacts with Pol I and recruits it to rDNA promoters (58). SIRT7 deacetylates PAF53, which acts as a signal to recruit RNA polymerase I to rDNA promoters and activate RNA Pol I-mediated transcription. Under low glucose conditions, the redistribution of SIRT7 from the nucleoli to the nucleoplasm permits PAF53 hyper-acetylation. This hyper-acetylation impairs the interaction between PAF53 and Pol I and decreases Pol I activity, thus leading to rDNA transcription inhibition (12). Sun et al. also showed that glucose starvation induces SIRT7 redistribution via AMPK-directed SIRT7 phosphorylation. This effect causes REGγ-proteasome-dependent degradation, thereby reducing rDNA transcription to avoid cell death (44).

Recent studies have provided insight on the role of SIRT7 in glycolysis. SIRT7 deacylates phosphoglycerate kinase 1 (PGK1), a key enzyme in glycolysis pathway, and suppresses PGK1 enzymatic activity in liver cancer cells (15). We also reported that SIRT7 regulates gluconeogenesis by modulating G6PC expression via USP7-mediated deubiquitination (45). SIRT7 also suppresses HIF1 and HIF2, which repress glucose oxidation through the tricarboxylic acid cycle (59). Taken together, these findings implicate SIRT7 in glucose metabolism.

Lipid Metabolism

The evidence supporting a role for SIRT7 in lipid metabolism in the liver is conflicting (60). Yoshizawa et al. found that SIRT7 knockout mice (generated by deleting exons 4–9), are resistant to high-fat diet (HFD)-induced fatty liver, glucose intolerance and obesity (61). They also showed that liver-specific SIRT7 knockout mice have reduced hepatic triglyceride accumulation (61). SIRT7 activates Cd36 expression, which is vital for fatty-acid uptake, as well as Mogat that incorporates fatty acids into triglycerides, and Cidea and Cidec that are involved in lipid storage and lipid droplet formation. The expression levels of these four genes were all reduced in the livers of the SIRT7 knockout mice fed a HFD (61). Mechanistically, an interaction between the E3 ubiquitin ligase complex (DDB1-CUL4-associated factor 1 (DCAF1)/damage-specific DNA binding protein 1 (DDB1)/cullin 4B (CUL4B) complex) and TR4 (a nuclear receptor involved in lipid metabolism) promotes TR4 degradation. However, SIRT7 binding to the DCAF1/DDB1/CUL4B complex inhibits TR4 degradation and activates TR4 target genes to increase fatty-acid uptake and triglyceride synthesis and storage. Consequently, the expression level of TR4 and its target genes are reduced in liver-specific SIRT7 knockout mice and lipid synthesis and storage is decreased to resist hepatic steatosis (61).

Two other groups have reported opposing results to Yoshizawa et al. finding that SIRT7 knockout mice instead suffer hepatic steatosis (13, 38). Shin et al. found that SIRT7 knockout mice (generated by replacing exons 4–11 with a LacZ gene), have a fatty liver without obesity (38). They showed that loss of SIRT7 increases lipogenic gene expression, liver triglyceride levels and inflammatory markers, indicating progression to steatohepatitis. These mice also exhibited low levels of plasma triglycerides compared to wild-type controls, due to reduced very-low-density lipoprotein (VLDL) secretion. Importantly, liver steatosis was reversed in these animals by reintroducing SIRT7 specifically in the liver (38). At the mechanistic level, it seems that SIRT7 prevents the development of fatty liver disease by suppressing ER stress. Consequently, SIRT7 knockout mice fail to relieve ER stress such that the UPR pathway is activated causing apoptosis, inflammation, increased lipogenesis and reduced VLDL secretion specifically in the liver (38).

Ryu et al. also described that SIRT7 knockout mice (generated by deleting exons 6–9) exhibited hepatic microvesicular steatosis, and increased plasma levels of triglycerides and free fatty acids. These mice also showed signs of multi-systemic mitochondrial dysfunction due to GABPβ1 hyperacetylation in the absence of SIRT7, including increased blood lactate levels and reduced exercise performance. As discussed, SIRT7 mediates mitochondrial function by deacetylating GABPβ1 (a regulator of multiple nuclear-encoded mitochondrial genes) to promote the formation and activation of the GABP complex that induces mitochondrial gene expression and contributes to mitochondrial homeostasis (13).

Although they used the same mice strain (C57BL/6J), the contradiction of the roles of SIRT7 in lipid metabolism discussed in these three studies may be due to the differences in the genetic background of and construction of SIRT7 knockout mice (60). Further studies with more sample size and parallel experiments are required to clarify this picture.

Cioffi et al. found that SIRT7 induces differentiation and maturation of early adipocyte precursors to promote adipogenesis (39). Consistently, SIRT7 knockdown resulted in reduced Oil Red O staining and adipogenesis marker (FABP4, PPARγ, C/ebpα, adipoq) expression. The researchers also found that miR-93 prevents adipogenesis by inhibiting SIRT7: adipogenesis was enhanced in mir-25-93-106b$^{-/-}$ mice but repressed in miR-93-reintroduced mice. Interestingly, SIRT7 expression was enhanced in the mir-25-93-106b$^{-/-}$ mice while nuclear SIRT7 expression was reduced upon injection of miR-93 mimics into the visceral fat pads of leptin-deficient (ob/ob) mice (39). Despite these preliminary findings, the definitive mechanism underlying how miR-93 regulates SIRT7 and how SIRT7 promotes adipogenesis remains unclear. Fang et al. demonstrated that SIRT7 can promote adipogenesis by binding to SIRT1 and inhibiting its activity by preventing its auto-deacetylation. SIRT1 is reported to repress PPARγ through interaction with nuclear receptor corepressor 1 (NCoR1, PPARγ corepressor) to inhibit adipogenesis (62). As such, SIRT7 knockout mice possess a notably diminished proportion of white fat due to enhanced SIRT1 activity, which blocks PPARγ and adipocyte differentiation (63). SIRT1 activity depletion restores adipogenesis in Sirt7 knockout mice (63). These data implicate a potential cross-regulatory network within the sirtuin family.

SIRT7 in Mitochondrial Metabolism

As discussed, the mitochondrion is a crucial organelle involved in regulating cellular energy homeostasis and thus cell survival. Mitochondria uptake energy from nutrients and then convert it into ATP by oxidative phosphorylation (OXPHOS) (64). In response to cellular stress, the mitochondrion has an armamentarium of quality-control mechanisms based on mitochondrial biosynthesis, mitophagy and mitochondrial unfolded protein responses, to maintain proper mitochondrial function. SIRT7 is an important regulator of mitochondrial homeostasis. As stated above, Ryu et al. found that SIRT7 knockout mice show multi-systemic mitochondrial dysfunction, including lactate accumulation in the blood and age-related hearing loss (13). Mechanistically, SIRT7 impacts on mitochondria function by deacetylating GABPβ1, which forms a hetero-tetramer complex with GABPα, occupies

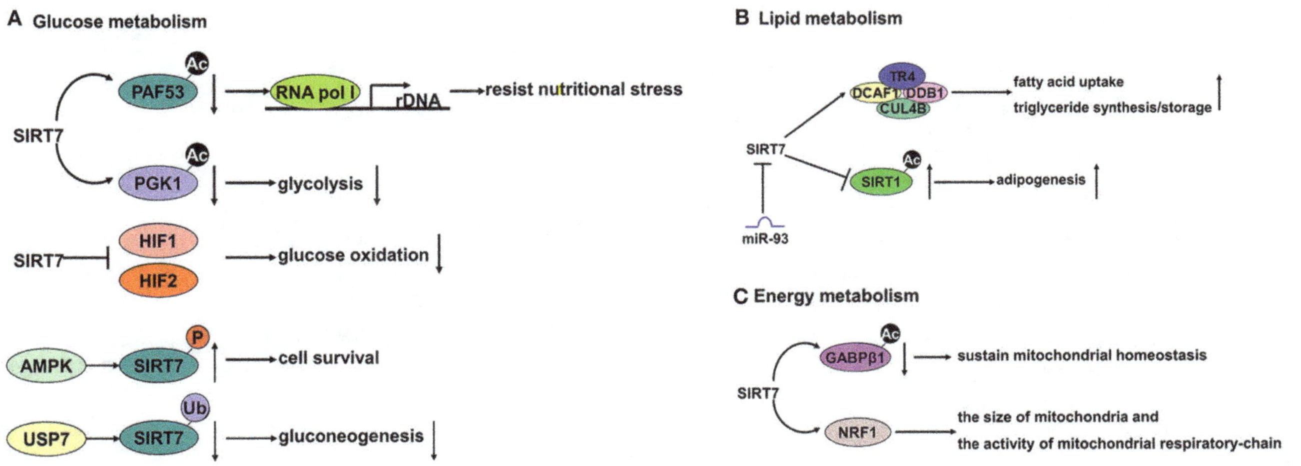

FIGURE 4 | The roles of SIRT7 in metabolism. **(A)** SIRT7 can deacetylate RNA polymerase I (Pol I)-associated factor PAF53 to resist nutritional stress and deacetylate Phosphoglycerate kinase-1 (PGK1) to affect glycolysis pathway. SIRT7 also suppresses the transcription factor Hypoxia-inducible factor-1 (HIF1) and HIF2 to influence glucose oxidation. In addition, SIRT7 can be modified by AMPK or USP7 to regulate glucose metabolism. **(B)** The interaction between SIRT7 and DCAF1/DDB1/CUL4B complex inhibits degradation of Testicular orphan nuclear receptor 4 (TR4) and activates TR4 target genes subsequently increasing fatty acid uptake and triglyceride synthesis/storage. SIRT7 also interacts with SIRT1 to promote adipogenesis. Besides, inhibition of SIRT7 by miR-93 represses adipogenesis. **(C)** SIRT7 can impact the mitochondria function by deacetylating GA-binding protein β1 (GABPβ1). Besides, the interaction of SIRT7 with Nuclear respiratory factor 1 (NRF1) regulates the size of mitochondria and the activity of mitochondrial respiratory-chain.

nuclear-encoded mitochondrial target genes and promotes their transcription. Further studies also found that SIRT7 deficiency affects OXPHOS in the heart and liver (13). Mohrin et al. also reported that SIRT7 interacts with NRF1 (a master regulator of mitochondria) to regulate mitochondria size and activity of the mitochondrial respiratory-chain (46).

Overall, SIRT7 has a vital role in metabolic homeostasis (**Figure 4**), but there remain many unresolved questions. The contradictory effect of SIRT7 on lipid metabolism also needs clarification. Future studies need to address these issues and determine whether SIRT7 may be a suitable therapeutic target in metabolic disorders.

Aging and Senescence

Consistent with the known functions of sirtuins in senescence and lifespan-extension, numerous studies have established a close relationship between SIRT7 and age-related processes (36). SIRT7-knockout mice have a shorter lifespan than control mice, and succumb to premature aging phenotypes around 1 year, with symptoms, such as kyphosis, decreased gonadal fat pad content, reduced IGF-1 plasma levels, hepatic steatosis, degenerative heart hypertrophy, reduced hearing and reduced hematopoietic stem cell-regenerative potential (13, 46, 65). SIRT7 expression gradually declines with age in mice, rat and several cells, including endothelial cells, fibroblasts, hepatocytes and HEK293FT cells (13, 14, 66–68). Kiran et al. found that SIRT7 over-expressing cells show a mostly normal morphology, with very few enlarged cells upon treatment with a low dose of doxorubicin (a cellular senescence inducing agent) (69). By contrast, control GFP expressing cells exhibit cell enlargement and multi-nucleation (typical features of cellular senescence) following doxorubicin exposure. The researchers also found that p53 and p21 senescence marker expression decreases in SIRT7 overexpressing cells upon doxorubicin treatment compared to control cells.

Lee et al. reported that the acetylation levels of nucleophosmin (NPM1) are increased while SIRT6 and SIRT7 levels are decreased in senescent cells. SIRT7 can deacetylate NPM1, which results in up-regulated p53 transcriptional activity in MEFs to induce cellular senescence (14, 70).

Telomeres have the potential to serve as the biomarker of biological cell age (71). Conomos et al. found that TR4 recruitment to the telomere can attribute to the ALT (alternative lengthening of telomeres) phenotype (72). SIRT7 positively regulates the protein level of TR4 (19), suggesting that SIRT7 might play an upstream role in DNA repair and telomere maintenance pathways.

A role for SIRT7 in aging and senescence has also been attributed to SIRT7-mediated regulation of mitochondrial ribosomal proteins (mRPs). SIRT7 interacts with NRF1 to repress mRPs, resulting in hematopoietic stem-cell longevity (46). Conversely, SIRT7-mediated GABPβ1 deacetylation promotes the formation and activation of the GABP complex to increase mRPs, resulting in hematopoietic stem-cell aging (13).

One study reported an interaction between SIRT7 with Tripeptidyl peptidase II (TPPII) that permits SIRT7 cytoplasmic localization (52). TPPII has regulatory effects on apoptosis and senescence, as observed in TPPII knockout mice that exhibit early immuno-senescence and have a shorter lifespan than controls (73). SIRT7 may, therefore, regulate aging and senescence by interacting with TPPII, but the underlying mechanisms need further study.

rDNA instability is common in premature aging syndromes. A recent study by Paredes et al. uncovered a critical role for

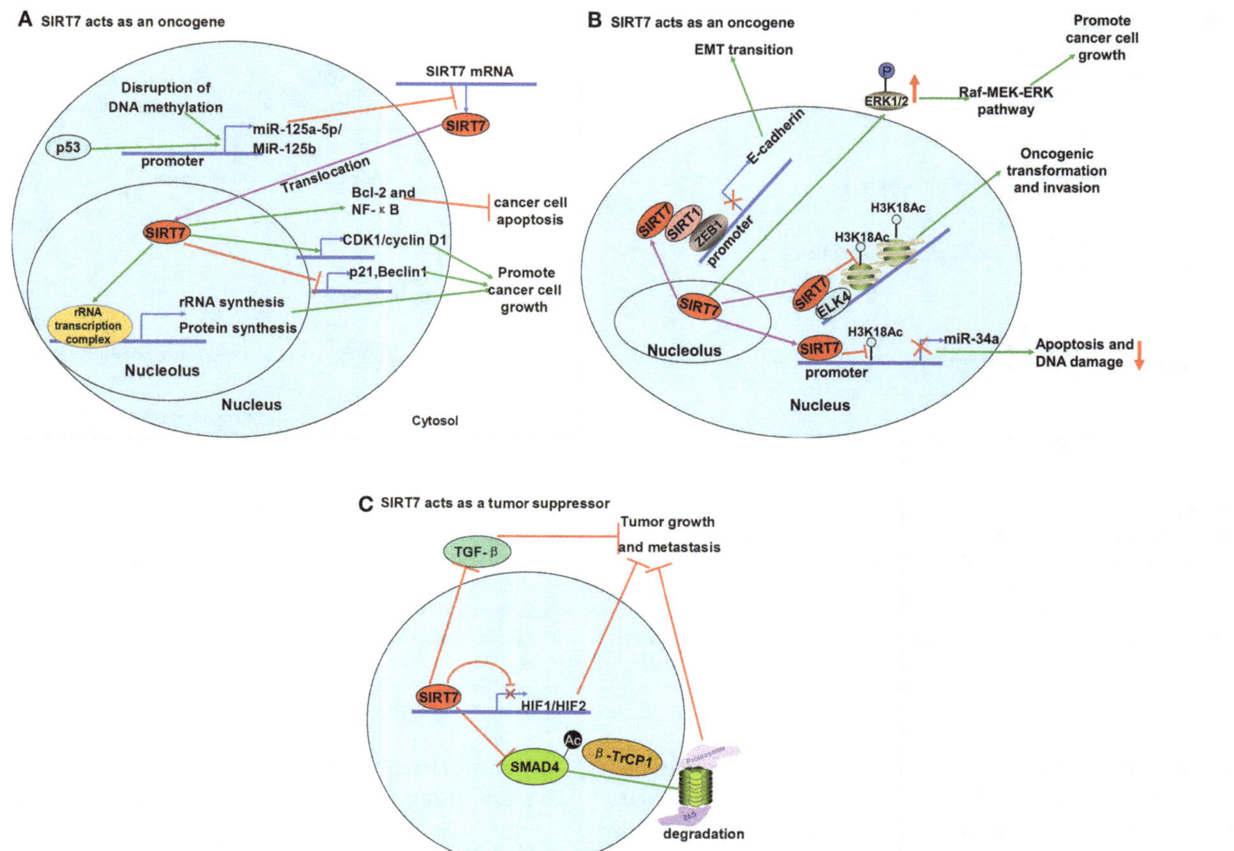

FIGURE 5 | The roles of SIRT7 in cancer. **(A,B)** SIRT7 acts as an oncogene. **(A)** The disruption of DNA methylation and p53 activates miR-125b and miR-125a-5p to inhibit the expression of SIRT7. Overexpression of SIRT7 upregulates the expression of CDK1/cyclin D1 while downregulates the level of p21 and Beclin1 as well as promotes rRNA and protein synthesis by interaction with rRNA transcription complex to promote cancer cell growth. In addition, overexpression of SIRT7 can also upregulate Bcl-2 and NF-κB to repress cancer cell apoptosis. **(B)** ETS-like transcription factor 4 (ELK4) targets SIRT7 to promoters of many tumor suppressor genes for H3K18 deacetylation and leads to cancer cell growth and metastasis eventually. SIRT7 induces ERK1/2 phosphorylation and activated the Raf-MEK-ERK pathway to promote cancer cell growth. SIRT7 also reduces miR-34a expression by deacetylating H3K18Ac to decrease cancer cell apoptosis and DNA damage. Besides, SIRT7 reduces expression of E-cadherin by interaction with SIRT1 to promote EMT transition. **(C)** SIRT7 acts as a tumor suppressor. SIRT7 inactivates TGF-β signaling and represses epithelial-to-mesenchymal transition. SIRT7 also negatively regulates HIF1 and HIF2 transcription. Moreover, SIRT7 deacetylates Mothers against decapentaplegic homolog 4 (SMAD4) and promotes β-transducin repeat–containing protein 1 (β-TrCP1)-dependent degradation to inhibit tumor growth and metastasis.

SIRT7 in protecting against cellular senescence by maintaining heterochromatin silencing and rDNA stability. Mechanistically, they found that SIRT7 acts as a scaffold to stabilize SNF2H at rDNA promoters for chromatin silencing (74). Taken together, SIRT7 might prevent aging-induced physiological changes and possibly extend lifespan via numerous pathways.

Cancer

Although ample evidence supports the involvement of SIRT7 in carcinogenesis, SIRT7 exhibits opposing roles in different cancer types (**Figure 5**). SIRT7 is up- regulated in the majority of cancers, including colorectal, gastric, thyroid, node-positive breast, bladder, ovarian and cervical cancers, hepatocellular and epithelial prostate carcinoma, where it acts as an oncogene (9, 40, 75–82). The exception is seen in pancreatic cancer, where SIRT7 is down-regulated and seems to act as a tumor suppressor (83) (**Table 2**).

As an oncogene, SIRT7 inhibition reduces cancer-cell growth, represses colony formation and cancer-cell metastasis and increases cancer-cell apoptosis. High SIRT7 expression is also considered a predictor of poor survival in various cancers (9, 40, 75–82). Many studies have reported mechanisms of action by which SIRT7 promotes cancer-cell growth (**Figure 5**). Yu et al. found that SIRT7 induces ERK1/2 phosphorylation and activates the Raf–MEK–ERK pathway to promote cancer-cell growth (81). Hypoacetylation of H3K18 is associated with oncogenic transformation, aggressive tumor phenotypes and poor prognosis and maintenance of essential human cancer-cell features, including anchorage-independent growth and escape from contact inhibition (84). As shown in prostate cancer, SIRT7 binds and maintains the deacetylated state of H3K18 at

TABLE 2 | SIRT7 related cancers.

Cancer	SIRT7 expression	Role/Impact
Colorectal cancer	Overexpression	Oncogene
Colorectal cancer	Downregulated	Induce radio-sensitivity; Enhance therapeutic effects
Gastric cancer	Overexpression	Oncogene
Thyroid cancer	Overexpression	Oncogene
Node-positive breast cancer	Overexpression	Oncogene
Breast cancer	Deficiency	Increase metastasis
Bladder cancer	Overexpression	Oncogene; promote cancer-cell growth
Ovarian cancer	Overexpression	Oncogene
Cervical cancer	Overexpression	Oncogene
Hepatocellular carcinoma	Overexpression	Oncogene; promote cancer-cell growth
Epithelial prostate cacinoma	Overexpression	Oncogene; maintaining cancer phenotypes; increase metastasis
Pancreatic cancer	Downregulated	Might be tumor suppressor
Liver cancer	Knockdown	Promote cancer-cell growth

the promoters of many tumor suppressor genes by interacting with the ELK4 transcription factor (85, 86). Thus, SIRT7 has a fundamental role in maintaining cancer phenotypes (6).

Zhang et al. found that SIRT7 knockdown promotes gastric cancer-cell apoptosis (82). Mechanically, SIRT7 prevents cellular apoptosis by down-regulating miR-34a via H3K18ac deacetylation. The miR-34 family is associated with cell-cycle arrest, senescence and apoptosis in cancers, and low miR-34a expression is associated with poor prognosis (82).

Another mechanism as to how SIRT7 promotes cancer-cell growth was identified by Kim et al. (9). They found that SIRT7 knockdown increases the number of liver cancer cells in G1/S phase and delays the cell-cycle transition: $p21^{WAF1/Cip1}$ expression was increased and cyclin D1 (a G1/S cell cycle regulator) was suppressed in SIRT7 knockdown cells. In patients with hepatocellular carcinoma, increased SIRT7 expression was attributed to p53 mutation or the endogenous hypermethylation of the microRNAs miR-125a-5p and miR-125b. Over-expression of SIRT7 led to $p21^{WAF1/Cip1}$ suppression and induction of cyclin D1 expression to promote cancer-cell growth (9). Han et al. also found that SIRT7 expression is regulated by hsa-miR-125b in bladder cancer. They observed that in bladder cancer, hsa-miR-125b and SIRT7 are inversely associated with the oncogenic long non-coding RNA MALAT1. Up-regulated hsa-miR-125b resulted in down-regulated SIRT7 and MALAT1; this effect inhibited bladder cancer cell growth, induced apoptosis, and decreased cell motility (40).

With regards to apoptosis, Wang et al. found that shRNA-mediated SIRT7 silencing reduced anti-apoptotic factor B-cell lymphoma 2 (Bcl-2) and nuclear factor kappa B (NF-κB) levels (80). The NF-κB signaling pathway is important in cellular proliferation, apoptosis and migration in malignant diseases (87). The researchers concluded that SIRT7 inhibits cancer-cell apoptosis by up-regulating Bcl-2 and NF-κB levels (80). The precise regulatory mechanisms remain to be identified.

SIRT7 also influences cancer-cell metastasis. High SIRT7 expression is associated with aggressive cancer phenotypes, metastatic diseases and poor patient prognosis; down-regulating SIRT7 reverses the metastatic properties of epithelial and mesenchymal cancer cells. In epithelial carcinomas, SIRT7 is associated with the EMT, a key process in metastatic progression. Malik et al., Yu et al., Zhang et al. focused on classic EMT regulatory factors and discovered that the expression of E-cadherin (an EMT regulatory factor) showed inverse correlation with SIRT7 *in vivo*. In SIRT7-deficient cells, E-cadherin and DAB2 interacting protein (DAB2IP; a tumor suppressor gene, whose loss promotes EMT and metastasis in prostate cancer) are significantly increased in mRNA level. These findings suggest a role for SIRT7 in cancer prevention and as prognostic factor (78, 81, 82). SIRT7 interacts with SIRT1 to enhance SIRT1-dependent prostate cancer cell metastatic properties and promotes E-cadherin transcriptional repression (88).

In non-epithelial cancers, SIRT7 may impact metastasis regulatory pathways to affect cellular metastatic properties. The expression levels of matrix metalloproteinase MMP16 and vascular endothelial growth factor (VEGF-A) are reduced in SIRT7-deficient HT1080 cells compared to control cells (78). Thus, SIRT7 may be of vital importance for cancer-cell metastasis (78).

As a tumor suppressor, low levels of SIRT7 are associated with aggressive tumor phenotypes and poor patient outcomes. One study found that patients with pancreatic cancer and high levels of nuclear SIRT7 had a longer lifespan (succumbed to disease later) than those with low levels of SIRT7. However, the precise mechanism underlying this association is unclear (83). Similar to the other sirtuins, SIRT7 has also been recognized as a tumor suppressor based on its negative regulation of HIF1 and HIF2 transcription (50, 89), as previously discussed.

The contradictory roles of SIRT7 in cancer may be related to its multiple interactions and functions in various cellular processes. First, SIRT7 deacetylates H3K18Ac, whose depletion is associated with highly malignant cancers and poor patient prognosis. Second, SIRT7 influences ribosome biogenesis to meet the high biosynthetic and metabolic needs of cancer cells. At the same time, although SIRT7 inactivates p53 by deacetylation, up to half of all tumors exhibit mutated p53, which may diminish the oncogenic role of SIRT7 and result in tumor suppressive characteristics (83, 90). Even though the definitive function of SIRT7 is uncertain, many consider SIRT7 as a cancer biomarker or a predictor of prognosis (73, 75, 81, 83). In sum, data suggest that SIRT7 may be a potential novel biomarker for prognosis in pancreatic cancer (83), a circulating marker in head and neck squamous cell carcinoma (73), and a predictive biomarker of pancreatic cancer (PCa) aggressiveness (91).

Our lab also found that down-regulation of SIRT7 after 5-FU exposure induces radio-sensitivity in human colorectal cancer and enhances therapeutic effects (92). Shi et al. found the microRNA-3666 induces SIRT7 inhibition, which in turn inhibits non-small cell lung cancer cell growth (41).

Recently, Tang et al. found that SIRT7 deficiency promotes breast cancer cell metastasis, while temporal expression of SIRT7 inhibits metastasis in a polyomavirus middle T antigen breast cancer model. Here, SIRT7 deacetylates SMAD4 and promotes β-TrCP1-dependent degradation. Finally, SIRT7 deficiency activates TGF-β signaling and enhances the EMT (21). Therefore, it can be assumed that SIRT7 is a worthwhile target to explore for cancer therapy.

CONCLUSIONS AND FUTURE PERSPECTIVES

The function of SIRT7 was ignored in the initial years of sirtuin-based research due to its localization in the nucleolus. However, major breakthroughs have been made over the past decade in SIRT7 biology. New substrates for SIRT7 deacetylase activity have been identified, which have highlighted new enzymatic activities that are critical for different cellular processes. SIRT7 has strong potential as a therapeutic target in various cancers, due to the identification of its up-regulation and activation in various cancer cells. SIRT7 is also considered a potential novel biomarker for prognosis in several cancers, such as pancreatic cancer. However, due to its complicated and controversial mechanism in the maintenance of cancers, future studies are needed to understand the precise molecular mechanism and downstream pathways of SIRT7 in the specific cancer types. The therapeutic uses of SIRT7 in cancers will rely on the further clinical trials. A recent report suggests a role for SIRT7 in the adaptive immune system and neurogenesis (93). This finding indicates that the roles and function of SIRT7 are still diversifying, and are wider than previously thought. Further studies are now needed to better understand and elucidate the molecular role of SIRT7, identify its substrate partners/cofactors, and delineate the intracellular pathways that regulate their activity in different disease models.

AUTHOR CONTRIBUTIONS

DW, YL, and KZ wrote the primary manuscript and revised the manuscript. HW and W-GZ conceived and designed the manuscript.

ACKNOWLEDGMENTS

The authors would like to thank Dr. Jessica Tamanini (Shenzhen University and ETediting) for editing the manuscript prior to submission.

REFERENCES

1. Imai S, Armstrong CM, Kaeberlein M, Guarente L. Transcriptional silencing and longevity protein Sir2 is an NAD-dependent histone deacetylase. *Nature* (2000) 403:795. doi: 10.1038/35001622
2. Landry J, Sutton A, Tafrov ST, Heller RC, Stebbins J, Pillus L, et al. The silencing protein SIR2 and its homologs are NAD-dependent protein deacetylases. *Proc Natl Acad Sci USA.* (2000) 97:5807–11. doi: 10.1073/pnas.110148297
3. Michishita E, Park JY, Burneskis JM, Barrett JC, Horikawa I. Evolutionarily conserved and nonconserved cellular localizations and functions of human SIRT proteins. *Mol Biol Cell* (2005) 16:4623–35. doi: 10.1091/mbc.e05-01-0033
4. Haigis MC, Sinclair DA. Mammalian sirtuins: biological insights and disease relevance. *Annu Rev Pathol.* (2010) 5:253–95. doi: 10.1146/annurev.pathol.4.110807.092250
5. Voelter-Mahlknecht S, Letzel S, Mahlknecht U. Fluorescence *in situ* hybridization and chromosomal organization of the human sirtuin 7 gene. *Int J Oncol.* (2006) 28:899–908. doi: 10.3892/ijo.28.4.899
6. Barber MF, Michishita-Kioi E, Xi Y, Tasselli L, Kioi M, Moqtaderi Z, et al. SIRT7 links H3K18 deacetylation to maintenance of oncogenic transformation. *Nature* (2012) 487:114–8. doi: 10.1038/nature 11043
7. Tsai Y, Greco TM, Boonmee A, Miteva Y, Cristea IM. Functional proteomics establishes the interaction of SIRT7 with chromatin remodeling complexes and expands its role in regulation of RNA polymerase I transcription. *Mol Cell Proteomics* (2011) 11:60–76. doi: 10.1074/mcp.A111.015156
8. Vakhrusheva O, Smolka C, Gajawada P, Kostin S, Boettger T, Kubin T, et al. SIRT7 increases stress resistance of cardiomyocytes and prevents apoptosis and inflammatory cardiomyopathy in mice. *Circ Res.* (2008) 102:703–10. doi: 10.1161/CIRCRESAHA.107.164558
9. Kim JK, Noh JH, Jung KH, Eun JW, Bae HJ, Kim MG, et al. Sirtuin7 oncogenic potential in human hepatocellular carcinoma and its regulation by the tumor suppressors MiR-125a-5p and MiR-125b. *Hepatology* (2013) 57:1055–67. doi: 10.1002/hep.26101
10. Nahalkova J. Novel protein-protein interactions of TPPII, p53, and SIRT7. *Mol Cell Biochem.* (2015) 409:13–22. doi: 10.1007/s11010-015-2507-y
11. Chen S, Blank MF, Iyer A, Huang B, Wang L, Grummt I, et al. SIRT7-dependent deacetylation of the U3-55k protein controls pre-rRNA processing. *Nat Commun.* (2016) 7:10734. doi: 10.1038/ncomms10734
12. Chen S, Seiler J, Santiago-Reichelt M, Felbel K, Grummt I, Voit R. Repression of RNA polymerase I upon stress is caused by inhibition of RNA-dependent deacetylation of PAF53 by SIRT7. *Mol Cell* (2013) 52:303–13. doi: 10.1016/j.molcel.2013.10.010
13. Ryu D, Jo YS, Lo Sasso G, Stein S, Zhang H, Perino A, et al. A SIRT7-dependent acetylation switch of GABPβ1 controls mitochondrial function. *Cell Metab.* (2014) 20:856–69. doi: 10.1016/j.cmet.2014.08.001
14. Lee N, Kim D, Kim E, Park SJ, Kwon J, Shin J, et al. Comparative interactomes of SIRT6 and SIRT7: implication of functional links to aging. *Proteomics* (2014) 14:1610–22. doi: 10.1002/pmic.201400001
15. Hu H, Zhu W, Qin J, Chen M, Gong L, Li L, et al. Acetylation of PGK1 promotes liver cancer cell proliferation and tumorigenesis. *Hepatology* (2016) 65:515–28. doi: 10.1002/hep.28887
16. Yu J, Qin B, Wu F, Qin S, Nowsheen S, Shan S, et al. Regulation of serine/threonine kinase Akt activation by NAD (+)-dependent deacetylase SIRT7. *Cell Rep.* (2017) 18:1229–40. doi: 10.1016/j.celrep.2017.01.009
17. Blank MF, Chen S, Poetz F, Schnölzer M, Voit R, Grummt I. SIRT7-dependent deacetylation of CDK9 activates RNA polymerase II transcription. *Nucleic Acids Res.* (2017) 45:2675–86. doi: 10.1093/nar/gkx053
18. Li Z, Bridges B, Olson J, Weinman SA. The interaction between acetylation and serine-574 phosphorylation regulates the apoptotic function of FOXO3. *Oncogene* (2016) 36:1887–98. doi: 10.1038/onc.2016.359

19. Karim MF, Yoshizawa T, Sobuz SU, Sato Y, Yamagata K. Sirtuin 7-dependent deacetylation of DDB1 regulates the expression of nuclear receptor TR4. *Biochem Biophys Res Commun.* (2017) 490:423–8. doi: 10.1016/j.bbrc.2017.06.057
20. Mo Y, Lin R, Liu P, Tan M, Xiong Y, Guan K, et al. SIRT7 deacetylates DDB1 and suppresses the activity of the CRL4 E3 ligase complexes. *FEBS J.* (2017) 284:3619–36. doi: 10.1111/febs.14259
21. Tang X, Shi L, Xie N, Liu Z, Qian M, Meng F, et al. SIRT7 antagonizes TGF-β signaling and inhibits breast cancer metastasis. *Nat Commun.* (2017) 8:318. doi: 10.1038/s41467-017-00396-9
22. Song C, Hotz-Wagenblatt A, Voit R, Grummt I. SIRT7 and the DEAD-box helicase DDX21 cooperate to resolve genomic R loops and safeguard genome stability. *Gene Dev.* (2017) 31:1370–81. doi: 10.1101/gad.300624.117
23. Zhang C, Zhai Z, Tang M, Cheng Z, Li T, Wang H, et al. Quantitative proteome-based systematic identification of SIRT7 substrates. *Proteomics* (2017) 17:1600395. doi: 10.1002/pmic.201600395
24. Li L, Shi L, Yang S, Yan R, Zhang D, Yang J, et al. SIRT7 is a histone desuccinylase that functionally links to chromatin compaction and genome stability. *Nat Commun.* (2016) 7:12235. doi: 10.1038/ncomms12235
25. Tsai Y, Greco TM, Cristea IM. Sirtuin 7 plays a role in ribosome biogenesis and protein synthesis. *Mol Cell Proteomics* (2013) 13:73–83. doi: 10.1074/mcp.M113.031377
26. Tanabe K, Liu J, Kato D, Kurumizaka H, Yamatsugu K, Kanai M, et al. LC–MS/MS-based quantitative study of the acyl group- and site-selectivity of human sirtuins to acylated nucleosomes. *Sci Rep.* (2018) 8:2656. doi: 10.1038/s41598-018-21060-2
27. Tong Z, Wang M, Wang Y, Kim DD, Grenier JK, Cao J, et al. SIRT7 is an RNA-activated protein lysine deacylase. *ACS Chem Biol.* (2016) 12:300–10. doi: 10.1021/acschembio.6b00954
28. Tong Z, Wang Y, Zhang X, Kim DD, Sadhukhan S, Hao Q, et al. SIRT7 is activated by DNA and deacetylates histone H3 in the chromatin context. *ACS Chem Biol.* (2016) 11:742–7. doi: 10.1021/acschembio.5b01084
29. Karim MF, Yoshizawa T, Sato Y, Sawa T, Tomizawa K, Akaike T, et al. Inhibition of H3K18 deacetylation of SIRT7 by Myb-binding protein 1a (Mybbp1a). *Biochem Biophys Res Commun.* (2013) 441:157–63. doi: 10.1016/j.bbrc.2013.10.020
30. Ford E, Voit R, Liszt G, Magin C, Grummt I, Guarente L. Mammalian Sir2 homolog SIRT7 is an activator of RNA polymerase I transcription. *Gene Dev.* (2005) 20:1075–80. doi: 10.1101/gad.1399706
31. Kiran S, Anwar T, Kiran M, Ramakrishna G. Sirtuin 7 in cell proliferation, stress and disease: rise of the Seventh Sirtuin!. *Cell Signal.* (2015) 27:673–82. doi: 10.1016/j.cellsig.2014.11.026
32. Wang W, Zhang X, Zheng K, Pei Y. Sirtuin 7 plays an oncogenic role in human osteosarcoma via downregulating CDC4 expression. *Am J Cancer Res.* (2017) 7:1788–803.
33. Li W, Sun Z, Chen C, Wang L, Geng Z, Tao J. Sirtuin7 has an oncogenic potential via promoting the growth of cholangiocarcinoma cells. *Biomed Pharmacother.* (2018) 100:257–66. doi: 10.1016/j.biopha.2018.02.007
34. Gong J, Wang H, Lou W, Wang G, Tao H, Wen H, et al. Associations of sirtuins with clinicopathological parameters and prognosis in non-small cell lung cancer. *Cancer Manag Res.* (2018) 10:3341–56. doi: 10.2147/CMAR.S166946
35. Armour SM, Bennett EJ, Braun CR, Zhang X, McMahon SB, Gygi SP, et al. A high-confidence interaction map identifies SIRT1 as a mediator of acetylation of USP22 and the SAGA coactivator complex. *Mol Cell Biol.* (2012) 33:1487–502. doi: 10.1128/MCB.00971-12
36. Blank MF, Grummt I. The seven faces of SIRT7. *Transcription* (2017) 8:67–74. doi: 10.1080/21541264.2016.1276658
37. Liu GF, Lu JY, Zhang YJ, Zhang LX, Lu GD, Xie ZJ, et al. C/EBPalpha negatively regulates SIRT7 expression via recruiting HDAC3 to the upstream-promoter of hepatocellular carcinoma cells. *Biochim Biophys Acta* (2016) 1859:348–54. doi: 10.1016/j.bbagrm.2015.12.004
38. Shin J, He M, Liu Y, Paredes S, Villanova L, Brown K, et al. SIRT7 represses Myc activity to suppress ER stress and prevent fatty liver disease. *Cell Rep.* (2013) 5:654–65. doi: 10.1016/j.celrep.2013.10.007
39. Cioffi M, Vallespinos-Serrano M, Trabulo SM, Fernandez-Marcos PJ, Firment AN, Vazquez BN, et al. MiR-93 controls adiposity via inhibition of SIRT7 and Tbx3. *Cell Rep.* (2015) 12:1594–605. doi: 10.1016/j.celrep.2015.08.006
40. Han Y, Liu Y, Zhang H, Wang T, Diao R, Jiang Z, et al. Hsa-miR-125b suppresses bladder cancer development by down-regulating oncogene SIRT7 and oncogenic long non-coding RNA MALAT1. *FEBS Lett.* (2013) 587:3875–82. doi: 10.1016/j.febslet.2013.10.023
41. Shi H, Ji Y, Zhang D, Liu Y, Fang P. MicroRNA-3666-induced suppression of SIRT7 inhibits the growth of non-small cell lung cancer cells. *Oncol Rep.* (2016) 36:3051–7. doi: 10.3892/or.2016.5063
42. Yu W, Cui X, Wan Z, Yu Y, Liu X, Jin L. Silencing forkhead box M1 promotes apoptosis and autophagy through SIRT7/mTOR/IGF2 pathway in gastric cancer cells. *J Cell Biochem.* (2018) 119:9090–8. doi: 10.1002/jcb.27168
43. Grob A, Roussel P, Wright JE, McStay B, Hernandez-Verdun D, Sirri V. Involvement of SIRT7 in resumption of rDNA transcription at the exit from mitosis. *J Cell Sci.* (2009) 122:489–98. doi: 10.1242/jcs.042382
44. Sun L, Fan G, Shan P, Qiu X, Dong S, Liao L, et al. Regulation of energy homeostasis by the ubiquitin-independent REGγ proteasome. *Nat Commun.* (2016) 7:12497. doi: 10.1038/ncomms12497
45. Jiang L, Xiong J, Zhan J, Yuan F, Tang M, Zhang C, et al. Ubiquitin-specific peptidase 7 (USP7)-mediated deubiquitination of the histone deacetylase SIRT7 regulates gluconeogenesis. *J Biol Chem.* (2017) 292:13296–311. doi: 10.1074/jbc.M117.780130
46. Mohrin M, Shin J, Liu Y, Brown K, Luo H, Xi Y, et al. Stem cell aging. A mitochondrial UPR-mediated metabolic checkpoint regulates hematopoietic stem cell aging. *Science* (2015) 347:1374–7. doi: 10.1126/science.aaa2361
47. Xu C, Bailly-Maitre B, Reed JC. Endoplasmic reticulum stress: cell life and death decisions. *J Clin Invest.* (2005) 115:2656–64. doi: 10.1172/JCI26373
48. Zhao Q, Wang J, Levichkin IV, Stasinopoulos S, Ryan MT, Hoogenraad NJ. A mitochondrial specific stress response in mammalian cells. *EMBO J.* (2002) 21:4411–9. doi: 10.1093/emboj/cdf445
49. Dioum EM, Chen R, Alexander MS, Zhang Q, Hogg RT, Gerard RD, et al. Regulation of hypoxia-inducible factor 2α signaling by the stress-responsive deacetylase sirtuin 1. *Science* (2009) 324:1289. doi: 10.1126/science.1169956
50. Hubbi ME, Hu H, Kshitiz Gilkes DM, Semenza GL. Sirtuin-7 inhibits the activity of hypoxia-inducible factors. *J Biol Chem.* (2013) 288:20768–75. doi: 10.1074/jbc.M113.476903
51. Lewinska A, Wnuk M, Grabowska W, Zabek T, Semik E, Sikora E, et al. Curcumin induces oxidation-dependent cell cycle arrest mediated by SIRT7 inhibition of rDNA transcription in human aortic smooth muscle cells. *Toxicol Lett.* (2015) 233:227–38. doi: 10.1016/j.toxlet.2015.01.019
52. Araki S, Izumiya Y, Rokutanda T, Ianni A, Hanatani S, Kimura Y, et al. SIRT7 contributes to myocardial tissue repair by maintaining transforming growth factor-β signaling pathway. *Circulation* (2015) 132:1081. doi: 10.1161/CIRCULATIONAHA.114.014821
53. Weber CE, Li NY, Wai PY, Kuo PC. Epithelial-mesenchymal transition, TGF-β, and osteopontin in wound healing and tissue remodeling after injury. *J Burn Care Res.* (2012) 33:311–8. doi: 10.1097/BCR.0b013e318240541e
54. Bosch-Presegue L, Vaquero A. Sirtuins in stress response: guardians of the genome. *Oncogene* (2014) 33:3764–75. doi: 10.1038/onc.2013.344
55. Vazquez BN, Thackray JK, Simonet NG, Kane Goldsmith N, Martinez Redondo P, Nguyen T, et al. SIRT7 promotes genome integrity and modulates non-homologous end joining DNA repair. *EMBO J.* (2016) 35:1488–503. doi: 10.15252/embj.201593499
56. Zhang P, Li G, Deng Z, Liu L, Chen L, Tang J, et al. Dicer interacts with SIRT7 and regulates H3K18 deacetylation in response to DNA damaging agents. *Nucleic Acids Res.* (2016) 44:3629–42. doi: 10.1093/nar/gkv1504
57. Mao Z, Hine C, Tian X, Van Meter M, Au M, Vaidya A, et al. SIRT6 promotes DNA repair under stress by activating PARP1. *Science* (2011) 332:1443–6. doi: 10.1126/science.1202723
58. Hanada K, Song CZ, Yamamoto K, Yano K, Maeda Y, Yamaguchi K, et al. RNA polymerase I associated factor 53 binds to the nucleolar transcription factor UBF and functions in specific rDNA transcription. *EMBO J.* (1996) 15:2217–26. doi: 10.1002/j.1460-2075.1996.tb00575.x
59. Kim J, Tchernyshyov I, Semenza GL, Dang CV. HIF-1-mediated expression of pyruvate dehydrogenase kinase: a metabolic switch required for cellular adaptation to hypoxia. *Cell Metab.* (2006) 3:177–85. doi: 10.1016/j.cmet.2006.02.002
60. Tang BL. SIRT7 and hepatic lipid metabolism. *Front Cell Dev Biol.* 3:1. doi: 10.3389/fcell.2015.00001

61. Yoshizawa T, Karim MF, Sato Y, Senokuchi T, Miyata K, Fukuda T, et al. SIRT7 controls hepatic lipid metabolism by regulating the ubiquitin-proteasome pathway. *Cell Metab.* (2014) 19:712–21. doi: 10.1016/j.cmet.2014.03.006
62. Picard F, Kurtev M, Chung N, Topark-Ngarm A, Senawong T, Machado De Oliveira R, et al. Sirtl promotes fat mobilization in white adipocytes by repressing PPAR-gamma. *Nature* (2004) 429:771–6. doi: 10.1038/nature 02583
63. Fang J, Ianni A, Smolka C, Vakhrusheva O, Nolte H, Krüger M, et al. SIRT7 promotes adipogenesis in the mouse by inhibiting autocatalytic activation of Sirtl. *Proc Natl Acad Sci USA.* (2017) 114:E8352–61. doi: 10.1073/pnas.1706945114
64. Poyton RO, McEwen JE. Crosstalk between nuclear and mitochondrial genomes. *Annu Rev Biochem.* (1996) 65:563–607. doi: 10.1146/annurev.bi.65.070196.003023
65. Vakhrusheva O, Braeuer D, Liu Z, Braun T, Bober E. SIRT7-dependent inhibition of cell growth and proliferation might be instrumental to mediate tissue integrity during aging. *J Physiol Pharmacol.* (2008) 59(Suppl. 9), 201–12.
66. Wronska A, Lawniczak A, Wierzbicki PM, Kmiec Z. Age-related changes in sirtuin 7 expression in calorie-restricted and refed rats. *Gerontology* (2016) 62:304–10. doi: 10.1159/000441603
67. Ghiraldini FG, Crispim ACV, Mello MLS. Effects of hyperglycemia and aging on nuclear sirtuins and DNA damage of mouse hepatocytes. *Mol Biol Cell* (2013) 24:2467–76. doi: 10.1091/mbc.e13-04-0186
68. Mortuza R, Chen S, Feng B, Sen S, Chakrabarti S. High glucose induced alteration of SIRTs in endothelial cells causes rapid aging in a p300 and FOXO regulated pathway. *PLoS ONE* (2013) 8:e54514. doi: 10.1371/journal.pone.0054514
69. Kiran S, Oddi V, Ramakrishna G. Sirtuin 7 promotes cellular survival following genomic stress by attenuation of DNA damage, SAPK activation and p53 response. *Exp Cell Res.* (2014) 331:123–41. doi: 10.1016/j.yexcr.2014.11.001
70. Colombo E, Marine J, Danovi D, Falini B, Pelicci PG. Nucleophosmin regulates the stability and transcriptional activity of p53. *Nat Cell Biol.* (2002) 4:529. doi: 10.1038/ncb814
71. Bojesen SE. Telomeres and human health. *J Intern Med.* (2013) 274:399–413. doi: 10.1111/joim.12083
72. Conomos D, Stutz MD, Hills M, Neumann AA, Bryan TM, Reddel RR, et al. Variant repeats re interspersed throughout the telomeres and recruit nuclear receptors in ALT cells. *J Cell Biol.* (2012) 199:893–906. doi: 10.1083/jcb.201207189
73. Lu CT, Hsu CM, Lin PM, Lai CC, Lin HC, Yang CH, et al. The potential of SIRT6 and SIRT7 as circulating markers for head and neck squamous cell carcinoma. *Anticancer Res.* (2014) 34:7137–43.
74. Paredes S, Angulo-Ibanez M, Tasselli L, Carlson SM, Zheng W, Li TM, et al. The epigenetic regulator SIRT7 guards against mammalian cellular senescence induced by ribosomal DNA instability. *J Biol Chem.* (2018) 293:11242–50. doi: 10.1074/jbc.AC118.003325
75. Geng Q, Peng H, Chen F, Luo R, Li R. High expression of SIRT7 served as a predictor of adverse outcome in breast cancer. *Int J Clin Exp Pathol.* (2015) 8:1938–45.
76. Aljada A, Saleh AM, Alkathiri M, Shamsa HB, Al-Bawab A, Nasr A. Altered sirtuin 7 expression is associated with early stage breast cancer. *Breast Cancer (Auckl).* (2015) 9:3–8. doi: 10.4137/BCBCR.S23156
77. Ashraf N, Zino S, MacIntyre A, Kingsmore D, Payne AP, George WD, et al. Altered sirtuin expression is associated with node-positive breast cancer. *Brit J Cancer* (2006) 95:1056–61. doi: 10.1038/sj.bjc.6603384
78. Malik S, Villanova L, Tanaka S, Aonuma M, Roy N, Berber E, et al. SIRT7 inactivation reverses metastatic phenotypes in epithelial and mesenchymal tumors. *Sci Rep.* (2015) 5:9841. doi: 10.1038/srep09841
79. Singh S, Kumar PU, Thakur S, Kiran S, Sen B, Sharma S, et al. Expression/localization patterns of sirtuins (SIRT1, SIRT2, and SIRT7) during progression of cervical cancer and effects of sirtuin inhibitors on growth of cervical cancer cells. *Tumor Biol.* (2015) 36:6159–71. doi: 10.1007/s13277-015-3300-y
80. Wang HL, Lu RQ, Xie SH, Zheng H, Wen XM, Gao X, et al. SIRT7 exhibits oncogenic potential in human ovarian cancer cells. *Asian Pac J Cancer Prev.* (2015) 16:3573–7. doi: 10.7314/APJCP.2015.16.8.3573
81. Yu H, Ye W, Wu J, Meng X, Liu RY, Ying X, et al. Overexpression of SIRT7 exhibits oncogenic property and serves as a prognostic factor in colorectal cancer. *Clin Cancer Res.* (2014) 20:3434–45. doi: 10.1158/1078-0432.CCR-13-2952
82. Zhang S, Chen P, Huang Z, Hu X, Chen M, Hu S, et al. SIRT7 promotes gastric cancer growth and inhibits apoptosis by epigenetically inhibiting miR-34a. *Sci Rep.* (2015) 5:9787. doi: 10.1038/srep09787
83. McGlynn LM, McCluney S, Jamieson NB, Thomson J, MacDonald AI, Oien K, et al. SIRT3 & SIRT7: potential novel biomarkers for determining outcome in pancreatic cancer patients. *PLoS ONE* (2015) 10:e131344. doi: 10.1371/journal.pone.0131344
84. Horwitz GA, Zhang K, McBrian MA, Grunstein M, Kurdistani SK, Berk AJ. Adenovirus small e1a alters global patterns of histone modification. *Science* (2008) 321:1084–5. doi: 10.1126/science.11 55544
85. Day BW, Stringer BW, Spanevello MD, Charmsaz S, Jamieson PR, Ensbey KS, et al. ELK4 neutralization sensitizes glioblastoma to apoptosis through downregulation of the anti-apoptotic protein Mcl-1. *Neuro Oncol.* (2011) 13:1202–12. doi: 10.1093/neuonc/nor119
86. Makkonen H, Jääskeläinen T, Pitkänen-Arsiola T, Rytinki M, Waltering KK, Mättö M, et al. Identification of ETS-like transcription factor 4 as a novel androgen receptor target in prostate cancer cells. *Oncogene* (2008) 27:4865. doi: 10.1038/onc.2008.125
87. Alvero AB. Recent insights into the role of NF-kappaB in ovarian carcinogenesis. *Genome Med.* (2010) 2:56. doi: 10.1186/gm177
88. Byles V, Zhu L, Lovaas JD, Chmilewski LK, Wang J, Faller DV, et al. SIRT1 induces EMT by cooperating with EMT transcription factors and enhances prostate cancer cell migration and metastasis. *Oncogene* (2012) 31:4619–29. doi: 10.1038/onc.2011.612
89. Gilkes DM, Xiang L, Lee SJ, Chaturvedi P, Hubbi ME, Wirtz D, et al. Hypoxia-inducible factors mediate coordinated RhoA-ROCK1 expression and signaling in breast cancer cells. *Proc Natl Acad Sci USA.* (2013) 111:E384–93. doi: 10.1073/pnas.1321510111
90. Paredes S, Villanova L, Chua KF. Molecular pathways: emerging roles of mammalian sirtuin SIRT7 in cancer. *Clin Cancer Res.* (2014) 20:1741–6. doi: 10.1158/1078-0432.CCR-13-1547
91. Haider R, Massa F, Kaminski L, Clavel S, Djabari Z, Robert G, et al. Sirtuin 7: a new marker of aggressiveness in prostate cancer. *Oncotarget* (2017) 8:77309–16. doi: 10.18632/oncotarget.20468
92. Tang M, Lu X, Zhang C, Du C, Cao L, Hou T, et al. Downregulation of SIRT7 by 5-fluorouracil induces radiosensitivity in human colorectal cancer. *Theranostics* (2017) 7:1346–59. doi: 10.7150/thno.18804
93. Burg N, Bittner S, Ellwardt E. Role of the epigenetic factor Sirt7 in neuroinflammation and neurogenesis. *Neurosci Res.* (2018) 131:1–9. doi: 10.1016/j.neures.2017.09.005

7

Sirt1 Promotes a Thermogenic Gene Program in Bone Marrow Adipocytes: From Mice to (Wo)Men

Hanna Artsi[1†], Irina Gurt[1†], Madi El-Haj[2], Ralph Müller[3], Gisela A. Kuhn[3], Gal Ben Shalom[1], Einav Cohen-Kfir[1‡], Eva Abramowitz[1], Leonid Kandel[2], Ori Safran[2] and Rivka Dresner-Pollak[1]*

[1] Division of Medicine, Department of Endocrinology and Metabolism, Faculty of Medicine, The Hadassah Medical Center, Hebrew University of Jerusalem, Jerusalem, Israel, [2] Department of Orthopedics, Faculty of Medicine, The Hadassah Medical Center, Hebrew University of Jerusalem, Jerusalem, Israel, [3] Department of Health Sciences and Technology, Institute for Biomechanics, ETH Zurich, Zurich, Switzerland

***Correspondence:**
Rivka Dresner-Pollak
rivkap@hadassah.org.il

[†] These authors have contributed equally to this work

[‡] Present Address:
Einav Cohen-Kfir, Institute of Medical Research Israel-Canada, Hebrew University-Hadassah Medical School, Jerusalem, Israel

Bone marrow adipose tissue (MAT) is influenced by nutritional cues, and participates in whole body energy metabolism. To investigate the role of Sirtuin1 (Sirt1), a key player in metabolism, in MAT, marrow adiposity was evaluated in inbred 5-month-old 129/Sv *Sirt1* haplo-insufficient (*Sirt1*$^{\Delta/+}$) and wild type (WT) mice. Decreased expression of the thermogenic genes: *Prdm16, Pgc1α, Foxc2, Dio2,* and *β3AR* was detected in whole tibiae derived from *Sirt1*$^{\Delta/+}$ compared to WT female mice. Similarly, decreased expression of *Prdm16* and *Pgc1α* was observed in primary bone marrow mesenchymal stem cell (BM-MSC) cultures obtained from *Sirt1*$^{\Delta/+}$ compared to WT female mice, suggesting a cell autonomous effect of Sirt1 in BM-MSCs. *In vitro*, Sirt1 over-expression in the mesenchymal embryonic fibroblast stem cell line C3HT101/2 increased Pgc1α and Prdm16 protein level. Similarly, pharmacologic activation of Sirt1 by SRT3025 increased *Foxc2, Pgc1α, Dio2, Tfam,* and *Cyc1* expression while inhibition of Sirt1 by EX527 down-regulated *UCP1* in C3HT101/2 cells. Importantly, in human femoral BM-MSCs obtained from female patients undergoing hip operations for fracture or osteoarthritis, Sirt1 activation by SRT3025 increased *PGC1α* mRNA and protein level. Blocking sclerostin, an inhibitor of the WNT pathway and a Sirt1 target, by the monoclonal humanized antibody (Sc-AbII), stimulated *β3AR, PRDM16,* and *UCP1* gene expression, and increased PGC1α protein level. These results show that Sirt1 stimulates a thermogenic gene program in marrow adipocytes in mice and humans via PGC1α activation and sclerostin inhibition. The implications of these findings to bone health, hematopoiesis and whole body energy metabolism remain to be investigated.

Keywords: sirtuin1, marrow adipose tissue, PGC1-alpha, bone marrow mesenchymal stem cells, thermogenic genes

INTRODUCTION

Adipose tissue consists of three main fat depots: visceral, subcutaneous, and marrow. Marrow adipose tissue (MAT) was initially thought to be metabolically inert and a filler only. Recent studies however have found that MAT responds to nutritional cues and exercise, and participates in whole body fat metabolism (1–4). Studies in mice and humans undergoing bone marrow transplantation have demonstrated trafficking of bone marrow (BM)-derived circulating progenitor cells to adipose tissue, their differentiation into subcutaneous adipocytes and increased representation in obesity (5, 6). Furthermore, MAT was shown to contribute to circulating adiponectin in mice subjected to calorie restriction and in humans undergoing anti-cancer therapy (1). Interestingly, MAT response to nutritional cues can be distinct than visceral and subcutaneous fat depots. Calorie restriction, anti-cancer therapy, type 1 diabetes mellitus and anorexia nervosa all lead to peripheral fat loss but are surprisingly associated with increased MAT volume (7). In addition, MAT volume is inversely related to bone mass and strength in postmenopausal osteoporosis, aging and glucocorticoid excess (8–11). Finally, marrow adipocytes negatively regulate hematopoiesis and support bone homing cancers (12, 13). Thus, elucidating the mechanisms that regulate MAT may reveal novel pathways that influence bone turnover, hematopoiesis and whole body energy metabolism.

Three types of adipocytes reside in fat depots: white, brown, and beige. Lipid rich white adipocytes expand with energy intake and store triglycerides. Mitochondria rich brown adipocyte arise from a muscle-like cell lineage (*Myf5*$^{+}$) and dissipate energy as heat, while beige adipocytes (brite) emerge in white fat depots, bear characteristics of brown adipocytes, but do not originate from the *Myf5*$^{+}$ lineage (14).

The origin of bone marrow adipocytes is still unknown, and tools to genetically manipulate it are limited. The prevailing model suggests that a self-renewing bone marrow (BM) mesenchymal stem cell (BM-MSC) exists within the bone marrow that gives rise to osteoblasts, adipocytes, chondrocytes and marrow stromal cells (15). This BM-MSC was identified as the bone marrow stromal stem cell (BMSC) that surrounds bone marrow sinusoids (16), and has *in vivo* osteogenic and adipogenic potential. The regulatory factors that are involved in BMSC commitment to the adipocyte lineage are starting to unravel. BMSCs that express the leptin receptor (LepR) have the capacity to differentiate into both adipocytes and osteoblasts, while LepR is not expressed by neither mature osteoblasts nor marrow adipocytes, suggesting that LepR in BMSCs influences lineage allocation (17). Consistently, Leptin signaling via the LepR induced by high-fat-diet failed to promote marrow adipogenesis in mice with LepR deletion in BMSCs but not in osteoblasts, confirming that the effect is restricted to BMSCs (18). Another hormonal pathway affecting the BMSC fate is the parathyroid hormone/parathyroid hormone related peptide (PTH/PTHrP) receptor signaling pathway. Genetic loss PTH/PTHrP receptor (PTH1R) in mesenchymal stem cells using the paired related homeobox transcription factor 1 (*Prx1*)-*Cre* driver was reported to induce marrow adipogenesis, while PTH administration reduced marrow fat in mice and male patients with idiopathic osteoporosis, suggesting that PTH inhibits the differentiation of adipocyte progenitors to the adipocyte lineage (19). On another level of complexity, region-specific variation in MAT development, regulation and phenotype was reported in mice, rats and humans (20).

Sirtuin1 (Sirt1), a member of the sirtuin family of NAD^{+}-dependent protein deacetylases, is a key cellular energy sensor and a mediator of the beneficial effects of calorie restriction in some animal models (21). Sirt1 regulates glucose and fat metabolism (22, 23). *In vitro*, Sirt1 inhibited the generation of white adipocytes in 3T3L-1 pre-adipocytes by down-regulating Pparγ, a master gene in white adipocytes differentiation (24). *In vivo*, adipose selective over-expression of a dominant negative Sirt1 resulted in dyslipidemia and ectopic lipid deposition (25). Targeted Sirt1 deficiency in mature adipocytes accelerated the onset of obesity-induced insulin resistance and glucose intolerance (26). On the other hand, Sirt1 gain-of-function induced a brown adipocyte-like phenotype in white adipocytes by deacetylating Pparγ and modulating its transcriptional activity (27).

Others and we have previously reported that Sirt1 directly regulates bone osteoblasts, osteoclasts and osteocytes (28–33). However, the role of Sirt1 in MAT is still largely unknown. *In vitro*, Sirt1 and its pharmacologic activation decreased adipogenesis of bone marrow MSCs (34–36). MSC-specific *Sirt1* knock-out mice using the *Prx1-Cre* driver (MSCKO mice) exhibited reduced subcutaneous fat with aging, but no significant change in marrow adipocyte size compared to young mice (37).

Marrow adipogenesis is influenced by the WNT signaling pathway (38, 39). We have previously reported that Sirt1 is a negative regulator of sclerostin, an inhibitor of the canonical WNT pathway in bone (28). Our findings were recently confirmed (40). Moreover, we have shown that the administration of the Sirt1 activator, SRT3025 reduced sclerostin in bone in mice *in vivo* (29), and in human femoral BM-MSCs *in vitro* (41). In the current study we investigated the role of Sirt1 in MAT, and discovered that it induces a thermogenic gene program, characteristic of brown adipocytes, in mouse and human BM-MSCs via PGC1α stimulation and sclerostin inhibition.

METHODS

Animals

Sirt1 haplo-insufficient mice (*Sirt1*$^{\Delta/+}$) lacking exon 4 of the *Sirt1* gene and their wild type (WT) littermates of 129/Sv background were a generous gift (see Acknowledgments), and were used for this study (42). Adult 5–7-month-old inbred *Sirt1*$^{\Delta/+}$ and WT female and male mice were studied. Animals were housed under specific pathogen free (SPF) conditions with free access to water and chow #2018 (Teklad Diets, Madison WI), containing 6.2% fat and energy density of 3.1 kCal/gr. Daily food intake was determined for each mouse for 3 weeks between age 5 and 6 months. Fasting (overnight) glucose was determined in blood collected from the tail vein by an automatic glucometer (Accuchek; Roche Diagnostics GmbH, Mannheim, Germany). For Glucose Challenge Test (GCT) mice were fasted overnight. Glucose 2 g/kg was injected intra-peritoneal, and blood was collected in 15 min intervals for 2 h. Mice were sacrificed using isoflurane inhalation (Minrad INC, USA). Whole tibia with marrow and L3–L5 were removed, immediately frozen in liquid nitrogen and stored in −80°C until analyzed. For bone fat volume determination tibiae were kept in 10% formalin for 48 h and then transferred to phosphate buffered saline (PBS) until analyzed. For bone histology tibiae were dehydrated in 50% and then in 70% EtOH and kept at 4°C. All experiments were performed with the approval of the Animal Study Committee of the Hebrew University-Hadassah Medical School (MD-12-13154-3).

Determination of Bone Marrow Fat

To determine tibiae bone marrow fat volume osmium tetroxide staining followed by micro-computed tomography (μCT) analysis was performed in WT and *Sirt1*$^{\Delta/+}$ female mice, as previously described (43). Briefly, tibiae were fixed in 10% formalin, decalcified in 0.5 M EDTA, soaked in a 1:1 solution of equal volumes of 2% aqueous osmium tetroxide (O_sO_4) and 5% potassium dichromate. The intact bones were scanned at 6 μm resolution using micro-focus conebeam X-ray computed tomography (μCT40 Scanco Medical AG Brüttisellen, Switzerland). The scanner was operated at 55 KVp, 144 μA, collecting 2,000 projections per rotation at 300 ms integration time. Total tibiae marrow fat volume as well as marrow fat volumes in the proximal and distal fourths were measured separately for each mouse. Histologic analysis was performed on 4 μm thick decalcified tibial sections from the proximal tibiae and stained with hematoxylin. Adipocytes were identified as empty oval structures and were manually counted, as previously described (44). Bone marrow fat area was determined as the fraction of adipocyte area per total area. Images were obtained with a DS-Fi camera attached to an Eclipse 80i microscope (Nikon, USA), and analyzed with ImageJ (National Institutes of Health, USA, https://imagej.nih.gov/ij/).

Primary Bone Marrow Cell Cultures

Bone marrow cells were harvested from femurs and tibiae of 6 month-old *Sirt1*$^{\Delta/+}$ and WT female mice. The femurs and tibiae were removed and cleaned of connective tissue, the ends were cut, and the marrow was flushed with α-MEM/15% fetal bovine serum. Single-cell suspensions were prepared in α-MEM by drawing the cells several times through graded needles. Cells collected from each mouse were plated in 100 mm plate. Non-adherent cells were removed after 3 days and the medium was changed every 3 days. Ten days later cells were harvested and plated in a density of 2x10^5 cells/well in six-well-plates. Adipogenesis was induced by 10 μg/ml insulin/50 μM dexamethasone/100 μM indomethacin/500 μM 3-isobutyl-1-methylxanthine administered on day 14 post plating at 70% confluence. RNA was isolated on day 3 post adipogenic induction.

Experiments in the Murine Mesenchymal Stem-Cell Line C3H10T1/2

The C3H10T1/2 (ATCC CCL-226) murine mesenchymal stem cell line is an established cell line model to investigate bone marrow adipocytes (45, 46). Sirt1 over-expressing C3H10T1/2 cells (*Sirt1-OE*) were previously generated and reported by us through stable retroviral infection with pBABE-*Sirt1* (28). Adipogenesis was induced in C3H10T1/2 and in *Sirt1-OE* cells with 10 μg/ml insulin/50 μM dexamethasone/100 μM indomethacin/500 μM 3-isobutyl-1-methylxanthine administered for 4 days followed by 10 μg/ml insulin/50 μM dexamethasone/5 μM rosiglitazone administration with medium changes twice a week (47). Protein was purified on day 7 post adipogenic induction. Adipogenesis was determined by oil-red-o staining on day 8–10 and was normalized to cell number determined by crystal violet staining (28, 48). In another set of experiments the Sirt1 activating compound SRT3025 (29, 49), kindly provided by SIRTRIS/GSK, was dissolved in dimethyl sulfoxide (DMSO) according to the manufacturer's instructions and was co-administered at a final concentration of 10 μM with the adipogenic medium to C3H10T1/2 cells. RNA was isolated on day 1. Oil-red-o staining and protein purification were conducted as described above.

The Sirt1 inhibiting compound Ex527 (6-Chloro-2,3,4,9-tetrahydro-1H-Carbazole-1-carboxamide; E7034, Sigma-Aldrich, Ukraine) (29, 50, 51) was dissolved in dimethyl sulfoxide (DMSO) according to the manufacturer's instructions and was co-administered at a final concentration of 10 μM with the adipogenic medium to C3H10T1/2 cells. RNA purification was conducted as described above.

Experiments in Human Bone Marrow Mesenchymal Stromal Cells

Human bone marrow mesenchymal stromal cells (hBM-MSCs) have the capacity to spontaneously differentiate into adipocytes in *ex vivo* cell cultures without the addition of an adipogenic medium (52). Fresh femoral bone marrow was harvested during femoral canal preparation from three female patients (age 68 ± 9.3 years) undergoing hip replacement for hip osteoarthritis or fractured head of femur (n = 4, age 81 ± 8.1), as part of an ongoing research project which was previously reported by us (41). None of the patients had diabetes or was treated with medications known to affect glucose, lipid or bone metabolism. The study was approved by the Hadassah-Hebrew University Medical Center ethics committee (HMO-0369-10), and informed consent was obtained from each patient prior to surgery. The bone marrow aspirate was collected in growing medium (GM) containing DMEM/5 mM glucose/10%FBS/100 Units/ml penicillin/100 mg/ml streptomycin sulfate/0.25 mg/ml amphotericin B, treated with Lymphoprep #1114544 (Ficoll, Axis-Shield PoC AS, Oslo, Norway), and centrifuged at 900 g for 30 min. Cells at the intermediate interface were collected and centrifuged again at 900 g for 10 min. The resulting mononuclear pellet was re-suspended in GM, plated at a density of 5 × 10^5 cells/35 mm dish and cultured in GM with a medium change twice a week (53). The Sirt1 activator SRT3025 at concentration of 5 μM or a vehicle was added upon confluence and with every medium change. RNA was collected 3 days following treatment initiation, while protein collection was carried out on day 10.

Gene Expression Analysis

Whole tibiae and vertebrae with marrow, primary cultures of BMSCs, C3H10T1/2 cells and human BM-MSCs were homogenized in TRIzol (Invitrogen, Carlsbad CA). Total RNA was extracted, converted to cDNA using the qScript kit (Quanta BioSciences, Inc. Gaithersburg, MD, USA). Gene expression analysis was performed using SYBR Green-based real-time-PCR (Kapa Syber, Kapa Biosystems (Pty) Ltd, Cape Town, South Africa). **Supplementary Table 1** provides all of the primer sequences used in this study. Relative gene expression was determined by the comparative CT method with *βActin* and *Polr2a* as controls in murine and cell line experiments (geometric mean). *βActin* was used as control for analysis of experiments conducted in human BM-MSCs. For experiments conducted in C3H10T1/2 cells gene expression was further normalized to the expression of *Adipoq*. For experiments conducted in human BM-MSCs data was further normalized to *PPARγ* expression.

Protein Analysis

Protein was extracted in Laemmli buffer (2% SDS/10% glycerol/5% 2-mercaptoethanol/ 0.01% bromphenol blue/60 mM Tris HCl). Antibodies for immunoblotting: Prdm16 (AbCam, ab106410), Pgc1α (Cell Signaling, #2178). α-Tubulin (AbCam, ab106375). Glyceraldehyde-3-phosphate dehydrogenase (GAPDH, Abcam, ab8245).

Statistical Analysis

Results are presented as Mean ± SEM. Data was analyzed by unpaired Student's *t*-test to compare group means. 1-way ANOVA followed by Holm-Sidak's analysis was used to compare three groups. Analysis was performed using GraphPad (San Diego, CA, USA) Prism version 6.01. Each experiment was conducted in triplicates and was repeated at least 3 times. $P < 0.05$ was considered statistically significant.

RESULTS

Reduced Expression of Thermogenic Genes in MAT of Sirt1$^{\Delta/+}$ Female Mice

Basal metabolic parameters including body weight, daily food intake, fasting glucose and the response to glucose load did not differ between WT and *Sirt1*$^{\Delta/+}$ mice of both genders (**Supplementary Figures 1A–H**). Previous work by others and us has demonstrated a sexual dimorphism with regard to the effects of Sirt1 deficiency in bone, showing a bone phenotype in female but not in male mice (28, 30, 31). We therefore conducted most of our studies in female mice. Whole tibiae bone marrow fat volume determined by osmium staining was not different between WT and *Sirt1*$^{\Delta/+}$ female mice (**Figure 1A**). Proximal and distal tibial marrow fat volume also did not differ between WT and *Sirt1*$^{\Delta/+}$ mice. In agreement with these results, tibial marrow adipocyte number and area was

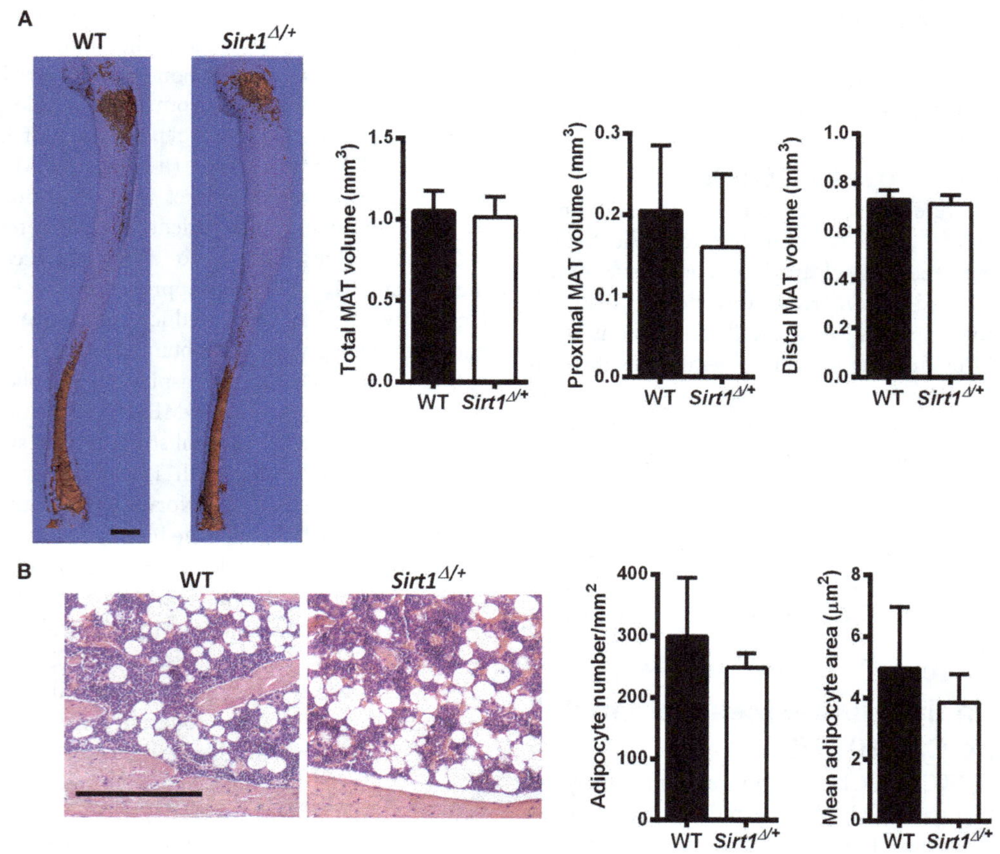

FIGURE 1 | Marrow adipose tissue (MAT) in *Sirt1*$^{\Delta/+}$ and WT female mice **(A)**. Osmium tetroxide staining of tibiae followed by µCT analysis; A representative image (left) and quantification (right). Data is presented as fat volume. Scale bar 1 mm ($n = 8$ mice/group). **(B)** Hematoxylin-stained histological sections of proximal tibiae. Scale bar 200 µm; ($n = 3$ mice/group). Results are Mean ± SEM.

similar in WT and $Sirt1^{\Delta/+}$ female mice (**Figure 1B**). Strikingly, gene expression analysis in tibial MAT revealed a dramatic decrease of ~50% in the thermogenic genes: *β3AR, FoxC2, Prdm16, Pgc1α,* and *Dio2* in $Sirt1^{\Delta/+}$ compared to WT female mice (**Figure 2A**). Importantly, *Prdm16* and *Pgc1α* mRNA expression was significantly decreased by over 2 fold in $Sirt1^{\Delta/+}$ compared to WT-derived primary BMSC cultures induced to adipogenesis (**Figure 2B**), indicating a cell autonomous effect of Sirt1 on the bone marrow adipocyte. No differences in tibial MAT gene expression were observed in $Sirt1^{\Delta/+}$ compared to WT male mice (**Figure 2C**). Thermogenic genes expression in vertebral MAT did not differ between genotypes in both genders (**Figures 3A,B**). Taken together, these results indicate that Sirt1 haplo-insufficiency leads to reduced thermogenic genes expression in tibial MAT in female mice.

We next asked if Sirt1 stimulation reciprocally increases the expression of a thermogenic genes program in BMSCs. To address this question three *in vitro* models were employed: (1) Sirt1 over-expressing C3H10T1/2 cells induced to adipogenesis. (2) Pharmacologic activation of Sirt1 by SRT3025 in C3H10T1/2 cells induced to adipogenesis. (3) Pharmacologic activation of Sirt1 in primary human femoral BM-MSCs.

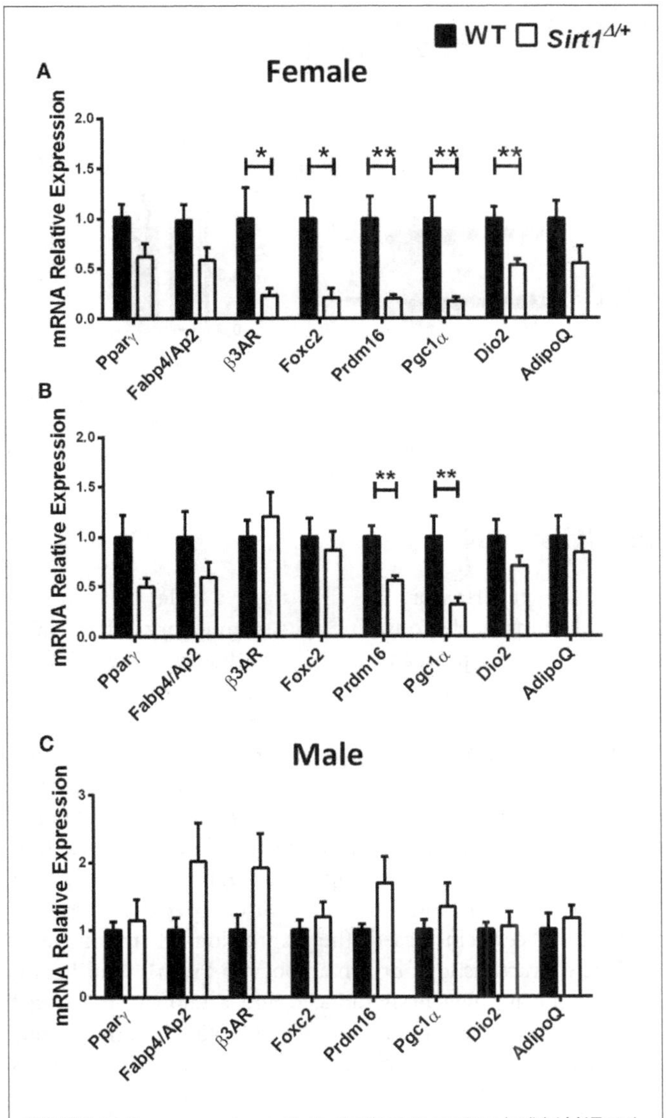

FIGURE 2 | Gene expression analysis of adipocyte markers in tibial MAT and primary bone marrow stromal cell cultures obtained from $Sirt1^{\Delta/+}$ and WT mice **(A)**. Gene expression analysis of adipocyte markers in tibial MAT obtained from 5-month old $Sirt1^{\Delta/+}$ and WT female mice ($n = 6$–9 mice/group). **(B)** Gene expression analysis of adipocyte markers in primary bone marrow stromal cell cultures induced to adipogenesis, derived from $Sirt1^{\Delta/+}$ and WT female mice ($n = 6$ mice/group). **(C)** Gene expression analysis of adipocyte markers in tibial MAT obtained from 5-month old $Sirt1^{\Delta/+}$ and WT male mice ($n = 6$–9 mice/group). Results are Mean ± SEM. $^{*}P < 0.05$; $^{**}P < 0.01$ vs. wild type mice (WT).

Increased Thermogenic Markers in Sirt1 Over-Expressing C3H10T1/2 cells

Decreased lipid accumulation was observed in *Sirt1 OE* compared to control C3H10T1/2 cells induced to adipogenesis (**Figure 4A**). Elevated Prdm16 and Pgc1α protein level was observed in *Sirt1 OE* compared to control cells (**Figures 4B,C**). Consistent with these results, pharmacologic activation of Sirt1 by SRT3025 reduced the generation of white adipocytes and stimulated the expression of *Pgc1α, Dio2, FoxC2, Tfam,* and *Cytochrome C* (**Figures 5A–C**). In contrast, Sirt1 inhibition by Ex527 significantly reduced the expression of *Ucp1* (**Figure 5D**).

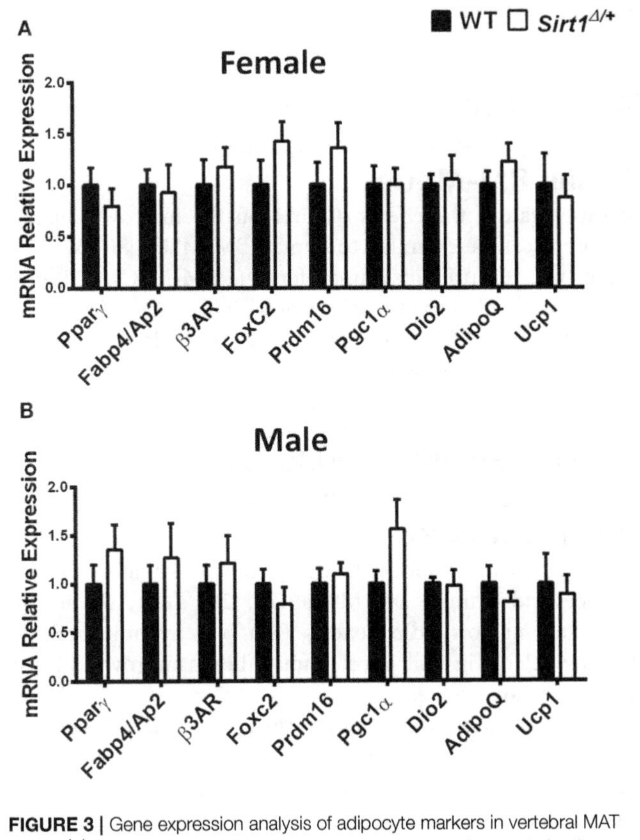

FIGURE 3 | Gene expression analysis of adipocyte markers in vertebral MAT in $Sirt1^{\Delta/+}$ and WT female and male mice, Gene expression analysis of adipocyte markers in vertebral MAT obtained from 5-month old $Sirt1^{\Delta/+}$ and WT female **(A)** and male **(B)** mice ($n = 10$ mice/group). Results are Mean ± SEM.

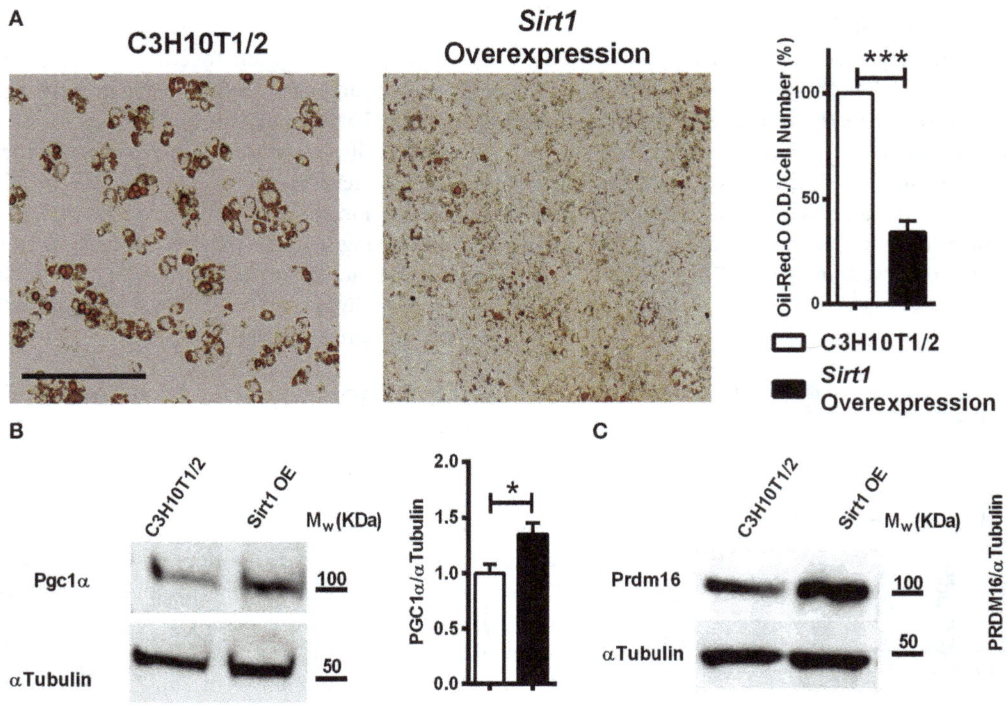

FIGURE 4 | The effect of *Sirt1* over-expression on adipogenesis in C3HT101/2 cells **(A)**. Oil-red-o staining in *Sirt1* over-expressing (*OE*) and C3H10T1/2 cells induced to adipogenesis. Data is presented as optical density (OD) corrected for cell number (crystal violet staining). Scale bar 500μm. **(B,C)** Immunoblot of Pgc1α and Prdm16 in *Sirt1 OE* and C3H10T1/2 cells 7 days post induction to adipogenesis. Results are Mean ± SEM. *$P < 0.05$; ***$P < 0.001$ vs. C3HT101/2 cells.

Sirt1 Activation by SRT3025 Promotes Thermogenic Genes Expression in Human BM-MSCs

To investigate if the effects of Sirt1 on the marrow adipocyte phenotype can be extended to human BM-MSCs, SRT3025 was administered to primary human femoral BM-MSCs. Strikingly, SRT3025-treated human BM-MSCs had increased mRNA expression of *PGC1α* (**Figure 6A**) accompanied by elevated PGC1α protein level (**Figure 6B**), suggesting that Sirt1 activates PGC1α in human femoral BM-MSCs.

Blocking Sclerostin Induces a Thermogenic Gene Program in Human BM-MSCs

We have previously shown that Sirt1 down-regulates sclersotin in mice and human BM-MSCs (28, 29, 41). As sclersotin stimulates marrow adipogenesis (54), we hypothesized that blocking sclerostin will affect human bone marrow adipocyte gene expression profile.

Indeed, blocking sclerostin with the monoclonal antibody Scl-AbII (55, 56) induced a marked increase in gene expression of: *PRDM16*, *β3AR*, *FOXC2*, and importantly an over 2-fold increase in *UCP1* expression, the hallmark of brown and beige adipocytes (**Figure 6C**). These effects were accompanied by a 2-fold increase in PGC1α protein level (**Figure 6D**). Taken together, this data indicate that blocking sclerostin stimulates a thermogenic genes signature in human femoral BM-MSCs.

DISCUSSION

This study reports for the first time a role for Sirt1 in MAT phenotype, demonstrating its stimulatory effect on a thermogenic gene program in marrow adipocytes. *Sirt1* haplo-insufficiency resulted in decreased expression of thermogenic gene markers in MAT in a gender- and site-specific manner. Reduced expression of *β3AR, FoxC2, Prdm16, Pgc1α,* and *Dio2* was found in tibial but not in vertebral MAT derived from adult female but not male $Sirt1^{\Delta/+}$ mice. Similar effects were noted in primary BM-MSC cultures derived from $Sirt1^{\Delta/+}$ mice, indicating a cell autonomous effect of Sirt1 on the BM-MSC. *In vitro*, Sirt1 over-expression in CH310T1/2 cells increased the expression of thermogenic markers characteristic of brown adipocytes Prdm16 and Pgc1α, a mitochondrial biogenesis inducer, and a known Sirt1 target (57). Importantly, in human femoral BM-MSCs pharmacologic Sirt1 activation and blocking its target, sclerostin, had a stimulatory effect on Pgc1α protein level and thermogenic genes expression.

Sirt1 was previously shown to directly deacetylase Pgc1α in liver and muscle, thereby promoting its phosphorylation by 5' adenosine monophosphate-activated protein kinase (AMPK), resulting in its activation (58, 59). The current study demonstrates for the first time that Sirt1 upregulates Pgc1α in murine and human BM-MSCs. Pgc1α was reported to increase thermogenic genes expression in white subcutaneous adipocytes (60) and brown adipocytes (61). Furthermore, Pgc1α is a master

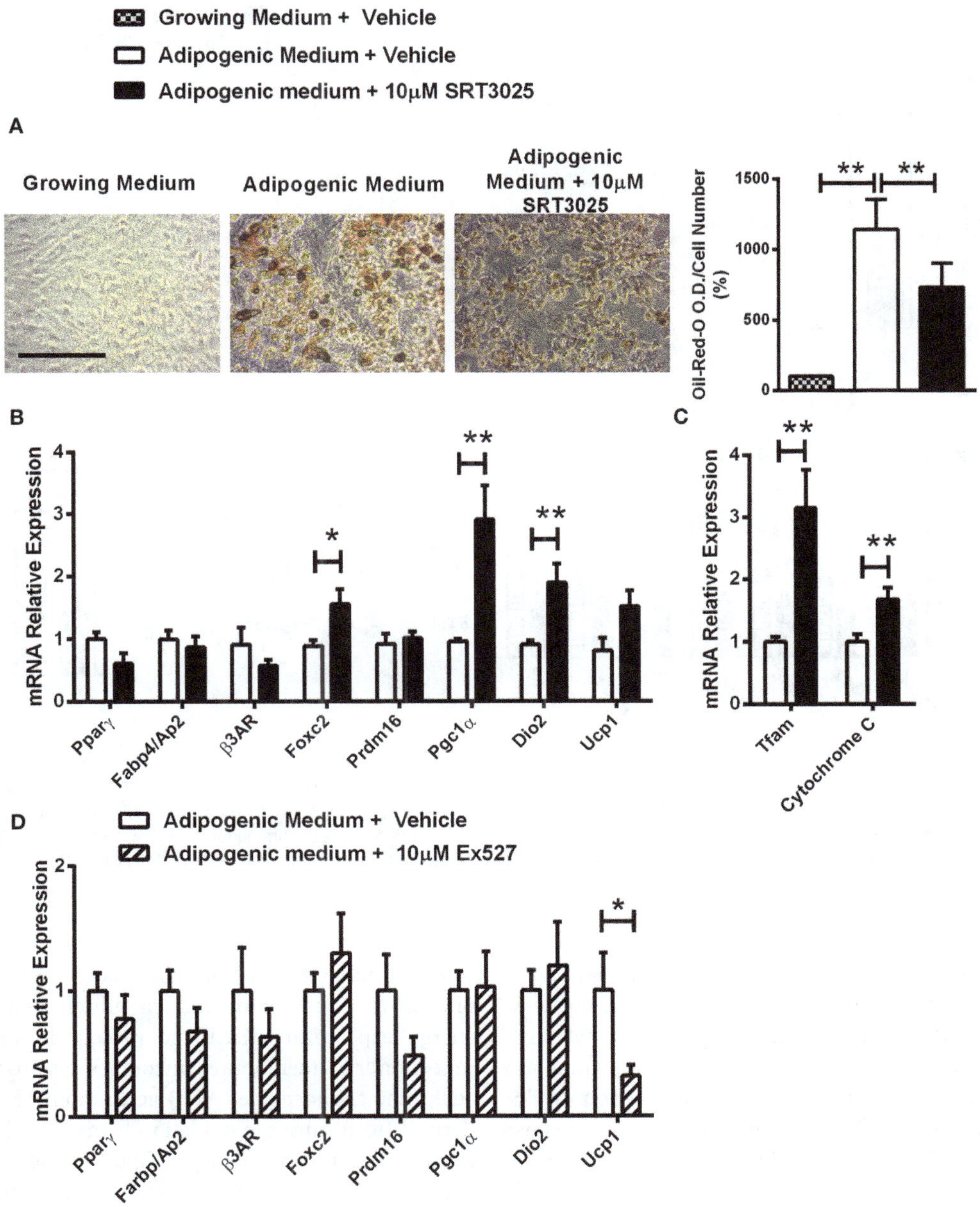

FIGURE 5 | The effects of Sirt1 pharmacologic activation and inhibition on adipogenic markers in C3HT101/2 cells **(A)**. Oil-red-o staining in C3H10T1/2 cells induced to adipogenesis and supplemented with SRT3025 or vehicle (DMSO). **(B,C)** Gene expression analysis of adipocyte **(B)** and mitochondrial markers **(C)** induced to adipogenesis and supplemented with SRT3025 or vehicle (DMSO). **(D)** Gene expression analysis of adipocyte markers induced to adipogenesis and supplemented with Ex527 or vehicle (DMSO). Results are Mean ± SEM. $^*P < 0.05$; $^{**}P < 0.01$ vs. vehicle-treated C3HT101/2 cells.

mitochondrial regulator, stimulating mitochondrial biogenesis and inducing the expression of components of the mitochondrial respiratory chain. Indeed, in our study gene expression of *Tfam*, a marker of mitochondrial biogenesis, and *Cytochrome C* was significantly increased with Sirt1 pharmacologic activation *in vitro*. The role of Pgc1α in bone and BM-MSCs was only recently revealed. *In vivo* and *in vitro* gain and loss-of-function studies demonstrated that Pgc1α regulates the skeletal stem cell fate, restraining marrow adipocyte differentiation and promoting osteogenesis (62). Our data indicate that Sirt1 stimulates Pgc1α expression in BM-MSCs thereby leading to induction of a thermogenic gene program.

Interestingly, Prdm16 was also consistently influenced by Sirt1 status in the various *in vivo* and *in vitro* models employed in this study. Prdm16 was significantly decreased in tibial MAT and in primary BM-MSC cultures derived from $Sirt1^{\Delta/+}$ compared to WT female mice. Along these lines, it was markedly increased with Sirt1 over-expression or activation *in vitro*. Prdm16 is an activator of Pgc1α expression and transcriptional function through direct protein interaction. It also induces *Pgc1α*, *Ucp1*,

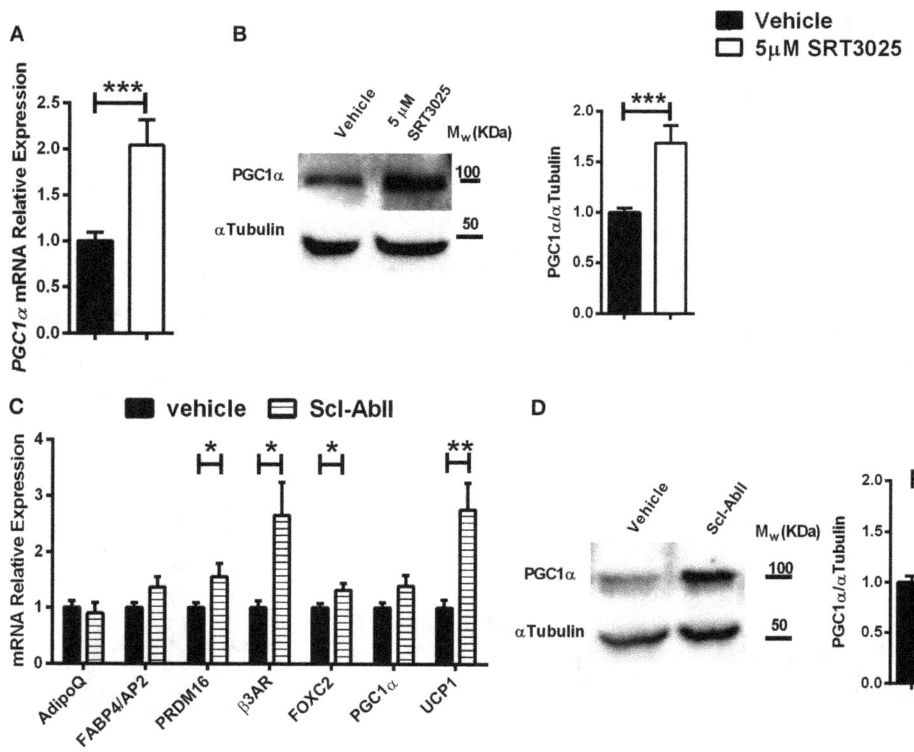

FIGURE 6 | The effects of SRT3025 and anti-Sclerostin antibody on adipogenic markers in human femoral bone marrow mesynchemal stem cells (hBM-MSCs) **(A)**. Gene expression analysis of PGC1α in SRT3025-treated hBM-MSCs. **(B)** Immunoblot of PGC1α. A representative image (left) and densitometry (right) with αTubulin as control. **(C)** Gene expression analysis of thermogenic genes in anti-Sclerostin AbII treated hBM-MSCs **(D)**. Immunoblot of PGC1α in hBM-MSCs treated with anti-Sclerostin AbII. A representative image (left) and densitometry (right) with αTubulin as control. Results are mean ± SEM. $^{*}P < 0.05$; $^{**}P < 0.01$; $^{***}P < 0.001$ vs. vehicle-treated hBM-MSCs.

and *Dio2* expression in adipocytes (63). However, regulation of Prdm16 by Sirt1 has not been described before. Only one study demonstrated that Sirt1-dependent Pparγ deacetylation allows Prdm16 recruitment to Pparγ thereby modulating its transcriptional activity, favoring BAT genes expression while repressing WAT genes (27). Thus, the underlying mechanisms governing the observed changes in Prdm16 in this study remain to be elucidated.

We have previously reported that Sirt1 down-regulates sclerostin by deacetylating histones 3 and 4 at its promoter, leading to inhibition of *Sost* gene expression (28). These results were recently confirmed by Stegen et al who demonstrated that conditional deletion of the oxygen sensor prolyl hydroxylase (PHD) 2 in osteocytes resulted in enhanced HIF-1α signaling that stimulated Sirt1-dependent deacetylation of the *Sost* promoter and reduced sclerostin expression (40). Sclerostin, an inhibitor of the WNT/β-catenin pathway, was reported to induce adipocyte differentiation in 3T3-L1 cells (64), primary murine BM-MSCs (54), and human BM-MSCs (54). Along these lines, lower levels of MAT were found in tibiae of sclerostin knock-out (SOST-KO) mice, while sclerostin neutralization with a neutralizing antibody significantly decreased MAT (54). Our results demonstrate for the first time that blocking sclerostin with a neutralizing antibody, currently under advanced investigation for the treatment of osteoporosis, induces a thermogenic gene program in human BM-MSCs, and increases the expression of *UCP1*, a driver of mitochondrial heat generation and energy expenditure. UCP1, a protein located on the inner mitochondrial membrane, uncouples electron transport from adenosine triphosphate (ATP) generation. The resulting energy derived from substrate oxidation is dissipated as heat. UCP1 is expressed in brown and beige adipocytes. Some previous studies failed to detect it in MAT, while others reported low expression levels (11, 44). The metabolic significance of inducing UCP1 in MAT by blocking sclerostin remains to be investigated.

Differences in MAT phenotype between $Sirt1^{\Delta/+}$ and WT female mice were detected in tibiae but not in lumbar MAT. Lumbar vertebrae is a skeletal site in the mouse that has little MAT, whereas proximal tibial MAT was shown to be metabolically responsive to cold exposure (20). Caudal vertebrae was previously shown to have characteristics of constitutive MAT (cMAT) that contains large adipocytes and does not respond to systemic challenges. Thus, lack of difference in vertebral MAT phenotype is not surprising. Of note, most of the studies investigating murine MAT have used the C57BL/6J and C3H/HeJ mouse strains, whereas data in 129/Sv used in this study, is lacking.

This study is not without its limitations. The physiologic significance of our findings could not be evaluated in the mouse model used in this study. Exposure of MSC-specific

Sirt1 knock-out mice to cold temperature or a high fat diet could have provided insight into the contribution of MAT Sirt1 to local and whole body energy metabolism and needs to be performed in future studies. Secondly, gene expression analyses were performed in whole tibiae and vertebrae extracts similar to previously published studies (4, 65), and introduce the bias of contamination by other cell types. However, consistent results were obtained in primary BM-MSCs cultures derived from $Sirt1^{\Delta/+}$ and WT mice, supporting the notion of a direct cell autonomous effect of Sirt1 on the marrow adipocyte phenotype. Thirdly, we did not account for regional differences in tibial MAT composition, as was previously suggested (66). Finally, additional Sirt1 targets beyond Pgc1α and sclerostin may have played a role in driving a brown-like adipocyte gene expression program in BM-MSCs.

Whether inducing a thermogenic gene program in marrow adipocytes is beneficial to bone health, hematopoiesis local and whole body energy metabolism begs further investigation. Reduced MAT expression of brown adipocyte markers was previously reported in diabetic and aged mice, conditions associated with both increased skeletal fragility and impaired energy metabolism (44). Due to its wide favorable physiologic effects, Sirt1 has been considered an attractive therapeutic target for drug discovery. Sirtuin1 activating compounds (STACs) were generated, amongst them SRT3025, used in this study. SRT3025 was previously shown by us to restore bone mass and strength in OVX mice (29), but also to have off-target effects (67). In humans SRT3025 was shown to prolong QTc and its development was discontinued (68). As NAD^+ is an indispensable co-substrate required for Sirt1 and other sirtuins activity, there has been an increasing interest in small molecules that raise NAD+ levels as a mechanism to stimulate sirtuins activity (69).

In conclusion, this study shows that Sirt1 regulates the bone marrow adipocyte phenotype inducing a thermogenic gene program in mouse and human BM-MSCs. Inducing BAT-like features in subcutaneous and visceral fat depots is a much desired goal in combating obesity. Whether browning of MAT by Sirt1 activation, sclerostin inhibition or other mechanisms is a plausible novel approach to serve this goal while improving skeletal health remains to be elucidated.

ETHICS STATEMENT

This study was carried out in accordance with the recommendations of IHC-GCP, Public Heath Regulation, the Governing regulations of Ministry of Health. The protocol was approved by The Ethics (Helsinki) Committee at Hadassah University Hospital. All subjects gave written informed consent in accordance with the Declaration of Helsinki.

AUTHOR CONTRIBUTIONS

HA designed and performed most of the experiments and analyzed the data. IG designed and conducted some of the *in vitro* experiments. ME-H, LK, and OS were responsible for studies in humans. ME-H obtained the human samples and performed the experiments. RM and GK designed and conducted the marrow fat μCT quantification studies. GB performed experiments in murine BM-MSCs. EC-K designed and performed the experiments in human BM-MSCs. EA performed some *in vitro* experiments with SRT3025. RD-P conceived and designed the study, prepared the manuscript, and takes full responsibility for the work as a whole.

ACKNOWLEDGMENTS

We thank Frederick W. Alt of Harvard University for providing the $Sirt1^{\Delta/+}$ mice, SIRTRIS/GSK and Amgen for providing SRT3025 and Scl-AbII, respectively. We thank the late Raymond Kaplan and the Bnai Brith Leo Baeck London Lodge for their support of osteoporosis research. The osmium tetroxide staining was performed at the SCOPEM (Scientific Center for Optical and Electron Microscopy), ETH, Zurich. We thank Dr. Stephan Preibisch SCOPEM for his assistance.

REFERENCES

1. Cawthorn WP, Scheller EL, Learman BS, Parlee SD, Simon BR, Mori H. et al. Bone marrow adipose tissue is an endocrine organ that contributes to increased circulating adiponectin during caloric restriction. *Cell Metab.* (2014) 20:368–75. doi: 10.1016/j.cmet.2014.06.003
2. Bredella MA, Fazeli PK, Miller KK, Misra M, Torriani M, Thomas BJ, et al. Increased bone marrow fat in anorexia nervosa. *J Clin Endocrinol Metab.* (2009) 94:2129–36. doi: 10.1210/jc.2008-2532
3. Tencerova M, Figeac F, Ditzel N, Taipaleenmaki H, Nielsen TK, Kassem M. High-fat diet-induced obesity promotes expansion of bone marrow adipose tissue and impairs skeletal stem cell functions in mice. *J Bone Miner Res.* (2018) 33:1154–65. doi: 10.1002/jbmr.3408
4. Styner M, Pagnotti GM, McGrath C, Wu X, Sen B, Uzer G, et al. Exercise decreases marrow adipose tissue through ss-oxidation in obese running mice. *J Bone Miner Res.* (2017) 32:1692–702. doi: 10.1002/jbmr.3159
5. Crossno JT Jr, Majka SM, Grazia T, Gill RG, Klemm DJ. Rosiglitazone promotes development of a novel adipocyte population from bone marrow-derived circulating progenitor cells. *J Clin Invest.* (2006) 116:3220–8. doi: 10.1172/JCI28510
6. Ryden M, Uzunel M, Hard JL, Borgstrom E, Mold JE, Arner E, et al. Transplanted bone marrow-derived cells contribute to human adipogenesis. *Cell Metab.* (2015) 22:408–17. doi: 10.1016/j.cmet.2015.06.011
7. Fazeli PK, Horowitz MC, MacDougald OA, Scheller EL, Rodeheffer MS, Rosen

CJ, et al. Marrow fat and bone-new perspectives. *J Clin Endocrinol Metab.* (2013) 98:935–45. doi: 10.1210/jc.2012-3634
8. Rosen CJ, Bouxsein ML. Mechanisms of disease: is osteoporosis the obesity of bone? *Nat Clin Pract Rheumatol.* (2006) 2:35–43. doi: 10.1038/ncprheum0070
9. Scheller EL, Rosen CJ. What's the matter with MAT? marrow adipose tissue, metabolism, and skeletal health. *Ann N Y Acad Sci.* (2014) 1311:14–30. doi: 10.1111/nyas.12327
10. Georgiou KR, Hui SK, Xian CJ. Regulatory pathways associated with bone loss and bone marrow adiposity caused by aging, chemotherapy, glucocorticoid therapy and radiotherapy. *Am J Stem Cells.* (2012) 1:205–24.
11. Ambrosi TH, Scialdone A, Graja A, Gohlke S, Jank AM, Bocian C, et al. Adipocyte accumulation in the bone marrow during obesity and aging impairs stem cell-based hematopoietic and bone regeneration. *Cell Stem Cell.* (2017) 20:771–84 e6. doi: 10.1016/j.stem.2017.02.00
12. Naveiras O, Nardi V, Wenzel PL, Hauschka PV, Fahey F, Daley GQ. Bone-marrow adipocytes as negative regulators of the haematopoietic microenvironment. *Nature.* (2009) 460:259–63. doi: 10.1038/nature08099
13. Morris EV, Edwards CM. Bone marrow adipose tissue: a new player in cancer metastasis to bone. *Front Endocrinol.* 7:90. doi: 10.3389/fendo.2016.00090
14. Kajimura S, Spiegelman BM, Seale P. Brown and beige fat: physiological roles beyond heat generation. *Cell Metab.* (2015) 22:546–559. doi: 10.1016/j.cmet.2015.09.007
15. Bianco P, Robey PG. Skeletal stem cells. *Development.* (2015) 142:1023–7. doi: 10.1242/dev.102210
16. Bianco P, Cao X, Frenette PS, Mao JJ, Robey PG, Simmons PJ, et al. The meaning, the sense and the significance: translating the science of mesenchymal stem cells into medicine. *Nat Med.* (2013) 19:35–42. doi: 10.1038/nm.3028
17. Zhou BO, Yue R, Murphy MM, Peyer JG, Morrison SJ. Leptin-receptor-expressing mesenchymal stromal cells represent the main source of bone formed by adult bone marrow. *Cell Stem Cell.* (2014) 15:154–68. doi: 10.1016/j.stem.2014.06.008
18. Yue R, Zhou BO, Shimada IS, Zhao Z, Morrison SJ. Leptin receptor promotes adipogenesis and reduces osteogenesis by regulating mesenchymal stromal cells in adult bone marrow. *Cell Stem Cell.* (2016) 18:782–96. doi: 10.1016/j.stem.2016.02.015
19. Fan Y, Hanai JI, Le PT, Bi R, Maridas D, DeMambro V, et al. Parathyroid hormone directs bone marrow mesenchymal cell fate. *Cell Metab.* (2017) 25:661–72. doi: 10.1016/j.cmet.2017.01.001
20. Scheller EL, Doucette CR, Learman BS, Cawthorn WP, Khandaker S, Schell B, et al. Region-specific variation in the properties of skeletal adipocytes reveals regulated and constitutive marrow adipose tissues. *Nat Commun.* (2015) 6:7808. doi: 10.1038/ncomms8808
21. Guarente L, Picard F. Calorie restriction-the SIR2 connection. *Cell.* (2005) 120:473–82. doi: 10.1016/j.cell.2005.01.029
22. Haigis MC, Guarente LP. Mammalian sirtuins-emerging roles in physiology, aging, and calorie restriction. *Genes Dev.* (2006) 20:2913–21. doi: 10.1101/gad.1467506
23. Bordone L, Cohen D, Robinson A, Motta MC, van Veen E, Czopik A, et al. SIRT1 transgenic mice show phenotypes resembling calorie restriction. *Aging Cell.* (2007) 6:759–67. doi: 10.1111/j.1474-9726.2007.00335.x
24. Picard F, Kurtev M, Chung N, Topark-Ngarm A, Senawong T, Machado De Oliveira R, et al. Sirt1 promotes fat mobilization in white adipocytes by repressing PPAR-gamma. *Nature.* (2004) 429:771–6. doi: 10.1038/nature02583
25. Xu C, Cai Y, Fan P, Bai B, Chen J, Deng HB, et al. Calorie restriction prevents metabolic aging caused by abnormal SIRT1 function in adipose tissues. *Diabetes.* (2015) 64:1576–90. doi: 10.2337/db14-1180
26. Hui X, Zhang M, Gu P, Li K, Gao Y, Wu D, et al. Adipocyte SIRT1 controls systemic insulin sensitivity by modulating macrophages in adipose tissue. *EMBO Rep.* (2017) 18:645–57. doi: 10.15252/embr.201643184
27. Qiang L, Wang L, Kon N, Zhao W, Lee S, Zhang Y, et al. Brown remodeling of white adipose tissue by SirT1-dependent deacetylation of Ppargamma. *Cell.* (2012) 150:620–32. doi: 10.1016/j.cell.2012.06.027
28. Cohen-Kfir E, Artsi H, Levin A, Abramowitz E, Bajayo A, Gurt I, et al. Sirt1 is a regulator of bone mass and a repressor of Sost encoding for sclerostin, a bone formation inhibitor. *Endocrinology.* (2011) 152:4514–24. doi: 10.1210/en.2011-1128
29. Artsi H, Cohen-Kfir E, Gurt I, Shahar R, Bajayo A, Kalish N, et al. The Sirtuin1 activator SRT3025 down-regulates sclerostin and rescues ovariectomy-induced bone loss and biomechanical deterioration in female mice. *Endocrinology.* (2014) 155:3508–15. doi: 10.1210/en.2014-1334
30. Edwards JR, Perrien DS, Fleming N, Nyman JS, Ono K, Connelly L, et al. Silent information regulator (Sir)T1 inhibits NF-kappaB signaling to maintain normal skeletal remodeling. *J Bone Miner Res.* (2013) 28:960–9. doi: 10.1002/jbmr.1824
31. Iyer S, Han L, Bartell SM, Kim HN, Gubrij I, de Cabo R, et al. Sirtuin1 (Sirt1) promotes cortical bone formation by preventing beta-catenin sequestration by FoxO transcription factors in osteoblast progenitors. *J Biol Chem.* (2014) 289:9–78. doi: 10.1074/jbc.M114.56180
32. Zainabadi K, Liu CJ, Caldwell AL, Guarente L. SIRT1 is a positive regulator of *in vivo* bone mass and a therapeutic target for osteoporosis. *PLoS ONE.* (2017) 12:e0185236. doi: 10.1371/journal.pone.0185236
33. Zainabadi K, Liu CJ, Guarente L. SIRT1 is a positive regulator of the master osteoblast transcription factor, RUNX2. *PLoS ONE.* (2017) 12:e0178520. doi: 10.1371/journal.pone.0178520
34. Backesjo CM, Li Y, Lindgren U, Haldosen LA. Activation of Sirt1 decreases adipocyte formation during osteoblast differentiation of mesenchymal stem cells. *J Bone Miner Res.* (2006) 21:993–1002. doi: 10.1359/jbmr.060415
35. Li Y, He X, Li Y, He J, Anderstam B, Andersson G, et al. Nicotinamide phosphoribosyltransferase (Nampt) affects the lineage fate determination of mesenchymal stem cells: a possible cause for reduced osteogenesis and increased adipogenesis in older individuals. *J Bone Miner Res.* (2011) 26:2656–64. doi: 10.1002/jbmr.480
36. Peltz L, Gomez J, Marquez M, Alencastro F, Atashpanjeh N, Quang T, et al. Resveratrol exerts dosage and duration dependent effect on human mesenchymal stem cell development. *PLoS ONE.* (2012) 7:e37162. doi: 10.1371/journal.pone.0037162
37. Simic P, Zainabadi K, Bell E, Sykes DB, Saez B, Lotinun S, et al. SIRT1 regulates differentiation of mesenchymal stem cells by deacetylating beta-catenin. *EMBO Mol Med.* (2013) 5:430–40. doi: 10.1002/emmm.201201606
38. Kennell JA, MacDougald OA. Wnt signaling inhibits adipogenesis through beta-catenin-dependent and -independent mechanisms. *J Biol Chem.* (2005) 280:24004–10. doi: 10.1074/jbc.M501080200
39. Qiu W, Andersen TE, Bollerslev J, Mandrup S, Abdallah BM, Kassem M. Patients with high bone mass phenotype exhibit enhanced osteoblast differentiation and inhibition of adipogenesis of human mesenchymal stem cells. *J Bone Miner Res.* (2007) 22:1720–31. doi: 10.1359/jbmr.070721
40. Stegen S, Stockmans I, Moermans K, Thienpont B, Maxwell PH, Carmeliet P, et al. Osteocytic oxygen sensing controls bone mass through epigenetic regulation of sclerostin. *Nat Commun.* (2018) 9:2557. doi: 10.1038/s41467-018-04679-7
41. El-Haj M, Gurt I, Cohen-Kfir E, Dixit V, Artsi H, Kandel L, et al. Reduced Sirtuin1 expression at the femoral neck in women who sustained an osteoporotic hip fracture. *Osteoporos Int.* (2016) 27:2373–8. doi: 10.1007/s00198-016-3536-4
42. Cheng HL, Mostoslavsky R, Saito S, Manis JP, Gu Y, Patel P, et al. Developmental defects and p53 hyperacetylation in Sir2 homolog (SIRT1)-deficient mice. *Proc Natl Acad Sci USA.* (2003) 100:10794–9. doi: 10.1073/pnas.1934713100
43. Clinthorne JF, Adams DJ, Fenton JI, Ritz BW, Gardner EM. Short-term re-feeding of previously energy-restricted C57BL/6 male mice restores body weight and body fat and attenuates the decline in natural killer cell function after primary influenza infection. *J Nutr.* (2010) 140:1495–501. doi: 10.3945/jn.110.122408
44. Krings A, Rahman S, Huang S, Lu Y, Czernik PJ, Lecka-Czernik B. *Bone* marrow fat has brown adipose tissue characteristics, which are attenuated with aging and diabetes. *Bone.* (2012) 50:546–52. doi: 10.1016/j.bone.2011.06.016
45. Lee N, Kim I, Park S, Han D, Ha S, Kwon M, et al. Creatine inhibits adipogenesis by downregulating insulin-induced activation of the phosphatidylinositol 3-kinase signaling pathway. *Stem Cells Dev.* (2015) 24:983–94. doi: 10.1089/scd.2014.0130

46. Beg M, Chauhan P, Varshney S, Shankar K, Rajan S, Saini D, et al. A withanolide coagulin-L inhibits adipogenesis modulating Wnt/beta-catenin pathway and cell cycle in mitotic clonal expansion. *Phytomedicine.* (2014) 21:406–14. doi: 10.1016/j.phymed.2013.10.009
47. Moisan A, Rivera MN, Lotinun S, Akhavanfard S, Coffman EJ, Cook EB, et al. The WTX tumor suppressor regulates mesenchymal progenitor cell fate specification. *Dev Cell.* (2011) 20:583–96. doi: 10.1016/j.devcel.2011.03.013
48. Scragg MA, Ferreira LR. Evaluation of different staining procedures for the quantification of fibroblasts cultured in 96-well plates. *Anal Biochem.* (1991) 198:80–5. doi: 10.1016/0003-2697(91)90509-R
49. Gilbert RE, Thai K, Advani SL, Cummins CL, Kepecs DM, Schroer SA, et al. SIRT1 activation ameliorates hyperglycaemia by inducing a torpor-like state in an obese mouse model of type 2 diabetes. *Diabetologia.* (2015) 58:819–27. doi: 10.1007/s00125-014-3485-4
50. Gertz M, Fischer F, Nguyen GT, Lakshminarasimhan M, Schutkowski M, Weyand M, et al. Ex-527 inhibits Sirtuins by exploiting their unique NAD+-dependent deacetylation mechanism. *Proc Natl Acad Sci USA.* (2013) 110, E2772–81. doi: 10.1073/pnas.1303628110
51. Yang H, Yang T, Baur JA, Perez E, Matsui T, Carmona JJ, et al. Nutrient-sensitive mitochondrial NAD+ levels dictate cell survival. *Cell.* (2007) 130:1095–107. doi: 10.1016/j.cell.2007.07.035
52. Amable PR, Teixeira MV, Carias RB, Granjeiro J, Borojevic R. Gene expression and protein secretion during human mesenchymal cell differentiation into adipogenic cells. *BMC Cell Biol.* (2014) 15:46. doi: 10.1186/s12860-014-0046-0
53. Mackay DL, Tesar PJ, Liang LN, Haynesworth SE. Characterizing medullary and human mesenchymal stem cell-derived adipocytes. *J Cell Physiol.* (2006) 207:722–8. doi: 10.1002/jcp.20617
54. Fairfield H, Falank C, Harris E, Demambro V, McDonald M, Pettitt JA, et al. The skeletal cell-derived molecule sclerostin drives bone marrow adipogenesis. *J Cell Physiol.* (2018) 233:1156–67. doi: 10.1002/jcp.25976
55. Li X, Ominsky MS, Warmington KS, Morony S, Gong J, Cao J, et al. Sclerostin antibody treatment increases bone formation, bone mass, and bone strength in a rat model of postmenopausal osteoporosis. *J Bone Miner Res.* (2009) 24:578–88. doi: 10.1359/jbmr.081206
56. Li X, Warmington KS, Niu QT, Asuncion FJ, Barrero M, Grisanti M, et al. Inhibition of sclerostin by monoclonal antibody increases bone formation, bone mass, and bone strength in aged male rats. *J Bone Miner Res.* (2010) 25:2647–56. doi: 10.1002/jbmr.182
57. Iwabu M, Yamauchi T, Okada-Iwabu M, Sato K, Nakagawa T, Funata M, et al. Adiponectin and AdipoR1 regulate PGC-1alpha and mitochondria by Ca(2+) and AMPK/SIRT1. *Nature.* (2010) 464:1313–9. doi: 10.1038/nature08991
58. Rodgers JT, Lerin C, Haas W, Gygi SP, Spiegelman BM, Puigserver P. Nutrient control of glucose homeostasis through a complex of PGC-1alpha and SIRT1. *Nature.* (2005) 434:113–8. doi: 10.1038/nature03354
59. Amat R, Planavila A, Chen SL, Iglesias R, Giralt M, Villarroya F. SIRT1 controls the transcription of the peroxisome proliferator-activated receptor-gamma co-activator-1alpha (PGC-1alpha) gene in skeletalmuscle through the PGC-1alpha autoregulatory loop and interaction with MyoD. *J Biol Chem.* (2009) 284:21872–880. doi: 10.1074/jbc.M109.022749
60. Tiraby C, Tavernier G, Lefort C, Larrouy D, Bouillaud F, Ricquier D, et al. Acquirement of brown fat cell features by human white adipocytes. *J Biol Chem.* (2003) 278:33370–6. doi: 10.1074/jbc.M305235200
61. Uldry M, Yang W, St-Pierre J, Lin J, Seale P, Spiegelman BM. Complementary action of the PGC-1 coactivators in mitochondrial biogenesis and brown fat differentiation. *Cell Metab.* (2006) 3:333–41. doi: 10.1016/j.cmet.2006.04.002
62. Yu B, Huo L, Liu Y, Deng P, Szymanski J, Li J, et al. PGC-1alpha controls skeletal stem cell fate and bone-fat balance in osteoporosis and skeletal aging by inducing TAZ. *Cell Stem Cell.* (2018) 23:193–209.e5. doi: 10.1016/j.stem.2018.09.001
63. Seale P, Kajimura S, Yang W, Chin S, Rohas LM, Uldry M, et al. Transcriptional control of brown fat determination by PRDM16. *Cell Metab.* (2007) 6:38–54. doi: 10.1016/j.cmet.2007.06.001
64. Ukita M, Yamaguchi T, Ohata N, Tamura M. Sclerostin enhances adipocyte differentiation in 3T3-L1 cells. *J Cell Biochem.* (2016) 117:1419–28. doi: 10.1002/jcb.25432
65. Styner M, Pagnotti GM, Galior K, Wu X, Thompson WR, et al. Exercise regulation of marrow fat in the setting of PPARgamma agonist treatment in female C57BL/6 mice. *Endocrinology.* (2015) 156:2753–61. doi: 10.1210/en.2015-1213
66. Lecka-Czernik B, Stechschulte LA, Czernik PJ, Sherman SB, Huang S, Krings A. Marrow adipose tissue: skeletal location, sexual dimorphism, and response to sex steroid deficiency. *Front Endocrinol.* (2017) 8:188. doi: 10.3389/fendo.2017.00188
67. Gurt I, Artsi H, Cohen-Kfir E, Hamdani G, Ben-Shalom G, Feinstein B, et al. The Sirt1 activators SRT2183 and SRT3025 inhibit RANKL-induced osteoclastogenesis in bone marrow-derived macrophages and down-regulate Sirt3 in Sirt1 null cells. *PLoS ONE.* (2015) 10:e0134391. doi: 10.1371/journal.pone.0134391
68. Dai H, Sinclair DA, Ellis JL, Steegborn C. Sirtuin activators and inhibitors: promises, achievements, and challenges. *Pharmacol Ther.* (2018) 188:140–54. doi: 10.1016/j.pharmthera.2018.03.004
69. Martens CR, Denman BA, Mazzo MR, Armstrong ML, Reisdorph N, McQueen MB, et al. Chronic nicotinamide riboside supplementation is well-tolerated and elevates NAD(+) in healthy middle-aged and older adults. *Nat Commun.* (2018) 9:1286. doi: 10.1038/s41467-018-03421-7

8

SIRT1 is a Potential Drug Target for Treatment of Diabetic Kidney Disease

Yifei Zhong[1]*, *Kyung Lee*[2] *and John Cijiang He*[2,3]*

[1] Division of Nephrology, Longhua Hospital, Shanghai University of Traditional Chinese Medicine, Shanghai, China, [2] Division of Nephrology, Department of Medicine, Icahn School of Medicine at Mount Sinai, New York City, NY, United States, [3] Renal Section, James J. Peters VA Medical Center, Bronx, NY, United States

***Correspondence:**
Yifei Zhong
yifeililly@126.com
John Cijiang He
cijiang.he@mssm.edu

Multiple studies have demonstrated a critical role of Sirtuin-1 (SIRT1) deacetylase in protecting kidney cells from cellular stresses. A protective role of SIRT1 has been reported in both podocytes and renal tubular cells in multiple kidney disease settings, including diabetic kidney disease (DKD). We and others have shown that SIRT1 exerts renoprotective effects in DKD in part through the deacetylation of transcription factors involved in the disease pathogenesis, such as p53, FOXO, RelA/p65NF-κB, STAT3, and PGC1α/PPARγ. Recently we showed that the podocyte-specific overexpression of SIRT1 attenuated proteinuria and kidney injury in an experimental model of DKD, further confirming SIRT1 as a potential target to treat kidney disease. Known agonists of SIRT1 such as resveratrol diminished diabetic kidney injury in several animal models. Similarly, we also showed that puerarin, a Chinese herbal medicine compound, activates SIRT1 to provide renoprotection in mouse models of DKD. However, as these are non-specific SIRT1 agonists, we recently developed a more specific and potent SIRT1 agonist (BF175) that significantly attenuated diabetic kidney injury in type 1 diabetic OVE26 mice. We also previously reported that MS417, a bromodomain inhibitor that disrupts the interaction between the acetyl-residues of NF-κB and bromodomain-containing protein 4 (BRD4) also attenuates DKD. These results suggest that SIRT1 agonists and bromodomain inhibitors could be potential new therapuetic treatments against DKD progression.

Keywords: SIRT1, acetylation, diabetic kidney disease, bromodomain inhibitor, podocytes

INTRODUCTION

Sirtuin family of nicotinamide adenine dinucleotide (NAD^+)-dependent deacetylases, a homolog of yeast Sir2 (silent mating type information regulation 2), has been shown to play an important role in a variety of cellular functions. The mammalian Sir2 ortholog, Sirtuin-1 (SIRT1) is upregulated by caloric restriction and mediates the longevity effect of calorie restriction by regulation of glucose and lipid metabolism (1, 2). At the cellular level, SIRT1 regulates variety of processes including autophagy (3), energetic homeostasis (2), mitochondrial biogenesis (4), and apoptosis (5). A large body of evidence suggests that SIRT1 plays a major role in various kidney diseases by providing protection against cellular stresses associated with kidney injury (6–8). Here, we provide an overview of the role of SIRT1 in kidney cells in the context of diabetic kidney disease (DKD), with a focus on its role on the regulation of transcription factor activation. The review also discusses the potential new therapies by targeting SIRT1 pathway for DKD.

ROLE OF SIRT1 IN REGULATION OF TRANSCRIPTION FACTOR ACETYLATION

Recent evidence suggests that transcription factor activation is regulated not only by protein phosphorylation, but also by acetylation. SIRT1 exerts biological effects not only through deacetylation of histones, but also deacetylation of various transcription factors that include p53, FOXO, RelA/p65, STAT3, PGC1α, and PPAR-γ (9), thereby leading to transcription repression. SIRT1 regulates p53 activity through deacetylation (10–13) and promotes cell survival through suppression of p53-dependent apoptosis in response to DNA damage and oxidative stress (5). SIRT1 was also shown to regulate the activities of FOXO family of transcription factors through deacetylation (14). Deacetylation of FOXO3 by SIRT1 enhances its ability to induce cell cycle arrest and resistance to oxidative stress, while inhibiting its ability to induce cell death (14, 15). We also showed that SIRT1 inhibits podocyte apoptosis through deacetylation of FOXO4 (16, 17). Several studies suggest that the transcriptional activity of signal transducer and activator of transcription 3 (STAT3) is also negatively regulated by SIRT1 (18–20). SIRT1 was found to cause the deacetylation and inactivation of STAT3 during caloric restriction (21). SIRT1 also exerts anti-inflammatory effects through the inhibition of NF-κB pathway. It was shown that the duration of nuclear NF-κB action is highly regulated by reversible acetylation (22, 23), and that SIRT1 inhibits the NF-κB signaling pathway through deacetylation of p65 (24). In addition, SIRT1 modulates cellular response to hypoxia via deacetylation of hypoxia-induced factor 1α (HIF-1α) (25–27). All these highlight an important transcription modulatory function by SIRT1 activity.

SIRT1 PROVIDES RENOPROTECTION AGAINST DKD

Diabetic kidney disease (DKD) is the leading cause of chronic kidney disease and end-stage renal failure in the US (28). Even with optimal therapy, the incidence of DKD remains high, as none of the currently available therapy can reverse or completely forestall the progression of DKD. Therefore, development of more effective treatment for DKD is urgently required. The important role of SIRT1 in DKD has been demonstrated by number of studies (**Table 1**). We have previous shown that SIRT1 expression is significantly reduced in human kidney with DKD and that its reduction is more pronounced in the glomerular compartment than in the tubular compartment (17). An association between single nucleotide polymorphisms within *SIRT1* gene and DKD was observed in Japanese subjects with type 2 diabetes (40). However, the exact mechanism of regulation of SIRT1 expression in DKD remains unclear. On the cellular level, SIRT1 has been shown to regulate autophagy (41, 42) and oxidative stress response in the diabetic kidneys (35). Resveratrol was shown to attenuate DKD through activation of AMPK/SIRT1 pathway (29, 31) and by modulating angiogenesis (43). Studies have demonstrated a clear role of SIRT1 in renal tubular cells in the setting of acute kidney injury (6, 44). In diabetic kidneys, it was shown that reduced proximal renal tubular SIRT1 expression contributes to albuminuria by upregulation of the tight junction protein Claudin-1 in podocytes (32). Interestingly, reduction in *Sirt1* expression in tubular cells induced hypomethylation of the *claudin-1* gene in podocytes to promote its expression, while overexpression of *Sirt1* in tubular cells induced hypermethylation of *claudin-1* and downregulated expression in podocytes, indicating an important cross-talk between the two cell types and epigenetic regulation of Claudin-1 expression by SIRT1. Work from our laboratory also demonstrated a critical role of SIRT1 in podocyte injury in DKD. We showed that either knockdown or knockout of *Sirt1* specifically in podocytes aggravated DKD injury in type 2 diabetic *db/db* mice (33) and in STZ-induced diabetic mice (34). Importantly, our recent study demonstrated that the podocyte-specific overexpression of SIRT1 was sufficient to significantly attenuate podocyte injury and to impede DKD progression in typel diabetic OVE26 mice. Together, these studies clearly demonstrate a protective role of SIRT1 against DKD in experimental models of both type 1 and type 2 diabetes.

RENOPROTECTIVE MECHANISMS OF SIRT1 IN DKD

As the cellular and molecular mechanisms of SIRT1 has been recently reviewed (42, 45, 46), as well as the role and mechanism of other sirtuins in kidney disease (47), this review is focused primarily on its modulation of transcription factor through deacetylation in the setting of DKD.

Effects of SIRT1 in Inflammation in Diabetic Kidneys Through NF-κB and STAT3 Deacetylation

Many studies suggest that SIRT1 regulates activity of several transcription factors that regulate kidney cell homeostasis and are involved in pathogenesis of DKD through deacetylation. Systems biology analysis of microarray data suggests that JAK-STAT and NF-κB are key inflammatory pathways activated in diabetic kidneys (48, 49). Recently, we showed that the acetylation of STAT3 and RelA/p65 is increased in kidneys from diabetic patients and mouse models (33). More importantly, we demonstrated that the podocyte-specific knockout of *Sirtl* in *db/db* mice led to higher levels of p65 and STAT3 acetylation and resulted in greater degree of proteinuria and kidney injury than in control *db/db* mice, implicating SIRT1 as a key inhibitor of the NF-κB- and STAT3-induced inflammatory responses in DKD (33). In addition, we found that expression of the key pro-inflammatory factors mediated by NF-kB and Stat3 were also increased in the kidney of Sirtl knockout *db/db* mice, further confirming a key role of Sirtl in regulation of inflammation in the diabetic kidney.

Effects of SIRT1 in Cell Death in Diabetic Kidneys Through p53 and FOXO4 Deacetylation

Several lines of evidence indicate that p53 mediates apoptosis of both podocytes and tubular epithelial cells in DKD (50–52). SIRT1 has been shown to promote cell survival by suppressing p53-dependent apoptosis in response to DNA damage and

TABLE 1 | Summary of the *in vivo* studies of SIRT1 in DKD.

Approaches	Animal models	Tissue/Cell types	Mechanisms regulated	References
Dietary restriction	Diabetic Wistar fatty (fa/fa) rats	Whole kidney	Inflammatory; autophagy	(29)
Resveratrol	db/db mice	Whole kidney	Oxidative stress	(30)
Resveratrol	db/db mice	Whole kidney	AMPK/PGC1a; Oxidative stress	(31)
nicotinamide mononucleotide	STZ-induced diabetic and db/db mice	Tubule/podocyte crosstalk	Epigenetics, Claudin-1	(32)
Sirt1 knockout	Db/db mice	Podocytes	Inflammation; apoptosis	(33)
Pyridoxamine				
Sirt1 knockdown	STZ-induced diabetic mice	Podocytes	Mitochondria; senescence	(34)
hnRNP F	db/db mice	Tubular cells	Oxidative stress	(35)
Glycyrrhizic Acid	db/db mice	Whole kidney	AMPK/PGC-1a	(36)
Puerarin	STZ-induced diabetic eNOS-null mice	Podocytes	Oxidative stress; inflammation	(37)
Tangshen formula	STZ-induced diabetic rats	Whole kidney	NF-kB/inflammation	(38)
Sirt1 overexpression; agonists	OVE26 mice	Podocytes	Mitochondrial function; apoptosis	(39)

oxidative stress (5). The interplay of SIRT1-p53 pathway also controls cellular senescence (53–55). We reported previously that advanced glycation endproducts (AGEs) induce podocyte apoptosis through FOXO4-mediated Bim expression and that acetylation of FOXO4 is critical for mediating this effect (17). Overexpression of SIRT1 inhibited AGE-induced FOXO4 acetylation and podocyte apoptosis.

Effects of SIRT1 in Mitochondrial Dysfunction and Fibrosis in Diabetic Kidneys Through of PGC-1α and Smad3 Deacetylation

SIRT1 has also been shown to regulate PGC-1α activity and to play an important role for maintenance of mitochondrial function in podocytes (56). The PGC-1α in regulation of mitochondrial function has been well described for neurodegenerative disorders (57). Both mitochondrial injury and cellular senescence are key pathological processes mediating kidney injury (58–60). Consistent with this, we have shown recently SIRT1 deficiency in podocytes aggravates aging-related kidney disease through enhanced cells senescence and mitochondrial dysfunction (61). Although the effects of SIRT1 on Smad3 acetylation remain to be determined, resveratrol was shown to affect acetylation but not phosphorylation of Smad3 to inhibit TGF-β1-induced up-regulation of collagen IV and fibronectin mRNA levels *in vitro* and renal fibrosis in the model of unilateral ureteral obstruction (UUO) *in vivo* (62). Therefore, it is plausible that increased SIRT1 activity may also attenuate renal fibrosis in DKD. Taken together, these studies suggest that SIRT1, as a negative regulator of inflammation, cellular senescence and mitochondrial dysfunction, is a key repressor of DKD pathogenesis.

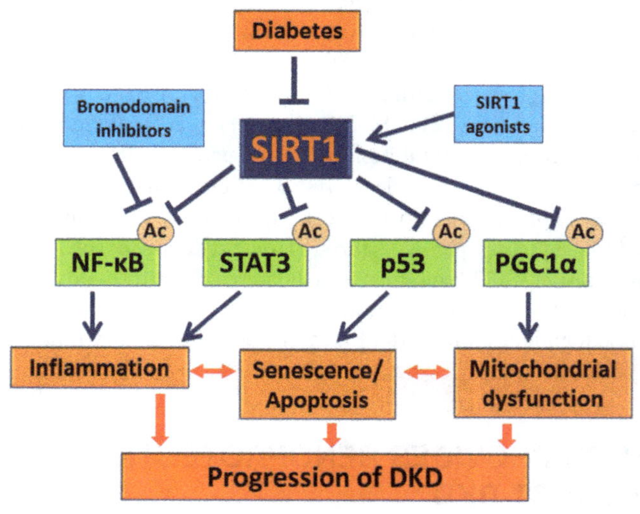

FIGURE 1 | Role of SIRT1 in DKD pathogenesis. This schema summarizes how Sirt1 mediates podocyte injury in DKD. The data suggest that Sirt1 expression is reduced in the diabetic glomeruli including podocytes. Reduced SIRT1 expression leads to increased acetylation and activation of transcription factors, such as NF-κB, STAT3, p53, and PGC1α, leading to exacerbated inflammation, senescence/apoptosis, and mitochondrial dysfunction of kidney cells such as podocytes (shown in blue arrows). All these processes interact each other and contribute to the progression of DKD (shown in red arrows). Therefore, SIRT1 agonists or inhibition of transcription factor acetylation through use of bromodomain inhibitors will reverse these diseased processes and could be developed to treat DKD. (⟶): stimulation; (⊣): inhibition; (⟷): interaction.

SIRT1 IS A POTENTIAL DRUG TARGET FOR TREATMENT OF DKD

Given that SIRT1 is a key mediator in thwarting the progression of DKD and other kidney diseases, development of therapeutic strategies to specifically restore SIRT1 activity is warranted. In support of this, we recently demonstrated that increased SIRT1 expression in podocytes attenuated albuminuria and glomerular injury in OVE26 diabetic mice (39). As SIRT1 expression is reduced in diseased kidneys, identifying the molecular basis of its suppression in diabetic kidneys and to interfere in this process may be an avenue of therapeutic approach. We previously showed that increased advanced glycation endproducts (AGEs) in in the diabetic milieu contribute to reduced SIRT1 expression in podocytes (17). Inhibition of AGE formation by pyridoxamine *in vivo* restored SIRT1 expression the glomeruli of *db/db* mice and attenuated podocyte injury and progression of DKD (17). Similar observations of SIRT1 reduction by AGEs were made in mesangial cells *in vitro* (63).

Another approach would be to stimulate SIRT1 activity through SIRT1 agonists. Resveratrol is a well-known SIRT1 agonist that has shown to improve DKD in several animal models (30, 31). However, recent reports indicate that resveratrol may not be a SIRT1-specific (64), nor are other purported SIRT1 agonists, such as SRT1720, SRT2183, and SRT1460 (65). We also showed that puerarin, an extract from a Chinese herbal medicine, attenuates diabetic kidney injury through activation of SIRT1 and suppression of NOX4 expression in podocytes in experimental diabetic mouse model (62). Other herbal medicines or compounds have also been reported to improve DKD through activation of SIRT1 (36, 38). Metformin is reported to improve podocyte function by activating SIRT1 (66). However, SIRT1-independent effects on podocytes or in DKD by non-specific SIRT1 agonists or metformin cannot be ruled out. Recently, we developed a new potent and selective SIRT1 agonist, BF175 (39). In cultured podocytes BF175 increased SIRT1-mediated activation of PGC1-α and protected against high glucose-mediated mitochondrial injury. *In vivo*, administration of BF175 for 6 weeks in type 1 diabetic OVE26 mice resulted in a marked reduction in albuminuria and in glomerular injury in a manner similar to podocyte-specific SIRT1 overexpression. BT175 treatment also attenuated diabetes-induced podocyte loss and reduced oxidative stress in glomeruli of OVE26 mice. Therefore, BT175 and its analogs could be developed as novel therapeutic strategy to treat DKD. However, these approaches of targeting SIRT1 are not without limitations. As discussed above, the specificity of the SIRT1 agonists remains a concern. Given the heterogeneity of SIRT1 function, the ever expanding list of its substrates, and the different effects of deacetylation on its target protein functions, it's possible that the beneficial effects of SIRT1 are mixed with potentially pernicious side effects.

As SIRT1 exerts its renoprotective effects through deacetylation of key transcription factors (TFs) involved in DKD, another therapeutic approach may be to directly regulate the transcription factor acetylation through bromodomain inhibitors (BrDi). Acetylated lysines of the key TFs involved in DKD pathogenesis such as p65 NF-κB interact with proteins containing bromodomains (67), and BrDi could suppress their acetylation in a more specific manner. For instance, NF-κB transcriptional activity is dependent upon its acetylation at lysine 310 (Lys310), and Lys310-acetylated p65 NF-κB recruits the BET protein BRD4 in complex with positive transcription elongation factor b (p-TEFb) and RNA polymerase II that together form a productive transcriptional machinery complex (68). We reported that a BET-specific BrDi MS417 suppresses TNF-α-induced acetylation of p65 NF-κB and the expression of NF-κB target genes in kidney cells *in vitro* and attenuates proteinuria and glomerulosclerosis in a mouse model of HIV-associated nephropathy *in vivo*. MS417 also inhibited AGE-induced acetylation of p65 NF-κB in podocytes *in vitro* and mitigated proteinuria in diabetic *db/db* mice. Therefore, MS417 or other BrDi might be another class of potential drug candidates to treat DKD patients.

In summary, SIRT1 has significant renoprotective effects against podocyte injury in DKD (**Figure 1**), and SIRT1 agonists and bromodomain inhibitors are promising candidates as therapeutic approach in treatment of DKD patients.

Clinical Perspectives

Since a large amount of evidence suggest that Sirtl is a key molecule involving in the pathogenesis of DKD and the expression of Sirtl is suppressed in human diabetic kidney, enhancing the SIRT1-induced transcription factor deacetylation via SIRT1 agonists or bromodomain inhibitors may serve as potential therapies for human DKD.

AUTHOR CONTRIBUTIONS

All authors listed have made a substantial, direct and intellectual contribution to the work, and approved it for publication.

ACKNOWLEDGMENTS

YZ is supported by National Natural Science Foundation of China (2015-81573768), Shanghai Shuguang Scholar (2016-6SG37), Shanghai Three Years' Pilot Project (ZY3-CCCX-2-1002, ZY3-CCCX-3-2001), and Award from Chen Yiping's National Research Studio for Famous Chinese Medicine Practitioners; KL is supported by NIH 1R01DK117913; and JH is supported by NIH 1R01DK078897, NIH 1R01DK088541.

REFERENCES

1. Moynihan KA, Grimm AA, Plueger MM, Bernal-Mizrachi E, Ford E, Cras-Meneur C, et al. Increased dosage of mammalian Sir2 in pancreatic beta cells enhances glucose-stimulated insulin secretion in mice. *Cell Metab.* (2005) 2:105–17. doi: 10.1016/j.cmet.2005.07.001
2. Rodgers JT, Lerin C, Haas W, Gygi SP, Spiegelman BM, Puigserver P. Nutrient control of glucose homeostasis through a complex of PGC-1alpha and SIRT1. *Nature* (2005) 434:113–8. doi: 10.1038/nature03354
3. Salminen A, Kaarniranta K. SIRT1: regulation of longevity via autophagy. *Cell Signal* (2009) 21:1356–60. doi: 10.1016/j.cellsig.2009.02.014
4. Scarpulla RC. Metabolic control of mitochondrial biogenesis through the PGC-1 family regulatory network. *Biochim Biophys Acta* (2011) 1813:1269–78. doi: 10.1016/j.bbamcr.2010.09.019
5. Luo J, Nikolaev AY, Imai S, Chen D, Su F, Shiloh A, et al. Negative control of p53 by Sir2alpha promotes cell survival under stress. *Cell* (2001) 107:137–48. doi: 10.1016/S0092-8674(01) 00524-4
6. Hasegawa K, Wakino S, Yoshioka K, Tatematsu S, Hara Y, Minakuchi H, et al. Kidney-specific overexpression of Sirtl protects against acute kidney injury by retaining peroxisome function. *J Biol Chem.* (2010) 285:13045–56. doi: 10.1074/jbc.M109.067728

7. He W, Wang Y, Zhang MZ, You L, Davis LS, Fan H, et al. Sirt1 activation protects the mouse renal medulla from oxidative injury. *J Clin Invest.* (2010) 120:1056–68. doi: 10.1172/JCI41563
8. Kume S, Uzu T, Horiike K, Chin-Kanasaki M, Isshiki K, Araki S, et al. Calorie restriction enhances cell adaptation to hypoxia through Sirt1-dependent mitochondrial autophagy in mouse aged kidney. *J Clin Invest.* (2010) 120:1043–55. doi: 10.1172/JCI41376
9. Nakagawa T, Guarente L. Sirtuins at a glance. *J Cell Sci.* (2011) 124:833–8. doi: 10.1242/jcs.081067
10. Vaziri H, Dessain SK, Ng Eaton E, Imai SI, Frye RA, Pandita TK, et al. hSIR2(SIRT1) functions as an NAD-dependent p53 deacetylase. *Cell* (2001) 107:149–59. doi: 10.1016/S0092-8674(01)00527-X
11. Jang SY, Kim SY, Bae YS. p53 deacetylation by SIRT1 decreases during protein kinase CKII downregulation-mediated cellular senescence. *FEBS Lett.* (2011) 585:3360–6. doi: 10.1016/j.febslet.2011.09.027
12. Milner J, Allison SJ. SIRT1, p53 and mitotic chromosomes. *Cell Cycle* (2011) 10:3049. doi: 10.4161/cc.10.18.16994
13. Shah ZH, Ahmed SU, Ford JR, Allison SJ, Knight JR, Milner J. A deacetylase-deficient SIRT1 variant opposes full-length SIRT1 in regulating tumor suppressor p53 and governs expression of cancer-related genes. *Mol Cell Biol.* (2012) 32:704–16. doi: 10.1128/MCB.06448-11
14. Brunet A, Sweeney LB, Sturgill JF, Chua KF, Greer PL, Lin Y, et al. Stress-dependent regulation of FOXO transcription factors by the SIRT1 deacetylase. *Science* (2004) 303:2011–5. doi: 10.1126/science.1094637
15. Motta MC, Divecha N, Lemieux M, Kamel C, Chen D, Gu W, et al. Mammalian SIRT1 represses forkhead transcription factors. *Cell* (2004) 116:551–63. doi: 10.1016/S0092-8674(04)00126-6
16. Chuang PY, Yu Q, Fang W, Uribarri J, He JC. Advanced glycation endproducts induce podocyte apoptosis by activation of the FOXO4 transcription factor. *Kidney Int.* (2007) 72:965–76. doi: 10.1038/sj.ki.5002456
17. Chuang PY, Dai Y, Liu R, He H, Kretzler M, Jim B, et al. Alteration of forkhead box O (foxo4) acetylation mediates apoptosis of podocytes in diabetes mellitus. *PLoS ONE* (2011) 6:e23566. doi: 10.1371/journal.pone.0023566
18. Bernier M, Paul RK, Martin-Montalvo A, Scheibye-Knudsen M, Song S, He HJ, et al. Negative regulation of STAT3 protein-mediated cellular respiration by SIRT1 protein. *J Biol Chem.* (2011) 286:19270–9. doi: 10.1074/jbc.M110.200311
19. Nie Y, Erion DM, Yuan Z, Dietrich M, Shulman GI, Horvath TL, et al. STAT3 inhibition of gluconeogenesis is downregulated by SirT1. *Nat Cell Biol.* (2009) 11:492–500. doi: 10.1038/ncb1857
20. Sestito R, Madonna S, Scarponi C, Cianfarani F, Failla CM, Cavani A, et al. STAT3-dependent effects of IL-22 in human keratinocytes are counterregulated by sirtuin 1 through a direct inhibition of STAT3 acetylation. *FASEB J.* (2011) 25:916–27. doi: 10.1096/fj.10-172288
21. Schenk S, Mccurdy CE, Philp A, Chen MZ, Holliday MJ, Bandyopadhyay GK, et al. Sirt1 enhances skeletal muscle insulin sensitivity in mice during caloric restriction. *J Clin Invest.* (2011) 121:4281–8. doi: 10.1172/JCI58554
22. Chen L, Fischle W, Verdin E, Greene WC. Duration of nuclear NF-kappaB action regulated by reversible acetylation. *Science* (2001) 293:1653–7. doi: 10.1126/science.1062374
23. Greene WC, Chen LF. Regulation of NF-kappaB action by reversible acetylation. *Novartis Found Symp.* (2004) 259:208–17; discussion 218–225. doi: 10.1002/0470862637.ch15
24. Yang XD, Tajkhorshid E, Chen LF. Functional interplay between acetylation and methylation of the RelA subunit of NF-kappaB. *Mol Cell Biol.* (2010) 30:2170–80. doi: 10.1128/MCB.01343-09
25. Geng H, Harvey CT, Pittsenbarger J, Liu Q, Beer TM, Xue C, et al. HDAC4 protein regulates HIF1alpha protein lysine acetylation and cancer cell response to hypoxia. *J Biol Chem.* (2011) 286:38095–102. doi: 10.1074/jbc.M111.257055
26. Lim JH, Lee YM, Chun YS, Chen J, Kim JE, Park JW. Sirtuin 1 modulates cellular responses to hypoxia by deacetylating hypoxia-inducible factor 1alpha. *Mol Cell* (2010) 38:864–78. doi: 10.1016/j.molcel.2010.05.023
27. Chen R, Dioum EM, Hogg RT, Gerard RD, Garcia JA. Hypoxia increases sirtuin 1 expression in a hypoxia-inducible factor-dependent manner. *J Biol Chem.* (2011) 286:13869–78. doi: 10.1074/jbc.M110.175414
28. Usrds I. *Annual Data Report: Atlas of End-Stage-Renal-Disease in the United States.* (2011).
29. Kitada M, Takeda A, Nagai T, Ito H, Kanasaki K, Koya D. Dietary restriction ameliorates diabetic nephropathy through anti-inflammatory effects and regulation of the autophagy via restoration of Sirt1 in diabetic Wistar fatty (fa/fa) rats: a model of type 2 diabetes. *Exp Diabetes Res.* (2011b) 2011:908185. doi: 10.1155/2011/908185
30. Kitada M, Kume S, Imaizumi N, Koya D. Resveratrol improves oxidative stress and protects against diabetic nephropathy through normalization of Mn-SOD dysfunction in AMPK/SIRT1-independent pathway. *Diabetes* (2011a) 60:634–43. doi: 10.2337/db10-0386
31. Kim MY, Lim JH, Youn HH, Hong YA, Yang KS, Park HS, et al. Resveratrol prevents renal lipotoxicity and inhibits mesangial cell glucotoxicity in a manner dependent on the AMPK-SIRT1-PGC1alpha axis in db/db mice. *Diabetologia* (2013) 56:204–17. doi: 10.1007/s00125-012-2747-2
32. Hasegawa K, Wakino S, Simic P, Sakamaki Y, Minakuchi H, Fujimura K, et al. Renal tubular Sirt1 attenuates diabetic albuminuria by epigenetically suppressing Claudin-1 overexpression in podocytes. *Nat Med.* (2013) 19:1496–504. doi: 10.1038/nm.3363
33. Liu R, Zhong Y, Li X, Chen H, Jim B, Zhou MM, et al. Role of transcription factor acetylation in diabetic kidney disease. *Diabetes* (2014) 63:2440–53. doi: 10.2337/db13-1810
34. Chuang PY, Xu J, Dai Y, Jia F, Mallipattu SK, Yacoub R, et al. *In vivo* RNA interference models of inducible and reversible Sirt1 knockdown in kidney cells. *Am J Pathol.* (2014) 184:1940–56. doi: 10.1016/j.ajpath.2014.03.016
35. Lo CS, Shi Y, Chenier I, Ghosh A, Wu CH, Cailhier JF, et al. Heterogeneous nuclear ribonucleoprotein f stimulates sirtuin-1 gene expression and attenuates nephropathy progression in diabetic mice. *Diabetes* (2017) 66:1964–78. doi: 10.2337/db16-1588
36. Hou S, Zhang T, Li Y, Guo F, Jin X. Glycyrrhizic acid prevents diabetic nephropathy by activating AMPK/SIRT1/PGC-1alpha signaling in db/db mice. *J Diabetes Res.* (2017) 2017:2865912. doi: 10.1155/2017/2865912
37. Li X, Cai W, Lee K, Liu B, Deng Y, Chen Y, et al. Puerarin attenuates diabetic kidney injury through the suppression of NOX4 expression in podocytes. *Sci Rep.* (2017) 7:14603. doi: 10.1038/s41598-017-17925-7
38. Du YG, Zhang KN, Gao ZL, Dai F, Wu XX, Chai KF. Tangshen formula improves inflammation in renal tissue of diabetic nephropathy through SIRT1/NF-kappaB pathway. *Exp Ther Med.* (2018) 15:2156–64. doi: 10.3892/etm.2017.5621
39. Hong Q, Zhang L, Das B, Li Z, Liu B, Cai G, et al. Increased podocyte Sirtuin-1 function attenuates diabetic kidney injury. *Kidney Int.* (2018) 93:1330–43 doi: 10.1016/j.kint.2017.12.008
40. Maeda S, Koya D, Araki SI, Babazono T, Umezono T, Toyoda M, et al. Association between single nucleotide polymorphisms within genes encoding sirtuin families and diabetic nephropathy in Japanese subjects with type 2 diabetes. *Clin Exp Nephrol.* (2011) 15:381–90. doi: 10.1007/s10157-011-0418-0
41. Kume S, Thomas MC, Koya D. Nutrient sensing, autophagy, and diabetic nephropathy. *Diabetes* (2012) 61:23–9. doi: 10.2337/db11-0555
42. Kitada M, Ogura Y, Monno I, Koya D. Regulating autophagy as a therapeutic target for diabetic nephropathy. *Curr Diab Rep.* (2017) 17:53. doi: 10.1007/s11892-017-0879-y
43. Wen D, Huang X, Zhang M, Zhang L, Chen J, Gu Y, et al. Resveratrol attenuates diabetic nephropathy via modulating angiogenesis. *PLoS ONE* (2013) 8:e82336. doi: 10.1371/journal.pone.0082336
44. Fan H, Yang HC, You L, Wang YY, He WJ, Hao CM. The histone deacetylase, SIRT1, contributes to the resistance of young mice to ischemia/reperfusion-induced acute kidney injury. *Kidney Int.* (2013) 83:404–13. doi: 10.1038/ki.2012.394
45. Nakatani Y, Inagi R. Epigenetic regulation through SIRT1 in podocytes. *Curr Hypertens Rev.* (2016) 12:89–94. doi: 10.2174/1573402112666160302102515
46. Hao CM, Haase VH. Sirtuins and their relevance to the kidney. *J Am Soc Nephrol.* (2010) 21:1620–7. doi: 10.1681/ASN.2010010046
47. Morigi M, Perico L, Benigni A. Sirtuins in renal health and disease. *J Am Soc Nephrol.* (2018) 29:1799–809. doi: 10.1681/ASN.2017111218
48. Berthier CC, Zhang H, Schin M, Henger A, Nelson RG, Yee B, et al. Enhanced expression of Janus kinase-signal transducer and activator of transcription pathway members in human diabetic nephropathy. *Diabetes* (2009) 58:469–77. doi: 10.2337/db08-1328
49. Schmid H, Boucherot A, Yasuda Y, Henger A, Brunner B, Eichinger F, et al. Modular activation of nuclear factor-kappaB transcriptional

programs in human diabetic nephropathy. *Diabetes* (2006) 55:2993–3003. doi: 10.2337/db06-0477

50. Niranjan T, Bielesz B, Gruenwald A, Ponda MP, Kopp JB, Thomas DB, et al. The Notch pathway in podocytes plays a role in the development of glomerular disease. *Nat Med.* (2008) 14:290–8. doi: 10.1038/nm1731
51. Tikoo K, Tripathi DN, Kabra DG, Sharma V, Gaikwad AB. Intermittent fasting prevents the progression of type I diabetic nephropathy in rats and changes the expression of Sir2 and p53. *FEBS Lett.* (2007) 581:1071–8. doi: 10.1016/j.febslet.2007.02.006
52. Brezniceanu ML, Liu F, Wei CC, Tran S, Sachetelli S, Zhang SL, et al. Catalase overexpression attenuates angiotensinogen expression and apoptosis in diabetic mice. *Kidney Int.* (2007) 71:912–23. doi: 10.1038/sj.ki.5002188
53. Tran D, Bergholz J, Zhang H, He H, Wang Y, Zhang Y, et al. Insulin-like growth factor-1 regulates the SIRT1-p53 pathway in cellular senescence. *Aging Cell* (2014) 13:669–78. doi: 10.1111/acel.12219
54. Xiong S, Salazar G, Patrushev N, Ma M, Forouzandeh F, Hilenski L, et al. Peroxisome proliferator-activated receptor gamma coactivator-1alpha is a central negative regulator of vascular senescence. *Arterioscler Thromb Vasc Biol.* (2013) 33:988–98. doi: 10.1161/ATVBAHA.112.301019
55. Imai S, Guarente L. NAD+ and sirtuins in aging and disease. *Trends Cell Biol.* (2014) 24:464–71. doi: 10.1016/j.tcb.2014.04.002
56. Yuan Y, Huang S, Wang W, Wang Y, Zhang P, Zhu C, et al. Activation of peroxisome proliferator-activated receptor-gamma coactivator 1alpha ameliorates mitochondrial dysfunction and protects podocytes from aldosterone-induced injury. *Kidney Int.* (2012) 82:771–89. doi: 10.1038/ki.2012.188
57. Lv J, Jiang S, Yang Z, Hu W, Wang Z, Li T, et al. PGC-1alpha sparks the fire of neuroprotection against neurodegenerative disorders. *Ageing Res Rev.* (2018) 44:8–21. doi: 10.1016/j.arr.2018.03.004
58. Chen J, Xavier S, Moskowitz-Kassai E, Chen R, Lu CY, Sanduski K, et al. Cathepsin cleavage of sirtuin 1 in endothelial progenitor cells mediates stress-induced premature senescence. *Am J Pathol.* (2012) 180:973–83. doi: 10.1016/j.ajpath.2011.11.033
59. Portilla D. Apoptosis, fibrosis and senescence. *Nephron Clin Pract.* (2014) 127:65–9. doi: 10.1159/000363717
60. Clements ME, Chaber CJ, Ledbetter SR, Zuk A. Increased cellular senescence and vascular rarefaction exacerbate the progression of kidney fibrosis in aged mice following transient ischemic injury. *PLoS ONE* (2013) 8:e70464. doi: 10.1371/journal.pone.0070464
61. Chuang PY, Cai W, Li X, Fang L, Xu J, Yacoub R, et al. Reduction in podocyte SIRT1 accelerates kidney injury in aging mice. *Am J Physiol Renal Physiol.* (2017) 313:F621–8. doi: 10.1152/ajprenal.00255.2017
62. Li J, Qu X, Ricardo SD, Bertram JF, Nikolic-Paterson DJ. Resveratrol inhibits renal fibrosis in the obstructed kidney: potential role in deacetylation of Smad3. *Am J Pathol.* (2010) 177:1065–71. doi: 10.2353/ajpath.2010.090923
63. Huang KP, Chen C, Hao J, Huang JY, Liu PQ, Huang HQ. AGEs-RAGE system down-regulates Sirt1 through the ubiquitin-proteasome pathway to promote FN and TGF-beta1 expression in male rat glomerular mesangial cells. *Endocrinology* (2015) 156:268–79. doi: 10.1210/en.2014-1381
64. Beher D, Wu J, Cumine S, Kim KW, Lu SC, Atangan L, et al. Resveratrol is not a direct activator of SIRT1 enzyme activity. *Chem Biol Drug Des.* (2009) 74:619–24. doi: 10.1111/j.1747-0285.2009.00901.x
65. Pacholec M, Bleasdale JE, Chrunyk B, Cunningham D, Flynn D, Garofalo RS, et al. SRT1720, SRT2183, SRT1460, and resveratrol are not direct activators of SIRT1. *J Biol Chem.* (2010) 285:8340–51. doi: 10.1074/jbc.M109.088682
66. Rogacka D, Audzeyenka I, Rychlowski M, Rachubik P, Szrejder M, Angielski S, et al. Metformin overcomes high glucose-induced insulin resistance of podocytes by pleiotropic effects on SIRT1 and AMPK. *Biochim Biophys Acta* (2018) 1864:115–25. doi: 10.1016/j.bbadis.2017.10.014
67. Sanchez R, Meslamani J, Zhou MM. The bromodomain: from epigenome reader to druggable target. *Biochim Biophys Acta* (2014) 1839:676–85. doi: 10.1016/j.bbagrm.2014.03.011
68. Huang B, Yang XD, Zhou MM, Ozato K, Chen LF. Brd4 coactivates transcriptional activation of NF-kappaB via specific binding to acetylated RelA. *Mol Cell Biol.* (2009) 29:1375–87. doi: 10.1128/MCB.01365-08

9

Sirtuins and Type 2 Diabetes: Role in Inflammation, Oxidative Stress and Mitochondrial Function

Munehiro Kitada [1,2], Yoshio Ogura [1], Itaru Monno [1] and Daisuke Koya [1,2]*

[1] Department of Diabetology and Endocrinology, Kanazawa Medical University, Uchinada, Japan, [2] Division of Anticipatory Molecular Food Science and Technology, Medical Research Institute, Kanazawa Medical University, Uchinada, Japan

***Correspondence:**
Munehiro Kitada
kitta@kanazawa-med.ac.jp

The rising incidence of type 2 diabetes mellitus (T2DM) is a major public health concern, and novel therapeutic strategies to prevent T2DM are urgently needed worldwide. Aging is recognized as one of the risk factors for metabolic impairments, including insulin resistance and T2DM. Inflammation, oxidative stress, and mitochondrial dysfunction are closely related to both aging and metabolic disease. Calorie restriction (CR) can retard the aging process in organisms ranging from yeast to rodents and delay the onset of numerous age-related disorders, such as insulin resistance and diabetes. Therefore, metabolic CR mimetics may represent new therapeutic targets for insulin resistance and T2DM. Sirtuin 1 (SIRT1), the mammalian homolog of Sir2, was originally identified as a nicotinamide adenine dinucleotide (NAD^+)-dependent histone deacetylase. The activation of SIRT1 is closely associated with longevity under CR, and it is recognized as a CR mimetic. Currently, seven sirtuins have been identified in mammals. Among these sirtuins, SIRT1 and SIRT2 are located in the nucleus and cytoplasm, SIRT3 exists predominantly in mitochondria, and SIRT6 is located in the nucleus. These sirtuins regulate metabolism through their regulation of inflammation, oxidative stress and mitochondrial function via multiple mechanisms, resulting in the improvement of insulin resistance and T2DM. In this review, we describe the current understanding of the biological functions of sirtuins, especially SIRT1, SIRT2, SIRT3, and SIRT6, focusing on oxidative stress, inflammation, and mitochondrial function, which are closely associated with aging.

Keywords: SIRT1, SIRT2, SIRT3, SIRT6, Type 2 diabetes

INTRODUCTION

The rising incidence of type 2 diabetes mellitus (T2DM) has significantly increased worldwide in recent decades, and the development of better treatments for T2DM is urgently needed. Aging is a universal process that affects all organs. Age-related disruptions in cellular homeostasis result in the decline in the responsiveness to physiological stress, including oxidative stress and inflammation, which are implicated in the pathogenesis of metabolic diseases, including insulin resistance and T2DM. Additionally, mitochondria play a central role in energy production and responsiveness to nutrient availability, and they are one of the sources of reactive oxygen species (ROS) (1). Therefore, mitochondrial function decline is also closely related to the impairment of metabolic homeostasis (2) and oxidative stress (3, 4), contributing to the progression of insulin resistance and T2DM, which are associated with aging. Additionally, oxidative stress is closely linked to

TABLE 1 | Seven sirtuins in mammals.

Sirtuin	Catalytic activity	Localization
SIRT1	Deacetylase	Nucleus and cytoplasm
SIRT2	Deacetylase	Cytoplasm and nucleus
SIRT3	Deacetylase	Mitochondria
SIRT4	ADP-ribosyl transferase	Mitochondria
SIRT5	Deacetylase	Mitochondria
SIRT6	Deacetylase and ADP-ribosyl transferase	Nucleus
SIRT7	Deacetylase	Nucleus

inflammation (5, 6); therefore, the suppression of oxidative stress/inflammation and preservation of mitochondrial function should be therapeutic targets for insulin resistance and T2DM, as well as for anti-aging treatments.

Calorie restriction (CR) retards aging or extends the life spans of yeast, worms, flies, and rodents (7). The benefits of CR for the suppression of age-related diseases, including glucose intolerance, cardiovascular disease and cancer, have also been observed in rhesus monkeys or humans (8–10), by improving insulin sensitivity and reducing inflammation and oxidative stress. Sirtuins have received attention for their role in modifying lifespan, especially in relation to the benefits of CR. From the initial studies on aging in yeast, silent information regulator 2 (Sir2), a nicotinamide adenine dinucleotide (NAD^+)-dependent deacetylase, was identified as one of the possible molecules through which CR improves lifespan extension (11). Homologs of Sir2 in higher eukaryotic organisms are known as SIRT1, which may contribute to CR-induced longevity (12–14), and, currently, seven sirtuins, including SIRT1, have been identified in mammals (15, 16) (**Table 1**). Numerous previous reports have shown the multiple physiological roles of sirtuins, including SIRT1, SIRT2, SIRT3 and SIRT6, in cellular function, such as glucose metabolism, mitochondrial function and resistance against cellular stresses, including oxidative stress and inflammation (15–20). Thus, the modulation of sirtuin activity, as a CR mimetic, may be a novel drug target for insulin resistance and T2DM.

In this review, we describe the current understanding of the biological functions of sirtuins, especially SIRT1, SIRT2, SIRT3, and SIRT6, focusing on oxidative stress, inflammation and mitochondrial function, which are closely associated with aging. We also discuss their potential as pharmacological targets to prevent the development of metabolic diseases, such as insulin resistance and T2DM.

INFLAMMATION, OXIDATIVE STRESS, AND MITOCHONDRIAL DYSFUNCTION, WHICH ARE RELATED TO THE PATHOGENESIS OF INSULIN RESISTANCE AND TYPE 2 DIABETES

Chronic inflammation, oxidative stress and impaired mitochondrial function in skeletal muscle, adipose tissue or monocytes/macrophages (21, 22) are closely related to the pathogenesis of insulin resistance and T2DM. Additionally, inflammation and oxidative stress contribute to pancreatic β-cell dysfunction (23, 24), contributing to the progression of T2DM.

The activation of monocytes in the circulation, adipocytes and macrophages residing in adipose tissue leads to the release of various inflammatory mediators, including tumor necrosis factor-α (TNF-α), interleukin-6 (IL-6), and chemoattractant protein-1 (MCP-1), in insulin-resistant and diabetic states. These cytokines activate inflammatory signaling pathways, such as the inhibitor of IκB kinase (IKK) and c-Jun NH_2-terminal kinase (JNK) pathways, which impair the insulin signaling pathway by modulating phosphoinositide 3-kinase (PI3K) and Akt (25–27), and they play a crucial role in the pathogenesis of insulin resistance in adipose tissue and skeletal muscle. Oxidative stress also impairs insulin signaling, which contributes to insulin resistance in T2DM. In insulin-resistant or diabetic states, in addition to hyperglycemia, other metabolites, including free fatty acids (FFAs) and certain cytokines, such as TNF-α, induce the overproduction of ROS from mitochondria. ROS trigger the activation of serine/threonine kinases, such as p38 mitogen-activated protein kinase (p38 MAPK), JNK, and IKK, which induce the serine phosphorylation of insulin receptor substrate-1 (IRS-1), and then degrade IRS-1 and reduce IRS-1 tyrosine phosphorylation, leading to the suppression of insulin signaling (28–31), as well as inflammation. Inflammatory mediators and oxidative stress are also related to pancreatic β-cell dysfunction, resulting in the impairment of insulin production or excretion from β cells (23, 24).

The impairment of mitochondrial function in skeletal muscle is involved in the pathogenesis of insulin resistance and progression of T2DM, which may be associated with aging. Mitochondria play a central role in energy production and responsiveness to nutrient availability by regulating mitochondrial oxidative phosphorylation (OXPHOS) and fatty acid oxidation. However, previous studies have shown that the rate of mitochondrial OXPHOS is reduced and that intramyocellular lipid accumulation is increased in the skeletal muscle of patients with insulin resistance and T2DM and in elderly individuals (32–35). Aging is closely linked to the impairment of metabolic homeostasis, such as insulin resistance and T2DM, which are closely related to the decline in mitochondria function. Mitochondrial function decline generates excess ROS from mitochondria, and oxidative stress is linked to inflammation. Thus, there is a vicious cycle among oxidative stress, inflammation and mitochondrial dysfunction, and breaking this cycle may be a therapeutic target for the treatment of age-related insulin resistance and T2DM, focusing on SIRT1, SIRT2, SIRT3, and SIRT6 (**Figure 1**).

SIRT1

SIRT1 exists in the nucleus and cytoplasm, and it has NAD^+-dependent deacetylase activity (16). Numerous non-histone proteins, including transcription factors, transcriptional coregulatory proteins and histones, serve as substrates for SIRT1, which is associated with a wide variety of cellular processes (16). SIRT1 may play a crucial role in reducing inflammation and oxidative stress and improving mitochondrial function, resulting in both the protection of pancreatic β cells and amelioration of insulin resistance in insulin-sensitive tissues such as skeletal muscle and adipose tissue. Therefore, SIRT1 should be a pharmacological therapeutic target to treat insulin resistance and T2DM (17, 36).

Regulation of Inflammation

Accumulated evidence has demonstrated that SIRT1 suppresses inflammatory processes likely through interfering with nuclear factor kappa-B (NF-κB) signaling. Yeung et al. found that SIRT1 deacetylates the p65 subunit of NF-κB at lysine 310 and inhibits its transcriptional activity (37).

In adipocytes and macrophages, SIRT1 reduces inflammatory process through the deacetylation of NF-κB (p65), leading to improved glucose metabolism (38, 39) (**Figure 2A**). Additionally, myeloid cell-specific SIRT1 knockout (KO) mice that were fed a high-fat diet (HFD) exhibited macrophage activation and elevated expression of inflammatory mediators in the liver and adipose tissues, which was associated with the development of systemic insulin resistance (40). Furthermore, we previously reported another mechanism regarding SIRT1 inactivation-induced inflammation (**Figure 2A**): SIRT1 inactivation may enhance the NF-κB signaling pathway by the phosphorylation of NF-κB (p65) via the cellular accumulation of p62/Sqstm1 due to autophagy dysfunction, in THP-1 cells, cultured human monocytes (41). Moreover, SIRT1 inactivation resulted in increased activation of the mammalian target of rapamycin complex 1 (mTORC1) pathway and reduced 5′ AMP-activated kinase (AMPK) activation, possibly contributing to impairment in autophagy (41). In humans, reduction of SIRT1 expression levels in circulating monocytes is correlated with glucose intolerance, insulin resistance and metabolic syndrome in humans (42). Gillum et al. also demonstrated that SIRT1 expression is decreased in adipose tissues from obese males and that the mRNA expression of CD14, a macrophage marker, in adipose tissue is negatively correlated with SIRT1 expression (43).

Interestingly, adipocyte SIRT1 controls systemic glucose homeostasis and insulin sensitivity through cross talk with adipose-resident macrophages (44) (**Figure 2B**). Hui et al. recently reported that adipose-specific SIRT1 KO mice showed a higher susceptibility to HFD-induced insulin resistance, which is associated with an increased number of adipose-resident macrophages and their polarization toward the proinflammatory M1 subtype, overexpressing inflammatory mediators (44). SIRT1 in adipocytes modulates the expression and secretion of several adipokines, including adiponectin, MCP-1, TNF-α, and IL-4, which, in turn, alters the recruitment and polarization of macrophages in adipose tissues. In adipocytes, SIRT1 enhances IL-4 expression through deacetylating the transcription factor nuclear factor of activated T cells, cytoplasmic 1 (NFATc1), leading to polarization of the M2 subtype (44). Thus, SIRT1 may diminish inflammation in adipose tissues and monocytes/macrophages and may improve insulin resistance and T2DM.

In addition, SIRT1 protein expression is reduced in skeletal muscle and primary myotubes derived from T2DM

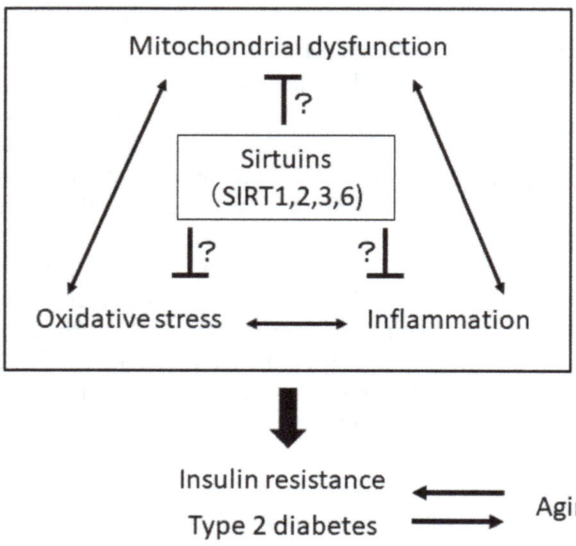

FIGURE 1 | A vicious cycle among oxidative stress, inflammation, and mitochondrial dysfunction is involved in the pathogenesis of insulin resistance, type 2 diabetes, and aging. Sirtuins, including SIRT1, 2, 3, and 6, may be a therapeutic target for the treatment of age-related insulin resistance and T2DM by breaking this vicious cycle.

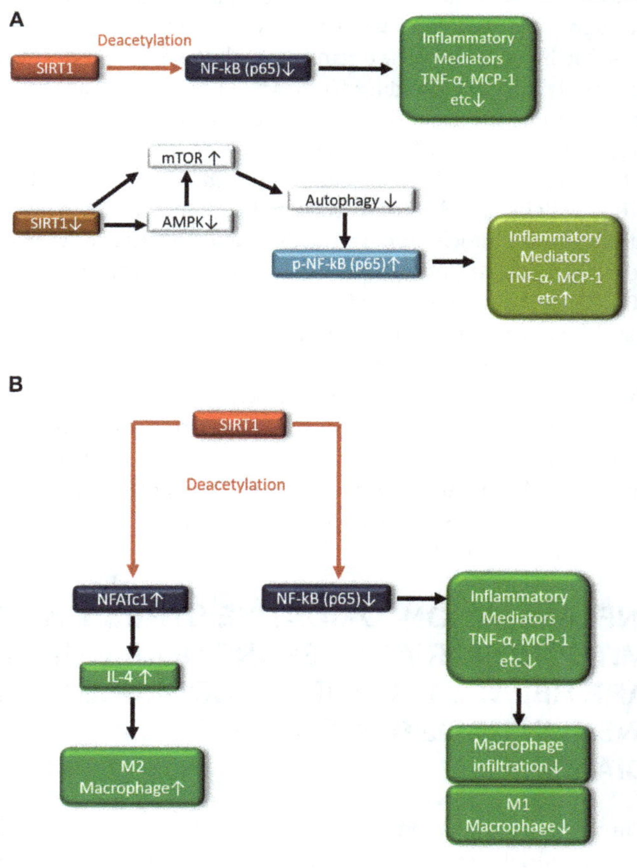

FIGURE 2 | continued

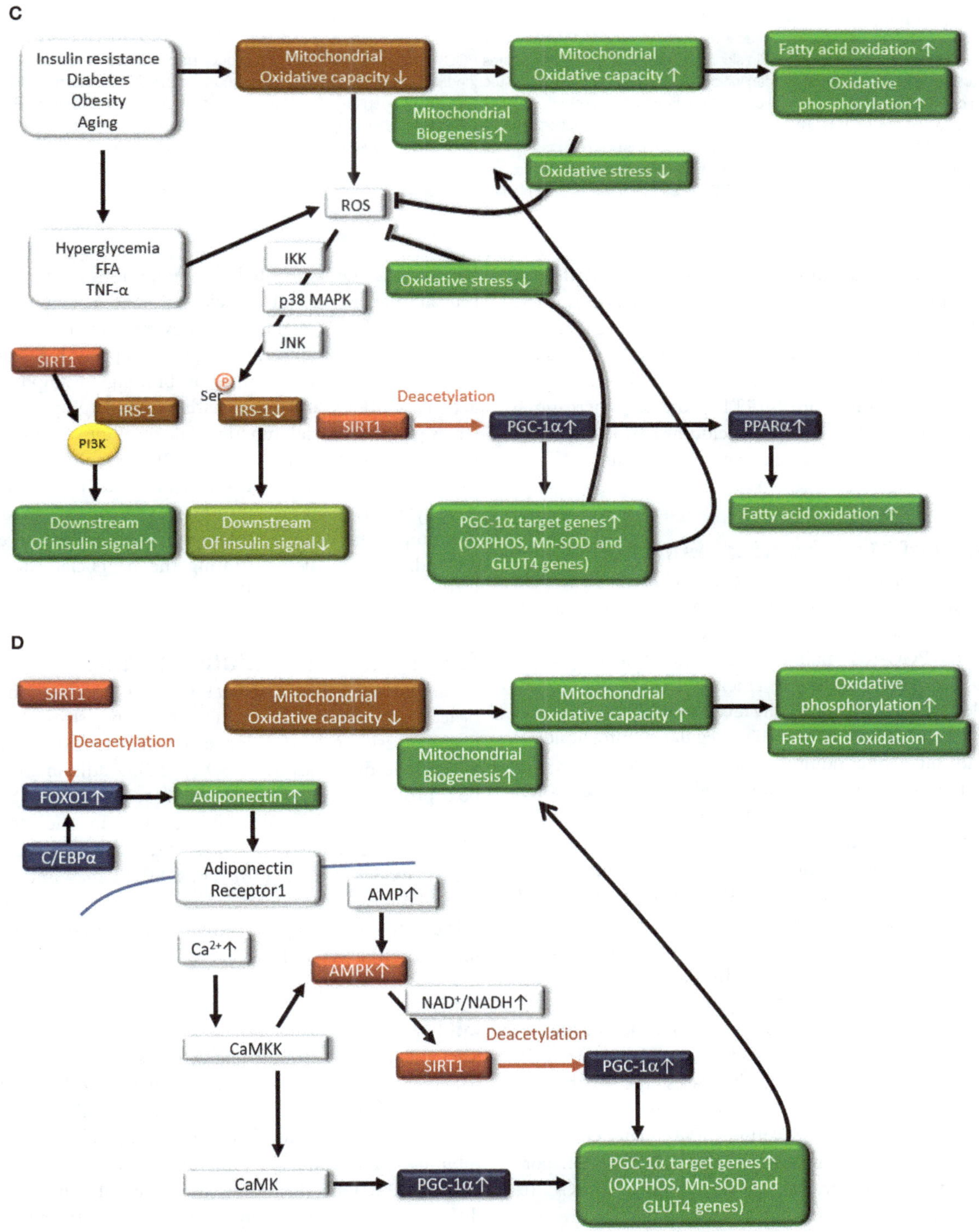

FIGURE 2 | (A) In monocytes/macrophages and adipocytes, SIRT1 deacetylates NF-κB(p65), resulting in reduced expression of inflammatory mediators such as TNF-α and MCP-1. SIRT1 inactivation also induces inflammation through the phosphorylation of the NF-κB pathway via impaired autophagy, which is associated with activation of mammalian target of rapamycin (mTOR) and reduced activation of AMP-activated kinase (AMPK). **(B)** In adipocytes, SIRT1 deacetylates nuclear factor-κB p65 subunit [NF-κB(p65)], resulting in reduced expression of inflammatory mediators such as tumor necrosis factor-α (TNF-α) and chemoattractant protein-1 (MCP-1), and decreased polarization to M1 macrophages and infiltration to adipose tissue. SIRT also induces polarization to M2 macrophages through increased expression of interleukin-4 (IL-4) expression via deacetylation of nuclear factor of activated T-cells 1 (NFATc1). **(C)** In skeletal muscle, SIRT1 increases mitochondrial biogenesis and fatty acid oxidation through acetylation and activation of the peroxisome proliferator-activated receptor (PPAR)-γ coactivator-1α (PGC-1α). Under conditions of insulin resistance, diabetes, obesity, or aging, mitochondrial oxidative capacity is decreased, contributing to the generation of reactive oxygen species

(Continued)

FIGURE 2 | (ROS) in mitochondria. Hyperglycemia, free fatty acids (FFAs) and TNF-α stimulate ROS production from the mitochondria, and increased levels of ROS lead to the serine-phosphorylation of insulin receptor substrate-1 (IRS-1), resulting in reduced insulin signaling. However, SIRT1 interacts with phosphoinositide 3-kinase (PI3K), leading to activation of insulin signaling. Additionally, SIRT1 activates PGC-1α transcriptional activity to induce mitochondrial biogenesis and the induction of antioxidative enzymes, which can inhibit the generation of ROS by mitochondria. Expression of glucose transporter 4 (GLUT4) is enhanced through deacetylation of PGC-1α by SIRT1. Moreover, SIRT1 activates peroxisome proliferator-activated receptor-α (PPAR-α), which induces fatty acid oxidation. **(D)** SIRT1 deacetylates Forkhead box protein O1 (FOXO1) and enhances its interaction with CCAAT/enhancer binding protein α (C/EBPα), resulting in the enhanced transcription of adiponectin in adipocytes. In skeletal muscle, adiponectin is involved in the regulation of Ca^{2+} signaling and PGC-1α expression through calcium/calmodulin-dependent protein kinase kinase (CaMKK) and calcium/calmodulin-dependent protein kinase (CaMK) activation. Adiponectin activates SIRT1 through AMPK activation, thereby deacetylating PGC-1α and resulting in mitochondrial biogenesis, increased fatty acid oxidation, and oxidative phosphorylation.

patients, suggesting that diminished SIRT1 contributes to insulin resistance induced by TNF-α in skeletal muscle (45). SIRT1 interacts with PI3K adaptor subunit p85 in an insulin-independent manner and activates insulin signaling at physiological insulin concentrations in skeletal muscle cells (45) (**Figure 2C**). Furthermore, SIRT1 protects pancreatic β cells against various toxic stresses, including oxidative stress and inflammatory cytokines, through suppressing NF-κB signaling (46).

Regulation of Mitochondrial Function

SIRT1 can be involved in the regulation of metabolism and insulin resistance through the modulation of mitochondrial function. Peroxisome proliferator-activated receptor-γ coactivator-1α (PGC-1α) maintains mitochondrial biogenesis and OXPHOS proteins, leading to efficient β oxidation of fatty acids in skeletal muscle. However, the levels of PGC-1α in skeletal muscle are decreased in T2DM. SIRT1 regulates mitochondrial function and metabolic homoeostasis, increases the oxygen consumption in skeletal muscle and leads to the expression of OXPHOS genes and mitochondrial biogenesis through the deacetylation of PGC-1α. SIRT1 knockdown largely prevents the upregulation of PGC-1α-induced genes that are involved in mitochondrial fatty acid utilization (47). Furthermore, SIRT1 can regulate peroxisome proliferator-activated receptor-α (PPAR-α) activation by PGC-1α deacetylation, resulting in increased fatty acid oxidation. Thus, the activation of SIRT1 may improve insulin resistance through promoting fatty acid oxidation and mitochondrial biogenesis via deacetylation of PGC-1α and PPAR-α activation in skeletal muscle (**Figure 2C**). Additionally, PGC-1α remarkably increases the expression of glucose transporter 4 (GLUT4) and activation of glucose transport in murine C2C12 myotubes (48). The effects of PGC-1α on GLUT4 gene expression leads to increased transport of glucose in myocytes, suggesting that the activation of PGC-1α by SIRT1 is involved in insulin sensitization (**Figure 2C**). Adiponectin has antidiabetic power (49), and the levels of plasma adiponectin are reduced in insulin resistance and T2DM (50, 51). Treatment with adiponectin can decrease glucose levels and ameliorate insulin resistance in mice (52). Mechanistically, adiponectin enhances insulin sensitivity through increasing fatty acid oxidation via AMPK and PPAR-α activation (49). Additionally, SIRT1 deacetylates Forkhead box protein O1 (FOXO1) and enhances its interaction with CCAAT/enhancer binding protein α (C/EBPα), resulting in enhanced transcription of the adiponectin gene in adipocytes (53) (**Figure 2D**). Iwabu et al. demonstrated that adiponectin signaling plays a crucial role in skeletal muscle cells and is implicated in the regulation of Ca^{2+} signaling and expression/activation of PGC-1α in muscle adiponectin receptor (adipoR) 1 KO mice (54). Adiponectin activates AMPK by binding to adipoR1, thereby activating SIRT1, and deacetylating PGC-1α improves oxidative stress, mitochondrial function, glucose/lipid metabolism, and exercise endurance (54) (**Figure 2D**), resulting in improved insulin resistance and T2DM. Thus, SIRT1-induced PGC-1α deacetylation leads to the improvement of mitochondrial function via mitochondrial biogenesis and induction of GLUT4 and adiponectin, demonstrating the beneficial effects against insulin resistance and T2DM.

Regulation of Oxidative Stress

In addition to mitochondrial function modulation, PGC-1α deacetylation by SIRT1 reduces oxidative stress through the overexpression of antioxidative enzymes, including manganese-superoxide dismutase (Mn-SOD) (55). Additionally, Forkhead box protein O3a (FOXO3a) is deacetylated by SIRT1 and translocates to the nucleus, resulting in the upregulation of other antioxidative enzymes and catalases and protection against oxidative stress (56). Thus, SIRT1 may improve insulin resistance and T2DM possibly through reducing oxidative stress (**Figure 2C**), inducing mitochondrial biogenesis, and increasing mitochondrial function.

SIRT2

SIRT2 is localized in both the cytoplasm and nucleus, and it is widely expressed in various tissues, including the brain, muscle, pancreas, liver, kidney, and adipose tissues. SIRT2 interacts with many histone and non-histone protein substrates, including tubulin and histone H4 (18). SIRT2 is involved in multiple cellular functions, including genomic integrity, cell growth, differentiation, and energy metabolism, and reduced SIRT2 activity has been implicated in cancer, neurodegeneration and metabolic diseases (18). Previous studies have demonstrated that SIRT2 plays an important role in various physiological processes in maintaining metabolic homeostasis, including inflammation, oxidative stress and mitochondrial function, as well as adipocyte differentiation, fatty acid oxidation, gluconeogenesis, and insulin sensitivity (18). A few reports have shown that SIRT2 exerts anti-inflammation and antioxidative stress effects and improves mitochondrial function in metabolic-related tissues, such as skeletal muscle.

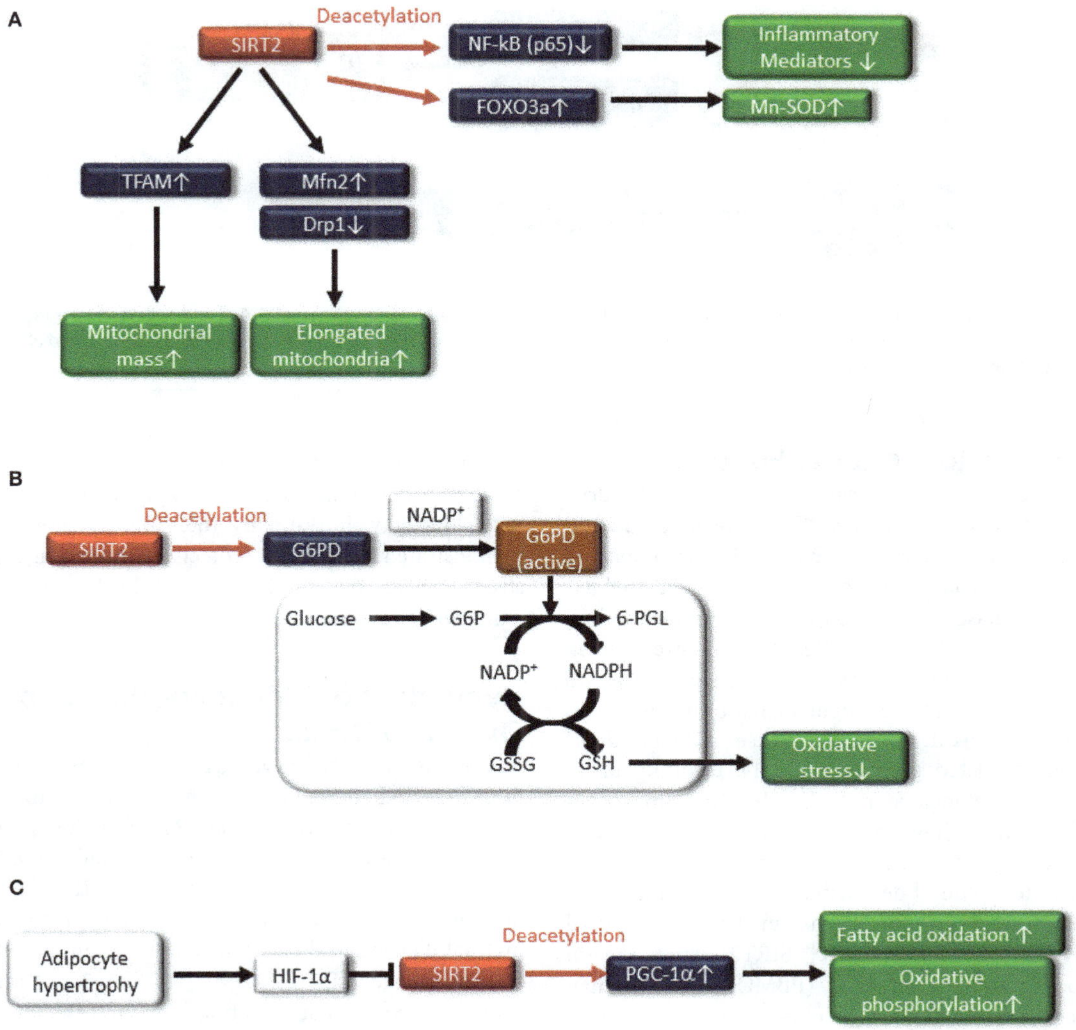

FIGURE 3 | (A) SIRT2 deacetylates nuclear factor-κB p65 subunit [NF-κB (p65)], resulting in decreased expression of inflammatory mediators. Sirt2 also induces Mn-SOD expression by deacetylating Forkhead box protein O3a (FOXO3a). Additionally, SIRT2 increases fusion-related protein mitofusion2 (Mfn2) and decreases mitochondrial-associated dynamin-related protein 1 (Drp1), resulting in an increased number of elongated mitochondria and improved mitochondrial function. SIRT2 also attenuates the downregulation of transcription factor A, mitochondrial (TFAM), a key mitochondrial deoxyribonucleic acid (mtDNA)-associated protein, leading to an increase in mitochondrial mass. **(B)** Glucose-6-phosphate dehydrogenase (G6PD) plays an important role in the oxidative stress response by producing nicotinamide adenine dinucleotide phosphate (NADPH) and the reduced form glutathione (GSH), which is associated with deacetylating G6PD and binding to nicotinamide adenine dinucleotide phosphate ($NADP^+$). **(C)** Hypoxia-inducible factor1α (HIF1α), which is accumulated in the adipocytes of hypertrophy, represses SIRT2 expression, resulting in decreased deacetylation of PGC-1α and the expression of β-oxidation and mitochondrial genes.

Regulation of Inflammation

SIRT2 regulates inflammation by deacetylating the NF-κB p65 subunit (57), similar to SIRT1. Pais et al. demonstrated that SIRT2 plays a crucial role as a major inhibitor of microglia-mediated inflammation and neurotoxicity through the deacetylation of NF-κB (p65) (58) (**Figure 2A**). In other experimental inflammatory disease models, the anti-inflammatory effect of SITR2 has been demonstrated through the suppression of the NF-κB signaling pathway (59, 60). However, further studies are necessary to elucidate whether this anti-inflammatory effect of SIRT2 may be exerted in metabolic diseases, including insulin resistance and T2DM.

Regulation of Oxidative Stress

SIRT2 regulates redox homeostasis in cells. SIRT2-dependent deacetylation of FOXO3a leads to increased expression of Mn-SOD to improve oxidative stress (61) (**Figure 3A**). In addition, glucose-6-phosphate dehydrogenase (G6PD) is a key enzyme in the pentose phosphate pathway (PPP) and plays a crucial role in the oxidative stress response by producing nicotinamide adenine dinucleotide phosphate (NADPH) and reduced form glutathione (GSH), the main intracellular reductant (**Figure 3B**). Wang et al. reported that SIRT2 activates G6PD through deacetylation on lysine 403 in G6PD, which plays an important role in maintaining the cellular redox status and protecting cells from oxidative damage (62).

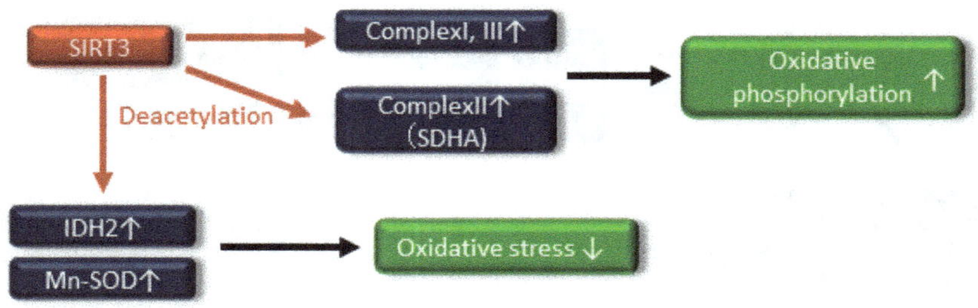

FIGURE 4 | SIRT3 deacetylates the electron transport chain complexes I, II [deacetylate succinate dehydrogenase (SDH) A] and III, leading to increased oxidative phosphorylation. SIRT3 also attenuates oxidative stress by enhancing the glutathione antioxidant defense system via deacetylation and activation of isocitrate dehydrogenase 2 (IDH2) and manganese superoxide dismutase (Mn-SOD).

Regulation of Mitochondrial Function

SIRT2 may be related to the regulation of mitochondrial function. Lemos et al. showed that SIRT2 is downregulated in insulin-resistant hepatocytes and the liver, and is accompanied by increased ROS production, activation of extracellular signal-regulated kinase (ERK1/2), and mitochondrial dysfunction in ob/ob mice (63). SIRT2 overexpression in insulin-resistant hepatocytes improved insulin sensitivity and reduced ROS production. SIRT2 might increase fusion-related protein mitofusion 2 (Mfn2) and decrease mitochondrial-associated dynamin-related protein 1 (Drp1), resulting in an increased number of elongated mitochondria and improving mitochondrial function (**Figure 3A**). SIRT2 also attenuated the downregulation of transcription factor A mitochondrial (TFAM), a key mitochondrial deoxyribonucleic acid (mtDNA)-associated protein, leading to an increase in the mitochondrial mass (63) (**Figure 3A**). Furthermore, SIRT2 expression in peripheral blood mononuclear cells (PBMCs) from human subjects was negatively correlated with obesity, insulin resistance and oxidative stress (63).

SIRT2 is most markedly expressed in adipocytes (61). Nutrient overload-induced adipose expansion enhances intra-adipose hypoxia, promoting the accumulation of adipocyte hypoxia-inducible factor 1α (HIF1α). HIF1α suppresses SIRT2 transcription through interaction at a cross-species conserved hypoxic response element (HRE) on the SIRT2 promoter. HIF1α accumulation in the adipocytes of human obese subjects correlates with low levels of SIRT2 in visceral adipose tissue, and reduced SIRT2 activity directly translates into decreased deacetylation of PGC-1α and expression of β-oxidation and mitochondrial genes. HIF-1α suppresses fatty acid catabolism in mitochondria by negatively regulating the SIRT2-PGC-1α axis (64) (**Figure 3C**).

SIRT3

Preservation of mitochondrial health is crucial to prevent insulin resistance and T2DM during aging. SIRT3 is localized primarily in the mitochondria. SIRT3 is a major mitochondrial deacetylase and plays a major role in deacetylating and modifying the enzymatic activities of several mitochondrial proteins (16). In humans, a polymorphism in the SIRT3 gene has been correlated with reduced enzymatic efficiency and the development of metabolic syndrome (65). SIRT3 is also recognized an anti-aging molecule, and high SIRT3 expression levels are associated with longevity in humans (66, 67). Previous studies have demonstrated that SIRT3 protects organisms against metabolic stress, cancer, the development of cardiac hypertrophy, and oxidative stress (16).

Regulation of Mitochondrial Function and Oxidative Stress

Numerous reports have exhibited that SIRT3 regulates mitochondrial function and maintains redox homeostasis; therefore, the impairment of SIRT3 function is implicated in the pathogenesis of insulin resistance and T2DM. Jing et al. demonstrated that decreased levels of SIRT3 in the skeletal muscle of streptozotocin (STZ)-induced diabetic mice and high-fat diet-induced obese mice were an important component of the pathogenesis of T2DM (68). SIRT3 KO mice exhibited decreased oxygen consumption and increased oxidative stress due to mitochondrial dysfunction via the hyperacetylation of complex I and III in OXPHOS, and these factors led to JNK activation and impaired insulin signaling. In addition, SIRT3 can directly deacetylate succinate dehydrogenase (SDH), a subunit of complex II and that succinate dehydrogenase activity is reduced in SIRT3 KO cells and brown adipose tissue (BAT) from SIRT3 KO mice (69). Thus, SIRT3 may induce mitochondrial oxidative phosphorylation through the deacetylation of complex I, III and SDHA of complex II (**Figure 4**).

A reduction in SIRT3 activity contributes to mitochondrial oxidative stress through decreasing the activation of antioxidative enzymes, such as isocitrate dehydrogenase 2 (IDH2) and Mn-SOD (70–72), by increasing the acetylation of antioxidative enzymes (**Figure 4**). SIRT3 protects pancreatic β cells against lipotoxicity by antagonizing oxidative stress-induced cell damage. Zhou et al. demonstrated that HFD feeding caused elevated oxidative stress accompanied by reduced SIRT3 expression in the pancreatic β cells of wild-type mice (73). Primary pancreatic islets of SIRT3 KO mice and murine pancreatic β-cell line MIN6 cells with downregulated SIRT3 expression showed increased Mn-SOD acetylation and reduced glucose-stimulated insulin secretion and glucose-stimulated ATP generation (73). On the other hand, SIRT3 overexpression,

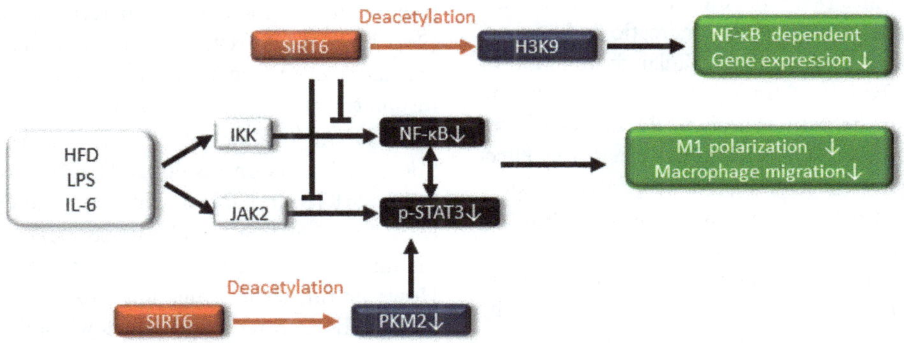

FIGURE 5 | SIRT6 also attenuates NF-κB signaling via histone H3K9 deacetylation at the chromatin level. SIRT6 suppresses the high-fat diet (HFD)-, LPS-, and IL-6-induced I-κ kinase (IKK)-nuclear factor-κB (NF-κB) pathway and Janus activating kinase 2 (JAK2)-signal transducer and activator of transcription 3 (STAT3) pathway, resulting in reduced M1 macrophage polarization and macrophage migration. Additionally, SIRT6 deacetylates pyruvate kinase M2 (PKM2), preventing STAT3 from phosphorylation.

using an adenoviral system, ameliorated palmitate-induced β-cell dysfunction including endoplasmic reticulum (ER) stress in pancreatic β-cell line NIT1 cells (74). In human, reduced expression of SIRT3 in pancreatic β cells from T2DM patients has been linked to impaired β-cell function (75). Thus, novel therapeutic approaches targeting SIRT3 activity may be important in providing new opportunities to treat insulin resistance and T2DM through maintaining mitochondrial health.

SIRT6

SIRT6 is located in the nucleus, and it acts as an adenosine diphosphate (ADP)-ribosyl transferase and NAD^+-dependent deacetylase (16). SIRT6 has been associated with longevity regulation. Kanfi et al. reported that the overexpression of SIRT6 extended the lifespan of male mice and was involved in decreased serum levels of insulin-like growth factor (IGF)-1 and increased levels of IGF-binding protein 1 (76). SIRT6 is implicated in DNA repair, telomere maintenance, genomic stability and cell senescence. SIRT6 also attenuates NF-κB signaling via histone H3K9 deacetylation at the chromatin level (77–79) (**Figure 5**).

Regulation of Inflammation, Oxidative Stress, and Mitochondrial Function

SIRT6 is involved in vascular inflammation and oxidative stress. Knockdown of SIRT6 in human umbilical vein endothelial cells (HUVECs) increases the expression of proinflammatory cytokines (80). Balestrieri et al. demonstrated that SIRT6 protein expression in atherosclerotic lesions of T2DM patients was downregulated, which was compared with SIRT6 protein expression in atherosclerotic lesions of non-diabetic patients, and the reduced SIRT6 expression was associated with increased oxidative stress and inflammation (81). Additionally, apolipoprotein E-deficient with SIRT6 knockdown using small hairpin RNA (shRNA) lentivirus-injected mice fed a high-cholesterol diet showed the promotion of atherosclerosis that was associated with increased inflammation in endothelial cells (82).

Regarding the relationship between SIRT6 and metabolic disease, SIRT6 levels increase in rats under the CR condition, and transgenic mice that overexpress SIRT6 are protected against HFD-induced several metabolic impairments, including glucose intolerance (83). By contrast, ablation of neural SIRT6 leads to obesity (84). Lee et al. demonstrated that myeloid-specific SIRT6 KO mice exhibit tissue inflammation and insulin resistance when fed an HFD (85). Myeloid SIRT6 deletion promoted proinflammatory M1 polarization of bone marrow macrophages and enhanced the migration potential of macrophages toward adipose-derived inflammatory mediators. SIRT6 deletion in macrophages facilitated activation of the IKK-NF-κB pathway and endogenous production of IL-6, leading to activation of the Janus activating kinase 2 (JAK2)-signal transducer and activator of transcription 3 (STAT3) pathway and positive feedback circuits for NF-κB stimulation; this cross talk expedited M1 polarization (85) (**Figure 5**). Furthermore, acetylated pyruvate kinase M2 (PKM2) phosphorylates STAT3 in the nucleus (86), PKM2 is deacetylated by SITR6 (87), and the study demonstrated that SIRT6 deacetylates PKM2, preventing STAT3 from being phosphorylated and leading to the suppression of M1 polarization in SIRT6-overexpressed intraperitoneal macrophages treated with LPS (**Figure 5**).

SIRT6 is involved in the regulation of mitochondrial function in skeletal muscle. Cui et al. demonstrated that muscle-specific SIRT6 KO mice impairs glucose homeostasis and insulin sensitivity, attenuates whole-body energy expenditure, and weakens exercise performance. Mechanistically, the deletion of SIRT6 in muscle decreased the expression of genes associated with glucose and lipid uptake, fatty acid oxidation, and mitochondrial OXPHOS in muscle cells caused by the reduced AMPK activity (88).

In pancreatic β cells, SIRT6 regulates insulin secretion in response to glucose stimulation. Xiong et al. demonstrated that the deletion of SIRT6 in pancreatic β-cells in mice leads to the impairment of glucose-stimulated insulin secretion (89, 90) and they further found that SIRT6 regulates insulin secretion by maintaining mitochondrial function and modulating intracellular Ca^{2+} dynamics (89, 90). Additionally, SIRT6 plays an important role in the protection of pancreatic β cells from lipotoxicity (palmitic acid, PA)-induced cellular dysfunction or even cell death (90). Oxidative stress generated by fatty acid oxidation is involved in the pathogenesis of PA-induced β-cell dysfunction and apoptosis (91). SIRT6 may exert the effect of antioxidative stress by coactivating NF-E2-related factor 2 (NRF2) (92). However, it is unclear whether SIRT6 plays a role in antioxidative stress in pancreatic β cells.

Thus, SIRT6 may have beneficial effects on glucose metabolism, including insulin resistance and T2DM, by reducing inflammation and improving mitochondrial function. Additionally, SIRT6 protects pancreatic β cells from lipotoxicity-induced cellular damage, through maintaining mitochondrial function and possibly antioxidative stress.

CONCLUDING REMARKS

The knowledge of sirtuins has expanded from the original description of a NAD^+-dependent deacetylase responsible for longevity in yeast, which is associated with CR. As described above, sirtuin family members, such as SIRT1, 2, 3, and 6, may induce beneficial effects in glucose metabolism, partially through improving inflammation, oxidative stress, and maintaining mitochondrial function. Therefore, pharmacological modulation of sirtuins may represent a novel therapeutic tool to improve insulin resistance and T2DM. Among the sirtuins, several SIRT1 activators, such as resveratrol and synthesized activators, have been evaluated for their antidiabetic effects in animal models (93). In humans, several small trials have shown that SIRT1 activators exert beneficial effects on glucose metabolism and insulin resistance, which resemble the effect of CR (94). However, there is still insufficient clinical data regarding the effect of SIRT1 activators on insulin resistance and T2DM. In addition, SIRT2, SIRT3, and SIRT6, which are induced by CR, play crucial roles in regulating cellular processes, including metabolism, inflammation, oxidative stress and mitochondrial function. However, further investigation into the targets and functions of SIRT1, SIRT2, SIRT3, and SIRT6 will aid in the development of new strategies to treat insulin resistance and T2DM. In addition to SIRT1, SIRT2, SIRT3, and SIRT6, other sirtuins, such as SIRT4, SIRT5, and SIRT7, play crucial roles in cellular homeostasis and functions, including redox homeostasis, anti-inflammation, cell survival, and mitochondrial quality control (95–100), which may be involved in the pathogenesis of insulin resistance and T2DM. However, further basic studies are necessary to elucidate the detailed molecular mechanisms.

AUTHOR CONTRIBUTIONS

MK and DK designed the manuscript, wrote and edited the manuscript. YO, IM, and DK contributed to the discussion. DK is the guarantor of this work.

REFERENCES

1. Murphy MP. How mitochondria produce reactive oxygen species. *Biochem J.* (2009) 417:1–13. doi: 10.1042/BJ20081386
2. McBride HM, Neuspiel M, Wasiak S. Mitochondria: more than just a powerhouse. *Curr Biol.* (2006) 16:R551–560. doi: 10.1016/j.cub.2006.06.054
3. Balaban RS, Nemoto S, Finkel T. Mitochondria, oxidants, and aging. *Cell.* (2005) 120:483–95. doi: 10.1016/j.cell.2005.02.001
4. Raha S, Robinson BH. Mitochondria, oxygen free radicals, disease and ageing. *Trends Biochem Sci.* (2000) 25:502–8. doi: 10.1016/S0968-0004(00)01674-1
5. Garg AK, Aggarwal BB. Reactive oxygen intermediates in TNF signaling. *Mol Immunol.* (2002) 39:509–17. doi: 10.1016/S0161-5890(02)00207-9
6. Janssen-Heininger YM, Poynter ME, Baeuerle PA. Recent advances towards understanding redox mechanisms in the activation of nuclear factor kappaB. *Free Radic Biol Med.* (2000) 28:1317–27. doi: 10.1016/S0891-5849(00)00218-5
7. Fontana L, Partridge L, Longo VD. Extending healthy life span–from yeast to humans. *Science.* (2010) 328:321–6. doi: 10.1126/science.1172539
8. Colman RJ, Anderson RM, Johnson SC, Kastman EK, Kosmatka KJ, Beasley TM, et al. Caloric restriction delays disease onset and mortality in rhesus monkeys. *Science.* (2009) 325:201–4. doi: 10.1126/science.1173635
9. Fontana L, Meyer TE, Klein S, Holloszy JO. Long-term calorie restriction is highly effective in reducing the risk for atherosclerosis in humans. *Proc Natl Acad Sci USA.* (2004) 101:6659–63. doi: 10.1073/pnas.0308291101
10. Meyer TE, Kovács SJ, Ehsani AA, Klein S, Holloszy JO, Fontana L. Long-term caloric restriction ameliorates the decline in diastolic function in humans. *J Am Coll Cardiol.* (2006) 47:398–402. doi: 10.1016/j.jacc.2005.08.069
11. Imai S, Armstrong CM, Kaeberlein M, Guarente L. Transcriptional silencing and longevity protein Sir2 is an NAD-dependent histone deacetylase. *Nature.* (2000) 403:795–800. doi: 10.1038/35001622
12. Cohen HY, Miller C, Bitterman KJ, Wall NR, Hekking B, Kessler B, et al. Calorie restriction promotes mammalian cell survival by inducing the SIRT1 deacetylase. *Science.* (2004) 305:390–2. doi: 10.1126/science.1099196
13. Bordone L, Cohen D, Robinson A, Motta MC, van Veen E, Czopik A, et al. SIRT1 transgenic mice show phenotypes resembling calorie restriction. *Aging Cell.* (2007) 6:759–67. doi: 10.1111/j.1474-9726.2007.00335.x
14. Boily G, Seifert EL, Bevilacqua L, He XH, Sabourin G, Estey C, et al. SirT1 regulates energy metabolism and response to caloric restriction in mice. *PLoS ONE.* (2008) 3:e1759. doi: 10.1371/journal.pone.0001759
15. Michan S, Sinclair D. Sirtuins in mammals: insights into their biological function. *Biochem J.* (2007) 404:1–13. doi: 10.1042/BJ20070140
16. Guarente L. Franklin H. Epstein lecture: sirtuins, aging, and medicine. *N Engl J Med.* (2011) 364:2235–44. doi: 10.1056/NEJMra1100831
17. Kitada M, Kume S, Kanasaki K, Takeda-Watanabe A, Koya D. Sirtuins as possible drug targets in type 2 diabetes. *Curr Drug Targets.* (2013) 14:622–36. doi: 10.2174/1389450111314060002
18. Gomes P, Fleming Outeiro T, Cavadas C. Emerging role of Sirtuin 2 in the regulation of mammalian metabolism. *Trends Pharmacol Sci.* (2015) 36:756–68. doi: 10.1016/j.tips.2015.08.001

19. McDonnell E, Peterson BS, Bomze HM, Hirschey MD. SIRT3 regulates progression and development of diseases of aging. *Trends Endocrinol Metab.* (2015) 26:486–92. doi: 10.1016/j.tem.2015.06.001
20. Kuang J, Chen L, Tang Q, Zhang J, Li Y, He J. The role of Sirt6 in obesity and diabetes. *Front Physiol.* (2018) 9:135. doi: 10.3389/fphys.2018.00135
21. Schenk S, Saberi M, Olefsky JM. Insulin sensitivity: modulation by nutrients and inflammation. *J Clin Invest.* (2008) 118:2992–3002. doi: 10.1172/JCI34260
22. de Luca C, Olefsky JM. Inflammation and insulin resistance. *FEBS Lett.* (2008) 582:97–105. doi: 10.1016/j.febslet.2007.11.057
23. Gerber PA, Rutter GA. The role of oxidative stress and hypoxia in pancreatic beta-cell dysfunction in diabetes mellitus. *Antioxid Redox Signal.* (2017) 26:501–18. doi: 10.1089/ars.2016.6755
24. Morgan D, Oliveira-Emilio HR, Keane D, Hirata AE, Santos da Rocha M, Bordin S, et al. Glucose, palmitate and pro-inflammatory cytokines modulate production and activity of a phagocyte-like NADPH oxidase in rat pancreatic islets and a clonal beta cell line. *Diabetologia.* (2007) 50:359–69. doi: 10.1007/s00125-006-0462-6
25. Arkan MC, Hevener AL, Greten FR, Maeda S, Li ZW, Long JM, et al. IKK-beta links inflammation to obesity-induced insulin resistance. *Nat Med.* (2005) 11:191–8. doi: 10.1038/nm1185
26. Olefsky JM, Glass CK. Macrophages, inflammation, and insulin resistance. *Annu Rev Physiol.* (2010) 72:219–46. doi: 10.1146/annurev-physiol-021909-135846
27. Solinas G, Karin M. JNK1 and IKKbeta: molecular links between obesity and metabolic dysfunction. *FASEB J.* (2010) 24:2596–611. doi: 10.1096/fj.09-151340
28. Archuleta TL, Lemieux AM, Saengsirisuwan V, Teachey MK, Lindborg KA, Kim JS, et al. Oxidant stress-induced loss of IRS-1 and IRS-2 proteins in rat skeletal muscle: role of p38 MAPK. *Free Radic Biol Med.* (2009) 47:1486–93. doi: 10.1016/j.freeradbiomed.2009.08.014
29. Evans JL, Maddux BA, Goldfine ID. The molecular basis for oxidative stress-induced insulin resistance. *Antioxid Redox Signal.* (2005) 7:1040–52. doi: 10.1089/ars.2005.7.1040
30. Evans JL, Goldfine ID, Maddux BA, Grodsky GM. Oxidative stress and stress-activated signaling pathways: a unifying hypothesis of type 2 diabetes. *Endocr Rev.* (2002) 23:599–622. doi: 10.1210/er.2001-0039
31. Bloch-Damti A, Bashan N. Proposed mechanisms for the induction of insulin resistance by oxidative stress. *Antioxid Redox Signal.* (2005) 7:1553–67. doi: 10.1089/ars.2005.7.1553
32. Petersen KF, Dufour S, Befroy D, Garcia R, Shulman GI. Impaired mitochondrial activity in the insulin-resistant offspring of patients with type 2 diabetes. *N Engl J Med.* (2004) 350:664–71. doi: 10.1056/NEJMoa031314
33. Morino K, Petersen KF, Dufour S, Befroy D, Frattini J, Shatzkes N, et al. Reduced mitochondrial density and increased IRS-1 serine phosphorylation in muscle of insulin-resistant offspring of type 2 diabetic parents. *J Clin Invest.* (2005) 115:3587–93. doi: 10.1172/JCI25151
34. Morino K, Petersen KF, Shulman GI. Molecular mechanisms of insulin resistance in humans and their potential links with mitochondrial dysfunction. *Diabetes.* (2006) 55(Suppl. 2):S9–15. doi: 10.2337/db06-S002
35. Petersen KF, Befroy D, Dufour S, Dziura J, Ariyan C, Rothman DL, et al. Mitochondrial dysfunction in the elderly: possible role in insulin resistance. *Science.* (2003) 300:1140–2. doi: 10.1126/science.1082889
36. Kitada M, Koya D. SIRT1 in type 2 diabetes: mechanisms and therapeutic potential. *Diabetes Metab J.* (2013) 37:315–25. doi: 10.4093/dmj.2013.37.5.315
37. Yeung F, Hoberg JE, Ramsey CS, Keller MD, Jones DR, Frye RA, et al. Modulation of NF-kappaB-dependent transcription and cell survival by the SIRT1 deacetylase. *EMBO J.* (2004) 23:2369–80. doi: 10.1038/sj.emboj.7600244
38. Yoshizaki T, Milne JC, Imamura T, Schenk S, Sonoda N, Babendure JL, et al. SIRT1 exerts anti-inflammatory effects and improves insulin sensitivity in adipocytes. *Mol Cell Biol.* (2009) 29:1363–74. doi: 10.1128/MCB.00705-08
39. Yoshizaki T, Schenk S, Imamura T, Babendure JL, Sonoda N, Bae EJ, et al. SIRT1 inhibits inflammatory pathways in macrophages and modulates insulin sensitivity. *Am J Physiol Endocrinol Metab.* (2010) 298:E419–428. doi: 10.1152/ajpendo.00417.2009
40. Schug TT, Xu Q, Gao H, Peres-da-Silva A, Draper DW, Fessler MB, et al. Myeloid deletion of SIRT1 induces inflammatory signaling in response to environmental stress. *Mol Cell Biol.* (2010) 30:4712–21. doi: 10.1128/MCB.00657-10
41. Takeda-Watanabe A, Kitada M, Kanasaki K, Koya D. SIRT1 inactivation induces inflammation through the dysregulation of autophagy in human THP-1 cells. *Biochem Biophys Res Commun.* (2012) 427:191–6. doi: 10.1016/j.bbrc.2012.09.042
42. de Kreutzenberg SV, Ceolotto G, Papparella I, Bortoluzzi A, Semplicini A, Dalla Man C, et al. Downregulation of the longevity-associated protein sirtuin 1 in insulin resistance and metabolic syndrome: potential biochemical mechanisms. *Diabetes.* (2010) 59:1006–15. doi: 10.2337/db09-1187
43. Gillum MP, Kotas ME, Erion DM, Kursawe R, Chatterjee P, Nead KT, et al. SirT1 regulates adipose tissue inflammation. *Diabetes.* (2011) 60:3235–45. doi: 10.2337/db11-0616
44. Hui X, Zhang M, Gu P, Li K, Gao Y, Wu D, et al. Adipocyte SIRT1 controls systemic insulin sensitivity by modulating macrophages in adipose tissue. *EMBO Rep.* (2017) 18:645–57. doi: 10.15252/embr.201643184
45. Fröjdö S, Durand C, Molin L, Carey AL, El-Osta A, Kingwell BA, et al. Phosphoinositide 3-kinase as a novel functional target for the regulation of the insulin signaling pathway by SIRT1. *Mol Cell Endocrinol.* (2011) 335:166–76. doi: 10.1016/j.mce.2011.01.008
46. Lee JH, Song MY, Song EK, Kim EK, Moon WS, Han MK, et al. Overexpression of SIRT1 protects pancreatic beta-cells against cytokine toxicity by suppressing the nuclear factor-kappaB signaling pathway. *Diabetes.* (2009) 58:344–51. doi: 10.2337/db07-1795
47. Gerhart-Hines Z, Rodgers JT, Bare O, Lerin C, Kim SH, Mostoslavsky R, et al. Metabolic control of muscle mitochondrial function and fatty acid oxidation through SIRT1/PGC-1alpha. *EMBO J.* (2007) 26:1913–23. doi: 10.1038/sj.emboj.7601633
48. Michael LF, Wu Z, Cheatham RB, Puigserver P, Adelmant G, Lehman JJ, et al. Restoration of insulin-sensitive glucose transporter. (GLUT4). gene expression in muscle cells by the transcriptional coactivator PGC-1. *Proc Natl Acad Sci USA.* (2001) 98:3820–5. doi: 10.1073/pnas.061035098
49. Kadowaki T, Yamauchi T, Kubota N, Hara K, Ueki K, Tobe K. Adiponectin and adiponectin receptors in insulin resistance, diabetes, and the metabolic syndrome. *J Clin Invest.* (2006) 116:1784–92. doi: 10.1172/JCI29126
50. Daimon M, Oizumi T, Saitoh T, Kameda W, Hirata A, Yamaguchi H, et al. Decreased serum levels of adiponectin are a risk factor for the progression to type 2 diabetes in the Japanese Population: the Funagata study. *Diabetes Care.* (2003) 26:2015–20. doi: 10.2337/diacare.26.7.2015
51. Spranger J, Kroke A, Möhlig M, Bergmann MM, Ristow M, Boeing H, et al. Adiponectin and protection against type 2 diabetes mellitus. *Lancet.* (2003) 361:226–8. doi: 10.1016/S0140-6736(03)12255-6
52. Yamauchi T, Kamon J, Waki H, Terauchi Y, Kubota N, Hara K, et al. The fat-derived hormone adiponectin reverses insulin resistance associated with both lipoatrophy and obesity. *Nat Med.* (2001) 7:941–6. doi: 10.1038/90984
53. Qiao L, Shao J. SIRT1 regulates adiponectin gene expression through Foxo1-C/enhancer-binding protein alpha transcriptional complex. *J Biol Chem.* (2006) 281:39915–24. doi: 10.1074/jbc.M607215200
54. Iwabu M, Yamauchi T, Okada-Iwabu M, Sato K, Nakagawa T, Funata M, et al. Adiponectin and AdipoR1 regulate PGC-1alpha and mitochondria by Ca (2+) and AMPK/SIRT1. *Nature* . (2010) 464:1313–9. doi: 10.1038/nature08991
55. St-Pierre J, Drori S, Uldry M, Silvaggi JM, Rhee J, Jäger S, et al. Suppression of reactive oxygen species and neurodegeneration by the PGC-1 transcriptional coactivators. *Cell.* (2006) 127:397–408. doi: 10.1016/j.cell.2006.09.024
56. Hasegawa K, Wakino S, Yoshioka K, Tatematsu S, Hara Y, Minakuchi H, et al. Sirt1 protects against oxidative stress-induced renal tubular cell apoptosis by the bidirectional regulation of catalase expression. *Biochem Biophys Res Commun.* (2008) 372:51–6. doi: 10.1016/j.bbrc.2008.04.176
57. Rothgiesser KM, Erener S, Waibel S, Lüscher B, Hottiger MO. SIRT2 regulates NF-kappaB dependent gene expression through deacetylation of p65 Lys310. *J Cell Sci.* (2010) 123:4251–8. doi: 10.1242/jcs.073783
58. Pais TF, Szego EM, Marques O, Miller-Fleming L, Antas P, Guerreiro P, et al. The NAD-dependent deacetylase sirtuin 2 is a suppressor of

microglial activation and brain inflammation. *EMBO J.* (2013) 32:2603–16. doi: 10.1038/emboj.2013.200

59. Lo Sasso G, Menzies KJ, Mottis A, Piersigilli A, Perino A, Yamamoto H, et al. SIRT2 deficiency modulates macrophage polarization and susceptibility to experimental colitis. *PLoS ONE.* (2014) 9:e103573. doi: 10.1371/journal.pone.0103573
60. Lin J, Sun B, Jiang C, Hong H, Zheng Y. Sirt2 suppresses inflammatory responses in collagen-induced arthritis. *Biochem Biophys Res Commun.* (2013) 441:897–903. doi: 10.1016/j.bbrc.2013.10.153
61. Wang F, Nguyen M, Qin FX, Tong Q. SIRT2 deacetylates FOXO3a in response to oxidative stress and caloric restriction. *Aging Cell.* (2007) 6:505–14. doi: 10.1111/j.1474-9726.2007.00304.x
62. Wang YP, Zhou LS, Zhao YZ, Wang SW, Chen LL, Liu LX, et al. Regulation of G6PD acetylation by SIRT2 and KAT9 modulates NADPH homeostasis and cell survival during oxidative stress. *EMBO J.* (2014) 33:1304–20. doi: 10.1002/embj.201387224
63. Lemos V, de Oliveira RM, Naia L, Szegö É, Ramos E, Pinho S, et al. The NAD+-dependent deacetylase SIRT2 attenuates oxidative stress and mitochondrial dysfunction and improves insulin sensitivity in hepatocytes. *Hum Mol Genet.* (2017) 26:4105–17. doi: 10.1093/hmg/ddx298
64. Krishnan J, Danzer C, Simka T, Ukropec J, Walter KM, Kumpf S, et al. Dietary obesity-associated Hif1alpha activation in adipocytes restricts fatty acid oxidation and energy expenditure via suppression of the Sirt2-NAD+ system. *Genes Dev.* (2012) 26:259–70. doi: 10.1101/gad.180406.111
65. Hirschey MD, Shimazu T, Goetzman E, Jing E, Schwer B, Lombard DB, et al. SIRT3 regulates mitochondrial fatty-acid oxidation by reversible enzyme deacetylation. *Nature.* (2010) 464:121–5. doi: 10.1038/nature08778
66. Bellizzi D, Rose G, Cavalcante P, Covello G, Dato S, De Rango F, et al. A novel VNTR enhancer within the SIRT3 gene, a human homologue of SIR2, is associated with survival at oldest ages. *Genomics.* (2005) 85:258–63. doi: 10.1016/j.ygeno.2004.11.003
67. Rose G, Dato S, Altomare K, Bellizzi D, Garasto S, Greco V, et al. Variability of the SIRT3 gene, human silent information regulator Sir2 homologue, and survivorship in the elderly. *Exp Gerontol.* (2003) 38:1065–70. doi: 10.1016/S0531-5565(03)00209-2
68. Jing E, Emanuelli B, Hirschey MD, Boucher J, Lee KY, Lombard D, et al. Sirtuin-3 (Sirt3) regulates skeletal muscle metabolism and insulin signaling via altered mitochondrial oxidation and reactive oxygen species production. *Proc Natl Acad Sci USA.* (2011) 108:14608–13. doi: 10.1073/pnas.1111308108
69. Finley LW, Haas W, Desquiret-Dumas V, Wallace DC, Procaccio V, Gygi SP, et al. Succinate dehydrogenase is a direct target of sirtuin 3 deacetylase activity. *PLoS ONE.* (2011) 6:e23295. doi: 10.1371/journal.pone.0023295
70. Someya S, Yu W, Hallows WC, Xu J, Vann JM, Leeuwenburgh C, et al. Sirt3 mediates reduction of oxidative damage and prevention of age-related hearing loss under caloric restriction. *Cell.* (2010) 143:802–12. doi: 10.1016/j.cell.2010.10.002
71. Qiu X, Brown K, Hirschey MD, Verdin E, Chen D. Calorie restriction reduces oxidative stress by SIRT3-mediated SOD2 activation. *Cell Metab.* (2010) 12:662–7. doi: 10.1016/j.cmet.2010.11.015
72. Ogura Y, Kitada M, Monno I, Kanasaki K, Watanabe A, Koya D. Renal mitochondrial oxidative stress is enhanced by the reduction of Sirt3 activity, in Zucker diabetic fatty rats. *Redox Rep.* (2018) 23:153–9. doi: 10.1080/13510002.2018.1487174
73. Zhou Y, Chung ACK, Fan R, Lee HM, Xu G, Tomlinson B, et al. Sirt3 deficiency increased the vulnerability of pancreatic beta cells to oxidative stress-induced dysfunction. *Antioxid Redox Signal.* (2017) 27:962–76. doi: 10.1089/ars.2016.6859
74. Kim M, Lee JS, Oh JE, Nan J, Lee H, Jung HS, et al. SIRT3 overexpression attenuates palmitate-induced pancreatic beta-cell dysfunction. *PLoS ONE.* (2015) 10:e0124744. doi: 10.1371/journal.pone.0124744
75. Caton PW, Richardson SJ, Kieswich J, Bugliani M, Holland ML, Marchetti P, et al. Sirtuin 3 regulates mouse pancreatic beta cell function and is suppressed in pancreatic islets isolated from human type 2 diabetic patients. *Diabetologia.* (2013) 56:1068–77. doi: 10.1007/s00125-013-2851-y
76. Kanfi Y, Naiman S, Amir G, Peshti V, Zinman G, Nahum L, et al. The sirtuin SIRT6 regulates lifespan in male mice. *Nature.* (2012) 483:218–21. doi: 10.1038/nature10815
77. Michishita E, McCord RA, Berber E, Kioi M, Padilla-Nash H, Damian M, et al. SIRT6 is a histone H3 lysine 9 deacetylase that modulates telomeric chromatin. *Nature.* (2008) 452:492–6. doi: 10.1038/nature06736
78. Michishita E, McCord RA, Boxer LD, Barber MF, Hong T, Gozani O, et al. Cell cycle-dependent deacetylation of telomeric histone H3 lysine K56 by human SIRT6. *Cell Cycle.* (2009) 8:2664–6. doi: 10.4161/cc.8.16.9367
79. Kawahara TL, Michishita E, Adler AS, Damian M, Berber E, Lin M, et al. SIRT6 links histone H3 lysine 9 deacetylation to NF-kappaB-dependent gene expression and organismal life span. *Cell.* (2009) 136:62–74. doi: 10.1016/j.cell.2008.10.052
80. Lappas M. Anti-inflammatory properties of sirtuin 6 in human umbilical vein endothelial cells. *Med Inflamm.* (2012) 2012:597514. doi: 10.1155/2012/597514
81. Balestrieri ML, Rizzo MR, Barbieri M, Paolisso P, D'Onofrio N, et al. Sirtuin 6 expression and inflammatory activity in diabetic atherosclerotic plaques: effects of incretin treatment. *Diabetes.* (2015) 64:1395–406. doi: 10.2337/db14-1149
82. Liu Z, Wang J, Huang X, Li Z, Liu P. Deletion of sirtuin 6 accelerates endothelial dysfunction and atherosclerosis in apolipoprotein E-deficient mice. *Transl Res.* (2016) 172:18–29. doi: 10.1016/j.trsl.2016.02.005
83. Kanfi Y, Peshti V, Gil R, Naiman S, Nahum L, Levin E, et al. SIRT6 protects against pathological damage caused by diet-induced obesity. *Aging Cell.* (2010) 9:162–73. doi: 10.1111/j.1474-9726.2009.00544.x
84. Schwer B, Schumacher B, Lombard DB, Xiao C, Kurtev MV, Gao J, et al. Neural sirtuin 6 (Sirt6) ablation attenuates somatic growth and causes obesity. *Proc Natl Acad Sci USA.* (2010) 107:21790–4. doi: 10.1073/pnas.1016306107
85. Lee Y, Ka SO, Cha HN, Chae YN, Kim MK, Park SY, et al. Myeloid Sirtuin 6 deficiency causes insulin resistance in high-fat diet-fed mice by eliciting macrophage polarization toward an M1 phenotype. *Diabetes.* (2017) 66:2659–68. doi: 10.2337/db16-1446
86. Lv L, Xu YP, Zhao D, Li FL, Wang W, Sasaki N, et al. Mitogenic and oncogenic stimulation of K433 acetylation promotes PKM2 protein kinase activity and nuclear localization. *Mol Cell.* (2013) 52:340–52. doi: 10.1016/j.molcel.2013.09.004
87. Bhardwaj A, Das S. SIRT6 deacetylates PKM2 to suppress its nuclear localization and oncogenic functions. *Proc Natl Acad Sci USA.* (2016) 113:E538–547. doi: 10.1073/pnas.1520045113
88. Cui X, Yao L, Yang X, Gao Y, Fang F, Zhang J, et al. SIRT6 regulates metabolic homeostasis in skeletal muscle through activation of AMPK. *Am J Physiol Endocrinol Metab.* (2017) 313:E493–E505. doi: 10.1152/ajpendo.00122.2017
89. Xiong X, Wang G, Tao R, Wu P, Kono T, Li K, et al. Sirtuin 6 regulates glucose-stimulated insulin secretion in mouse pancreatic beta cells. *Diabetologia.* (2016) 59:151–60. doi: 10.1007/s00125-015-3778-2
90. Xiong X, Sun X, Wang Q, Qian X, Zhang Y, Pan X, et al. SIRT6 protects against palmitate-induced pancreatic beta-cell dysfunction and apoptosis. *J Endocrinol.* (2016) 231:159–65. doi: 10.1530/JOE-16-0317
91. Janikiewicz J, Hanzelka K, Kozinski K, Kolczynska K, Dobrzyn A. Islet beta-cell failure in type 2 diabetes–Within the network of toxic lipids. *Biochem Biophys Res Commun.* (2015) 460:491–6. doi: 10.1016/j.bbrc.2015.03.153
92. Pan H, Guan D, Liu X, Li J, Wang L, Wu J, et al. SIRT6 safeguards human mesenchymal stem cells from oxidative stress by coactivating NRF2. *Cell Res.* (2016) 26:190–205. doi: 10.1038/cr.2016.4
93. Milne JC, Lambert PD, Schenk S, Carney DP, Smith JJ, Gagne DJ, et al. Small molecule activators of SIRT1 as therapeutics for the treatment of type 2 diabetes. *Nature.* (2007) 450:712–6. doi: 10.1038/nature06261
94. Smoliga JM, Baur JA, Hausenblas HA. Resveratrol and health–a comprehensive review of human clinical trials. *Mol Nutr Food Res.* (2011) 55:1129–41. doi: 10.1002/mnfr.201100143
95. Tao Y, Huang C, Huang Y, Hong L, Wang H, Zhou Z, et al. SIRT4 suppresses inflammatory responses in human umbilical vein endothelial cells. *Cardiovasc Toxicol.* (2015) 15:217–23. doi: 10.1007/s12012-014-9287-6

96. Lang A, Anand R, Altinoluk-Hambüchen S, Ezzahoini H, Stefanski A, Iram A, et al. SIRT4 interacts with OPA1 and regulates mitochondrial quality control and mitophagy. *Aging.* (2017) 9:2163–89. doi: 10.18632/aging.101307
97. Singh CK, Chhabra G, Ndiaye MA, Garcia-Peterson LM, Mack NJ, Ahmad N. The role of sirtuins in antioxidant and redox signaling. *Antioxid Redox Signal.* (2018) 28:643–61. doi: 10.1089/ars.2017.7290
98. Zhou L, Wang F, Sun R, Chen X, Zhang M, Xu Q, et al. SIRT5 promotes IDH2 desuccinylation and G6PD deglutarylation to enhance cellular antioxidant defense. *EMBO Rep.* (2016) 17:811–22. doi: 10.15252/embr.201541643
99. Wang Y, Liu Q, Huan Y, Li R, Li C, Sun S, et al. Sirtuin 5 overexpression attenuates glucolipotoxicity-induced pancreatic β cells apoptosis and dysfunction. *Exp Cell Res.* (2018) 371:205–13. doi: 10.1016/j.yexcr.2018.08.011
100. Ma Y, Fei X. SIRT5 regulates pancreatic β-cell proliferation and insulin secretion in type 2 diabetes. *Exp Ther Med.* (2018) 16:1417–25. doi: 10.3892/etm.2018.6301

10

The Roles of Mitochondrial SIRT4 in Cellular Metabolism

Zheying Min [1,2†], Jiangman Gao [1†] and Yang Yu [1]*

[1] Beijing Key Laboratory of Reproductive Endocrinology and Assisted Reproductive Technology and Key Laboratory of Assisted Reproduction, Ministry of Education, Department of Obstetrics and Gynecology, Center for Reproductive Medicine, Peking University Third Hospital, Beijing, China, [2] Peking-Tsinghua Center for Life Sciences, Academy for Advanced Interdisciplinary Studies, Peking University, Beijing, China

Correspondence:
Yang Yu
yuyang5012@hotmail.com

† These authors have contributed equally to this work

Sirtuins comprise a family of nicotinamide adenine dinucleotide (NAD^+)-dependent lysine deacylases that regulate the life span, aging, and metabolism. Seven sirtuin family members (SIRT1-7) have been identified in mammals, including humans. Despite the indispensable role of mitochondrial sirtuin 4 (SIRT4) in metabolic regulation, the primary enzymatic activity of SIRT4 remains enigmatic. SIRT4 possesses ADP-ribosyltransferase, lipoamidase and deacylase activities. Interestingly, the enzymatic activities and substrates of SIRT4 vary in different tissues and cells. SIRT4 inhibits insulin secretion in pancreatic β cells and regulates insulin sensitivity as a deacylase in the pancreas. SIRT4 represses fatty acid oxidation (FAO) in muscle and liver cells differently. SIRT4 has also been identified as a mitochondrial-localized tumor suppressor. A comprehensive understanding of the enzymology of SIRT4 in metabolism is essential for developing novel therapeutic agents for human metabolic diseases. This review will update the roles of SIRT4 in cellular and organismal metabolic homeostasis.

Keywords: SIRT4, mitochondrial, enzymatic activities, insulin secretion, fatty acid metabolism, tumor suppressor

INTRODUCTION

Sirtuins include β-NAD^+-dependent deacylases and ADP-ribosyltransferases involved with metabolism and aging (1, 2). Sirtuins (SIRT1-7) can be divided into nuclear (SIRT1, SIRT6, and SIRT7), mitochondrial (SIRT3, SIRT4, and SIRT5) and cytosolic (SIRT2) forms, and some sirtuins are found in more than one compartment (**Figure 1B**). The mitochondrial sirtuins are involved in metabolic regulation and antioxidative defense. In contrast to other members of SIRT, the enzymatic activities of SIRT4 have remained unclear (3, 4). SIRT4 is critical for cellular metabolism and DNA damage responses in mitochondria. SIRT4 contains an N-terminal mitochondrial signal sequence that directs of its localization to mitochondria (4). SIRT4 has the requisite amino acids to participate in deacylase reactions (5), namely, a homologous sirtuin deacylase domain, a conserved catalytic histidine, and a Rossmann fold/NAD^+-binding motif (aa 62–82, 143–146, 260–262, and 286–288) (**Figure 1A**). Previous genetic studies divide human sirtuins into four classes. SIRT4 belongs to the class II human sirtuins (**Figure 1C**). SIRT4 mRNA and protein are detected in human muscle, kidney, testis, and liver cells (6). This expression pattern is consistent with the functions of SIRT4. In this review, we summarize the roles of SIRT4 in cellular metabolic homeostasis, including the regulation of insulin secretion and fatty acid oxidation and the effect on tumor cells of different tissues (**Table 1**).

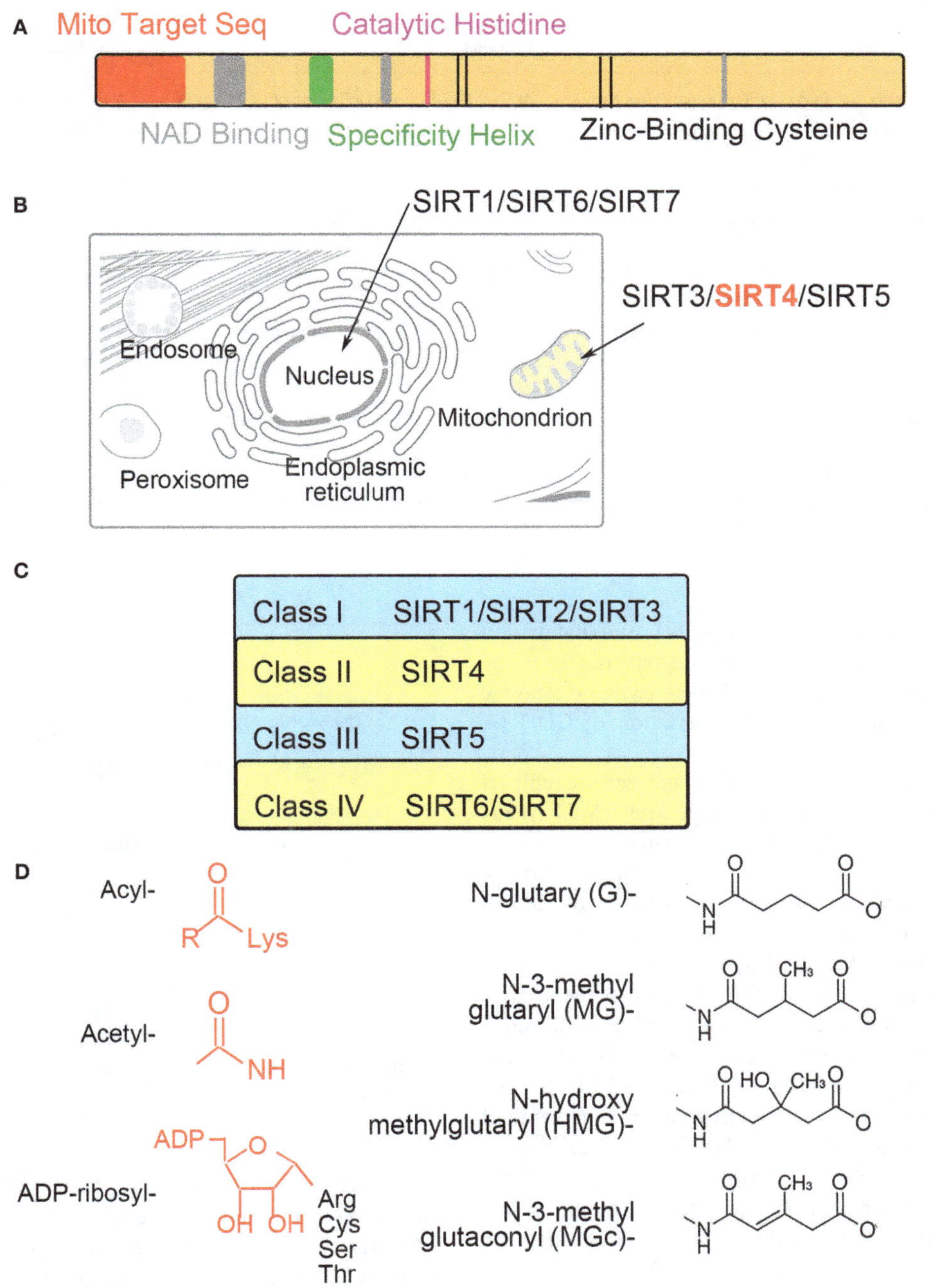

FIGURE 1 | The characteristics of mitochondrial SIRT4 **(A).** Sequence analyses show the amino acid sequence of the mitochondrial localization, NAD^{+}-binding, substrate specificity, catalytic and Zn^{2+}-binding domains **(B)**. SIRT4 is localized in the mitochondrion **(C)**. SIRT4 is belong to a class II human sirtuins **(D)**. Structure of groups catalyzed by SIRT4.

SIRT4 INHIBITS INSULIN SECRETION IN PANCREATIC β CELLS

SIRT4 was initially found to reduce glutamate dehydrogenase (GDH) activity, thereby inhibiting insulin secretion in pancreatic β cells (7, 9). GDH is known to facilitate glutamine metabolism and ATP production, thus inducing insulin secretion (19, 20). GDH is ADP-ribosylated and inhibited by SIRT4, subsequently repressing leucine-mediated insulin secretion (7, 21). The depletion of SIRT4 in insulinoma cells could activate GDH, thus increasing amino acid-stimulated insulin secretion. Pancreatic β cells derived from SIRT4 knockout mice and those from mice on calorie restriction (CR) as a dietary regimen show a similar effect of insulin secretion (8, 22). Phosphodiesterase (PDE) can be used as a probe for ADP-ribosylation because it cleaves the ADP-ribose and can relieve inhibition. GDH from

TABLE 1 | Summary of roles of SIRT4 in celluar metabolism.

Genotype	Phenotype	Process	Activities	References
SIRT4 OE cells	Inhibition of insulin secretion in pancreas β cells	ADP-ribosylation and inhibition of GDH	ADP-ribosylation	(6–8)
SIRT4 KO cells	Activation of GDH and stimulation of insulin secretion in insulinoma cells	Activation of GDH	ADP-ribosylation	
SIRT4 KO mice	Increased insulin secretion,	Activation of GDH	ADP-ribosylation	
SIRT4 KO mice	Deregulated lecuine metabolism and aging induced IR	Dysregulated leucine oxidation	deacylation	(9–11)
SIRT4 OE cells	Increased lipogenesis and decreased FAO in adipocyte and myocyte cell	Deacetylation of MCD	deacetylation	(12–15)
SIRT4 KO cells	Increased FAO in muscle and WAT cells	Activation of MCD and decreased malony-CoA	Deacetylation	
SIRT4 KO mice	Elevated FAO and resistance to obesity and exercise	Activation of GDH	Deacetylation	
SIRT4 OE cells	Depressed FAO in liver cells	Repression of PPARα transcriptional activation by SIRT1	–	(12, 16–18)
SIRT4 KO cells	Increased FAO rate	Activation of PPARα	–	
SIRT4 KO mice	Increased FAO rate and PPARα pathway	Activation of FAO by PPARα and SIRT1	–	

OE, over expression; KO, knock out.

SIRT4-deficient mice is insensitive to (PDE), and incubation with PDE increases the GDH activity of wild-type lysates to the KO samples. It indicates the absence of the enzymatic cleavage of ADP-ribose would decrease ADP-ribosylation of GDH (6, 8).

A recent study demonstrated that SIRT4 catalyzed the removal of novel lysine modifications: methylglutaryl (MG)-lysine, hydroxymethylglutaryl (HMG)-lysine, and 3-methylglutaconyl (MGc)-lysine (10, 11). SIRT4 participates in leucine oxidation by removing these modifications sequentially. These modifications were discovered and characterized through phylogenetic and structural analysis (**Figure 1D**). The α-helical region containing the catalytic pocket of SIRT4 was associated with an interaction with negatively charged acyl- modifications (23, 24). In a complementary study, a recombinant SIRT4 protein could remove glutaryl-, MG-, HMG-, and MGc-lysine modifications. Further, SIRT4 overexpression in cells resulted in decreased glutaryl-, MG-, and HMG-lysine expression levels. The methylcrotonyl-CoA carboxylase complex (MCCC) associated with leucine catabolism and interacting with SIRT4 was marked with these new modifications *in vivo* (10). The absence of SIRT4 increased and destabilized MCCC acylation, leading to decreased leucine flux. The level of a key allosteric GDH activator, leucine, was changed due to the repression of GDH activity and glutamine metabolism by SIRT4 (25, 26). Knowledge about these new modifications provided new insights into SIRT4 function in further metabolism studies (**Figure 2**).

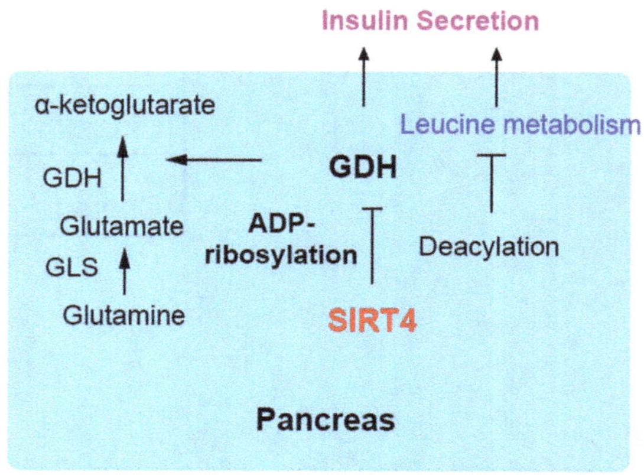

FIGURE 2 | SIRT4 regulates insulin secretion in pancreatic β cells. GDH is ADP-ribosylated and inhibited by SIRT4, repressing insulin secretion.

SIRT4 INHIBITS FATTY ACID OXIDATION IN MUSCLE AND FAT CELLS

The repressive effect of SIRT4 against FAO in muscle cells is regulated by the deacetylation and inhibition of the activity of mitochondrial malonyl-CoA decarboxylase (MCD), leading to an increase in malonyl-CoA (12, 13, 27). Malonyl CoA is a key metabolite that inhibits fat catabolism and promotes fat synthesis (28). There are two enzymes that regulate cellular malonyl-CoA levels. MCD catalyzes the conversion of malonyl-CoA to acetyl-CoA, while acetyl-CoA carboxylase (ACC) converts acetyl-CoA back to malonyl-CoA via a reaction regulated by the phosphorylation of AMPK (14, 29). Cytosolic fatty acids transported into the mitochondrial matrix cross the outer and inner mitochondrial membranes for β-oxidation, and this key step is catalyzed by carnitine palmitoyltransferase (CPT1), which is inhibited by accumulated malonyl-CoA (30, 31). During the nutritional rich state (Fed), when the metabolic intermediates funnel into fat synthesis and energy storage, the steady state is increased malonyl-CoA. This suppresses entry of fatty acids into mitochondria and weakens FAO sequentially (15). Conversely, in the fasted state, the malonyl-CoA is decreased and the FAO is evaluated for energy production (**Figure 3**). Therefore, SIRT4 regulates malonyl-CoA levels of muscle and WAT of mice in

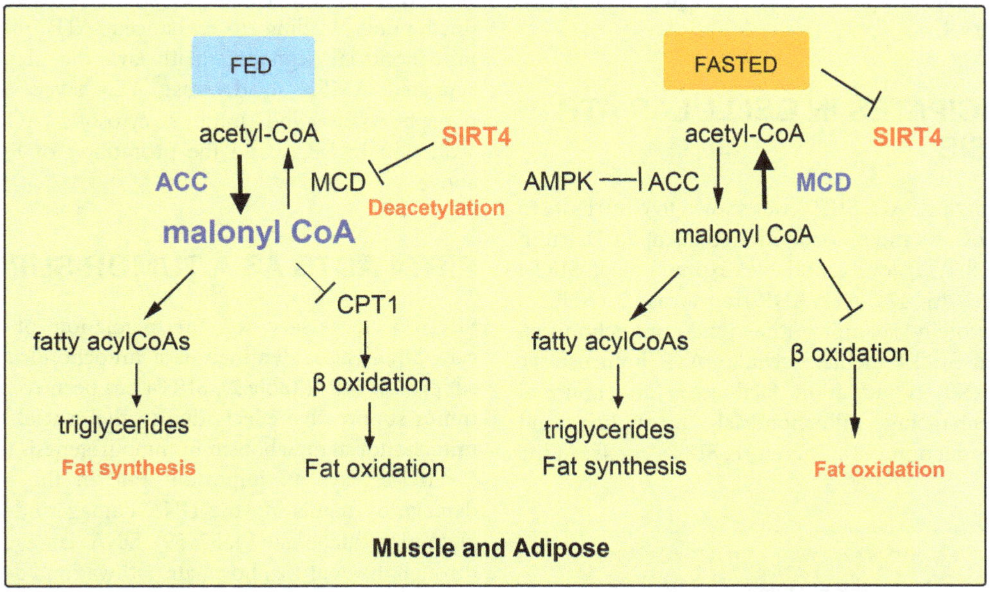

FIGURE 3 | SIRT4 mediates fatty acid oxidation in muscle and adipose cells. In fed state, SIRT4 decreases the activity of the mitochondrial malonyl-CoA decarboxylase (MCD), which can increase malonyl-CoA levels, thus inhibiting FAO. In fasted state, the level malonyl-CoA of is decreased conversely.

the fed and fasted state. In addition, as a unit of fatty acid synthesis, the accumulated malonyl-CoA promotes and provides a carbon skeleton for fatty acid biosynthesis in white adipose tissue (WAT) (32, 33). A previous study reported that SIRT4 overexpression increased lipogenesis and decreased fatty acid oxidation, while SIRT4 knockdown showed the opposite effect on lipid synthesis and catabolism in mouse adipocyte and myocyte cell lines (3, 34). Furthermore, the regulation pattern was confirmed in SIRT4 knockout mice, which showed elevated FAO associated with a resistance to diet-induced obesity and an increased exercise tolerance (24, 35, 36). Additionally, the interaction of MCD and SIRT4 in the mitochondrial matrix was demonstrated by coimmunoprecipitation. SIRT4 lacked detectable histone deacetylase activity, but it deacetylated MCD in a substrate-specific manner (37, 38). Further, mitochondrial located SIRT3 was confirmed and excluded the possibility of deacetylation activity, because interaction between SIRT3 and SIRT4. SIRT3 showed no detectable interaction with MCD indicating the specific function of SIRT4. SIRT4 coordinated lipid homeostasis by promoting lipid anabolism and repressing lipid catabolism (39, 40).

SIRT4 REPRESSES HEPATIC FAO IN LIVER CELLS

Liver plays a role in energy homeostasis by balancing lipid metabolism and energetic demands in organisms (12, 16). Under nutrient-rich conditions, hepatic lipogenesis, and lipoprotein secretion are activated. In contrast, during fasting, hepatic FAO is stimulated to provide the organism with ketone bodies as cellular energy fuel for the brain. One of the key mediators of the hepatic response to fasting is nuclear receptor peroxisome proliferation-activated receptor α (PPARα). SIRT4 negatively mediated fatty acid oxidation in liver cells by suppressing the transcriptional activity of PPARα (17, 41). More specifically, the interaction of SIRT1 and PPARα was disrupted by SIRT4, thus attenuating the activation of PPARα transcriptional activity via SIRT1 to inhibit FAO (18). In normal liver cells, by interacting with PPARα, SIRT1 is recruited to the PPARα response element (PPRE), which catalyzes the N^{ε}-acetyl-lysine deacetylation of the transcriptional coactivator peroxisome proliferator-activated receptor gamma coactivator 1-alpha (PGC-1α) to promote FAO (42). Additionally, SIRT4 competes with other sirtuins including SIRT1 for β-NAD^+, leading to decreased SIRT1 activity and a reduced effect of SIRT1 on both the transcriptional activity of PPARα and FAO (43, 44). During fasting, FAO is promoted as a source of cellular energy. The decreased SIRT4 levels in liver cells demonstrate the inhibitory effect of SIRT4 on liver FAO (45).

The roles of SIRT4 in liver cells were supported by knockout and overexpression experiments in cellular and animal models. In SIRT4 knockdown and knockout primary hepatocytes, the expression of mitochondrial and fatty acid metabolism enzyme genes was increased significantly (17). Consistent with increased FAO gene expression, SIRT4 knockdown hepatocytes exhibited higher rates of FAO than wild-type cells. The increase in FAO gene expression in SIRT4 knockout mice was consistent with the results in primary hepatocytes (12). Additionally, SIRT1 mRNA and protein levels were also evaluated both *in vitro* and *in vivo* by the knockdown of SIRT4. In SIRT4/SIRT1 double-knockdown hepatocytes, there was not an increase in FAO compared with that induced by SIRT4 knockdown only (17). These results suggested that SIRT4-modulated FAO was dependent on SIRT1 in primary hepatocytes (22, 46). Moreover, SIRT4 overexpression repressed SIRT1 activation of PPARα and consequently inhibited hepatic FAO (**Figure 4**).

SIRT4 PARTICIPATES IN CELLULAR ATP HOMEOSTASIS

In addition to regulating FAO, SIRT4 was shown to contribute to cellular ATP homeostasis and mitochondrial biogenesis. Deletion of SIRT4 decreased ATP levels, and overexpression of SIRT4 increased ATP levels (3, 47). ATP/ADP translocase 2 (ANT2a, transmembrane protein spanning the inner mitochondrial membrane) helped SIRT4 mediate cellular ATP homeostasis. Mechanistically, ANT N^{ε}-acylation facilitated mitochondrial respiration by enhancing mitochondrial uncoupling and decreasing ATP production (48). Therefore, SIRT4 catalyzed the N^{ε}-acyl-lysine deacylation of ANT2 to reduce mitochondrial uncoupling, leading to enhanced ATP production. In the mitochondrial signaling pathway, the depletion of SIRT4 activated AMPK to decrease ATP levels. Activated AMPK phosphorylates and inhibits cytosolic ACC, leading to a reduction in MCA and the promotion of FAO as mentioned above.

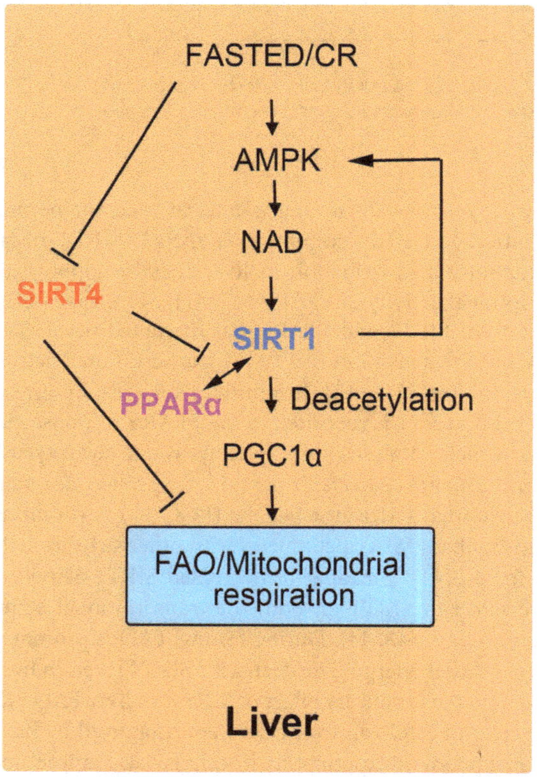

FIGURE 4 | SIRT4 mediates fatty acid oxidation in liver cells. The interaction of SIRT1 and PPARα is blocked by SIRT4, leading to a decrease in FAO.

SIRT4 ACTS AS A TUMOR SUPPRESSOR

SIRT4 is necessary for the regulation of FAO in normal cells but is also identified as a mitochondrial-localized tumor suppressor (49) (**Table 2**). SIRT4 has been recognized to possess tumor-suppressive effects due to the crucial regulatory role of mitochondrial metabolism in tumourigenesis (34, 50).

SIRT4 plays an important role in the response to DNA damage by regulating the DNA damage-induced inhibition of glutamine catabolism (4, 57, 59). DNA damage increases the flux through the pentose phosphate pathway and decreases glutamine uptake and the levels of TCA cycle intermediates. Mitochondrial glutaminase can catabolize glutamine to form glutamate via mitochondrial GDH and aspartate aminotransferase activity (60). Previous research showed that SIRT4 ADP-ribosylated and inhibited GDH and was thus involved in DNA damage-induced inhibition of glutamine metabolism and anaplerosis (33, 39).

SIRT4 possesses a tumor suppressive effect because of its inhibitory effect on glutamine catabolism and its antiproliferative

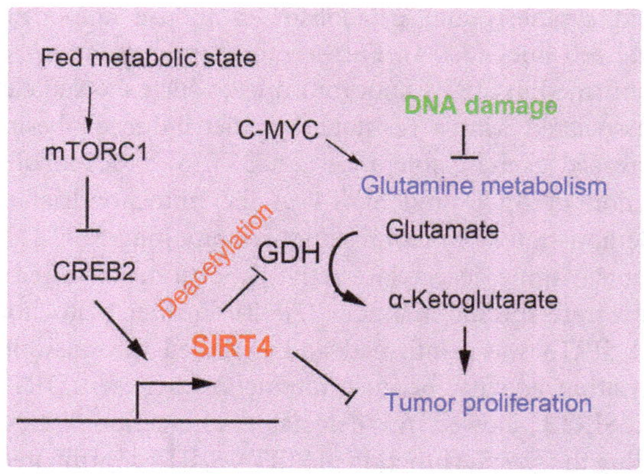

FIGURE 5 | SIRT4 plays a role in tumor suppression. SIRT4 suppresses tumor proliferation by inhibiting glutamine metabolism and DNA damage repair.

TABLE 2 | Summary tumor repressor roles of SIRT4.

Phenotype	Type of tumor	Roles	References
SIRT4 is decreased	Acute myeloid leukemia	Inhibiting proliferation of tumor	(50, 51)
SIRT4 is decreased	Burkitt lymphoma	Inhibiting proliferation of tumor	(52, 53)
SIRT4 is decreased	Colorectal cancer	Inhibiting proliferation and migration of tumor	(54, 55)
SIRT4 is decreased	Gastric cancer	Inhibiting proliferation and migration of tumor	(56)
SIRT4 is decreased	Lung tumor	Inhibiting proliferation and migration of tumor	(57, 58)

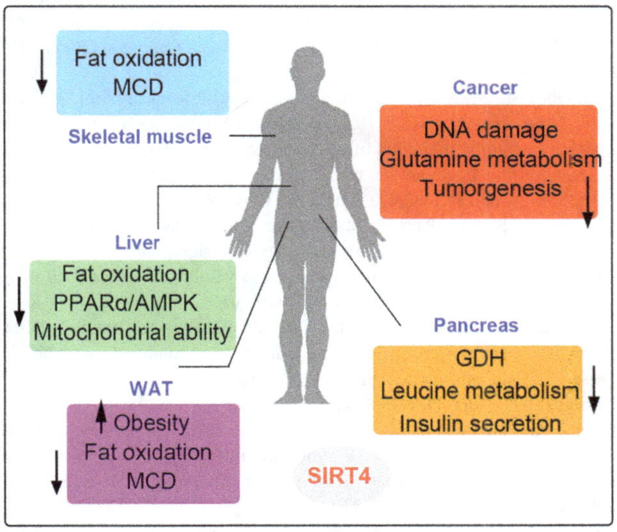

FIGURE 6 | The metabolic roles of SIRT4 in various organs. SIRT4 is mainly involved in the metabolism of muscle, liver, fat, pancreatic, and cancer cells. The up arrows indicate the increased regulation pathways and the down arrows indicate the decreased regulation pathways induced by SIRT4.

effect on cells with DNA damage (61, 62). Indeed, SIRT4 expression is upregulated by DNA damage and is downregulated in many types of human tumor tissues and cells (44). SIRT4 depletion leads to both elevated glutamine-dependent proliferation and stress-induced genomic instability, resulting in tumourigenic phenotypes. SIRT4 inhibits glutamine catabolism, especially replenishment into the citric acid cycle, creating a cellular state promoting DNA damage repair (63). In the absence of SIRT4, DNA damage results in delayed DNA repair and increased chromosomal aneuploidies, suggesting that SIRT4 could protect cells from spontaneous damage. Furthermore, SIRT4 null mice spontaneously develop lung tumors (19, 64).

SIRT4 can specifically repress the growth of B cells induced by the transcriptional factor c-Myc through inhibiting glutamine metabolism induced by the abnormal activation of c-Myc in c-Myc-dependent cancers (52, 65). In human Burkitt lymphoma cells, the overexpression of SIRT4 repressed glutamine metabolism and glutamine-dependent cell proliferation, as observed in cells treated with glycolysis inhibitors, promoting cell death (66). Consistent with these findings, the depletion of SIRT4 resulted in increased glutamine-absorbing and GDH enzymic activity in a mouse model of Burkitt lymphoma induced by c-Myc dysregulation. Additionally, SIRT4 suppressed Burkitt lymphoma driven by c-Myc, independent of c-Myc activity. Furthermore, SIRT4 was found to be overexpressed in colorectal cancer cell lines and to increase E-cadherin expression, which resulted in the suppression of cell proliferation and invasion (59). During the development of colorectal cancer invasion, SIRT4 expression was decreased. The suppressive role of SIRT4 is also mediated by inhibiting glutamine metabolism in colorectal cancer (54). Moreover, SIRT4 could enhance the sensitivity of colorectal cancer cells to the chemical drug 5-fluorouracil by inhibiting the cell cycle, thus showing the antiproliferative effect of SIRT4 overexpression (55). Recent reports have demonstrated that mammalian target of rapamycin complex1 (mTORC1) is correlated with increased nutrient uptake and metabolism. mTORC1 promotes glutamine supplement by activating GDH required transcriptional repression of SIRT4. Specifically mTORC1 suppresses SIRT4 by destabilizing of cAMP-responsive element binding 2 (CREB2) (67). Overexpression of SIRT4 decreases cell growth, transformation and development of tumor. Furthermore, leucine is an important positive regulator of mTORC1, which activity may be regulated by SIRT4 by reducing intracellular leucine levels (**Figure 5**). Therefore, as a glutamine steward, SIRT4 acts as a necessary component of the DNA damage response pathway that manages the metabolic blockade of glutamine metabolism, the cell cycle, and tumor suppression.

CONCLUSION

In this review, we summarize different roles of SIRT4 in terms of enzymatic activities and functions in specific tissues and cells. SIRT4 possesses ADP-ribosyltransferase, lipoamidase and deacylase activities (46, 68, 69). Importantly, the enzymatic activities, and substrates of SIRT4 vary in different tissues and cells (**Figure 6**). SIRT4 inhibits insulin secretion as an ADP-ribosyltransferase and regulates insulin sensitivity as a deacylase in the pancreas. SIRT4 represses fatty acid oxidation (FAO) in the muscles and livers differently. SIRT4 has also been identified as a mitochondrial-localized tumor suppressor. SIRT4 is a less well-understood mammalian sirtuin, its cellular functions require further discovery. Knowledge of roles SIRT4 in cellular metabolism is helpful to provide new insights in the potential development of therapeutic agents for human diseases by targeting enzymatic activities (36).

AUTHOR CONTRIBUTIONS

ZM and JG draft the original manuscript. YY proofed and edited the finalized manuscript.

REFERENCES

1. Finkel T, Deng CX, Mostoslavsky R. Recent progress in the biology and physiology of sirtuins. *Nature* (2009) 460:587–91. doi: 10.1038/nature08197

2. Tan Y, Xu Z, Tao J, Ni J, Zhao W, Lu J, et al. A SIRT4-like auto ADP-ribosyltransferase is essential for the environmental growth of *Mycobacterium smegmatis. Acta Biochim Biophys Sin (Shanghai).* (2016) 48:145–52. doi: 10.1093/abbs/gmv121

3. Li Y, Zhou Y, Wang F, Chen X, Wang C, Wang J, et al. SIRT4 is the last puzzle of mitochondrial sirtuins. *Bioorg Med Chem.* (2018) 26:3861–5. doi: 10.1016/j.bmc.2018.07.031
4. van de Ven RAH, Santos D, Haigis MC. Mitochondrial sirtuins and molecular mechanisms of aging. *Trends Mol Med.* (2017) 23:320–331. doi: 10.1016/j.molmed.2017.02.005
5. Min J, Landry J, Sternglanz R, Xu R-M. Crystal structure of a SIR2 homolog–NAD complex. *Cell* (2001) 105:269–79. doi: 10.1016/S0092-8674(01)00317-8
6. Ahuja N, Schwer B, Carobbio S, Waltregny D, North BJ, Castronovo V, et al. Regulation of insulin secretion by SIRT4, a mitochondrial ADP-ribosyltransferase. *J Biol Chem.* (2007) 282:33583–92. doi: 10.1074/jbc.M705488200
7. Argmann C, Auwerx J. Insulin secretion: SIRT4 gets in on the act. *Cell* (2006) 126:837–9. doi: 10.1016/j.cell.2006.08.031
8. Haigis MC, Mostoslavsky R, Haigis KM, Fahie K, Christodoulou DC, Murphy AJ, et al. SIRT4 inhibits glutamate dehydrogenase and opposes the effects of calorie restriction in pancreatic beta cells. *Cell* (2006) 126:941–54. doi: 10.1016/j.cell.2006.06.057
9. Zaganjor E, Vyas S, Haigis MC. SIRT4 is a regulator of insulin secretion. *Cell Chem Biol.* (2017) 24:656–8. doi: 10.1016/j.chembiol.2017.06.002
10. Anderson KA, Huynh FK, Fisher-Wellman K, Stuart JD, Peterson BS, Douros JD, et al. SIRT4 is a lysine deacylase that controls leucine metabolism and insulin secretion. *Cell Metab.* (2017) 25:838–55 e815. doi: 10.1016/j.cmet.2017.03.003
11. Kumar S, Lombard DB. For certain, SIRT4 activities! *Trends Biochem Sci.* (2017) 42:499–501. doi: 10.1016/j.tibs.2017.05.008
12. Nasrin N, Wu X, Fortier E, Feng Y, Bare OC, Chen S, et al. SIRT4 regulates fatty acid oxidation and mitochondrial gene expression in liver and muscle cells. *J Biol Chem.* (2010) 285:31995–2002. doi: 10.1074/jbc.M110.124164
13. Acs Z, Bori Z, Takeda M, Osvath P, Berkes I, Taylor AW, et al. High altitude exposure alters gene expression levels of DNA repair enzymes, and modulates fatty acid metabolism by SIRT4 induction in human skeletal muscle. *Respir Physiol Neurobiol.* (2014) 196:33–7. doi: 10.1016/j.resp.2014.02.006
14. Koves TR, Ussher JR, Noland RC, Slentz D, Mosedale M, Ilkayeva O, et al. Mitochondrial overload and incomplete fatty acid oxidation contribute to skeletal muscle insulin resistance. *Cell Metab.* (2008) 7:45–56. doi: 10.1016/j.cmet.2007.10.013
15. Laurent G, German NJ, Saha AK, de Boer VCJ, Davies M, Koves TR, et al. SIRT4 coordinates the balance between lipid synthesis and catabolism by repressing malonyl CoA decarboxylase. *Molecular Cell* (2013) 50:686–98. doi: 10.1016/j.molcel.2013.05.012
16. Schirmer H, Pereira TC, Rico EP, Rosemberg DB, Bonan CD, Bogo MR, et al. Modulatory effect of resveratrol on SIRT1, SIRT3, SIRT4, PGC1alpha, and NAMPT gene expression profiles in wild-type adult zebrafish liver. *Mol Biol Rep.* (2012) 39:3281–9. doi: 10.1007/s11033-011-1096-4
17. Laurent G, de Boer VC, Finley LW, Sweeney M, Lu H, Schug TT, et al. SIRT4 represses peroxisome proliferator-activated receptor alpha activity to suppress hepatic fat oxidation. *Mol Cell Biol.* (2013) 33:4552–61. doi: 10.1128/MCB.00087-13
18. Lu M, Wan M, Leavens KF, Chu Q, Monks BR, Fernandez S, et al. Insulin regulates liver metabolism *in vivo* in the absence of hepatic Akt and Foxo1. *Nat Med.* (2012) 18:388–95. doi: 10.1038/nm.2686
19. Kim EA, Yang SJ, Choi SY, Lee WJ, Cho SW. Inhibition of glutamate dehydrogenase and insulin secretion by KHG26377 does not involve ADP-ribosylation by SIRT4 or deacetylation by SIRT3. *BMB Rep.* (2012) 45:458–63. doi: 10.5483/BMBRep.2012.45.8.040
20. Matsumoto M, Han S, Kitamura T, Accili D. Dual role of transcription factor FoxO1 in controlling hepatic insulin sensitivity and lipid metabolism. *J Clin Invest.* (2006) 116:2464–72. doi: 10.1172/JCI27047
21. Chen YR, Fang SR, Fu YC, Zhou XH, Xu MY, Xu WC. Calorie restriction on insulin resistance and expression of SIRT1 and SIRT4 in rats. *Biochem Cell Biol.* (2010) 88:715–22. doi: 10.1139/O10-010
22. Carrico C, Meyer JG, He W, Gibson BW, Verdin E. The mitochondrial acylome emerges: proteomics, regulation by sirtuins, and metabolic and disease implications. *Cell Metab.* (2018) 27:497–512. doi: 10.1016/j.cmet.2018.01.016
23. Pannek M, Simic Z, Fuszard M, Meleshin M, Rotili D, Mai A, et al. Crystal structures of the mitochondrial deacylase Sirtuin 4 reveal isoform-specific acyl recognition and regulation features. *Nat Commun.* (2017) 8:1513. doi: 10.1038/s41467-017-01701-2
24. Choubey SK, Prabhu D, Nachiappan M, Biswal J, Jeyakanthan J. Molecular modeling, dynamics studies and density functional theory approaches to identify potential inhibitors of SIRT4 protein from Homo sapiens : a novel target for the treatment of type 2 diabetes. *J Biomol Struct Dyn.* (2017) 35:3316–29. doi: 10.1080/07391102.2016.1254117
25. Newgard CB, An J, Bain JR, Muehlbauer MJ, Stevens RD, Lien LF, et al. A Branched-Chain amino acid-related metabolic signature that differentiates obese and lean humans and contributes to insulin resistance. *Cell Metab.* (2009) 9:565–6. doi: 10.1016/j.cmet.2009.05.001
26. Mathias RA, Greco TM, Cristea IM. Identification of sirtuin4 (SIRT4) protein interactions: uncovering candidate acyl-modified mitochondrial substrates and enzymatic regulators. *Methods Mol Biol.* (2016) 1436:213–39. doi: 10.1007/978-1-4939-3667-0_15
27. Zeng G, Liu H, Wang H. Amelioration of myocardial ischemia-reperfusion injury by SIRT4 involves mitochondrial protection and reduced apoptosis. *Biochem Biophys Res Commun.* (2018) 502:15–21. doi: 10.1016/j.bbrc.2018.05.113
28. Saha AK, Ruderman NB. Malonyl-CoA and AMP-activated protein kinase: an expanding partnership. *Mol Cell Biochem.* (2003) 253:65–70. doi: 10.1023/A:1026053302036
29. Liu B, Che W, Xue J, Zheng C, Tang K, Zhang J, et al. SIRT4 prevents hypoxia-induced apoptosis in H9c2 cardiomyoblast cells. *Cell Physiol Biochem.* (2013) 32:655–62. doi: 10.1159/000354469
30. Bugger H, Witt CN, Bode C. Mitochondrial sirtuins in the heart. *Heart Fail Rev.* (2016) 21:519–28. doi: 10.1007/s10741-016-9570-7
31. Luo YX, Tang X, An XZ, Xie XM, Chen XF, Zhao X, et al. SIRT4 accelerates Ang II-induced pathological cardiac hypertrophy by inhibiting manganese superoxide dismutase activity. *Eur Heart J.* (2017) 38:1389–98. doi: 10.1093/eurheartj/ehw138
32. Boulange CL, Claus SP, Chou CJ, Collino S, Montoliu I, Kochhar S, et al. Early metabolic adaptation in C57BL/6 mice resistant to high fat diet induced weight gain involves an activation of mitochondrial oxidative pathways. *J Proteome Res.* (2013) 12:1956–68. doi: 10.1021/pr400051s
33. Jokinen R, Pirnes-Karhu S, Pietilainen KH, Pirinen E. Adipose tissue NAD(+)-homeostasis, sirtuins and poly(ADP-ribose) polymerases - important players in mitochondrial metabolism and metabolic health. *Redox Biol.* (2017) 12:246–63. doi: 10.1016/j.redox.2017.02.011
34. Parik S, Tewary S, Ayyub C, Kolthur-Seetharam U. Loss of mitochondrial SIRT4 shortens lifespan and leads to a decline in physical activity. *J Biosci.* (2018) 43:243–7. doi: 10.1007/s12038-018-9754-5
35. Elkhwanky MS, Hakkola J. Extranuclear sirtuins and metabolic stress *Antioxid Redox Signal.* (2017) 28:662–76. doi: 10.1089/ars.2017.7270
36. George J, Ahmad N. Mitochondrial sirtuins in cancer: emerging roles and therapeutic potential *Cancer Res.* (2016) 76:2500–6. doi: 10.1158/0008-5472.CAN-15-2733
37. Wood JG, Schwer B, Wickremesinghe PC, Hartnett DA, Burhenn L, Garcia M, et al. Sirt4 is a mitochondrial regulator of metabolism and lifespan in *Drosophila melanogaster. Proc Natl Acad Sci USA.* (2018) 115:1564–9. doi: 10.1073/pnas.1720673115
38. Saltiel AR, Kahn CR. Insulin signalling and the regulation of glucose and lipid metabolism. *Nature* (2001) 414:799–806. doi: 10.1038/414799a
39. Hershberger KA, Martin AS, Hirschey MD. Role of NAD(+) and mitochondrial sirtuins in cardiac and renal diseases. *Nat Rev Nephrol.* (2017) 13:213–25. doi: 10.1038/nrneph.2017.5
40. Dolinsky VW. The role of sirtuins in mitochondrial function and doxorubicin-induced cardiac dysfunction. *Biol Chem.* (2017) 398:955–74. doi: 10.1515/hsz-2016-0316
41. Langlet F, Haeusler RA, Linden D, Ericson E, Norris T, Johansson A, et al. Selective inhibition of FOXO1 activator/repressor balance modulates hepatic glucose handling. *Cell* (2017) 171:824–35 e818. doi: 10.1016/j.cell.2017.09.045
42. Osborne B, Bentley NL, Montgomery MK, Turner N. The role of mitochondrial sirtuins in health and disease. *Free Radic Biol Med.* (2016) 100:164–74. doi: 10.1016/j.freeradbiomed.2016.04.197

43. Kulkarni SS, Canto C. Mitochondrial post-translational modifications and metabolic control: sirtuins and beyond. *Curr Diabetes Rev.* (2017) 13:338–51. doi: 10.2174/1573399812666160217122413
44. Shukla S, Sharma A, Pandey VK, Raisuddin S, Kakkar P. Concurrent acetylation of FoxO1/3a and p53 due to sirtuins inhibition elicit Bim/PUMA mediated mitochondrial dysfunction and apoptosis in berberine-treated HepG2 cells. *Toxicol Appl Pharmacol.* (2016) 291:70–83. doi: 10.1016/j.taap.2015.12.006
45. Banks AS, Kim-Muller JY, Mastracci TL, Kofler NM, Qiang L, Haeusler RA, et al. Dissociation of the glucose and lipid regulatory functions of FoxO1 by targeted knockin of acetylation-defective alleles in mice. *Cell Metab.* (2011) 14:587–97. doi: 10.1016/j.cmet.2011.09.012
46. Gertz M, Steegborn C. Using mitochondrial sirtuins as drug targets: disease implications and available compounds. *Cell Mol Life Sci.* (2016) 73:2871–96. doi: 10.1007/s00018-016-2180-7
47. Ho L, Titus AS, Banerjee KK, George S, Lin W, Deota S, et al. SIRT4 regulates ATP homeostasis and mediates a retrograde signaling via AMPK. *Aging (Albany NY)* (2013) 5:835–49. doi: 10.18632/aging.100616
48. Zeng J, Jiang M, Wu X, Diao F, Qiu D, Hou X, et al. SIRT4 is essential for metabolic control and meiotic structure during mouse oocyte maturation. *Aging Cell* (2018) 29:e12789. doi: 10.1111/acel.12789
49. Sun H, Huang D, Liu G, Jian F, Zhu J, Zhang L. SIRT4 acts as a tumor suppressor in gastric cancer by inhibiting cell proliferation, migration, and invasion. *Onco Targets Ther.* (2018) 11:3959–68. doi: 10.2147/OTT.S156143
50. Huang G, Zhu G. Sirtuin-4 (SIRT4), a therapeutic target with oncogenic and tumor-suppressive activity in cancer. *Onco Targets Ther.* (2018) 11:3395–400. doi: 10.2147/OTT.S157724
51. Bradbury CA, Khanim FL, Hayden R, Bunce CM, White DA, Drayson MT, et al. Histone deacetylases in acute myeloid leukaemia show a distinctive pattern of expression that changes selectively in response to deacetylase inhibitors. *Leukemia* (2005) 19:1751–9. doi: 10.1038/sj.leu.2403910
52. Jeong SM, Lee A, Lee J, Haigis MC. SIRT4 protein suppresses tumor formation in genetic models of Myc-induced B cell lymphoma. *J Biol Chem.* (2014) 289:4135–44. doi: 10.1074/jbc.M113.525949
53. Roth M, Chen WY. Sorting out functions of sirtuins in cancer. *Oncogene* (2014) 33:1609–20. doi: 10.1038/onc.2013.120
54. Miyo M, Yamamoto H, Konno M, Colvin H, Nishida N, Koseki J, et al. Tumour-suppressive function of SIRT4 in human colorectal cancer. *Br J Cancer* (2015) 113, 492–9. doi: 10.1038/bjc.2015.226
55. Zhu Y, Wang G, Li X, Wang T, Weng M, Zhang Y. Knockout of SIRT4 decreases chemosensitivity to 5-FU in colorectal cancer cells. *Oncol Lett.* (2018) 16:1675–81. doi: 10.3892/ol.2018.8850
56. Huang G, Cui F, Yu F, Lu H, Zhang M, Tang H, et al. Sirtuin-4 (SIRT4) is downregulated and associated with some clinicopathological features in gastric adenocarcinoma. *Biomed Pharmacother.* (2015) 72:135–9. doi: 10.1016/j.biopha.2015.04.013
57. Fu L, Dong Q, He J, Wang X, Xing J, Wang E, et al. SIRT4 inhibits malignancy progression of NSCLCs, through mitochondrial dynamics mediated by the ERK-Drp1 pathway. *Oncogene* (2017) 36:2724–36. doi: 10.1038/onc.2016.425
58. Garber ME, Troyanskaya OG, Schluens K, Petersen S, Thaesler Z, Pacyna-Gengelbach M, et al. Diversity of gene expression in adenocarcinoma of the lung. *Proc Natl Acad Sci USA.* (2001) 98:13784–9. doi: 10.1073/pnas.241500798
59. Wang L, Zhou H, Wang Y, Cui G, Di LJ. CtBP maintains cancer cell growth and metabolic homeostasis via regulating SIRT4. *Cell Death Dis.* (2015) 6:e1620. doi: 10.1038/cddis.2014.587
60. Komlos D, Mann KD, Zhuo Y, Ricupero CL, Hart RP, Liu AY, et al. Glutamate dehydrogenase 1 and SIRT4 regulate glial development. *Glia* (2013) 61:394–408. doi: 10.1002/glia.22442
61. Jeong SM, Xiao C, Finley LW, Lahusen T, Souza AL, Pierce K, et al. SIRT4 has tumor-suppressive activity and regulates the cellular metabolic response to DNA damage by inhibiting mitochondrial glutamine metabolism. *Cancer Cell* (2013) 23:450–63. doi: 10.1016/j.ccr.2013.02.024
62. Potthast AB, Heuer T, Warneke SJ, Das AM. Alterations of sirtuins in mitochondrial cytochrome c-oxidase deficiency. *PLoS ONE* (2017) 12:e0186517. doi: 10.1371/journal.pone.0186517
63. Fernandez-Marcos PJ, Serrano M. Sirt4: the glutamine gatekeeper. *Cancer Cell* (2013) 23:427–8. doi: 10.1016/j.ccr.2013.04.003
64. Germain D. Sirtuins and the estrogen receptor as regulators of the mammalian mitochondrial UPR in cancer and aging. *Adv Cancer Res.* (2016) 130:211–56. doi: 10.1016/bs.acr.2016.01.004
65. Gao P, Tchernyshyov I, Chang TC, Lee YS, Kita K, Ochi T, et al. c-Myc suppression of miR-23a/b enhances mitochondrial glutaminase expression and glutamine metabolism. *Nature* (2009) 458:762–5. doi: 10.1038/nature07823
66. de Moura MB, Uppala R, Zhang YX, Van Houten B, Goetzman ES. Overexpression of mitochondrial sirtuins alters glycolysis and mitochondrial function in HEK293 cells. *PLoS ONE* (2014) 9:e106028. doi: 10.1371/journal.pone.0106028
67. Csibi A, Fendt SM, Li C, Poulogiannis G, Choo AY, Chapski DJ, et al. The mTORC1 pathway stimulates glutamine metabolism and cell proliferation by repressing SIRT4. *Cell* (2013) 153:840–54. doi: 10.1016/j.cell.2013.04.023
68. Celichowski P, Jopek K, Szyszka M, Tyczewska M, Malendowicz LK, Rucinski M. Mitochondrial sirtuins in the rat adrenal gland: location within the glands of males and females, hormonal and developmental regulation of gene expressions. *Folia Histochem Cytobiol.* (2017) 55:190–202. doi: 10.5603/FHC.a2017.0020
69. Mathias RA, Greco TM, Oberstein A, Budayeva HG, Chakrabarti R, Rowland EA, et al. Sirtuin 4 is a lipoamidase regulating pyruvate dehydrogenase complex activity. *Cell* (2014) 159:1615–25. doi: 10.1016/j.cell.2014.11.046

11

Brain SIRT1 Mediates Metabolic Homeostasis and Neuroprotection

Jing Xu [1,2], *Charlie W. Jackson* [1,2], *Nathalie Khoury* [1,2], *Iris Escobar* [1,2] *and Miguel A. Perez-Pinzon* [1,2*]

[1] *Cerebral Vascular Disease Research Laboratories, Department of Neurology, Leonard M. Miller School of Medicine, University of Miami, Miami, FL, United States,* [2] *Department of Neurology, Leonard M. Miller School of Medicine, University of Miami, Miami, FL, United States*

Correspondence:
Miguel A. Perez-Pinzon
perezpinzon@med.miami.edu

Sirtuins are evolutionarily conserved proteins that use nicotinamide adenine dinucleotide (NAD^+) as a co-substrate in their enzymatic reactions. There are seven proteins (SIRT1-7) in the human sirtuin family, among which SIRT1 is the most conserved and characterized. SIRT1 in the brain, in particular, within the hypothalamus, plays crucial roles in regulating systemic energy homeostasis and circadian rhythm. Apart from this, SIRT1 has also been found to mediate beneficial effects in neurological diseases. In this review, we will first summarize how SIRT1 in the brain relates to obesity, type 2 diabetes, and circadian synchronization, and then we discuss the neuroprotective roles of brain SIRT1 in the context of cerebral ischemia and neurodegenerative disorders.

Keywords: Sirt1, obesity, type 2 diabetes mellitus, circadian rhythms, cerebral ischemia, Alzheimer's disease, Parkinson's disease

INTRODUCTION

Sirtuins are homologs of yeast silent information regulator 2 (Sir2). Sir2 has attracted the attention of researchers given its involvement in longevity (1). The mammalian sirtuins (SIRT1-7) have different subcellular localizations. SIRT1, SIRT6, and SIRT7 are mainly localized in the nucleus, whereas SIRT1 is also reported to translocate in the cytoplasm. SIRT2 is predominantly cytoplasmic and shuttles to the nucleus transiently. The mitochondrial sirtuins are SIRT3, SIRT4, and SIRT5 (2). In terms of enzymatic activities, sirtuins share a conserved nicotinamide adenine dinucleotide (NAD^+) binding site and remove acetyl groups from target proteins in an NAD^+-dependent manner. Additionally, some sirtuins have been reported to exhibit demyristoylase (SIRT2), ADP-ribosyltransferase (SIRT4 and SIRT6), and demanlonylase and desuccinylase (SIRT5) activities (2).

The Role of SIRT1 as a Metabolic Sensor

Among all sirtuins, SIRT1 is the most extensively studied and well-characterized. As mentioned above, SIRT1 is an NAD^+ dependent deacetylase that removes the acetyl groups from protein substrates to add to the ADP-ribose, a product from the cleavage of NAD^+. NAD^+ is a dinucleotide with one nucleotide contains an adenine and the other contains nicotinamide (3). In addition to be the rate-limiting co-substrate for NAD^+ dependent enzymes, NAD^+ can be used a coenzyme in the metabolic redox reactions. NAD^+ exists in two forms, the oxidized form as NAD^+, and the reduced form as NADH. NAD^+/NADH plays a critical role in glycolysis and cellular respiration for ATP production. In glycolysis, NAD^+ is reduced to NADH. In oxidative phosphorylation and cellular respiration, NADH is oxidized to NAD^+ by electron transport chain (ETC) (1). As such, NAD^+ concentrations fluctuate with cellular metabolic status and nutrient availability.

NAD^+ levels increased during the energetic crisis, such as calorie restriction and decreased under conditions of high-energy load, such as high-fat diets. The fact that Sirt1 enzymatic activity depends upon NAD^+ levels allows Sirt1 to act as a metabolic sensor that couples cellular metabolic status to regulatory responses (1).

SIRT1 in Metabolism

SIRT1 is widely distributed in the body and plays diverse roles in metabolism in different organs including liver, pancreas, muscle, and adipose tissue (4–6). One of the important aspects associated with increased SIRT1 activity is the caloric restriction (CR) (7, 8). CR has been extensively studied, where it has been demonstrated that SIRT1 plays a central role in CR-induced longevity (8–11). As mentioned, it has been suggested that SIRT1, as a metabolic sensor, coordinates the transcriptional networks with the restricted metabolic status (8, 12, 13). During times of energy reduction, NAD^+ concentrations increase, thereby enhancing the NAD^+ deacetylase activity of SIRT1. The SIRT1 mediates deacetylation of a broad range of protein substrates. Proteins that regulate mitochondrial biogenesis, glucose homeostasis, inflammation, and apoptosis have been identified as SIRT1 substrates (14–16). These biological functions are linked to energy homeostasis and eventually extend lifespan.

SIRT1 in the Brain

SIRT1 is widely expressed in the adult brain. Most of the SIRT1 is localized in the neuronal nuclei. However, SIRT1 is also found in the glial cells of post-mortem human brains, and in neural stem cells, microglia, and astrocytes in culture (17). In the hypothalamus, the control center for homeostasis, SIRT1 mRNA is highly expressed in the arcuate, ventromedial, dorsomedial and paraventricular nuclei of the hypothalamus, which suggests an important role for brain SIRT1 in regulating metabolic status (18). Another function of brain SIRT1 is the regulation of the central circadian clock in the suprachiasmatic nucleus (SCN) of the hypothalamus. In the SCN of the hypothalamus, SIRT1 regulates circadian clock gene expressions by mediating the acetylation status of circadian genes (19). Besides the physiological functions of SIRT1 in the hypothalamus, SIRT1 is reported to exert neuroprotection in neurological dysfunctions (20). In this review, we will focus on the roles of SIRT1 in the brain in metabolism, circadian rhythm, and SIRT1 function in the context of cerebral ischemia and neurodegenerative disorders (**Figure 1**).

SIRT1 AND MITOCHONDRIAL FUNCTIONS

Mitochondrial is one of the most important sources for cellular energy in eukaryotes, producing up to 95% of the ATP through oxidative phosphorylation (21). This provides great significance into the roles of the mitochondrial in the brain, where it is estimated to take up to 20% of the total oxygen consumption of the body energy (22). As such, this dysfunction could affect metabolic efficiency, thus linking to a common pathology ranging from metabolic disorders to neurological diseases (21).

SIRT1 can regulate the transcription of mitochondrial genes encoded in the nucleus that are involved in vital mitochondrial processes related to longevity and aging. While SIRT1 is mainly localized in the nucleus, levels have also been detected in the mitochondrion where it may interact with different substrates (23). In this section, we will discuss SIRT1's involvement in important mitochondrial functions including mitochondrial biogenesis, mitophagy, and energy metabolism.

Regulation of Insulin Secretion by SIRT1 Via UCP2

Uncoupling protein 2 (UCP2) is an inner mitochondrial membrane protein that can uncouple oxidative phosphorylation from respiration/ATP production. This is done via dissipation of the proton gradient, in which protons are returned to the mitochondrial matrix. UCP2 is found in many different tissues, including the brain, and has been shown to be involved in energy balance (24), homeostasis, and longevity (25). SIRT1 has been found to positively regulate insulin production by means of repressing UCP2 (26–28). As a result, cells express higher ATP levels after glucose stimulation, which is essential for inducing insulin secretion (26). In this manner, levels of insulin are regulated commensurate to levels of food intake and if impaired may contribute to obesity-induced diabetes (26). In this respect, SIRT1 can respond to nutrients available in the environment and promote transcriptional changes that may enhance energy metabolism.

PGC-1α and SIRT1 Interact to Induce Mitochondrial Biogenesis and Metabolic Processes

Peroxisome proliferator-activated receptor γ (PPARγ) coactivator-1α (PGC-1α) is a transcriptional coactivator and major regulator of mitochondrial biogenesis and several metabolic processes (29). Studies have shown that SIRT1 interacts with PGC-1α to induce its transcriptional activity via deacetylation (16, 30–32). PGC-1α may activate a wide array of transcription factors (TFs) that include both DNA-binding TFs, such as nuclear respiratory factor 1 (NRF-1), and nuclear hormone receptors, such as PPARγ, thyroid hormone receptors, retinoic acid receptors, glucocorticoid receptors, and estrogen receptors (33, 34).

NRF-1, specifically, can regulate the activation of the nuclear-encoded mitochondrial transcription factor A (TFAM), which can bind to mtDNA and stimulate mitochondrial DNA replication and increase the expression of mitochondrial genes (35). As a result, NRF-1 induces the expression of mitochondrial transporters, components of oxidative phosphorylation, and ribosomal proteins (36). Aquilano et al. found that SIRT1 and PGC-1α also interact with TFAM within the mitochondria (23). In either case, the subsequent increased expression of mitochondrial genes promotes mitochondrial biogenesis—an essential process important for maintaining oxidative capacity and levels of energy production. In some instances, SIRT1 activity is required to stimulate mitochondrial biogenesis, as reported in pulmonary arteriolar smooth muscle cells (37); however, whether

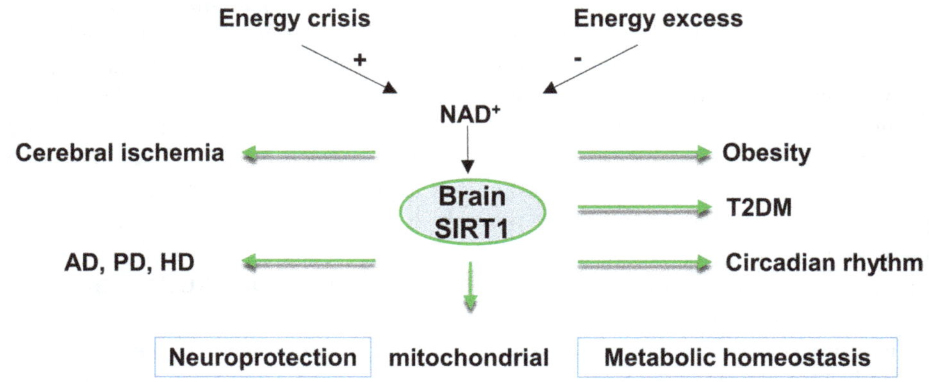

FIGURE 1 | An overview of brain SIRT1 in metabolic and neurological disorders. Brain SIRT1 activity is dependent on NAD^+ levels, which increases under energy crisis, and decline with high energy load. Any dysregulation of brain SIRT1 activity can have devastating consequences in terms of mitochondrial function, metabolic homeostasis, circadian synchronization, and neurological function. A proper function of brain SIRT1 is protective against obesity, diabetes, circadian dysregulation. In addition, brain SIRT1 exerts neuroprotection against ischemic injury and neurodegenerative disorders, such as Alzheimer's disease (AD), Parkinson's disease (PD), and Huntington's disease (HD). T2DM, type 2 diabetes, NAD^+, nicotinamide adenine dinucleotide.

SIRT1 is necessary for mitochondrial biogenesis to occur has recently become controversial (38).

The increase of mitochondrial gene expression also stimulates several metabolic processes depending on the tissue type (33, 36). In the brain and heart, PGC-1α functions as an important regulator of the metabolism of reactive oxygen species (ROS) under normal physiological conditions and certain states of oxidative stress (36). In conditional liver-specific SIRT1 KO mice, PPARα signaling activated by PGC-1α was impaired (39). This lead to a decrease in fatty acid oxidation and ketogenesis, suggesting a vital role for SIRT1 in regulating hepatic lipid homeostasis (39). Dysregulation of any of these processes may contribute to both aging and age-associated metabolic diseases.

SIRT1 and Mitophagy

Maintaining quality mitochondrial pools is essential for cell health and viability. Mitochondrial components are typically damaged by the accumulation of ROS—a byproduct of the mitochondrial electron transport chain—which typically occurs during conditions of stress. Due to its close proximity, ROS overproduction damages mtDNA that may ultimately contribute to neurodegenerative disorders, stroke, cancer, and age-related diseases (40–42). Constant mitochondrial turnover is important to maintain a healthy mitochondrial population. Thus, a quality control mechanism is required to eliminate and replace dysfunctional mitochondria with new and more efficient mitochondria. To achieve this specialized form of homeostasis in response to stress, cells utilize a process known as mitophagy for the selective degradation of mitochondrial components. This elimination process is balanced with mitochondrial biogenesis. While the exact mechanism for mitophagy has yet to be elucidated, some studies indicate PINK1/PARKIN as the key pathway involved (43, 44). As discussed above, SIRT1 is essential for promoting mitochondrial biogenesis; however, it also plays an important role in autophagy.

Several studies have shown that SIRT1 interacts with components of the autophagy machinery including Forkhead box O3 (FOXO3)—a transcription factor heavily associated with autophagy induction (45–47). In the aged kidney, the mitochondrial damage was associated with deficiencies in SIRT1, and under hypoxic conditions, SIRT1 was able to promote cell adaptation by deacetylation of FOXO3 (46). Another study demonstrated that SIRT1 is essential for fully activating autophagy under conditions of starvation (48). Additionally, SIRT1 deficient embryos and neonatal mice displayed an accumulation of abnormal organelles, especially mitochondria, and impaired autophagy (48). PGC-1α is also involved in mitophagy as it regulates the expression of transcription factor EB (TFEB)—a well-known master regulator of autophagy and lysosomal biogenesis (49). It may be possible that SIRT1 may also influence mitophagy given its interaction with PGC-1α. Taken together, SIRT1 is involved in diverse mechanisms for the regulation of mitochondrial functions (**Figure 2**). The regulation of SIRT1 in mitochondrial functions may underlie its importance in regulating energy metabolism and in so doing, may be part of its neuroprotective role.

BRAIN SIRT1 AND OBESITY

The hypothalamus is the control center for homeostasis. In the arcuate nucleus of the hypothalamus, the proopiomelanocortin (POMC) neurons suppress appetite while the activation of agouti-related peptide/neuropeptide Y (AgRP/NPY) neurons stimulate appetite (50). The ventromedial nucleus (VMN) is another nucleus involved in satiety as VMN lesions lead to an increase in food intake and obesity (51). In recent years, a substantial number of studies demonstrated that the hypothalamic SIRT1 is crucially important for the central regulation of food intake and energy expenditure.

SIRT1 in the POMC neurons is required to protect against high calorie-induced obesity. When challenged with a hypercaloric diet, POMC-SIRT1 mutant mice showed reduced energy expenditure and increased body weight (52). Interestingly,

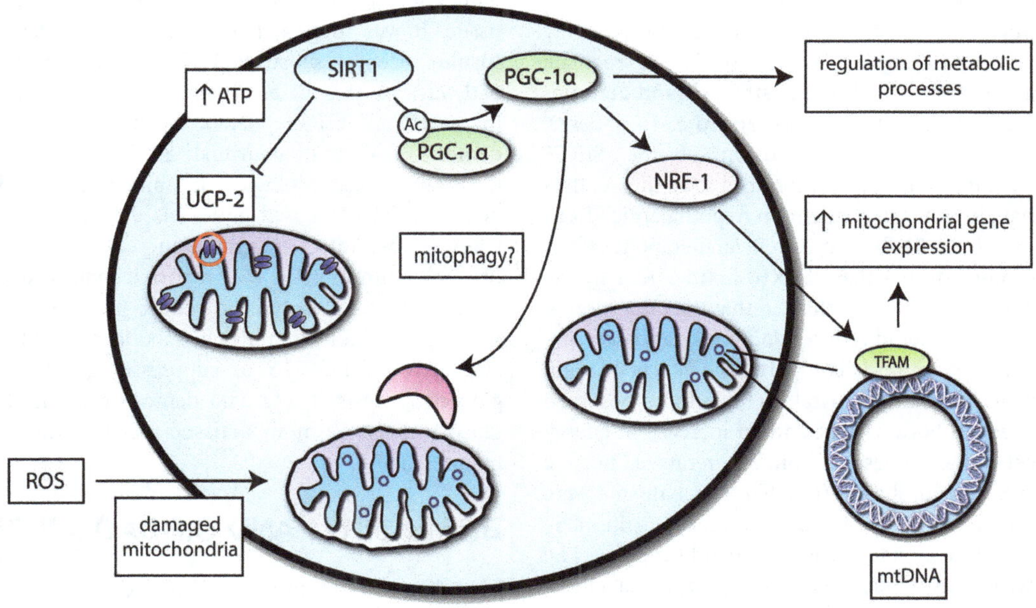

FIGURE 2 | A simplified overview of mitochondrial functions mediated by SIRT1 activity. SIRT1 may interact with transcription factors or mitochondrial proteins to induce different effects related to mitochondrial function—a select few of these proteins are highlighted. SIRT1 can suppress Uncoupling protein 2 (UCP-2) in the inner mitochondrial membrane to increase levels of ATP, which is important for energy metabolism. SIRT1 may also deacetylate Peroxisome proliferator-activated receptor γ (PPARγ) coactivator-1α (PGC-1α) to induce its activation and augment mitochondrial biogenesis by increasing mitochondrial gene expression via Nuclear respiratory factor 1 (NRF-1) and Nuclear-encoded mitochondrial transcription factor A (TFAM). PGC-1α itself can regulate different metabolic processes and may potentially play a role in mitophagy.

these metabolic changes were not due to hypoactivity, as the mutant mice showed unaltered levels of daily activities compared to their control counterparts (52). The reduction in energy expenditure could be explained by a reduction in sympathetic nerve activity in the adipose tissue of the mutant mice (52). Conversely, mice with overexpressed SIRT1 in the POMC neurons exhibited a leaner phenotype compared to their wild-type littermates (53). Age-related weight gain was absent in the POMC-SIRT1 overexpressed mice. The leaner phenotype was attributed to increased sympathetic activity in the adipose tissue with consequently enhanced energy expenditure (53).

Another mechanism in which SIRT1 modulates systemic homeostasis is through deacetylation of Forkhead box protein O1 (FoxO1). FoxO1 is a downstream transcription factor in the insulin signaling pathway. Hypothalamic FoxO1 activation or overexpression inhibits the anorexigenic effects of insulin (54), increases adiposity, and leads to weight gain (55). The overexpression of SIRT1 in POMC neurons was able to rescue FoxO1 activation induced obesity (55). These effects occurred through decreased acetylation and expression of FoxO1 by POMC-SIRT1 overexpression (55). Similarly, FoxO1 mediated hyperphagia was blunted by hypothalamic SIRT1 overexpression (56).

Hypothalamic SIRT1 is also implicated in the leptin-mediated regulation of metabolism. Leptin is a hormone secreted by the adipose tissue that suppresses body weight. In the hypothalamus, leptin binds to its receptor (Ob-Rb) and activates the signal transducer and activator of transcription 3 (STAT3), which further regulates gene expressions to affect energy homeostasis. The leptin-induced protective mechanisms against obesity are dependent on SIRT1 in the POMC neurons. In POMC-SIRT1 deficient mice, leptin-mediated activation of the phosphatidylinositol-4,5-bisphosphate 3-kinase (PI3K) signaling pathway and the suppression of food intake were disrupted (52). In addition, when SIRT1 is overexpressed in the hypothalamus, either in POMC or AgRP neurons, non-obese mice exhibited increased sensitivity to leptin, as demonstrated by increased phosphorylation of STAT3 as well as reduced food intake (53). Interestingly, these phenotypes were blunted in mice consuming a high-fat diet, due to decreased expression of SIRT1 and NAD^+ levels in the hypothalamus, suggesting that the metabolic status could influence the function of hypothalamic SIRT1 (53). In support of this, the hypothalamic SIRT1 expression is induced upon feeding in the standard fed mice, whereas diet-induced obesity abrogated this induction (56). In addition to the arcuate nucleus, SIRT1 in steroidogenic factor 1 (SF1) neurons of the VMN also contributes to the physiological function of leptin. The lack of SIRT1 in the SF1 neurons predisposed mice to dietary-induced obesity. SF1-SIRT1 mutant mice exhibited diminished energy expenditure and impaired leptin sensitivity (57). In contrast, SIRT1 overexpression in the SF1 neurons restored oxygen consumption, increased leptin sensitivity and protected mice against high-calorie diet induced weight gain (57).

In the aforementioned studies, the activation of hypothalamic SIRT1 negatively regulated energy balance and protected against obesity. Contrary to these findings, studies also reported a positive energy regulation by brain SIRT1. Apart from leptin, ghrelin is another peptide released peripherally and acts on the central nervous system (CNS) to regulate metabolism. Ghrelin is produced by the stomach and activates AMPK in the hypothalamus to increase appetite. In rodents, the intracerebroventricular (ICV) infusion of the SIRT1 inhibitor, EX-527, blunted the ghrelin-induced food intake, thus demonstrating that ghrelin is dependent on hypothalamic SIRT1 to stimulate appetite (58, 59). Similar beneficial metabolic effects were seen in two other studies that blocked brain SIRT1 by the ICV infusion of EX-527. One study showed that the inhibition of brain SIRT1 in fasted rats could reduce food intake and decrease weight gain (60). The other study compared the effects of brain SIRT1 inhibition in obese and lean rats. The authors observed a significant decrease in body weight and an increase in energy expenditure in diet-induced obese rats, but not in rats fed normal chow upon brain SIRT1 inhibition (61). The mechanisms were attributed to increased activity of the hypothalamic-pituitary-thyroid axis, resulting in enhanced energy expenditure (61). The discrepancy between the hypophagia and hyperphagia effects by SIRT1 activation may be due to the different animal models used in these studies (i.e., ICV infusion of EX-527 and genetic deletion of SIRT1 in a specific population of neurons). Despite the controversies, these studies demonstrated a crucial role for brain SIRT1 in the systematic regulation of energy homeostasis (**Figure 3**).

BRAIN SIRT1 AND TYPE 2 DIABETES

Obesity is a leading risk factor for type 2 diabetes (T2DM). The accumulation of fat, especially visceral fat, progressively enhances insulin resistance and eventually leads to T2DM (62, 63). Given the crucial role of SIRT1 in obesity, it is no surprise that emerging evidence suggests SIRT1 within the brain controls the systematic regulation of glucose/insulin homeostasis. Mentioned briefly above, SIRT1 in SF1 neurons is required for the defense against dietary-induced obesity. In addition to this, insulin activated PI3K signaling was blunted in the skeletal muscle of SF1-neuron-SIRT1 deleted mice. Conversely, SIRT1 overexpression in SF1 neurons enhanced skeletal muscle insulin sensitivity in these mice (57).

Resveratrol is a potent SIRT1 activator that improves glucose homeostasis. Studies demonstrate that brain SIRT1 at least partially contributes to the resveratrol-mediated glucose balance (64). ICV infusion of resveratrol rescued the hyperglycemia phenotype in diet-induced obese and diabetic mice (64). In support of the former data, hypothalamic or systemic administration of resveratrol increased hepatic insulin sensitivity, which was blunted by the inhibition of SIRT1 in the hypothalamus (65). Collectively, these data suggest SIRT1 activation within the brain is likely to improve insulin resistance and combat against diabetes. In such cases, brain SIRT1 activation leads to suppressed peripheral glucose production.

Two studies that investigated the cell type-specific role of neuronal SIRT1 in glucose metabolism suggested a different regulatory mechanism. Neuronal SIRT1-deficient mice exhibited higher insulin sensitivity in the hypothalamus and peripheral tissue. It was suggested that SIRT1 deacetylates and represses Insulin receptor substrate 1 (IRS-1) and the insulin signaling pathway. In this case, central PI3K signaling was enhanced in neuronal SIRT1 deficient mice (66). Another study demonstrated that neuronal SIRT1 mediates glycolysis in the brain. Pharmacological inhibition or genetic mutation of neuronal SIRT1 caused glycolysis deficits *in vitro* and *in vivo*, whereas resveratrol treatment increased the glycolysis rate in primary neurons (67). It is reported that, in peripheral tissues, SIRT1 inhibits glycolysis to reduce glucose consumption (68). For example, in liver, under metabolic stress, SIRT1 deacetylates and activates PGC-1α to suppresses glycolysis and promote gluconeogenesis. These data demonstrate that SIRT1 regulates glucose metabolism in a tissue-specific and cell type-specific manner (16).

BRAIN SIRT1 AND CIRCADIAN RHYTHM

The circadian rhythm is a 24 h endogenous cycle that allows organisms to synchronize their physiology and behavior to the daily cycle of daylight and darkness (69, 70). The circadian clock is entrainable by internal and external zeitgebers "time givers." In mammals, the circadian clock is found across different tissues, yet the central clock is found in the SCN of the hypothalamus from which it entrains peripheral clocks to regulate oscillatory functions, such as metabolism and the sleep/wakefulness cycle (69, 70).

The molecular mechanism of the circadian rhythm consists of a set of transcriptional activators and repressors involved in positive and negative autoregulatory feedback loops (69, 71). In mammals, the core clock genes are the acetyltransferase CLOCK (Circadian Locomotor Output Cycles Kaput) and its heterodimer BMAL1 (Brain and muscle Arnt-like protein-1). When dimerized, the CLOCK-BMAL1 complex translocates to the nucleus and induces the expression of several downstream genes. Among these genes are their own negative regulators period (PER1, PER2, PER3) and cryptochrome (CRY1 and CRY2) proteins (69, 70). Over the course of the day, PER and CRY start to accumulate and together with the casein kinase 1δ (CK1δ) and CK1ε translocate to the nucleus to repress their own transcription (70). As repression progresses, PER and CRY levels decline and transcription by CLOCK-BMAL1 re-initiates a new cycle (70). PER and CRY are also eliminated by post-translational modifications and degradation (69, 70). The CLOCK-BMAL1 complex also regulates the downstream retinoic acid-related orphan receptors (RORα, RORβ) and the nuclear receptors (Rev-Erbα, Rev-Erbβ), which compete for the regulation of the BMAL1 promoter and reinforce the oscillation (70).

SIRT1 in the Peripheral Clocks

SIRT1 has been shown to be an important regulator of the circadian clock genes in both the central and peripheral clocks (**Figure 4**). In 2008, two independent studies using peripheral tissues were the first to link SIRT1 to the regulation of the clock genes. Using mouse hepatocytes and cultured fibroblasts, it was shown that the protein levels of SIRT1 cycle in a

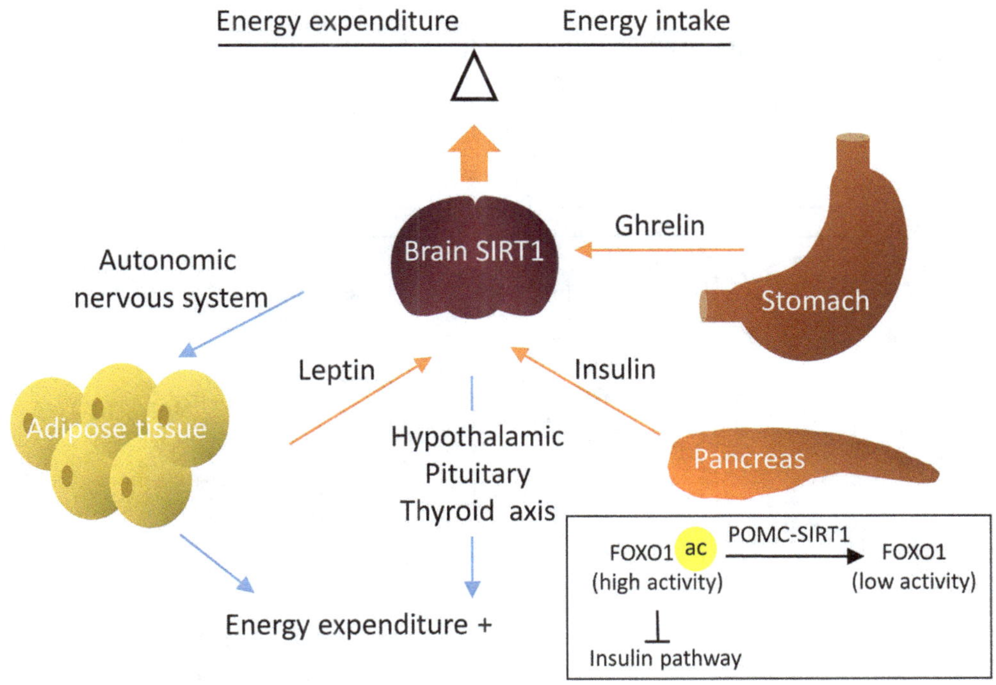

FIGURE 3 | Regulative mechanisms of brain SIRT1 in metabolic homeostasis. Brain SIRT1 increases energy expenditure via the hypothalamic pituitary thyroid axis and increased sympathetic nerve activity in the adipose tissue. In addition, hormones, such as leptin, insulin, and ghrelin through brain SIRT1 to balance energy expenditure and energy intake. For example, SIRT1 in POMC neurons deacetylate Forkhead box protein O1 (FOXO1) to increase the insulin signal pathway.

circadian manner, in turn, is required to promote the circadian transcription of Bmal1, Rorγ, Per2, and Cry1 (19). This study also showed that the binding of SIRT1 to the CLOCK-BMAL1 complex is rhythmic and promotes the deacetylation and degradation of the PER2 protein (19). In the second study using fibroblasts and liver tissues, SIRT1 was reported to be a negative regulator of the CLOCK-BMAL1 complex (72). By antagonizing the acetyltransferase activity of CLOCK, SIRT1 removes acetyl-marks from histone H3 and BMAL1, preventing the CLOCK-BMAL1 heterodimer from activating circadian promoters. This study also revealed that SIRT1's activity rather than levels is regulated in a circadian manner (72). Subsequent studies then revealed that the rhythmic activity of SIRT1 is due to the oscillatory patterns of NAD^+ levels regulated by its rate-limiting enzyme NAMPT, which is positively regulated by the core clock genes CLOCK-BMAL1 (73, 74). The activation of SIRT1 through this NAMPT-mediated NAD^+ biosynthetic pathway, in turn, inhibits the activity of CLOCK-BMAL1, thus forming a negative feedback loop (73, 74). These studies revealed a crucial role for SIRT1 in coupling metabolism to the circadian cycle through its reliance on NAD^+ as a cofactor. Supporting this observation, studies have shown that high-fat diets can disrupt the rhythmicity of circadian clock genes in several tissues and that the administration of SIRT1 activators such resveratrol, can reverse these effects and restore the rhythmicity to the circadian genes (75, 76). Additionally, several other studies have attributed different functions to SIRT1 in the regulation of the circadian clock genes in peripheral tissues thus adding additional levels of complexity to its function (77–79).

SIRT1 in the Central Clock

In the SCN of the hypothalamus, SIRT1 was reported to activate the transcription of the circadian genes BMAL1 and CLOCK through PGC-1α (80) (**Figure 4**). Interestingly, this study also showed that aging reduces the levels of SIRT1 in the SCN, which coincided with reduced BMAL1 and PER2 levels. This, in turn, leads to a longer intrinsic period and disruption in the activity patterns and entrainment of mice to the light schedule. Furthermore, the knockout of *Sirt1* from young mice brains was able to phenocopy these age-dependent disruptions in the circadian cycle, while its overexpression protected old mice from the age-dependent effects (80). Thus, this study revealed a crucial role for SIRT1 in the activation of the central pacemaker and maintenance of robust circadian control in young animals. It also suggested that the age-dependent reduction in SIRT1 led to the observed disruptions in the circadian cycle with aging (80). Another interesting study showed that SIRT1 from the ventromedial hypothalamus (VMH) sends nutrient-time information to the central clock through efferent signals to synchronize the central clock to feeding cues (81). SIRT1 ablation from the SF1 neurons of the VMH disrupted the connection between food intake and circadian rhythm as revealed by deregulated activity behaviors and circadian gene expression in the SCN (81). This study strongly supports the role of SIRT1 as a nutrient sensor that couples metabolism to the circadian rhythm of the central clock.

The regulation of the circadian genes by SIRT1 in the central clock has also been reported to be disrupted in a

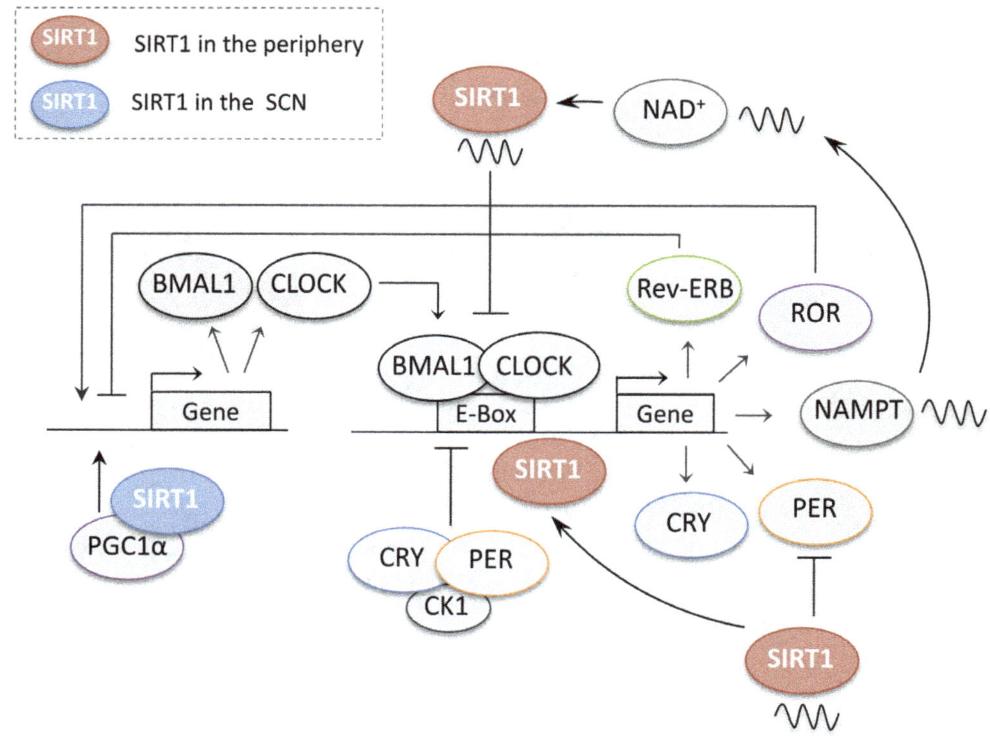

FIGURE 4 | The regulation of central and peripheral clock genes by SIRT1. When dimerized, the core clock genes CLOCK and BMAL1 promote the expression of several downstream genes including their own negative regulators periods (PER) and cryptochromes (CRY). PER and CRY accumulate during the day and together with casein kinase 1 (CK1) then repress their own transcription. The CLOCK-BMAL1 complex also regulates the retinoic acid-related orphan receptors (ROR) and the nuclear receptors (Rev-Erb), which compete for the regulation of the BMAL1 promoter. In the peripheral clocks, SIRT1 regulates the circadian genes at different levels. SIRT1 protein levels cycle in a circadian manner, and through its rhythmic binding to the CLOCK-BMAL1 complex SIRT1 promotes the circadian transcription of Bmal1, Rorγ, Per2, and Cry1. SIRT1 also promotes the deacetylation and degradation of the PER2 protein. SIRT1 activity has also been reported to cycle in a circadian manner owing to the rhythmic expression of NAMPT, a crucial enzyme for NAD^+ biosynthesis, by the CLOCK-BMAL1 complex. In turn, SIRT1 also acts as a negative regulator of the CLOCK-BMAL1 complex thus preventing the activation of circadian promoters. In the suprachiasmatic nucleus (SCN), SIRT1 activates the transcription of the circadian genes BMAL1 and CLOCK through PGC-1α.

number of neurological diseases (**Figure 5**). It was shown that Apolipoprotein E knockout ($ApoE^{-/-}$) mice, a model of Alzheimer's disease, exhibit disruptions in the circadian locomotor activity under dim light and constant darkness along with impairments in re-entrainment to phase change schedules (82). These mice also exhibit an alteration in the expression of SIRT1 and circadian clock genes in the SCN (82). Interestingly, the supplementation with fat or ketone bodies or the intraperitoneal administration of nicotinamide can rescue the circadian clock in these mice by restoring their locomotor rhythmicity and circadian expression of SIRT1 and clock genes (82). Additionally, in triple transgenic Alzheimer's disease (3 × Tg-AD) mice, the patterns of expression of circadian clock genes were also reported to be disrupted in the SCN in response to daylight and darkness. Consistently, these mice also exhibited significantly higher levels of SIRT1 in the SCN compared to non-transgenic after a 12 h exposure to darkness (83). Thus, these studies combined suggest that SIRT1 may be a relevant therapeutic target for the restoration of the circadian rhythm in the SCN, which is disrupted in both aging and neurological disorders.

SIRT1 AND CEREBRAL ISCHEMIA

Researchers have established different roles for brain SIRT1 in different neurological diseases. Evidence from preclinical studies established a neuroprotective role for SIRT1 in ischemic injury. SIRT1 deficient mice, compared to their wild-type littermates, exhibited significantly larger infarct volume and increased impairment of neurological functions after permanent middle cerebral artery occlusion (pMCAO) (84). In a similar line of evidence, pharmacological blockade of SIRT1 activity by SIRT1 inhibitor sirtinol increased the infarct volume following pMCAO (84). In contrast, SIRT1-overexpression protected the brain from cerebral ischemic injury. In a bilateral common carotid artery stenosis (BCAS) model that causes chronic cerebral hypoperfusion, wild-type mice displayed white matter deficits and spatial memory impairments following BCAS (85). Conversely, SIRT1 overexpressed mice showed preserved histological outcome of the corpus callosum and restored spatial working memory (85). Additionally, increased SIRT1 activity by Activator 3, a specific SIRT1 activator, reduced infarct volume in mice (84).

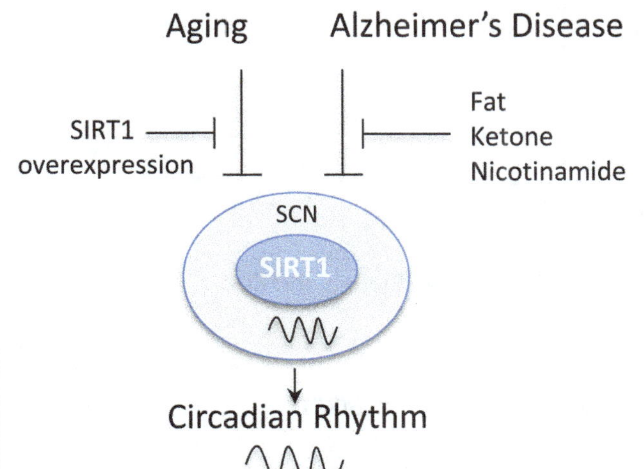

FIGURE 5 | SIRT1 levels in the suprachiasmatic nucleus (SCN) are disrupted by aging and Alzheimer's disease. The rhythmic expression of SIRT1 in the SCN has been reported to be disrupted in animal models of aging and Alzheimer's disease. This, in turn, disrupts the circadian expression of clock genes causing a disruption in the activity patterns of mice and their entrainment to light. The overexpression of SIRT1 protected mice from these age-dependent effects. Similarly, the administration of fat, ketone bodies, or nicotinamide rescued the circadian expression of clock genes in Alzheimer's disease mouse models and restored their locomotor rhythmicity.

The neuroprotection against cerebral ischemia by SIRT1 is achieved through multiple mechanisms. Following ischemia, stressors, such as DNA damage and oxidative stress activate the tumor suppressor gene, p53, which mediates apoptosis (86). Ischemia-induced activation of p53 triggers the mitochondrial apoptotic pathway and facilitates neuronal cell death (86, 87). Inhibition of p53 blocks apoptosis, promotes a survival signaling pathway, and protects neurons against ischemic-induced cell death (88, 89). Genetic deletion or pharmacological inhibition of SIRT1 increased the acetylation of p53 in the peri-infarct area (84). In contrast, SIRT1 activation deacetylated p53 and reduced p53-dependent neuronal apoptosis (90).

SIRT1 dependent endothelial nitric oxide synthase (eNOS) modulation is another beneficial mechanism. Nitric oxide (NO) is a vasodilatory factor that is produced by endothelial nitric oxide synthase (eNOS) in endothelial cells. Acetylated eNOS was significantly increased at 2 h after BCAS in wild-type mice, whereas in SIRT1-Tg mice, the acetylation of eNOS was not observed (85). Increased deacetylation of eNOS is suggested to increase NO production, regulating the vascular tone of blood vessels, and helping to maintain cerebral blood flow during chronic hypoperfusion (85). Consistent with this, in a global cerebral ischemia model of bilateral common carotid artery occlusion (BCAO), SIRT1-Tg mice showed significantly preserved cerebral blood flow during BCAO, which was absent in their wild-type littermates. Similar to the former, pharmacological activation of SIRT1 by resveratrol treatment 1 h after MCAO increased plasma NO and decreased infarction volumes in an eNOS dependent manner (91).

As briefly mentioned above, SIRT1 can also mediate protection by retaining the integrity of white matter (85). White matter lesions are commonly seen in elderly people. One study, which enrolled 1,077 subjects, revealed only 5% were completely free of white matter lesions (92). The prevalence of white matter lesions increased with aging and is associated with cognitive defects. Moreover, the cerebral white matter is highly vulnerable to ischemic injuries (93, 94). Of note, evidence also showed that the degree of white matter lesions relates to infarct volumes and predicts future ischemic incidence after the first stroke attack in patients (95). Supporting the white matter protection by SIRT1 in ischemic stroke, studies in other neurological models demonstrate a similar SIRT1 mediated benefit. In neonatal brain injury, SIRT1 regulates glial progenitor cells to promote white matter regeneration (96). Similarly, SIRT1 mediates neuronal protection in an autoimmune model of white matter injury (97).

Importantly, Sirtl is required in the neuroprotection elicited by ischemic preconditioning (IPC) or resveratrol preconditioning (RPC) (1, 17, 67). IPC develops when a brief period of sublethal ischemia is followed by a period of recovery. It exerts a neuroprotective state against lethal ischemia in different organs of the body including the brain. Furthermore, IPC has shown promising prophylactic potential in diminishing cerebral ischemic injury as shown in recent translational research studies (98, 99). Similar to IPC, resveratrol treatment is able to protect the brain from a following cerebral ischemic attack (1, 17, 67). Collectively, the evidence gathered here demonstrates the pivotal role SIRT1 plays against cerebral ischemia (**Figure 6**).

SIRT1 AND NEURODEGENERATIVE DISORDERS

In addition to providing neuroprotection against cerebral ischemia, the activation of SIRT1 has been shown to confer protection against neurodegenerative diseases, such as Alzheimer's disease (AD), Parkinson's disease (PD) and Huntington's disease (HD) (20, 100). These diseases are substantial burdens to society and can be debilitating to afflicted individuals, making it imperative to investigate potential therapeutic factors, like SIRT1.

The benefits of SIRT1 in neurodegenerative diseases was first reported by Graff et al. in a CR model (101). Graff et al. studied an inducible neurodegenerative mouse model, called CK-p25. These mice exhibited a substantial neuronal loss, deficits in synaptic density and plasticity, as well as learning and memory impairments under the induction of doxycycline. CK-p25 mice underwent 3 months of CR and after the sixth week of CR the neurodegeneration was induced. The CR group showed preserved synaptic density, synaptic plasticity, and memory capacities. CR neuroprotection was mediated by SIRT1 activation, shown by the deacetylation of p53, in the CR but not control group. Furthermore, the use of a small SIRT1 activator, as well as SIRT1 overexpression, recapitulated the CR neuroprotection (101). This evidence shows SIRT1's neuroprotective capacity against neurodegenerative effects on synaptic function and memory capacities. In this way, SIRT1

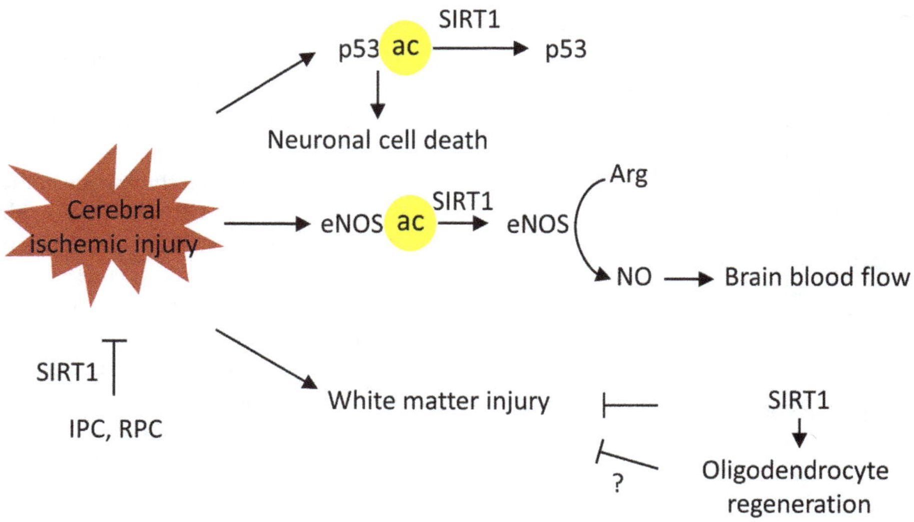

FIGURE 6 | SIRT1 protects against cerebral ischemic injury in multiple mechanisms. SIRT1 deacetylate p53 to block the p53-induced apoptotic pathway, thus, promoting neuronal survival. SIRT1 deacetylates endothelial nitric oxide synthase (eNOS) to regulate vascular tone and maintain brain blood flow. SIRT1protects against white matter injury in ischemic injury, possible via promoting the oligodendrocyte regeneration. Finally, SIRT1 is required for ischemic preconditioning (IPC) and resveratrol preconditioning (RPC) induced ischemic neuroprotection. Arg, L-arginine, NO, nitric oxide.

activation, or perhaps overexpression, may protect against synaptic dysfunction in common forms of neurodegeneration.

Alzheimer's Disease and the Therapeutic Potential of SIRT1

AD is a neurodegenerative disease that can be either early-onset or late-onset. Early-onset is associated with a genetic contribution to the disease's etiology, while the late onset etiology is more complicated and likely multifactorial (102). In the more common, late-onset form of the disease, neuritic senile plaques (NSP) and neurofibrillary tangles (NFT) contribute to neuronal toxicity and death. NSPs originate from the buildup of a protein called β-amyloid (Aβ). β-secretase and γ-secretase are enzymes that cleaves the amyloid precursor protein (APP) to produce Aβ, which is then secreted into the extracellular space, eventually forming toxic aggregates. NFT's are tangles of the cytoskeletal protein tau that receive an aberrant post-translational modification. A common pathological modification of tau is phosphorylation, which forms the toxic p-tau (103). The formation of NSP's and NFT's are pivotal steps in AD pathology.

Recent evidence has linked SIRT1 activity with the interference of the factors and-or processes that produce NSP's and NFT's (**Figure 7**). CR in mice was shown to reduce the expression of β-secretase in part due to the activation of SIRT1 (104). This effect was through the AMPK-SIRT1-PGC-1α pathway in which the transcription factor PGC-1α became upregulated and reciprocally downregulated β-secretase. PGC-1α required SIRT1 deacetylase activity for its transcriptional repression of β-secretase. Thus, CR induced activation of SIRT1 promotes AD neuroprotection through changes in transcription factor activity. As stated before p-tau can contribute to AD. The acetylation of p-tau (acetylated-tau, ac-tau) prevents its degradation and promotes pathological accumulation (105). The overexpression of SIRT1 in HEK293T cells expressing human tau showed a reduction of ac-tau, while SIRT1 deletion results in hyperacetylation. Furthermore, a GST pull-down assay showed a direct interaction of SIRT1 and tau (105). SIRT1 has the capacity to deacetylate ac-tau, which in turn, allows for the degradation of tau and p-tau, potentially reducing the formation of NFT's in AD pathology.

In an oxidative stress model of neuroblastoma SK-N-BE cells, the SIRT1 activator resveratrol was administered to determine its effect on neurodegenerative oxidative stress and protein aggregation (106). Resveratrol treatment prevented toxicity from hydrogen peroxide-induced oxidative stress and prevented Aβ aggregation (106). When applying sirtinol, a non-specific SIRT1 inhibitor, the protection afforded by resveratrol against oxidative stress was lost but not the prevention of Aβ accumulation (106). This evidence indicates that oxidative stress that accompanies AD can be protected against through SIRT1 activation, however, resveratrol protection of Aβ accumulation is SIRT1-independent. SIRT1 overexpression in a transgenic mouse model of AD was investigated by Corpas et al. (107). They studied the CA1 region of the hippocampus to determine if SIRT1 is protective against memory loss and cognitive decline in AD. In the transgenic AD mouse, 6 months of SIRT1 overexpression preserved learning and memory (107). SIRT1 overexpression heavily reduced the presence of Aβ and p-tau in the AD model while increasing the expression of neurotrophic factors, such as brain-derived neurotrophic factor (BDNF) (107). Interestingly, in wild-type mice, SIRT1 overexpression enhanced cognitive function (107). Overexpression of SIRT1 provided protection against pathological protein aggregation and cognitive decline in an AD model while improving cognitive function in the wild-type control (107). SIRT1 is a robust candidate for AD therapies as it has been shown to prevent the accumulation of NSP's and

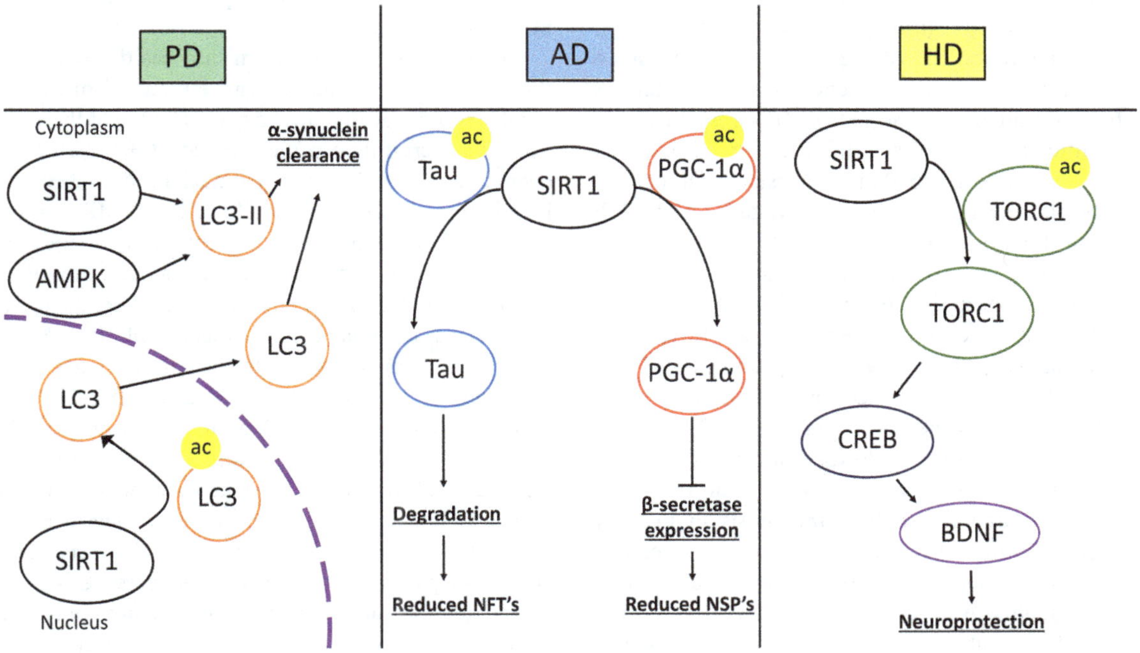

FIGURE 7 | Therapeutic mechanisms of SIRT1 in neurodegenerative disease. The left panel represents SIRT1 in Parkinson's disease (PD). SIRT1 deacetylates microtubule-associated protein 1A/1B-light chain 3 (LC3) in the nucleus which induces the translocation of LC3 into the cytoplasm. In the cytoplasm, SIRT1 and AMP-activated Protein Kinase (AMPK) coordinate to activate LC3-phosphatidylethanolamine (LC3-II). These mechanisms lead to increased autophagic clearance of α-synuclein, reducing α-synuclein deposits. In the middle panel, SIRT1's role in Alzheimer's disease (AD) is represented. SIRT1 can directly deacetylate acetylated-tau protein, increasing its susceptibility to degradation and prevent tau from forming neurofibrillary tangles. SIRT1 can also deacetylate peroxisome proliferator-activated receptor γ (PPARγ) coactivator-1α (PGC-1α), which increases its transcriptional regulation activity. After being deacetylated, PGC-1α can instill transcriptional repression of β-secretase, which in turn can reduce the level of amyloid-β production and neuritic senile plaque accumulation. The right panel represents Huntington's disease (HD). SIRT1 deacetylates CREB-regulated transcription coactivator 1 (TORC1), which allows TORC1 to activate cAMP response element-binding protein (CREB). CREB then transcriptionally upregulates brain-derived neurotrophic factor (BDNF). The increase in BDNF promotes neurotrophic and neuroprotective mechanisms against HD pathology.

NFT's, reduce AD-related oxidative stress, and protect against the cognitive deficits that result from AD pathology. Further investigation into SIRT1's role in AD protection may provide endogenous targets for treating, and potentially preventing, the disease.

Parkinson's Disease and the Therapeutic Potential of SIRT1

PD is a neurodegenerative disease that causes the early and large-scale death of dopaminergic neurons (DA) in the substantia nigra pars compacta (SNpc) (108). The loss of these dopaminergic neurons results in motor deficits and other quality of life diminishing symptoms (109). PD pathology is not exclusive to dopaminergic neurons or the SNpc; thus, making PD therapies difficult to design. DA neuronal death in PD typically results from the aggregation of the protein α-synuclein which forms inclusions called Lewy bodies and Lewy neurites (108). The inclusions of α-synuclein are formed in some familial cases of PD due to mutations in the *SNCA* gene which produces the protein in a misfolded state (110). Another prominent aspect of PD is inflammation and reactive gliosis, both of which may have the capacity to be harmful and protective (111). Overall, the current therapies and understanding of pathology for PD are lacking, making PD a pressing focus of future investigation.

Once again, SIRT1 may play a protective role in neurodegenerative disorders, PD included. There is evidence that suggests there may be genetic correlations between SIRT1 and PD, SIRT1-activated anti-PD signaling, and SIRT1-dependent neuroprotection in various models. Extracellular α-synuclein accumulation leads to mitochondrial dysfunction and a reduction of SIRT1 expression (112). The downregulation of SIRT1 facilitated pathological mechanisms, such as apoptotic cell death. In a genetic study with PD patients and healthy controls, the sequence of the SIRT1 promoter and associated regulatory regions were analyzed to determine if there is a mutational connection between the factor and the disease. Three heterozygous sequence variants within the SIRT1 promoter were identified in PD patients, but not controls (113). These variants may alter the transcription of the SIRT1 gene and could potentially link SIRT1-associated mutations to PD risk. These lines of evidence suggest that the loss or mutation of SIRT1 facilitates PD pathology which highlights SIRT1 as a protective target.

There is evidence that shows that cellular signaling resultant from SIRT1 activation, or pathways that include SIRT1, are involved in the reduction of α-synuclein and promotion of DA neuron survival (**Figure 7**). The application of an activator for the PPARγ, called GW1929, to an *in vitro* human DA neuronal culture conferred resilience when the cultures were subjected to oxidative stress (114). This resilience was attributed to antioxidant signaling and PGC-1α stimulation. GW1929 treatment increased SIRT1 expression and protein levels. GW1929 also resulted in phosphorylated cyclic-AMP response element binding protein 1 (CREB), a pro-survival transcription factor, which then activated SIRT1 (114). Ultimately, upregulation and activation of SIRT1 activated PGC-1α to confer DA neuron protection against oxidative stress (114). In this way, SIRT1 is indirectly upregulated and activated by PPARγ activation in DA neurons suggesting a key role for SIRT1 in DA neuron vitality. In PD, PGC-1α activity may be altered resulting in downregulation of its target genes (115). A study looked at how resveratrol treatment would affect PGC-1α and metabolic homeostasis in primary fibroblasts from early-onset PD. The treatment of resveratrol helped to regulate metabolic homeostasis through AMPK-SIRT1-PGC-1α signaling. An increase in PGC-1α transcription and improvement in mitochondrial function was observed (115). Again, activated SIRT1, in this study through resveratrol treatment, conferred protection against a PD model by activating PGC-1α. In a mouse model of PD induced by 1-methyl-4-phenyl-1,2,3,6-tetrahydropyridine (MPTP), the transgenic overexpression of PGC-1α conferred DA neuronal protection against oxidative stress. Resveratrol treatment recapitulated the protective effects of PGC-1α overexpression in the mouse PD model (116). In a PC12 PD model, the treatment of EGCG, a polyphenol, protected against toxicity through an upregulation of PGC-1α, via SIRT1 activity (117). It is clear that SIRT1 signaling can result in the activation of PGC-1α which is protective against oxidative stress and PD pathology. The evidence supports SIRT1 as a target for future therapeutic approaches in PD treatment due to its induction of neuroprotective cell signaling. Further investigation will provide a greater depth of understanding for PD pathology.

Inflammation within the CNS can exacerbate or potentially initiate PD pathology (118). The cell signaling that occurs from increased inflammation and reactive nitrogen species enhances the dysfunction of neurons and promotes cell death (119). A study looked at how inducible nitric oxide synthase (iNOS), which produces NO that can modify proteins through S-nitrosylation, effects inflammatory signaling in neurodegenerative diseases. S-nitrosylation of SIRT1 inhibits its deacetylase activity. In a rodent model of PD with systemic inflammation, S-nitrosylation of SIRT1 correlated with an increase in p53 and NF-κB acetylation, thereby increasing their activity and promoting further inflammation (119). In SH-SY5Y cells, SIRT1 was shown to directly deacetylate histone residue H3K9 of the p53 promoter, eventually resulting in reduced expression and protecting against apoptosis (120). Additionally, resveratrol-activated SIRT1 regulated p53 and protected against dopaminergic neurodegeneration induced by rotenone, a complex I inhibitor (120). As an inflammatory regulator in PD and potentially other neurodegenerative diseases, SIRT1's deacetylase activity protects against pro-apoptotic inflammatory signaling.

The removal of α-synuclein in a healthy DA neuron entails the use of a few cellular clearance mechanisms, most of which involve some type of autophagy (121). One of these mechanisms utilizes a recruitment protein called LC3, which helps to drive degradation of misfolded α-synuclein that is present in the LC3 bound autophagosome (122). In an MPTP-mouse model, resveratrol or EX-527 were administered to study their effects on motor impairments and autophagic clearance of α-synuclein (122). Resveratrol treatment attenuated MPTP effects on motor deficits and autophagic impairment while EX-527 exacerbated them (122). Furthermore, the beneficial effects of resveratrol treatment were shown to be SIRT1 dependent. SIRT1 was shown to deacetylate nuclear LC3 allowing for its translocation to the cytosol from the nucleus and initiate autophagic clearance (122). Thus, SIRT1 deacetylase activity mediates clearance of α-synuclein through LC3 mediated autophagy to protect against PD pathology. In addition, activation of the AMPK-SIRT1-autophagy pathway was shown to increase LC3-II and enhance α-synuclein clearance after resveratrol treatment (123). Increased clearance of α-synuclein is yet another mechanism by which SIRT1 confers protection against PD pathology.

Considering the multitude of evidence supporting SIRT1's neuroprotective potential against PD and the dynamic range of mechanisms in which that protection is enacted, SIRT1 appears to be an optimal target for the therapeutic treatment of PD. However, recent attempts to enhance SIRT1 expression or activity directly, not through activators, has not shown the same robust results. A study utilized a CNS SIRT1 overexpression mouse model to study the MPTP model of PD. As compared to controls the SIRT1 overexpression mouse did not confer protection against acute toxicity of MPTP in nigrostriatal DA neurons (124). Additionally, in a study that looked at the modulation of SIRT1 expression in multiple human neurodegenerative diseases, there was no significant change found in the SIRT1 expression of patient samples of PD and Lewy bodies dementia (125). This contradictory evidence suggests SIRT1 must operate in a network of cellular signaling and deacetylase activity to confer is neuroprotection against PD pathology.

Huntington's Disease and the Therapeutic Potential of SIRT1

Another neurodegenerative disease in which SIRT1 has been investigated is HD. HD is a genetically autosomal dominant disease in which the HD gene produces a mutant version of the protein. Extended CAG-repeats in the HD gene results in the translated protein acquiring a pathological conformation, affecting its solubility and promoting aggregations (126). Aggregations of the pathological Huntington's protein commonly occur in the axons of neurons, predominantly within the striatum. These axonal aggregations are considered to block anterograde and retrograde axonal transport in affected cells. Post-mortem tissue of HD patients showed cytological features of ballooned cells and shrunken cells within the affected brain regions (127). The blockage of axonal transport is suggested to result in pathological localization of mitochondria and mitochondrial dysfunction. The combination the cytological aberrations and mitochondrial dysfunction are implicated as leading reasons for neuronal death in HD pathology (128).

Like other neurodegenerative diseases, the role of SIRT1 has been investigated in the context of HD pathology. In the R6/2 mouse model of HD, the levels of metabolic and cell cycle regulators were assessed. SIRT1 mRNA and protein were increased in this model but this increase did not correlate to increased activity as shown by no significant change in p53 acetylation (129). This change in SIRT1 expression suggests that SIRT1 levels are altered as a result of HD pathology. In the same model of HD, treatment with β-Lapachone, a natural compound found in the Lapacho tree's bark, was shown to increase the expression of SIRT1 (130). Increased SIRT1 resulted in PGC-1α deacetylation and CREB phosphorylation, which correlated with reduced reactive oxygen species and improvement of rota-rod performance. β-Lapachone thus showed therapeutic potential for HD, enacted through SIRT1 activation. There may be specific contexts in which increased SIRT1 is therapeutic rather than a feature of HD pathology and this is likely related to increased SIRT1 activity.

Many studies have intentionally augmented SIRT1 in the contexts of HD to elucidate whether it is part of the pathology or potentially therapeutic. In an HD mouse model, SIRT1 was overexpressed, improving motor functions and pathological metabolic functioning (131). SIRT1 overexpression was shown to alleviate the HD associated reduction in BDNF concentrations (**Figure 7**). BDNF signaling via its TrkB receptor was shown to be rescued as well. Interestingly, this study also suggests that mutant HD protein inhibits deacetylase activity of SIRT1, as shown by the hyperacetylation of SIRT1-specific targets in the presence of HD mutant protein (131). Another study looked at the effects of SIRT1 absence in HD pathology by using a brain-specific KO of SIRT1 in a mouse model of HD (132). The loss of SIRT1 exacerbated pathological features of HD. These mice had acceleration of motor deficits and increased mutant HD protein aggregation compared to the HD mice with SIRT1 (132). This study also investigated SIRT1 overexpression, which afforded neuroprotection against HD. SIRT1 neuroprotection was dependent on CREB-regulated transcription coactivator 1 (TORC1), which is deacetylated by SIRT1. This interaction increases BDNF and in the presence of the mutant HD protein, the SIRT1-TORC1 interaction is inhibited, repressing BDNF (132).

The role of SIRT1 in HD certainly warrants further investigation. Though there are pathological increases in SIRT1 in neurons suffering from HD pathology, this may be a compensatory mechanism due to the inhibition of SIRT1 by the mutant HD protein. In studies overexpressing SIRT1, HD pathology has been ameliorated and this protection is dependent on SIRT1's activity. Taken together, these lines of evidence suggest that SIRT1 is inhibited in HD pathology and there may be an increase in its expression for compensatory reasons. Furthermore, the loss of SIRT1 deacetylation activity may contribute to HD pathology and restoration of SIRT1 activity likely possess therapeutic potential against the disease.

CONCLUSIONS

In summary, any dysregulation of brain SIRT1 activity can have devastating consequences in terms of metabolism, circadian synchronization, and neurological function. Given that SIRT1 is highly specialized distributed in the hypothalamic nuclei, it is no surprise that brain SIRT1 is a major contributor to the systemic network of metabolic homeostasis. It should be noted that, nowadays, accumulated evidence supports a reciprocal relationship between brain and peripheral tissues in metabolic benefits, circadian oscillations and neurological functions (133, 134). Although we only discussed SIRT1 in the brain, SIRT1 in various peripheral organs also mediates metabolism and circadian rhythms through sensing environmental cues and feeding back into the homeostatic network (13, 133). Therefore, pharmacological agents that target SIRT1 and its relevant signal pathway in one system could potentially provide pleiotropic benefits.

Although most studies discussed above have used resveratrol as the SIRT1 activator, limitations remain for the resveratrol-induced SIRT1 activation. One study reported the activation of AMPK by high-dose resveratrol, suggesting the indirect effects of SIRT1 through AMPK pathway as well as the off-target effects of resveratrol (135). As a polyphenol activator, resveratrol is poorly water-soluble. Thus, the bioavailability of resveratrol also needs to be taken into consideration, especially when applied in clinical trials. To improve the bioavailability, targeted delivery of resveratrol, such as nanoparticles has been developed (136, 137).

In addition to resveratrol, another promising target to activate SIRT1 is the NAD^+ pathway. As mentioned before, NAD^+ is the rate-limiting co-substrate for SIRT1. Thus, increased NAD^+ levels is presumably to activate SIRT1. So far, to supplement NAD^+ precursor and boost NAD biosynthesis has been the main approaches to alter NAD^+ levels. Experimental studies have reported beneficial effects of NAD^+ precursor supplementation (138–140). Current information from clinical studies is still lacking. One recent study reported promising result that chronic nicotinamide riboside, a NAD^+ precursor, effectively increased NAD^+ levels in elders (141). Again, it is difficult to tell whether the beneficial phenotypes are produced by NAD^+ or NAD^+-induced SIRT1 activation. Therefore, pharmacological agents that are ligand-specific and tissue-specific are warranted to further clarify the functions of SIRT1 in biological and pathological events.

AUTHOR CONTRIBUTIONS

JX, CJ, NK, IE, and MP-P cooperated to write the article and revised the content. MP-P and JX outlined the manuscript. MP-P supervised the work.

REFERENCES

1. Khoury N, Koronowski KB, Young JI, Perez-Pinzon MA. The NAD(+)-dependent family of sirtuins in cerebral ischemia and preconditioning. *Antioxid Redox Signal* (2018) 28:691–710. doi: 10.1089/ars.2017.7258
2. Gomes P, Fleming Outeiro T, Cavadas C. Emerging role of sirtuin 2 in the regulation of mammalian metabolism. *Trends Pharmacol Sci.* (2015) 36:756–68. doi: 10.1016/j.tips.2015.08.001
3. Verdin E. NAD(+) in aging, metabolism, and neurodegeneration. *Science* (2015) 350:1208–13. doi: 10.1126/science.aac4854
4. Ding RB, Bao J, Deng CX. Emerging roles of SIRT1 in fatty liver diseases. *Int J Biol Sci.* (2017) 13:852–67. doi: 10.7150/ijbs.19370
5. Sun C, Zhang F, Ge X, Yan T, Chen X, Shi X, et al. SIRT1 improves insulin sensitivity under insulin-resistant conditions by repressing PTP1B. *Cell Metab.* (2007) 6:307–19. doi: 10.1016/j.cmet.2007.08.014
6. Wang Y, Xu C, Liang Y, Vanhoutte PM. SIRT1 in metabolic syndrome: where to target matters. *Pharmacol Ther.* (2012) 136:305–18. doi: 10.1016/j.pharmthera.2012.08.009
7. Bordone L, Guarente L. Calorie restriction, SIRT1 and metabolism: understanding longevity. *Nat Rev Mol Cell Biol.* (2005) 6:298–305. doi: 10.1038/nrm1616
8. Cantó C, Auwerx J. Caloric restriction, SIRT1 and longevity. *Trends Endocrinol Metab.* (2009) 20:325–31. doi: 10.1016/j.tem.2009.03.008
9. Morselli E, Maiuri MC, Markaki M, Megalou E, Pasparaki A, Palikaras K, et al. Caloric restriction and resveratrol promote longevity through the Sirtuin-1-dependent induction of autophagy. *Cell Death Dis.* (2010) 1:e10. doi: 10.1038/cddis.2009.8
10. Cohen DE, Supinski AM, Bonkowski MS, Donmez G, Guarente LP. Neuronal SIRT1 regulates endocrine and behavioral responses to calorie restriction. *Genes Dev.* (2009) 23:2812–7. doi: 10.1101/gad.1839209
11. Satoh A, Brace CS, Ben-Josef G, West T, Wozniak DF, Holtzman DM, et al. SIRT1 promotes the central adaptive response to diet restriction through activation of the dorsomedial and lateral nuclei of the hypothalamus. *J Neurosci.* (2010) 30:10220–32. doi: 10.1523/JNEUROSCI.1385-10.2010
12. Guarente L. Calorie restriction and sirtuins revisited. *Genes Dev.* (2013) 27:2072–85. doi: 10.1101/gad.227439.113
13. Chalkiadaki A, Guarente L. Guarente L. Sirtuins mediate mammalian metabolic responses to nutrient availability. *Nat Rev Endocrinol.* (2012) 8:287–96. doi: 10.1038/nrendo.2011.225
14. Gerhart-Hines Z, Rodgers JT, Bare O, Lerin C, Kim SH, Mostoslavsky R, et al. Metabolic control of muscle mitochondrial function and fatty acid oxidation through SIRT1/PGC-1alpha. *EMBO J.* (2007) 26:1913–23. doi: 10.1038/sj.emboj.7601633
15. Wang P, Xu TY, Guan YF, Tian WW, Viollet B, Rui YC, et al. Nicotinamide phosphoribosyltransferase protects against ischemic stroke through SIRT1-dependent adenosine monophosphate-activated kinase pathway. *Ann Neurol.* (2011) 69:360–74. doi: 10.1002/ana.22236
16. Rodgers JT, Lerin C, Haas W, Gygi SP, Spiegelman BM, Puigserver P. Nutrient control of glucose homeostasis through a complex of PGC-1alpha and SIRT1. *Nature* (2005) 434:113–8. doi: 10.1038/nature03354
17. Koronowski KB, Perez-Pinzon MA. Perez-Pinzon MA. Sirt1 in cerebral ischemia. *Brain Circ.* (2015) 1:69–78. doi: 10.4103/2394-8108.162532
18. Ramadori G, Lee CE, Bookout AL, Lee S, Williams KW, Anderson J, et al. Brain SIRT1: anatomical distribution and regulation by energy availability. *J Neurosci.* (2008) 28:9989–96. doi: 10.1523/JNEUROSCI.3257-08.2008
19. Asher G, Gatfield D, Stratmann M, Reinke H, Dibner C, Kreppel F, et al. SIRT1 regulates circadian clock gene expression through PER2 deacetylation. *Cell* (2008) 134:317–28. doi: 10.1016/j.cell.2008.06.050
20. Zhang F, Wang S, Gan L, Vosler PS, Gao Y, Zigmond MJ, et al. Protective effects and mechanisms of sirtuins in the nervous system. *Prog Neurobiol.* (2011) 95:373–95. doi: 10.1016/j.pneurobio.2011.09.001
21. Tzameli I. The evolving role of mitochondria in metabolism. *Trends Endocrinol Metab.* (2012) 23:417–9. doi: 10.1016/j.tem.2012.07.008
22. Raichle ME, Gusnard DA. Appraising the brain's energy budget. *Proc Natl Acad Sci USA.* (2002) 99:10237–9. doi: 10.1073/pnas.172399499
23. Aquilano K, Vigilanza P, Baldelli S, Pagliei B, Rotilio G, Ciriolo MR. Peroxisome proliferator-activated receptor gamma co-activator 1alpha (PGC-1alpha) and sirtuin 1 (SIRT1) reside in mitochondria: possible direct function in mitochondrial biogenesis. *J Biol Chem.* (2010) 285:21590–9. doi: 10.1074/jbc.M109.070169
24. Bechmann I, Diano S, Warden CH, Bartfai T, Nitsch R, Horvath TL. Brain mitochondrial uncoupling protein 2 (UCP2): a protective stress signal in neuronal injury. *Biochem Pharmacol.* (2002) 64:363–7. doi: 10.1016/S0006-2952(02)01166-8
25. Andrews ZB. Uncoupling protein-2 and the potential link between metabolism and longevity. *Curr Aging Sci.* (2010) 3:102–12. doi: 10.2174/1874609811003020102
26. Bordone L, Motta MC, Picard F, Robinson A, Jhala US, Apfeld J, et al. Sirt1 regulates insulin secretion by repressing UCP2 in pancreatic beta cells. *PLoS Biol.* (2006) 4:e31. doi: 10.1371/journal.pbio.0040295
27. Bordone L, Motta MC, Picard F, Robinson A, Jhala US, Apfeld J, et al. Correction: Sirt1 Regulates Insulin Secretion by Repressing UCP2 in Pancreatic beta Cells. *PLoS Biol.* (2015) 13:e1002346. doi: 10.1371/journal.pbio.1002346
28. Moynihan KA, Grimm AA, Plueger MM, Bernal-Mizrachi E, Ford E, Cras-Méneur C, et al. Increased dosage of mammalian Sir2 in pancreatic beta cells enhances glucose-stimulated insulin secretion in mice. *Cell Metab.* (2005) 2:105–17. doi: 10.1016/j.cmet.2005.07.001
29. Yuan Y, Cruzat VF, Newsholme P, Cheng J, Chen Y, Lu Y. Regulation of SIRT1 in aging: roles in mitochondrial function and biogenesis. *Mech Ageing Dev.* (2016) 155:10–21. doi: 10.1016/j.mad.2016.02.003
30. Nemoto S, Fergusson MM, Finkel T. SIRT1 functionally interacts with the metabolic regulator and transcriptional coactivator PGC-1{alpha}. *J Biol Chem.* (2005) 280:16456–60. doi: 10.1074/jbc.M501485200
31. Amat R, Planavila A, Chen SL, Iglesias R, Giralt M, Villarroya F. SIRT1 controls the transcription of the peroxisome proliferator-activated receptor-gamma Co-activator-1alpha (PGC-1alpha) gene in skeletal muscle through the PGC-1alpha autoregulatory loop and interaction with MyoD. *J Biol Chem.* (2009) 284:21872–80. doi: 10.1074/jbc.M109.022749
32. Cantó C, Gerhart-Hines Z, Feige JN, Lagouge M, Noriega L, Milne JC, et al. AMPK regulates energy expenditure by modulating NAD+ metabolism and SIRT1 activity. *Nature* (2009) 458:1056–60. doi: 10.1038/nature07813
33. Puigserver P, Spiegelman BM. Peroxisome proliferator-activated receptor-gamma coactivator 1 alpha (PGC-1 alpha): transcriptional coactivator and metabolic regulator. *Endocr Rev.* (2003) 24:78–90. doi: 10.1210/er.2002-0012
34. Teyssier C, Ma H, Emter R, Kralli A, Stallcup MR. Activation of nuclear receptor coactivator PGC-1alpha by arginine methylation. *Genes Dev.* (2005) 19:1466–73. doi: 10.1101/gad.1295005
35. Campbell CT, Kolesar JE, Kaufman BA. Mitochondrial transcription factor A regulates mitochondrial transcription initiation, DNA packaging, and genome copy number. *Biochim Biophys Acta* (2012) 1819:921–9. doi: 10.1016/j.bbagrm.2012.03.002
36. Lin J, Handschin C, Spiegelman BM. Metabolic control through the PGC-1 family of transcription coactivators. *Cell Metab.* (2005) 1:361–70. doi: 10.1016/j.cmet.2005.05.004
37. Li P, Liu Y, Burns N, Zhao KS, Song R. SIRT1 is required for mitochondrial biogenesis reprogramming in hypoxic human pulmonary arteriolar smooth muscle cells. *Int J Mol Med.* (2017) 39:1127–36. doi: 10.3892/ijmm.2017.2932
38. Tang BL. Sirt1 and the mitochondria. *Mol Cells* (2016) 39:87–95. doi: 10.14348/molcells.2016.2318
39. Purushotham A, Schug TT, Xu Q, Surapureddi S, Guo X, Li X. Hepatocyte-specific deletion of SIRT1 alters fatty acid metabolism and results in hepatic steatosis and inflammation. *Cell Metab.* (2009) 9:327–38. doi: 10.1016/j.cmet.2009.02.006
40. Tanaka A. Parkin-mediated selective mitochondrial autophagy, mitophagy: parkin purges damaged organelles from the vital mitochondrial network. *FEBS Lett.* (2010) 584:1386–92. doi: 10.1016/j.febslet.2010.02.060
41. Wallace DC. A mitochondrial paradigm of metabolic and degenerative diseases, aging, and cancer: a dawn for evolutionary medicine. *Annu Rev Genet.* (2005) 39:359–407. doi: 10.1146/annurev.genet.39.110304.095751
42. Singh G, Pachouri UC, Khaidem DC, Kundu A, Chopra C, Singh P. Mitochondrial DNA damage and diseases. *F1000Res.* (2015) 4:176. doi: 10.12688/f1000research.6665.1

43. Jin SM, Youle RJ. PINK1- and Parkin-mediated mitophagy at a glance. *J Cell Sci.* (2012) 125(Pt 4):795–9. doi: 10.1242/jcs.093849
44. Whitworth AJ, Pallanck LJ. PINK1/Parkin mitophagy and neurodegeneration-what do we really know *in vivo*? *Curr Opin Genet Dev.* (2017) 44:47–53. doi: 10.1016/j.gde.2017.01.016
45. Brunet A, Sweeney LB, Sturgill JF, Chua KF, Greer PL, Lin Y, et al. Stress-dependent regulation of FOXO transcription factors by the SIRT1 deacetylase. *Science* (2004) 303:2011–5. doi: 10.1126/science.1094637
46. Kume S, Uzu T, Horiike K, Chin-Kanasaki M, Isshiki K, Araki S, et al. Calorie restriction enhances cell adaptation to hypoxia through Sirt1-dependent mitochondrial autophagy in mouse aged kidney. *J Clin Invest.* (2010) 120:1043–55. doi: 10.1172/JCI41376
47. Tan S, Wong E. Mitophagy Transcriptome: mechanistic insights into polyphenol-mediated mitophagy. *Oxid Med Cell Longev.* (2017) 2017:9028435. doi: 10.1155/2017/9028435
48. Lee IH, Cao L, Mostoslavsky R, Lombard DB, Liu J, Bruns NE, et al. A role for the NAD-dependent deacetylase Sirt1 in the regulation of autophagy. *Proc Natl Acad Sci USA.* (2008) 105:3374–9. doi: 10.1073/pnas.0712145105
49. Tsunemi T, Ashe TD, Morrison BE, Soriano KR, Au J, Roque RA, et al. PGC-1alpha rescues Huntington's disease proteotoxicity by preventing oxidative stress and promoting TFEB function. *Sci Transl Med.* (2012) 4:142ra97. doi: 10.1126/scitranslmed.3003799
50. Sohn JW. Network of hypothalamic neurons that control appetite. *BMB Rep.* (2015) 48:229–33. doi: 10.5483/BMBRep.2015.48.4.272
51. King BM. The rise, fall, and resurrection of the ventromedial hypothalamus in the regulation of feeding behavior and body weight. *Physiol Behav.* (2006) 87:221–44. doi: 10.1016/j.physbeh.2005.10.007
52. Ramadori G, Fujikawa T, Fukuda M, Anderson J, Morgan DA, Mostoslavsky R, et al. SIRT1 deacetylase in POMC neurons is required for homeostatic defenses against diet-induced obesity. *Cell Metab.* (2010) 12:78–87. doi: 10.1016/j.cmet.2010.05.010
53. Sasaki T, Kikuchi O, Shimpuku M, Susanti VY, Yokota-Hashimoto H, Taguchi R, et al. Hypothalamic SIRT1 prevents age-associated weight gain by improving leptin sensitivity in mice. *Diabetologia* (2014) 57:819–31. doi: 10.1007/s00125-013-3140-5
54. Kim MS, Pak YK, Jang PG, Namkoong C, Choi YS, Won JC, et al. Role of hypothalamic Foxo1 in the regulation of food intake and energy homeostasis. *Nat Neurosci.* (2006) 9:901–6. doi: 10.1038/nn1731
55. Susanti VY, Sasaki T, Yokota-Hashimoto H, Matsui S, Lee YS, Kikuchi O, et al. Sirt1 rescues the obesity induced by insulin-resistant constitutively-nuclear FoxO1 in POMC neurons of male mice. *Obesity* (2014) 22:2115–9. doi: 10.1002/oby.20838
56. Sasaki T, Kim HJ, Kobayashi M, Kitamura YI, Yokota-Hashimoto H, Shiuchi T, et al. Induction of hypothalamic Sirt1 leads to cessation of feeding via agouti-related peptide. *Endocrinology* (2010) 151:2556–66. doi: 10.1210/en.2009-1319
57. Ramadori G, Fujikawa T, Anderson J, Berglund ED, Frazao R, Michán S, et al. SIRT1 deacetylase in SF1 neurons protects against metabolic imbalance. *Cell Metab.* (2011) 14:301–12. doi: 10.1016/j.cmet.2011.06.014
58. Velásquez DA, Martínez G, Romero A, Vázquez MJ, Boit KD, Dopeso-Reyes IG, et al. The central Sirtuin 1/p53 pathway is essential for the orexigenic action of ghrelin. *Diabetes* (2011) 60:1177–85. doi: 10.2337/db10-0802
59. Dietrich MO, Antunes C, Geliang G, Liu ZW, Borok E, Nie Y, et al. Agrp neurons mediate Sirt1's action on the melanocortin system and energy balance: roles for Sirt1 in neuronal firing and synaptic plasticity. *J Neurosci.* (2010) 30:11815–25. doi: 10.1523/JNEUROSCI.2234-10.2010
60. Cakir I, Perello M, Lansari O, Messier NJ, Vaslet CA, Nillni EA. Hypothalamic Sirt1 regulates food intake in a rodent model system. *PLoS ONE* (2009) 4:e8322. doi: 10.1371/journal.pone.0008322
61. Cyr NE, Steger JS, Toorie AM, Yang JZ, Stuart R, Nillni EA. Central Sirt1 regulates body weight and energy expenditure along with the POMC-derived peptide alpha-MSH and the processing enzyme CPE production in diet-induced obese male rats. *Endocrinology* (2015) 156:961–74. doi: 10.1210/en.2014-1970
62. Barnes AS. The epidemic of obesity and diabetes: trends and treatments. *Tex Heart Inst J.* (2011) 38:142–4.
63. Golay A, Ybarra J. Link between obesity and type 2 diabetes. *Best Pract Res Clin Endocrinol Metab.* (2005) 19:649–63. doi: 10.1016/j.beem.2005.07.010
64. Ramadori G, Gautron L, Fujikawa T, Vianna CR, Elmquist JK, Coppari R. Central administration of resveratrol improves diet-induced diabetes. *Endocrinology* (2009) 150:5326–33. doi: 10.1210/en.2009-0528
65. Knight CM, Gutierrez-Juarez R, Lam TK, Arrieta-Cruz I, Huang L, Schwartz G, et al. Mediobasal hypothalamic SIRT1 is essential for resveratrol's effects on insulin action in rats. *Diabetes* (2011) 60:2691–700. doi: 10.2337/db10-0987
66. Lu M, Sarruf DA, Li P, Osborn O, Sanchez-Alavez M, Talukdar S, et al. Neuronal Sirt1 deficiency increases insulin sensitivity in both brain and peripheral tissues. *J Biol Chem.* (2013) 288:10722–35. doi: 10.1074/jbc.M112.443606
67. Koronowski KB, Khoury N, Saul I, Loris ZB, Cohan CH, Stradecki-Cohan HM, et al. Neuronal SIRT1 (Silent Information Regulator 2 Homologue 1) regulates glycolysis and mediates resveratrol-induced ischemic tolerance. *Stroke.* (2017) 48:3117–25. doi: 10.1161/STROKEAHA.117.018562
68. Ye X, Li M, Hou T, Gao T, Zhu WG, Yang Y. Sirtuins in glucose and lipid metabolism. *Oncotarget* (2017) 8:1845–59. doi: 10.18632/oncotarget.12157
69. Gallego M, Virshup DM. Post-translational modifications regulate the ticking of the circadian clock. *Nat Rev Mol Cell Biol.* (2007) 8:139–48. doi: 10.1038/nrm2106
70. Takahashi JS. Transcriptional architecture of the mammalian circadian clock. *Nat Rev Genet.* (2017) 18:164–79. doi: 10.1038/nrg.2016.150
71. Takahashi JS. Molecular architecture of the circadian clock in mammals. In: Sassone-Corsi P, Christen Y. editors *A Time for Metabolism and Hormones*, Cham: Springer. (2016) p. 13–24. doi: 10.1007/978-3-319-27069-2_2
72. Nakahata Y, Kaluzova M, Grimaldi B, Sahar S, Hirayama J, Chen D, et al. The NAD+-dependent deacetylase SIRT1 modulates CLOCK-mediated chromatin remodeling and circadian control. *Cell* (2008) 134:329–40. doi: 10.1016/j.cell.2008.07.002
73. Nakahata Y, Sahar S, Astarita G, Kaluzova M, Sassone-Corsi P. Circadian control of the NAD+ salvage pathway by CLOCK-SIRT1. *Science* (2009) 324(5927):654–7. doi: 10.1126/science.1170803
74. Ramsey KM, Yoshino J, Brace CS, Abrassart D, Kobayashi Y, Marcheva B, et al. Circadian clock feedback cycle through NAMPT-mediated NAD+ biosynthesis. *Science* (2009) 324:651–4. doi: 10.1126/science.1171641
75. Tong X, Zhang D, Arthurs B, Li P, Durudogan L, Gupta N, et al. Palmitate inhibits SIRT1-Dependent BMAL1/CLOCK interaction and disrupts circadian gene oscillations in hepatocytes. *PLoS ONE* (2015) 10:e0130047. doi: 10.1371/journal.pone.0130047
76. Sun L, Wang Y, Song Y, Cheng XR, Xia S, Rahman MR, et al. Resveratrol restores the circadian rhythmic disorder of lipid metabolism induced by high-fat diet in mice. *Biochem Biophys Res Commun.* (2015) 458:86–91. doi: 10.1016/j.bbrc.2015.01.072
77. Zhou B, Zhang Y, Zhang F, Xia Y, Liu J, Huang R, et al. CLOCK/BMAL1 regulates circadian change of mouse hepatic insulin sensitivity by SIRT1. *Hepatology* (2014) 59:2196–206. doi: 10.1002/hep.26992
78. Aguilar-Arnal L, Katada S, Orozco-Solis R, Sassone-Corsi P. NAD(+)-SIRT1 control of H3K4 trimethylation through circadian deacetylation of MLL1. *Nat Struct Mol Biol.* (2015) 22:312–8. doi: 10.1038/nsmb.2990
79. Wang RH, Zhao T, Cui K, Hu G, Chen Q, Chen W, et al. Negative reciprocal regulation between Sirt1 and Per2 modulates the circadian clock and aging. *Sci Rep.* (2016) 6:28633. doi: 10.1038/srep28633
80. Chang HC, Guarente L. SIRT1 mediates central circadian control in the SCN by a mechanism that decays with aging. *Cell* (2013) 153:1448–60. doi: 10.1016/j.cell.2013.05.027
81. Orozco-Solis R, Ramadori G, Coppari R, Sassone-Corsi P. SIRT1 Relays nutritional inputs to the circadian clock through the Sf1 neurons of the ventromedial hypothalamus. *Endocrinology* (2015) 156:2174–84. doi: 10.1210/en.2014-1805
82. Zhou L, Gao Q, Nie M, Gu JL, Hao W, Wang L, et al. Degeneration and energy shortage in the suprachiasmatic nucleus underlies the circadian rhythm disturbance in ApoE(-/-) mice: implications for Alzheimer's disease. *Sci Rep.* (2016) 6:36335. doi: 10.1038/srep36335
83. Bellanti F, Iannelli G, Blonda M, Tamborra R, Villani R, Romano A, et al. Alterations of clock gene RNA expression in brain regions of a triple transgenic model of Alzheimer's disease. *J Alzheimers Dis.* (2017) 59:615–31. doi: 10.3233/JAD-160942

84. Hernández-Jiménez M, Hurtado O, Cuartero MI, Ballesteros I, Moraga A, Pradillo JM, et al. Silent information regulator 1 protects the brain against cerebral ischemic damage. *Stroke* (2013) 44:2333–7. doi: 10.1161/STROKEAHA.113.001715
85. Hattori Y, Okamoto Y, Maki T, Yamamoto Y, Oishi N, Yamahara K, et al. Silent information regulator 2 homolog 1 counters cerebral hypoperfusion injury by deacetylating endothelial nitric oxide synthase. *Stroke* (2014) 45:3403–11. doi: 10.1161/STROKEAHA.114.006265
86. Hong LZ, Zhao XY, and Zhang HL, p53-mediated neuronal cell death in ischemic brain injury. *Neurosci Bull.* (2010) 26:232–40. doi: 10.1007/s12264-010-1111-0
87. Wang DB, Kinoshita C, Kinoshita Y, Morrison RS. p53 and mitochondrial function in neurons. *Biochim Biophys Acta* (2014) 1842:1186–97. doi: 10.1016/j.bbadis.2013.12.015
88. Plesnila N, von Baumgarten L, Retiounskaia M, Engel D, Ardeshiri A, Zimmermann R, et al. Delayed neuronal death after brain trauma involves p53-dependent inhibition of NF-kappaB transcriptional activity. *Cell Death Differ* (2007) 14:1529–41. doi: 10.1038/sj.cdd.4402159
89. Culmsee C, Zhu X, Yu QS, Chan SL, Camandola S, Guo Z, et al. A synthetic inhibitor of p53 protects neurons against death induced by ischemic and excitotoxic insults, and amyloid beta-peptide. *J Neurochem.* (2001) 77:220–8. doi: 10.1046/j.1471-4159.2001.t01-1-00220.x
90. Shi X, Pi L, Zhou S, Li X, Min F, Wang S, et al. Activation of sirtuin 1 attenuates high glucose-induced neuronal apoptosis by deacetylating p53. *Front Endocrinol.* (2018) 9:274. doi: 10.3389/fendo.2018.00274
91. Tsai SK, Hung LM, Fu YT, Cheng H, Nien MW, Liu HY, et al. Resveratrol neuroprotective effects during focal cerebral ischemia injury via nitric oxide mechanism in rats. *J Vasc Surg.* (2007) 46:346–53. doi: 10.1016/j.jvs.2007.04.044
92. de Leeuw FE, de Groot JC, Achten E, Oudkerk M, Ramos LMP, Heijboer R, et al. Prevalence of cerebral white matter lesions in elderly people: a population based magnetic resonance imaging study. The Rotterdam Scan Study. *J Neurol Neurosurg Psychiatry* (2001) 70:9–14. doi: 10.1136/jnnp.70.1.9
93. Pantoni L, Garcia JH, Gutierrez JA. Cerebral white matter is highly vulnerable to ischemia. *Stroke* (1996) 27:1641–6; discussion 1647. doi: 10.1161/01.STR.27.9.1641
94. Wang Y, Liu G, Hong D, Chen F, Ji X, Cao G. White matter injury in ischemic stroke. *Prog Neurobiol.* (2016) 141:45–60. doi: 10.1016/j.pneurobio.2016.04.005
95. Fu JH, Lu CZ, Hong Z, Dong Q, Luo Y, Wong KS. Extent of white matter lesions is related to acute subcortical infarcts and predicts further stroke risk in patients with first ever ischaemic stroke. *J Neurol Neurosurg Psychiatry.* (2005) 76:793–6. doi: 10.1136/jnnp.2003.032771
96. Jablonska B, Gierdalski M, Chew LJ, Hawley T, Catron M, Lichauco A, et al. Sirt1 regulates glial progenitor proliferation and regeneration in white matter after neonatal brain injury. *Nat Commun.* (2016) 7:13866. doi: 10.1038/ncomms13866
97. Nimmagadda VK, Bever CT, Vattikunta NR, Talat S, Ahmad V, Nagalla NK, et al. Overexpression of SIRT1 protein in neurons protects against experimental autoimmune encephalomyelitis through activation of multiple SIRT1 targets. *J Immunol.* (2013) 190:4595–607. doi: 10.4049/jimmunol.1202584
98. Meng R, Asmaro K, Meng L, Liu Y, Ma C, Xi C, et al. Upper limb ischemic preconditioning prevents recurrent stroke in intracranial arterial stenosis. *Neurology* (2012) 79:1853–61. doi: 10.1212/WNL.0b013e318271f76a
99. Jensen HA, Loukogeorgakis S, Yannopoulos F, Rimpiläinen E, Petzold A, Tuominen H, et al. Remote ischemic preconditioning protects the brain against injury after hypothermic circulatory arrest. *Circulation* (2011) 123:714–21. doi: 10.1161/CIRCULATIONAHA.110.986497
100. Donmez G, Outeiro TF. SIRT1 and SIRT2: emerging targets in neurodegeneration. *EMBO Mol Med.* (2013) 5:344–52. doi: 10.1002/emmm.201302451
101. Gräff J, Kahn M, Samiei A, Gao J, Ota KT, Rei D, et al. A dietary regimen of caloric restriction or pharmacological activation of SIRT1 to delay the onset of neurodegeneration. *J Neurosci.* (2013) 33:8951–60. doi: 10.1523/JNEUROSCI.5657-12.2013
102. Balin BJ, Hudson AP. Etiology and pathogenesis of late-onset Alzheimer's disease. *Curr Allergy Asthma Rep.* (2014) 14:417. doi: 10.1007/s11882-013-0417-1
103. Barañano AE, Keane PA, Ruiz-Garcia H, Walsh AC, Sadda SR. Impact of scanning density on spectral domain optical coherence tomography assessments in neovascular age-related macular degeneration. *Acta Ophthalmol.* (2012) 90:e274–80. doi: 10.1111/j.1755-3768.2012.02398.x
104. Wang R, Li JJ, Diao S, Kwak YD, Liu L, Zhi L, et al. Metabolic stress modulates Alzheimer's beta-secretase gene transcription via SIRT1-PPARgamma-PGC-1 in neurons. *Cell Metab.* (2013) 17:685–94. doi: 10.1016/j.cmet.2013.03.016
105. Lee JW, Zoumalan RA, Valenzuela CD, Nguyen PD, Tutela JP, Roman BR, et al. Regulators and mediators of radiation-induced fibrosis: Gene expression profiles and a rationale for Smad3 inhibition. *Otolaryngol Head Neck Surg.* (2010) 143:525–30. doi: 10.1016/j.otohns.2010.06.912
106. Albani D, Polito L, Batelli S, De Mauro S, Fracasso C, Martelli G, et al. The SIRT1 activator resveratrol protects SK-N-BE cells from oxidative stress and against toxicity caused by alpha-synuclein or amyloid-beta (1–42) peptide. *J Neurochem.* (2009) 110:1445–56. doi: 10.1111/j.1471-4159.2009.06228.x
107. Corpas R, Revilla S, Ursulet S, Castro-Freire M, Kaliman P, Petegnief V, et al. SIRT1 overexpression in mouse hippocampus induces cognitive enhancement through proteostatic and neurotrophic mechanisms. *Mol Neurobiol.* (2017) 54:5604–19. doi: 10.1007/s12035-016-0087-9
108. Kalia LV, Lang AE. Parkinson's disease. *Lancet* (2015) 386:896–912. doi: 10.1016/S0140-6736(14)61393-3
109. Dickson DW. Parkinson's disease and parkinsonism: neuropathology. *Cold Spring Harb Perspect Med.* (2012) 2:8. doi: 10.1101/cshperspect.a009258
110. Polymeropoulos MH, Lavedan C, Leroy E, Ide SE, Dehejia A, Dutra A, et al. Mutation in the alpha-synuclein gene identified in families with Parkinson's disease. *Science* (1997) 276:2045–7. doi: 10.1126/science.276.5321.2045
111. Phani S, Loike JD, Przedborski S. Neurodegeneration and inflammation in Parkinson's disease. *Parkinsonism Relat Disord.* (2012) 18(Suppl. 1):S207–9. doi: 10.1016/S1353-8020(11)70064-5
112. Motyl J, Wencel PL, Cieślik M, Strosznajder RP, Strosznajder JB. Alpha-synuclein alters differently gene expression of Sirts, PARPs and other stress response proteins: implications for neurodegenerative disorders. *Mol Neurobiol.* (2018) 55:727–40. doi: 10.1007/s12035-016-0317-1
113. Zhang A, Wang H, Qin X, Pang S, Yan B. Genetic analysis of SIRT1 gene promoter in sporadic Parkinson's disease. *Biochem Biophys Res Commun.* (2012) 422:693–6. doi: 10.1016/j.bbrc.2012.05.059
114. Mäkelä J, Tselykh TV, Kukkonen JP, Eriksson O, Korhonen LT, Lindholm D. Peroxisome proliferator-activated receptor-gamma (PPARgamma) agonist is neuroprotective and stimulates PGC-1alpha expression and CREB phosphorylation in human dopaminergic neurons. *Neuropharmacology* (2016) 102:266–75. doi: 10.1016/j.neuropharm.2015.11.020
115. Ferretta A, Gaballo A, Tanzarella P, Piccoli C, Capitanio N, Nico B, et al. Effect of resveratrol on mitochondrial function: implications in parkin-associated familiar Parkinson's disease. *Biochim Biophys Acta* (2014) 1842:902–15. doi: 10.1016/j.bbadis.2014.02.010
116. Mudò G, Mäkelä J, Di Liberto V, Tselykh TV, Olivieri M, Piepponen P, et al. Transgenic expression and activation of PGC-1alpha protect dopaminergic neurons in the MPTP mouse model of Parkinson's disease. *Cell Mol Life Sci.* (2012) 69:1153–65. doi: 10.1007/s00018-011-0850-z
117. Ye Q, Ye L, Xu X, Huang B, Zhang X, Zhu Y, et al. Epigallocatechin-3-gallate suppresses 1-methyl-4-phenyl-pyridine-induced oxidative stress in PC12 cells via the SIRT1/PGC-1alpha signaling pathway. *BMC Complement Altern Med.* (2012) 12:82. doi: 10.1186/1472-6882-12-82
118. Deleidi M, Gasser T. The role of inflammation in sporadic and familial Parkinson's disease. *Cell Mol Life Sci.* (2013) 70:4259–73. doi: 10.1007/s00018-013-1352-y
119. Shinozaki S, Chang K, Sakai M, Shimizu N, Yamada M, Tanaka T, et al. Inflammatory stimuli induce inhibitory S-nitrosylation of the deacetylase SIRT1 to increase acetylation and activation of p53 and p65. *Sci Signal* (2014) 7:ra106. doi: 10.1126/scisignal.2005375
120. Feng Y, Liu T, Dong SY, Guo YJ, Jankovic J, Xu H, et al. Rotenone affects p53 transcriptional activity and apoptosis via targeting SIRT1 and

H3K9 acetylation in SH-SY5Y cells. *J Neurochem.* (2015) 134:668–76. doi: 10.1111/jnc.13172
121. Lopes da Fonseca T, Villar-Pique A, Outeiro TF. The interplay between alpha-synuclein clearance and spreading. *Biomolecules* (2015) 5:435–71. doi: 10.3390/biom5020435
122. Guo YJ, Dong SY, Cui XX, Feng Y, Liu T, Yin M, et al. Resveratrol alleviates MPTP-induced motor impairments and pathological changes by autophagic degradation of alpha-synuclein via SIRT1-deacetylated LC3. *Mol Nutr Food Res.* (2016) 60:2161–2175. doi: 10.1002/mnfr.201600111
123. Coelho V, Shankland A. Making the right to health a reality for Brazil's indigenous peoples: innovation, decentralization and equity. *MEDICC Rev.* (2011) 13:50–3. doi: 10.1590/S1555-79602011000300012
124. Kitao Y, Ageta-Ishihara N, Takahashi R, Kinoshita M, Hori O. Transgenic supplementation of SIRT1 fails to alleviate acute loss of nigrostriatal dopamine neurons and gliosis in a mouse model of MPTP-induced parkinsonism. *F1000Res.* (2015) 4:130. doi: 10.12688/f1000research.6386.1
125. Pallàs M, Pizarro JG, Gutierrez-Cuesta J, Crespo-Biel N, Alvira D, Tajes M., et al. Modulation of SIRT1 expression in different neurodegenerative models and human pathologies. *Neuroscience* (2008) 154:1388–97. doi: 10.1016/j.neuroscience.2008.04.065
126. Rüb U, Seidel K, Heinsen H, Vonsattel JP, den Dunnen WF, Korf HW. Huntington's disease (HD): the neuropathology of a multisystem neurodegenerative disorder of the human brain. *Brain Pathol.* (2016) 26:726–740. doi: 10.1111/bpa.12426
127. Rüb U, Hoche F, Brunt ER, Heinsen H, Seidel K, Del Turco D, et al. Degeneration of the cerebellum in Huntington's disease (HD): possible relevance for the clinical picture and potential gateway to pathological mechanisms of the disease process. *Brain Pathol.* (2013) 23:165–77. doi: 10.1111/j.1750-3639.2012.00629.x
128. Gil JM, Rego AC. Mechanisms of neurodegeneration in Huntington's disease. *Eur J Neurosci.* (2008) 27:2803–20. doi: 10.1111/j.1460-9568.2008.06310.x
129. Reynolds RH, Petersen MH, Willert CW, Heinrich M, Nymann N, Dall M, et al. Perturbations in the p53/miR–34a/SIRT1 pathway in the R6/2 Huntington's disease model. *Mol Cell Neurosci.* (2018) 88:118–29. doi: 10.1016/j.mcn.2017.12.009
130. Lee M, Ban JJ, Chung JY, Im W, Kim M. Amelioration of Huntington's disease phenotypes by Beta-Lapachone is associated with increases in Sirt1 expression, CREB phosphorylation and PGC-1alpha deacetylation. *PLoS ONE* (2018) 13:e0195968. doi: 10.1371/journal.pone.0195968
131. Jiang M, Wang J, Fu J, Du L, Jeong H, West T, et al. Neuroprotective role of Sirt1 in mammalian models of Huntington's disease through activation of multiple Sirt1 targets. *Nat Med.* (2011) 18:153–8. doi: 10.1038/nm.2558
132. Jeong H, Cohen DE, Cui L, Supinski A, Savas JN, Mazzulli JR, et al. Sirt1 mediates neuroprotection from mutant huntingtin by activation of the TORC1 and CREB transcriptional pathway. *Nat Med.* (2011) 18:159–65. doi: 10.1038/nm.2559
133. Mohawk JA, Green CB, Takahashi JS. Central and peripheral circadian clocks in mammals. *Annu Rev Neurosci.* (2012) 35:445–62. doi: 10.1146/annurev-neuro-060909-153128
134. Chauhan R, Chen KF, Kent BA, Crowther DC. Central and peripheral circadian clocks and their role in Alzheimer's disease. *Dis Model Mech.* (2017) 10:1187–1199. doi: 10.1242/dmm.030627
135. Price NL, Gomes AP, Ling AJ, Duarte FV, Martin-Montalvo A, North BJ, et al. SIRT1 is required for AMPK activation and the beneficial effects of resveratrol on mitochondrial function. *Cell Metab.* (2012) 15:675–90. doi: 10.1016/j.cmet.2012.04.003
136. Neves AR, Queiroz JF, Reis S. Brain-targeted delivery of resveratrol using solid lipid nanoparticles functionalized with apolipoprotein E. *J Nanobiotechnol.* (2016) 14:27. doi: 10.1186/s12951-016-0177-x
137. Sinico C, Pireddu R, Pini E, Valenti D, Caddeo C, Fadda AM, et al. Enhancing topical delivery of resveratrol through a nanosizing approach. *Planta Med.* (2017) 83:476–81. doi: 10.1055/s-0042-103688
138. Zhang H, Ryu D, Wu Y, Gariani K, Wang X, Luan P, et al. NAD(+) repletion improves mitochondrial and stem cell function and enhances life span in mice. *Science* (2016) 352:1436–43. doi: 10.1126/science.aaf2693
139. Cantó C, Houtkooper RH, Pirinen E, Youn DY, Oosterveer MH, Cen Y, et al. The NAD(+) precursor nicotinamide riboside enhances oxidative metabolism and protects against high-fat diet-induced obesity. *Cell Metab.* (2012) 15:838–47. doi: 10.1016/j.cmet.2012.04.022
140. Khan NA, Auranen M, Paetau I, Pirinen E, Euro L, Forsström S, et al. Effective treatment of mitochondrial myopathy by nicotinamide riboside, a vitamin B3. *EMBO Mol Med.* (2014) 6:721–31. doi: 10.1002/emmm.201403943
141. Martens CR, Denman BA, Mazzo MR, Armstrong ML, Reisdorph N, McQueen MB, et al. Chronic nicotinamide riboside supplementation is well-tolerated and elevates NAD(+) in healthy middle-aged and older adults. *Nat Commun.* (2018) 9:1286. doi: 10.1038/s41467-018-03421-7

12

Survival and Clinicopathological Significance of SIRT1 Expression in Cancers

Min Sun[1,2†], *Mengyu Du*[2†], *Wenhua Zhang*[3], *Sisi Xiong*[4], *Xingrui Gong*[2], *Peijie Lei*[5], *Jin Zha*[2], *Hongrui Zhu*[2], *Heng Li*[1], *Dong Huang*[1*] and *Xinsheng Gu*[6*]

[1] *Department of General Surgery, Taihe Hospital, Hubei University of Medicine, Shiyan, China,* [2] *Department of Anesthesiology, Institute of Anesthesiology, Taihe Hospital, Hubei University of Medicine, Shiyan, China,* [3] *Department of Pharmaceutical Sciences, College of Pharmacy, Hubei University of Medicine, Shiyan, China,* [4] *School of Nursing, Hubei University of Medicine, Shiyan, China,* [5] *The First Clinical School, Hubei University of Medicine, Shiyan, China,* [6] *Department of Pharmacology, College of Basic Medical Sciences, Hubei University of Medicine, Shiyan, China*

***Correspondence:**
Dong Huang
hd_814@sohu.com
Xinsheng Gu
gu.xinsheng@gmail.com

† These authors have contributed equally to this work

Background: Silent information regulator 2 homolog 1 (SIRT1) is an evolutionarily conserved enzymes with nicotinamide adenine dinucleotide $(NAD)^{+}$-dependent deacetylase activity. SIRT1 is involved in a large variety of cellular processes, such as genomic stability, energy metabolism, senescence, gene transcription, and oxidative stress. SIRT1 has long been recognized as both a tumor promoter and tumor suppressor. Its prognostic role in cancers remains controversial.

Methods: A meta-analysis of 13,138 subjects in 63 articles from PubMed, EMBASE, and Cochrane Library was performed to evaluate survival and clinicopathological significance of SIRT1 expression in various cancers.

Results: The pooled results of meta-analysis showed that elevated expression of SIRT1 implies a poor overall survival (OS) of cancer patients [Hazard Ratio (HR) = 1.566, 95% CI: 1.293–1.895, $P < 0.0001$], disease free survival (DFS) (HR = 1.631, 95% CI: 1.250–2.130, $P = 0.0003$), event free survival (EFS) (HR = 2.534, 95% CI: 1.602–4.009, $P = 0.0001$), and progress-free survival (PFS) (HR = 3.325 95% CI: 2.762–4.003, $P < 0.0001$). Elevated SIRT1 level was associated with tumor stage [Relative Risk (RR) = 1.299, 95% CI: 1.114–1.514, $P = 0.0008$], lymph node metastasis (RR = 1.172, 95% CI: 1.010–1.360, $P = 0.0363$), and distant metastasis (RR = 1.562, 95% CI: 1.022–2.387, $P = 0.0392$). Meta-regression and subgroup analysis revealed that ethnic background has influence on the role of SIRT1 expression in predicting survival and clinicopathological characteristics of cancers. Overexpression of SIRT1 predicted a worse OS and higher TNM stage and lymphatic metastasis in Asian population especially in China.

Conclusion: Our data suggested that elevated expression of SIRT1 predicted a poor OS, DFS, EFS, PFS, but not for recurrence-free survival (RFS) and cancer-specific survival (CCS). SIRT1 overexpression was associated with higher tumor stage, lymph node metastasis, and distant metastasis. SIRT1-mediated molecular events and biological processes could be an underlying mechanism for metastasis and SIRT1 is a therapeutic target for inhibiting metastasis, leading to good prognosis.

Keywords: SIRT1, cancer, prognosis, clinicopathological significance, meta-analysis

INTRODUCTION

Silent information regulator 2 homolog 1 (SIRT1) is an evolutionarily conserved enzymes with nicotinamide adenine dinucleotide (NAD)$^+$-dependent deacetylase activity and a member of the mammalian sirtuin family. It is expressed in almost all human tissues and localized in both nuclei and cytoplasm (1). Its substrates include histones and non-histone proteins such as transcription factors (2–4). SIRT1 is involved in a large variety of cellular processes, such as genomic stability, energy metabolism, senescence, gene transcription, and oxidative stress (5). It has been shown to be involved in a spectrum of diseases, including cancer, diabetes, obesity, and neurodegenerative diseases (6–8). SIRT1 plays an important role in regulating glucose and lipid metabolism and regulates malignancy in tumors (9).

SIRT1 has long been recognized as both a tumor promoter and tumor suppressor (10–12). This is also shown in recent studies. SIRT1 promotes proliferation, migration, and invasion of breast cancer cell line MCF-7 (13). SIRT1 promotes proliferation and paclitaxel-resistance of human cervical cancer cells (14). Yang et al. found that SIRT1 levels are lower in non-small cell lung cancer (NSCLC) than the normal control group (15), but Gharabaghi et al. found that SIRT1 are over expressed in NSCLC (16). The role of SIRT1 in prognosis of cancer was also investigated in several studies. Over expression of SIRT1 suggests poor prognosis in luminal breast cancer (17) and serous epithelial ovarian cancer (EOC) (18), gastric cancer (19), high pathological stage and worse overall survival in the lung adenocarcinoma patients (20), decreased survival and increased relapse in breast cancer patients (3, 21), colorectal carcinoma patients (22), lymphangiogenesis, lymphovascular invasion, and prognosis in pN0 esophageal squamous cell carcinoma (23), soft tissue sarcomas (24), both operable triple-negative and non-triple-negative breast cancer (25), hepatocellular carcinoma (26), gastric carcinoma (27), diffuse large B-cell lymphoma (28). On the other hand, SIRT1 expression is found to be associated with good prognosis for head and neck squamous cell carcinoma patients (29), and colorectal cancer (30). Therefore, the prognostic and clinicopathological significance of SIRT1 abnormal expression in cancers remain to be elucidated.

Prognostic value and clinicopathological association of SIRT1 with cancers have been analyzed in previous meta-analysis (31–36). However, the studies included in these meta-analysis were limited to mostly Asian population, single or several cancer types, or they were published several years ago (31–36). In the present study, we conducted an updated and more comprehensive meta-analysis and subgroup analysis to reveal the prognostic value and clinicopathological association of SIRT1 abnormal expression in cancers.

Abbreviations: OS, overall survival; SIRT1, silent information regulator 1, sirtuin-1; HR, hazard ratio; RR, relative risk; CI, confidence interval; DFS, disease free survival; EFS, event free survival; PFS, progress-free survival; RFS, recurrence-free survival; CCS, cancer-specific survival; NAD, nicotinamide adenine dinucleotide; q-PCR, quantitative real-time polymerase chain reaction; IHC, immunohistochemistry; ISH, *in situ* hybridization; NA, not available; NOS, newcastle-ottawa scale; NSCLC, non-small cell lung cancer; EOC, epithelial ovarian cancer; TNM, tumor, node, metastasis; MOOSE, meta-analysis of observational Studies in Epidemiology.

METHODS

Search Strategy

We retrieved literature published in between 1966 and April 1st, 2018 by searching PubMed, EMBASE, and Cochrane Library with the keywords (1) "SIRT1" OR "sirtuin 1" OR "SIR2" OR "SIR2L1" OR "SIR2alpha" OR "silent mating type information regulation 2 homolog-1" AND (2) "tumor OR cancer OR carcinoma OR neoplasm" and using the search strategies as illustrated in **Supplementary Tables 1A–C**. We selected and evaluated all relevant studies and review articles about SIRT1 and inquired the authors for unpublished raw data. The search and selection of articles for the study were separately conducted based on a common set of criteria. The divergence in opinion were settled through discussion among ourselves.

Inclusion and Exclusion Criteria

This meta-analysis was conducted according to Meta-analysis of Observational Studies in Epidemiology (MOOSE) Checklist. Studies enrolled in this analysis satisfied the following requirements: (i) patients must be diagnosed with cancer via pathology; (ii) The expression of SIRT1 must be determined by quantitative real-time polymerase chain reaction (q-PCR), immunohistochemistry (IHC), or *in situ* hybridization (ISH); (iii) The correlation between SIRT1 expression and prognosis or clinicopathological features was investigated; (iv) The Hazard Ratio (HR) and its 95% confidence interval (CI) for survival indicator on the basis of SIRT1 expression level were readily available or could be calculated indirectly; (v) The most representative and most accurate study was adopted when a single sample source was used in multiple studies to avoid unnecessary cohort overlapping. Studies that have satisfied the abovementioned inclusion requirements were further ruled out if they had any of the following flaws: (i) duplicated articles or data; (ii) not human studies; (iii) review articles or letters; (iv) lack of sufficient data or information to get HR; (v) articles not written in English.

Quality Assessment of Included Studies

We used the Newcastle-Ottawa Scale (NOS) to assess the quality of each included study. Scores ≥ 7 were considered high quality. We used a "star system" for case-control studies (**Supplementary Table 2**).

Data Extraction

We extracted the following data from the full texts of eligible studies: (i) the first author; (ii) publication year; (iii) characteristics of the studies, which comprised of the patients' nationality, sample size, tumor type, and clinicopathological characteristics; (iv) the assay method and cut-off value of SIRT1; (v) HRs of SIRT1 expression for OS, disease-free survival (DFS), event-free survival (EFS), recurrence-free survival (RFS), cancer-specific survival (CCS), progression-free survival (PFS); (vi) if the HR for OS, DFS, EFS, RFS, CCS and PFS were

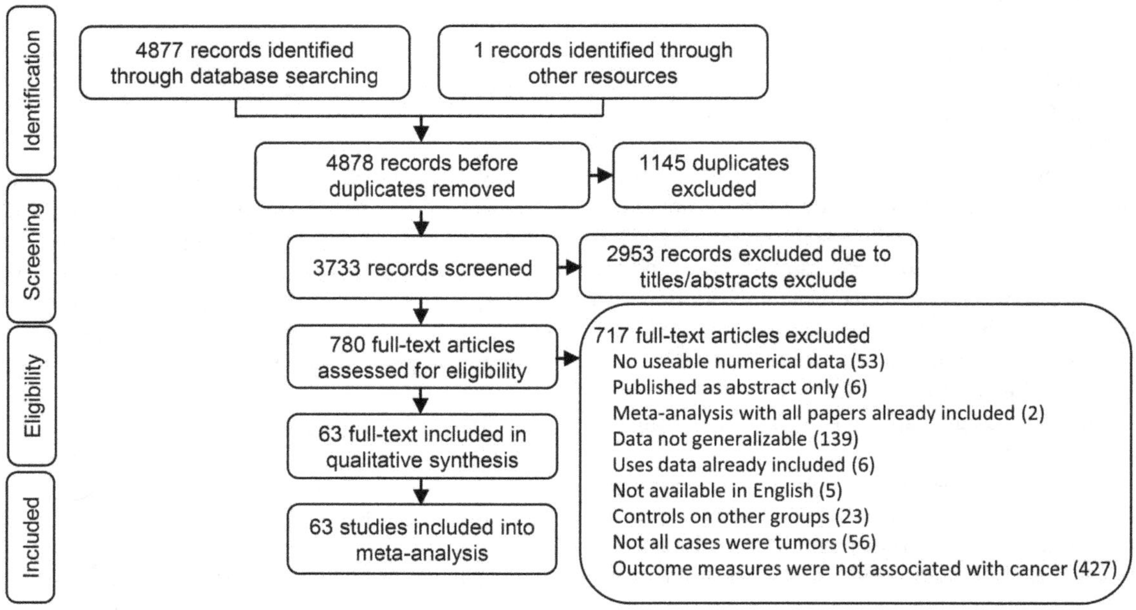

FIGURE 1 | Flow chart of the identification process for eligible studies.

calculated by both univariate and multivariate analyses, the latter was our first choice, given that these results were adjusted for confounding factors. If a study did not report the HR, we estimated HR and their corresponding 95% CI using the method described by Parmar et al. (37) and Tierney et al. (38). We recovered the data of Kaplan-Meier curves via the Engauge Digitizer version 9.8 (http://markummitchell.github.io/engauge-digitizer) and calculated the HR and its 95% CI. We repeated this process three times to reduce variability. Any divergence regarding the extraction and interpretation of all data was resolved by discussion among ourselves until consensus was reached.

Statistical Analysis

All the HRs and their 95% CIs were combined to evaluate the effect of SIRT1 high expression on prognosis. If the pooled HR < 1 and their 95% CI did not overlap the invalid line in the forest plot, the high expression of SIRT1 predicted a good OS. If the 95% CI overlapped the invalid line, the combined HR was considered insignificant. Otherwise, the combined HR predicted a poor OS. The heterogeneity of the pooled results was examined via Cochrane's Q test and Higgins' I-squared, and $P < 0.1$ or $I^2 \geq 25\%$ was considered high heterogeneity. If $P > 0.1$ and $I^2 < 25\%$, we ignored the influence of heterogeneity and pooled the overall result using a fixed effects model, otherwise employing the random effects model. The potential publication bias was assessed by a funnel plot, and Egger's test (39). $P < 0.05$ was considered significant. Statistical analysis was carried out using the "metafor" and "meta" packages of the R/BioConductor (version 3.5.1).

RESULTS

Search Results

We found 2,397 articles in PubMed, 2,460 articles in EMBASE, 20 articles in Cochrane library, and one articles through the references. We had a total of 3,733 articles after removing 1,145 duplicated articles. We then ruled out 2,953 articles which were review, letters, laboratory studies, or articles irrelevant to present research. We further excluded 717 full-text articles according to the inclusion and exclusion criteria of this study. The remaining 63 articles were finally eligible and included in this meta-analysis (**Figure 1**).

Study Demographics

The 63 eligible articles were published in between 2008 and 2017 with 63 studies that included a total of 13,138 participants from 9 countries who represented 16 cancer types and Asian and Caucasian ethnic groups (**Table 1**). The mean and median value were selected as the cut-off value in most articles. All studies measured SIRT1 expression in tumor tissue or serum via q-PCR, IHC, or ISH.

Correlation Between SIRT1 Expression and Prognosis

We performed meta-analysis of correlation between SIRT1 expression and OS, DFS, EFS, RFS, CCS, and PFS. The results and analysis of publication bias are presented in **Table 2**. The results showed that higher SIRT1 expression indicated an unfavorable OS ($n = 48$, HR: 1.566, 95% CI: [1.293, 1.895], $P < 0.0001$, $I^2 = 81.3\%$) (**Figure 2**), poor patient DFS ($n = 14$, HR: 1.631, 95% CI: [1.250–2.130], $P = 0.0003$, $I^2 = 72.6\%$, **Figure 3A**), poor

TABLE 1 | Main characteristics of 63 included studies.

References	Study design	Country	Case (N)	Type of Cancer	Disease stage	Follow-up (Mo.) median(range)	Race	Sample type	Survival end points	Adjusted variables	NOS score
Stenzinger et al. (40)	Retrospective	Germany	129	Pancreatic ductal adenocarcinoma	I–IV	54	Caucasian	Tissue	OS	Stage, grade	7
Li et al. (41)	Retrospective	China	91	Pancreatic ductal adenocarcinoma	I–IV	NA	Asian	Tissue	NA	NA	8
Teramae et al. (42)	Retrospective	Japan	62	Uterine cervical cancer	III	NA	Asian	Tissue	OS	NA	7
Asaka et al. (43)	Retrospective	Japan	108	Endometrial carcinoma	I–IV	NA	Asian	Tissue	OS, DFS	NA	8
Jang et al. (44)	Retrospective	Korea	64	Ovarian cancer	I–IV	29 (1–137)	Asian	Tissue	OS	Age, P53	6
Shuang et al. (18)	Retrospective	China	63	Ovarian cancer	I–IV	NA	Asian	Serum	OS	Age, grade, FIGO stage, lymphatic metastasis	6
Mvunta et al. (45)	Retrospective	Japan	68	Ovarian cancer	I–IV	74	Asian	Tissue	OS	Stage, lymphovascular space invasion	7
Zhang et al. (46)	Retrospective	China	22	Osteosarcoma	NA	NA	Asian	Tissue	OS	NA	7
Feng et al. (47)	Retrospective	China	89	Osteosarcoma	I–III	11 (3–83)	Asian	Tissue	OS	Stage, neoadjuvant chemotherapy	8
Kim et al. (24)	Retrospective	Korea	104	Soft tissue sarcoma	I–IV	NA	Asian	Tissue	OS, EFS	P53, β-catenin, stage, depth of tumor, tumor necrosis, distant metastasis	8
Noguchi et al. (29)	Retrospective	Japan	437	Head and neck squamous cell carcinoma	I–IV	46.6 (1–174)	Asian	Tissue	RFS, CSS	Age, gender, tumor site, tumor status, lymph node status, distant metastasis, pathologic grade	8
Yu et al. (48)	Retrospective	China	120	Laryngeal and hypopharyngeal carcinomas	I–IV	NA	Asian	Tissue	OS	NA	7
Batra et al. (49)	Retrospective	India	94	Retinoblastoma	I–IV	59	Asian	Tissue	NA	NA	7
Chen et al. (50)	Retrospective	China	206	Esophageal squamous cell carcinoma	I–II	55.9 (5–86)	Asian	Tissue	OS, DFS	Differentiation, T status, stage, VEGF-C, peritumoral lymphatic microvessel density	7
He et al. (51)	Retrospective	China	86	Esophageal squamous cell carcinoma	I–III	NA	Asian	Tissue	OS	Gender, clinical stage, histological grade, lymph node metastasis	7
Feng et al. (52)	Retrospective	China	34	Pelvis chondrosarcoma	I–III	37.7 vs. 53.8*	Asian	Tissue	OS	NA	8
Noh et al. (53)	Retrospective	Korea	200	Renal cell carcinoma	I–III	NA	Asian	Tissue	OS, RFS, CSS	NA	6
Jeh et al. (54)	Retrospective	Korea	102	Renal cell carcinoma	I–IV	73	Asian	Tissue	CSS	Age, T stage, grade, metastasis, karnofsky performance status	7
Jang et al. (28)	Retrospective	Korea	104	Diffuse large B cell lymphoma	I–IV	17.3 (1–135)	Asian	Tissue	OS, EFS	International prognostic index	8

(Continued)

TABLE 1 | Continued

References	Study design	Country	Case (N)	Type of Cancer	Disease stage	Follow-up (Mo.) median(range)	Race	Sample type	Survival end points	Adjusted variables	NOS score
Ren et al. (55)	Retrospective	China	45	Angioimmunoblastic T cell lymphoma	I–IV	NA	Asian	Tissue	PFS	P53, LDH, hemoglobin, γ-Globulin, sex, age, international prognostic index score, stage	8
Nosho et al. (56)	Retrospective	USA	485	Colorectal cancer	I–IV	NA	Caucasian	Tissue	OS, CSS	Age, year of diagnosis, sex, body Mass index, tumor location, stage, grade, microsatellite instability, the CpG island methylator phenotype	6
Jang et al. (2)	Retrospective	Korea	497	Colorectal cancer	I–IV	70.8	Asian	Tissue	OS, DFS	Histological grade, AJCC stage	8
Jung et al. (30)	Retrospective	Korea	349	Colorectal cancer	I–IV	55.3	Asian	Tissue	OS	Age, location, TNM stage, Histologic grade, β-catenin	8
Benard et al. (57)	Retrospective	Netherlands	254	Colorectal cancer	I–III	103.2	Caucasian	Tissue	OS	NA	7
Chen et al. (22)	Retrospective	China	102	Colorectal cancer	II–IV	NA	Asian	Tissue	OS	Gender, age, metastasis, TNM stage	8
Lv et al. (58)	Retrospective	China	120	Colorectal cancer	I–IV	53.3 (1–78)	Asian	Tissue	OS	NA	6
Lee et al. (59)	Retrospective	China	351	Colorectal cancer	I–IV	NA	Asian	Tissue	DFS, CSS	NA	7
Cheng et al. (60)	Retrospective	China	90	Colorectal cancer	I–III	NA	Asian	Tissue	OS	NA	8
Chen et al. (61)	Retrospective	China	172	Hepatocellular Carcinoma	I–III	125 (45–236)	Asian	Tissue	OS	NA	6
Jang et al. (62)	Retrospective	Korea	154	Hepatocellular Carcinoma	I–IV	NA	Asian	Tissue	OS, DFS	Stage, albumin, AFP, c-Myc, P53	8
Hao et al. (63)	Retrospective	China	99	Hepatocellular Carcinoma	I–IV	NA	Asian	Tissue	OS	NA	7
Cheng et al. (64)	Retrospective	China	148	Hepatocellular Carcinoma	I–III	NA	Asian	Tissue	OS	NA	8
Li et al. (65)	Retrospective	China	72	Hepatocellular Carcinoma	I–III	NA	Asian	Tissue	OS, DFS	NA	8
Liu et al. (66)	Retrospective	China	148	Hepatocellular Carcinoma	I–III	NA	Asian	Tissue	NA	NA	7
Cha et al. (27)	Retrospective	Korea	177	Gastric Cancer	I–IV	NA	Asian	Tissue	OS, RFS	TNM stage	7
Feng et al. (67)	Retrospective	China	176	Gastric Cancer	I–IV	NA	Asian	Tissue	OS	NA	6
Kang et al. (68)	Retrospective	Korea	452	Gastric Cancer	I–IV	53.3 (3–83)	Asian	Tissue	OS	Lymph node metastasis, depth of invasion, lymphatic invasion, histologic grade, DBC1, cytoplasmic β-catenin	7
Noguchi et al. (19)	Retrospective	Japan	557	Gastric Cancer	I–IV	69 (6–142)	Asian	Tissue	CSS	NA	7

(Continued)

TABLE 1 | Continued

References	Study design	Country	Case (N)	Type of Cancer	Disease stage	Follow-up (Mo.) median(range)	Race	Sample type	Survival end points	Adjusted variables	NOS score
Qiu et al. (69)	Retrospective	China	96	Gastric Cancer	I–IV	31.6 (6–78)	Asian	Tissue	OS, RFS	Lymph node metastasis, Beclin1 expression	8
Szász et al. (70)	Retrospective	Hungary	1065	Gastric Cancer	I–IV	NA	Caucasian	Tissue	OS	NA	8
Zhang et al. (71)	Retrospective	China	128	Gastric Cancer	I–IV	NA	Asian	Tissue	OS	NA	8
Zhang et al. (72)	Retrospective	China	176	Gastric Cancer	I–IV	NA	Asian	Tissue	OS	NA	6
Ren et al. (73)	Retrospective	USA	348	Colorectal cancer	I–IV	NA	Caucasian	Tissue	OS	NA	8
Shin et al. (74)	Retrospective	Korea	45	Ovarian cancer	NA	NA	Asian	Tissue	OS	NA	6
Zhang et al. (75)	Retrospective	China	50	Colorectal cancer	NA	NA	Asian	Tissue	NA	NA	7
Cao et al. (76)	Retrospective	China	150	Breast carcinoma	I–IV	161	Asian	Tissue	OS, DFS	Lymph node metastasis, TNM stage, ER status, PR status, Snail expression	8
Jin et al. (77)	Retrospective	Korea	319	Breast carcinoma	I–III	NA	Asian	Tissue	OS, DFS	AJCC stage, lymphatic invasion, DCIS	6
Kim et al. (78)	Retrospective	Korea	278	Breast carcinoma	NA	63.78 (2–74)	Asian	Tissue	DFS	T stage, caspase3, lymphovascular invasion	7
Lee et al. (21)	Retrospective	USA	142	Breast carcinoma	I–IV	NA	Caucasian	Tissue	OS, EFS	Stage, HER2 status, P53 expression	8
Chung et al. (79)	Retrospective	Korea	344	Breast carcinoma	I–III	NA	Asian	Tissue	OS, DFS	T stage, lymphatic invasion, DCIS	6
Derr et al. (3)	Retrospective	Netherlands	822	Breast carcinoma	I–III	11.8 (0.16–27.55)	Caucasian	Tissue	OS, DFS	NA	6
Wu et al. (25)	Retrospective	China	134	Breast carcinoma	I–III	154	Asian	Tissue	OS, DFS	Stages, P53, Lymph nodes status	8
Lee et al. (80)	Retrospective	Korea	688	Breast carcinoma	I–IV	190.8	Asian	Tissue	NA	NA	8
Chung et al. (81)	Retrospective	Korea	427	Breast carcinoma	I–III	NA	Asian	Tissue	DFS	NA	6
Zhang et al. (82)	Retrospective	China	149	Breast carcinoma	NA	101.03 vs. 88.38*	Asian	Tissue	OS	NA	6
Sung et al. (83)	Retrospective	Korea	28	Breast carcinoma	I-IV	NA	Asian	Tissue	NA	NA	6
Gharabaghi et al. (16)	Retrospective	Iran	40	NSCLC	NA	NA	Caucasian	Tissue	OS	Gender, age, histologic grade, T stage, lymph node metastasis, BIRC6 expression	6
Li et al. (20)	Retrospective	China	75	NSCLC	I–IV	NA	Asian	Tissue	OS	Age, TNM stage	7
Lin et al. (84)	Retrospective	China	260	NSCLC	NA	37.1 (0–128)	Asian	Tissue	OS	NA	8
Noh et al. (85)	Retrospective	Korea	144	NSCLC	NA	NA	Asian	Tissue	NA	NA	7
Zhang et al. (86)	Retrospective	China	295	NSCLC	III–IV	NA	Asian	Tissue	OS	Tumor stage, tumor differentiation	6
Chen et al. (23)	Retrospective	China	125	NSCLC	I–IV	NA	Asian	Tissue	NA	NA	8
Grbesa et al. (87)	Retrospective	Spain	179	NSCLC	I–IV	45	Asian	Tissue	OS, RFS	Stage	6

Mo., month; NSCLC, non-small cell lung cancer; NA, not available; NOS, newcastle-ottawa scale. FIGO, the international federation of gynecology and obstetrics; OS, overall survival; EFS, event-free survival; DFS, disease-free survival; CSS, cancer-specific survival; RFS, recurrence-free survival; LDH, lactate dehydrogenase; DBC1, deleted in breast cancer 1; ER, estrogen receptor; PR, progesterone receptor; DCIS, ductal carcinoma in situ; HER2, human epidermal growth factor receptor 2; BIRC6, Baculoviral IAP repeat-containing 6.

The median survival time of high expression group vs. low expression group.

TABLE 2 | Survival effects of SIRT1 overexpression and the prognosis of patients.

Outcome	No. of trials (patients)	HR (95%CI) Fixed-effect estimate	*P*-value of Fixed-effect Model	HR (95%CI) Random-effect estimate	*P* value of Random-effect Model	Heterogeneity I^2(%), *P*-value	*P*-value of Egger's test, Begg's test
OS	48 (9573)	1.259 (1.170–1.355)	<0.0001	***1.566 (1.293–1.895)***	***<0.0001***	81.3%, <0.0001	0.0043, 0.1884
DFS	14 (3982)	1.482 (1.308–1.679)	<0.0001	***1.631 (1.250–2.130)***	***0.0003***	72.6%, <0.0001	0.2234, 0.2503
EFS	3 (350)	***2.534 (1.602–4.009)***	***0.0001***	2.534 (1.602–4.009)	0.0001	0.0%, 0.8557	0.1174, 0.1172
RFS	5 (1089)	1.253 (0.996–1.575)	0.0542	1.936 (0.903–4.151)	0.0898	88.90%, <0.0001	0.0037, 0.3272
CCS	6 (2132)	1.097 (0.900–1.338)	0.3591	1.229 (0.757–1.994)	0.4037	77.3%, 0.0005	0.6331, 0.3476
PFS	2 (340)	***3.325 (2.762–4.003)***	***<0.0001***	3.325 (2.762–4.003)	<0.0001	0.0%, 0.9089	NA, NA

HR, hazard ratio; CI, confidence interval; OS, overall survival; DFS, disease free survival; EFS, event free survival; RFS, recurrence-free survival; CCS, cancer-specific survival; PFS, progress-free survival; NA, not available. I^2, index for assessing heterogeneity; value ≥25% indicates a moderate to high heterogeneity; Egger's test, P-value of Egger's regression for asymmetry assessment; Begg's test, P-value of Begg and Mazumdar rank correlation test for asymmetry assessment. Bold italics indicate statistically significant values ($P < 0.05$).

EFS ($n = 3$, HR: 2.534, 95% CI: [1.602, 4.009], $P = 0.0001$, $I^2 = 0\%$, **Figure 3B**), and poor PFS ($n = 2$, HR: 3.325, 95% CI: [2.762, 4.003], $P < 0.0001$, $I^2 = 0\%$, **Figure 3C**), but not correlated with RFS of the Asian or tissue ($n = 5$, HR: 1.936, 95% CI: [0.903 - 4.151], $P = 0.0898$, $I^2 = 88.9\%$) (**Figure 3D**) or CCS ($n = 6$, HR: 1.229, 95% CI: [0.757–1.994], $P = 0.4037$, $I^2 = 77.3\%$) (**Figure 3E**).

Correlation Between SIRT1 Expression and Prognosis of Cancer Types

Cancer type subgroup analysis showed that SIRT1 overexpression was associated with a worse OS in osteosarcoma ($n = 2$, HR: 1.661, 95% CI: [1.162, 2.372], $P = 0.0053$, $I^2 = 0\%$), esophageal squamous cell carcinoma ($n = 2$, HR: 1.781, 95% CI: [1.197, 2.652], $P = 0.0044$, $I^2 = 0\%$), hepatocellular carcinoma ($n = 5$, HR: 1.969, 95% CI: [1.539, 2.520], $P < 0.0001$, $I^2 = 0\%$), breast carcinoma ($n = 7$, HR: 1.744, 95% CI: [1.022, 2.978], $P < 0.0416$, $I^2 \doteq 70.18\%$), NSCLC ($n = 5$, HR: 1.929, 95% CI: [1.259, 2.957], $P < 0.0025$, $I^2 = 59.40\%$), whereas SIRT1 overexpression was not correlated with the OS in ovarian cancer ($n = 4$, HR: 1.971, 95% CI: [0.899, 4.323], $P = 0.0903$, $I^2 = 55.18\%$), colorectal carcinoma ($n = 8$, HR: 0.932, 95% CI: [0.636, 1.366], $P = 0.7198$, $I^2 = 82.96\%$), gastric carcinoma ($n = 7$, HR: 1.535, 95% CI: [0.864, 2.726], $P = 0.1436$, $I^2 = 87.90\%$) (**Supplementary Figure 1A**).

SIRT1 overexpression was associated with a worse DFS in colorectal cancer ($n = 3$, HR: 1.544, 95% CI: [1.061, 2.247], $P = 0.0233$, $I^2 = 68.69\%$), and breast carcinoma ($n = 7$, HR: 1.819, 95% CI: [1.026, 3.223], $P = 0.0404$, $I^2 = 84.59\%$), whereas it was not correlated with the DFS in hepatocellular carcinoma ($n = 2$, HR: 1.357, 95% CI: [0.872, 2.113], $P = 0.1758$, $I^2 = 9.41\%$) (**Supplementary Figure 2A**).

SIRT1 overexpression was correlated with RFS of Gastric Cancer ($n = 2$, HR: 2.734, 95% CI: [1.694, 4.413], $P < 0.0001$, $I^2 = 0\%$), Renal cell carcinoma ($n = 1$, HR: 2.233, 95% CI: [1.088, 4.583]), and NSCLC (HR: 2.698, 95% CI: [1.457, 4.996]), whereas SIRT1 overexpression was negatively correlated with RFS of head and neck squamous cell carcinoma (HR: 0.655, 95% CI: [0.478, 0.897], $P = 0.0084$) (**Supplementary Table 3**).

SIRT1 overexpression was correlated with CCS in head and neck squamous cell carcinoma ($n = 1$, HR: 0.640, 95% CI: [0.453, 0.905], $P = 0.0116$), gastric cancer ($n = 1$, HR: 1.450, 95% CI: [1.018, 2.066], $P = 0.0396$), and renal cell carcinoma ($n = 2$, HR: 1.478, 95% CI: [0.124, 17.621]), but not with CCS in colorectal cancer (HR: 1.344, 95% CI: [0.716, 2.521], $P = 0.3577$) (**Supplementary Table 3**).

Correlation Between SIRT1 Expression and Prognosis of Cancer in Different Countries

Analysis of country subgroups showed that high expression of SIRT1 was correlated with poor OS in China ($n = 24$, HR: 1.661, 95% CI: [1.339, 2.060], $P < 0.0001$, $I^2 = 63.03\%$), Korea ($n = 12$, HR: 1.902, 95% CI: [1.187, 3.047], $P = 0.0075$, $I^2 = 80.65\%$), Japan ($n = 3$, HR: 1.940, 95% CI: [1.029, 3.655], $P = 0.0405$, $I^2 = 0\%$), but not in USA ($n = 3$, HR: 1.043, 95% CI: [0.465, 2.338], $P = 0.9193$, $I^2 = 84.36\%$), or Netherlands ($n = 2$, HR: 1.003, 95% CI: [0.671, 1.498], $P = 0.9893$, $I^2 = 73.79\%$) (**Supplementary Figure 1B**).

SIRT1 overexpression was also correlated with poor DFS in China ($n = 6$, HR: 2.021, 95% CI: [1.612, 2.534], $P < 0.0001$, $I^2 = 0\%$), but not in Korea ($n = 6$, HR: 1.321, 95% CI: [0.773, 2.259]) (**Supplementary Figure 2B**).

SIRT1 overexpression was correlated with poor EFS in Korea ($n = 2$, HR: 2.714, 95% CI: [1.506, 4.894], $P = 0.0009$, $I^2 = 0\%$) and USA ($n = 1$, HR: 2.280, 95% CI: [1.098, 4.734]).

Correlation Between SIRT1 Expression and Prognosis of Cancer in Asian and Caucasian

Elevated SIRT1 expression predicted a significantly worse OS in Asian population with cancers (HR: 1.708, 95% CI: [1.406, 2.076], $P < 0.0001$, $I^2 = 69.59\%$) rather than in Caucasian population (HR: 1.04, 95% CI: [0.75, 1.45], $P < 0.01$, $I^2 = 81\%$) (**Supplementary Figure 1C**).

SIRT1 expression predicted a significantly worse DFS in Asian population with cancers ($n = 13$, HR: 1.683, 95% CI: [1.235, 2.294], $P < 0.0010$, $I^2 = 74.27\%$), whereas one article suggested that increased expression of SIRT1 is correlated with Caucasian patient DFS (HR: 1.344, 95% CI: [1.040; 1.736], $P = 0.0237$) (**Supplementary Figure 2C**).

Study	TE	seTE	HR	95%-CI	Weight (fixed)	Weight (random)
Stenzinger, 2013	0.50	0.2499	1.65	[1.01; 2.69]	2.3%	2.6%
Teramae, 2014	0.41	0.4894	1.51	[0.58; 3.94]	0.6%	1.7%
Asaka, 2015	0.08	0.8845	1.08	[0.19; 6.11]	0.2%	0.9%
Jang, 2009	−0.25	0.5397	0.78	[0.27; 2.25]	0.5%	1.6%
Shuang, 2015	0.36	0.4447	1.43	[0.60; 3.42]	0.7%	1.9%
Mvunta, 2016	1.10	0.4930	3.00	[1.14; 7.88]	0.6%	1.7%
Zhang, 2016	0.46	0.3127	1.59	[0.86; 2.93]	1.4%	2.3%
Feng, 2016	0.53	0.2238	1.70	[1.10; 2.63]	2.8%	2.6%
Kim, 2013	2.31	0.6434	10.06	[2.85; 35.51]	0.3%	1.3%
Yu, 2013	−0.58	0.4828	0.56	[0.22; 1.44]	0.6%	1.8%
Chen, 2014	0.54	0.2674	1.71	[1.01; 2.89]	2.0%	2.5%
He, 2015	0.63	0.3119	1.88	[1.02; 3.47]	1.4%	2.3%
Feng, 2017	0.20	0.9717	1.22	[0.18; 8.19]	0.1%	0.8%
Noh, 2013	1.33	0.4917	3.79	[1.45; 9.94]	0.6%	1.7%
Jang, 2008	1.56	0.6073	4.78	[1.45; 15.72]	0.4%	1.4%
Nosho, 2009	0.07	0.1768	1.07	[0.76; 1.51]	4.5%	2.8%
Jang, 2012	0.26	0.1602	1.30	[0.95; 1.78]	5.5%	2.8%
Jung, 2013	−0.62	0.2865	0.54	[0.31; 0.95]	1.7%	2.4%
Benard, 2014	−0.22	0.1746	0.80	[0.57; 1.13]	4.6%	2.8%
Chen, 2014	−0.90	0.3117	0.41	[0.22; 0.75]	1.4%	2.3%
Lv, 2014	0.76	0.2375	2.13	[1.34; 3.39]	2.5%	2.6%
Cheng, 2016	0.84	0.3785	2.31	[1.10; 4.85]	1.0%	2.1%
Chen, 2011	0.62	0.1954	1.85	[1.26; 2.71]	3.7%	2.7%
Jang, 2012	0.76	0.2693	2.14	[1.26; 3.63]	1.9%	2.5%
Hao, 2014	0.34	0.3671	1.41	[0.69; 2.90]	1.0%	2.1%
Cheng, 2016	0.82	0.2874	2.27	[1.29; 3.99]	1.7%	2.4%
Li, 2016	1.02	0.5288	2.77	[0.98; 7.81]	0.5%	1.6%
Cha, 2009	1.46	0.4289	4.32	[1.86; 10.01]	0.8%	1.9%
Feng, 2011	0.51	0.4346	1.66	[0.71; 3.89]	0.7%	1.9%
Kang, 2012	−0.40	0.2156	0.67	[0.44; 1.02]	3.0%	2.7%
Qiu, 2016	0.87	0.3221	2.39	[1.27; 4.50]	1.4%	2.3%
Szász, 2016	−0.45	0.0872	0.64	[0.54; 0.76]	18.5%	3.0%
Zhang, 2017	0.89	0.3585	2.43	[1.21; 4.91]	1.1%	2.2%
Zhang, 2013	0.54	0.4462	1.72	[0.72; 4.12]	0.7%	1.9%
Ren, 2017	−0.73	0.2458	0.48	[0.30; 0.78]	2.3%	2.6%
Shin, 2016	1.82	0.7170	6.19	[1.52; 25.23]	0.3%	1.2%
Cao, 2014	1.52	0.5229	4.55	[1.63; 12.68]	0.5%	1.6%
Jin, 2015	0.82	0.4243	2.26	[0.98; 5.19]	0.8%	1.9%
Lee, 2010	1.16	0.5421	3.18	[1.10; 9.20]	0.5%	1.6%
Chung, 2016	0.01	0.6397	1.01	[0.29; 3.54]	0.3%	1.3%
Derr, 2014	0.19	0.1177	1.21	[0.96; 1.52]	10.2%	2.9%
Wu, 2012	1.28	0.5005	3.59	[1.34; 9.57]	0.6%	1.7%
Zhang, 2016	−0.63	0.3871	0.53	[0.25; 1.13]	0.9%	2.1%
Gharabaghi, 2016	0.92	0.5012	2.51	[0.94; 6.70]	0.6%	1.7%
Li, 2015	−1.06	0.6193	0.35	[0.10; 1.17]	0.4%	1.4%
Lin, 2015	0.73	0.2568	2.07	[1.25; 3.42]	2.1%	2.5%
Zhang, 2013	0.91	0.1276	2.48	[1.93; 3.18]	8.6%	2.9%
Grbesa, 2015	0.79	0.3436	2.19	[1.12; 4.30]	1.2%	2.2%
Fixed effect model			**1.26**	**[1.17; 1.35]**	**100.0%**	**--**
Random effects model			**1.57**	**[1.29; 1.90]**	**--**	**100.0%**

Heterogeneity: $I^2 = 81\%$, $p < 0.01$

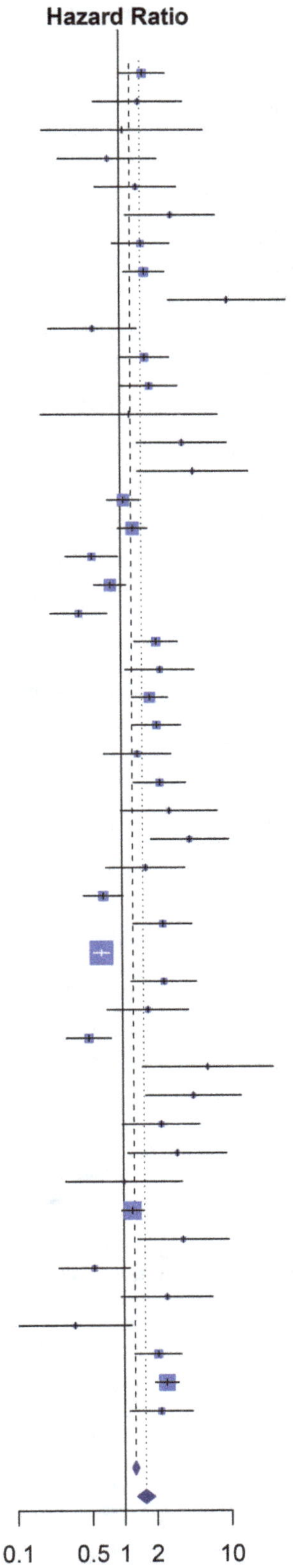

FIGURE 2 | Forest plot of SIRT1 expression and overall survival in various cancers.

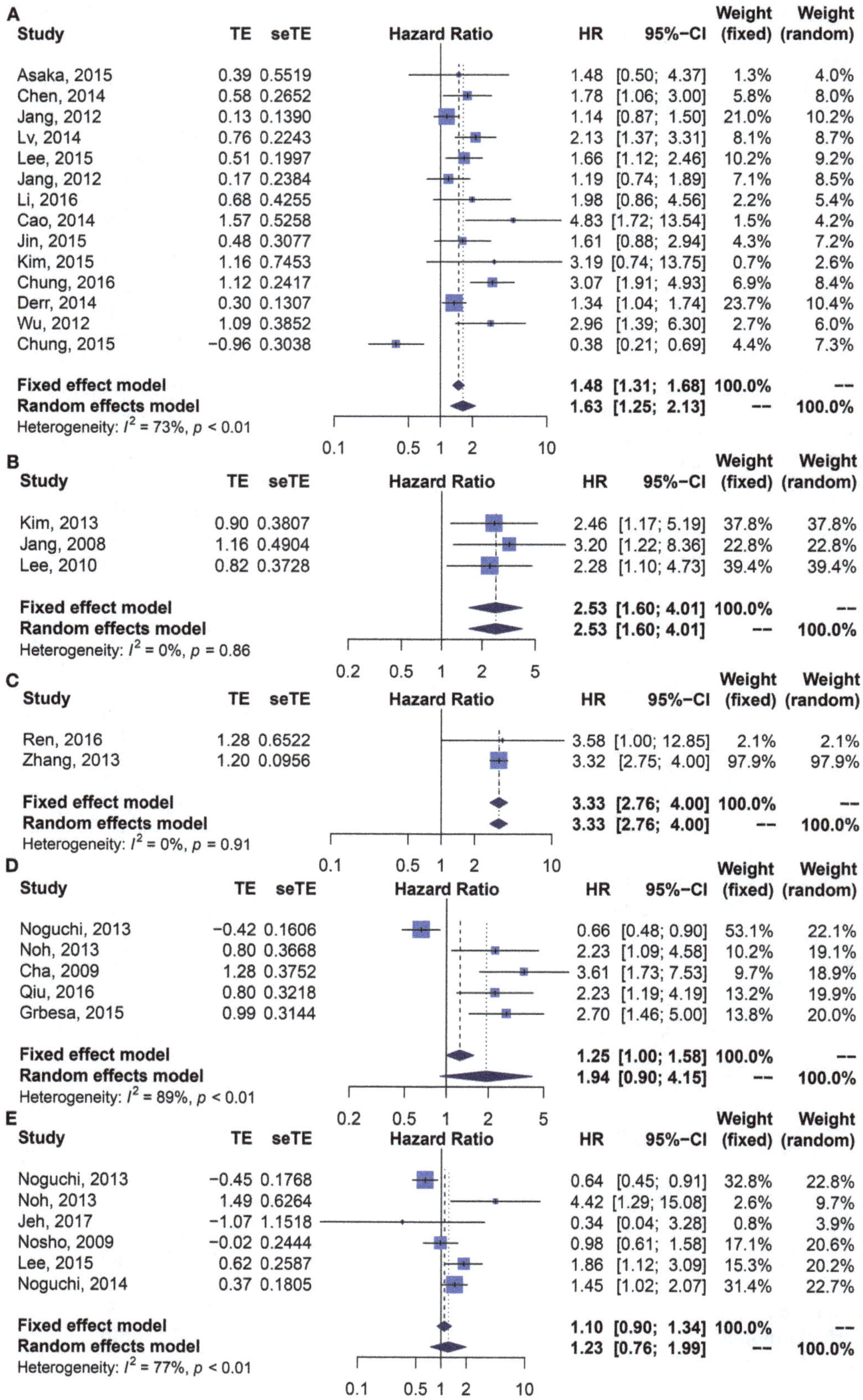

FIGURE 3 | Forest plots of main survival outcomes compared SIRT1 overexpression with underexpression. **(A)** DFS. **(B)** EFS. **(C)** PFS. **(D)** RFS. **(E)** CCS.

TABLE 3 | The associations of SIRT1 overexpression with the clinicopathological characteristics of the study patients.

Clinicopathological parameters	No. of trials (patients)	RR (95%CI) Fixed-effect estimate	*P*-value of Fixed-effect Model	RR (95%CI) Random-effect estimate	*P*-value of Random-effect Model	Heterogeneity I^2(%), *P*-value	*P*-value of Egger's test, Begg's test
Tumor stage	33 (5857)	1.133 (1.062–1.209)	0.0002	***1.299 (1.114–1.514)***	***0.0008***	77.4%, <0.0001	0.0070, 0.1827
Lymphatic metastasis	29 (6354)	1.046 (0.995–1.100)	0.0763	***1.172 (1.010–1.360)***	***0.0363***	86.3%, <0.0001	0.0637, 0.4308
Distant metastasis	14 (2632)	1.607 (1.312–1.968)	<0.0001	***1.562 (1.022–2.387)***	***0.0392***	71.0%, <0.0001	0.6780, 0.3520
Tumor size	21 (2469)	1.143 (1.050–1.245)	0.0021	1.101 (0.984–1.232)	0.0924	41.7%, 0.0241	0.1660, 0.2047
Depth of tumor invasion	19 (4689)	1.036 (0.982–1.093)	0.1912	1.113 (0.985–1.258)	0.0852	81.70%, <0.0001	0.0903, 0.1955
Differentiation	28 (5740)	1.010 (0.940–1.085)	0.7841	1.055 (0.931–1.196)	0.3996	63.10%, <0.0001	0.1170, 0.3847
Age	38 (7223)	1.052 (1.004–1.102)	0.0345	1.043 (0.973–1.118)	0.2373	43.50%, 0.0027	0.5651, 0.8308
Gender	34 (6129)	1.003 (0.967–1.040)	0.8739	0.991 (0.950–1.035)	0.6858	35.00%, 0.0247	0.1727, 0.3353

RR, relative risk; CI, confidence interval; I^2, index for assessing heterogeneity; value ≥25% indicates a moderate to high heterogeneity; Egger's test, P-value of Egger's regression for asymmetry assessment; Begg's test: P-value of Begg and Mazumdar rank correlation test for asymmetry assessment. Bold italics indicate statistically significant values ($P < 0.05$).

Correlation Between SIRT1 Expression and Clinicopathological Characteristics

We performed an analysis of the association of SIRT1 expression with clinicopathological characteristics (**Table 3**). The results showed that overexpression of SIRT1 was significantly correlated with TNM stage. Higher SIRT1 expression indicated high TNM stage for various malignancies ($n = 33$, RR: 1.299; 95% CI: [1.114, 1.514], $P = 0.0008$, $I^2 = 77.4\%$, **Figure 4**). SIRT1 expression was significantly correlated with lymphatic metastasis ($n = 29$, RR: 1.172, 95% CI: [1.010, 1.360], $P = 0.0363$, $I^2 = 86.3\%$, **Figure 5**), distant metastasis ($n = 14$, RR: 1.562, 95% CI: [1.022, 2.387], $P = 0.0392$, $I^2 = 71.0\%$, **Figure 6**), but not correlated with tumor size (RR:1.101, 95% CI [0.984-1.232], $I^2 = 41.7\%$), depth of tumor invasion (RR: 1.113, 95% CI [0.985–1.258], $I^2 = 81.7\%$), differentiation (RR: 1.055, 95% CI [0.931–1.196], $I^2 = 63.1\%$), gender (RR: 0.991, 95% CI [0.950–1.035], $I^2 = 35.0\%$), or age (RR: 1.043, 95% CI [0.973–1.118], $I^2 = 43.5\%$) (**Table 3, Supplementary Figure 3**).

Correlation Between SIRT1 Expression and Clinicopathological Characteristics of Cancers Types

We performed analysis of correlation between SIRT1 expression and clinicopathological characteristics of cancers types (**Supplementary Table 4**). The results showed that SIRT1 overexpression was associated with a higher TNM stage in hepatocellular carcinoma ($n = 6$, RR: 1.611, 95% CI: [1.185, 2.188], $P = 0.0023$, $I^2 = 55.30\%$), but not correlated with the TNM stage in pancreatic ductal adenocarcinoma ($n = 2$, RR: 2.275, 95% CI: [0.928, 5.579], $P = 0.0725$, $I^2 = 0\%$), ovarian cancer ($n = 2$, RR: 0.820, 95% CI: [0.561, 1.201], $P = 0.3082$, $I^2 = 3.18\%$), colorectal cancer ($n = 4$, RR: 1.146, 95% CI: [0.817, 1.608], $P = 0.4290$, $I^2 = 70.90\%$), gastric cancer ($n = 6$, RR: 1.264, 95% CI: [0.823, 1.942], $P = 0.2842$, $I^2 = 92.48\%$), breast carcinoma ($n = 5$, RR: 1.411, 95% CI: [0.846, 2.356], $P = 0.1873$, $I^2 = 65.10\%$), or NSCLC (n = 2, RR: 1.389, 95% CI: [0.661, 2.917], $P = 0.3853$, $I^2 = 16.51\%$) (**Supplementary Figure 4A**).

SIRT1 overexpression was associated with distant metastasis in pancreatic ductal adenocarcinoma ($n = 2$, RR: 2.046, 95% CI: [1.153, 3.631], $P = 0.0144$, $I^2 = 0\%$) and breast carcinoma ($n = 2$, RR: 3.257, 95% CI: [1.777, 5.970], $P = 0.0001$, $I^2 = 0\%$), but not in colorectal cancer ($n = 3$, RR: 1.140, 95% CI: [0.444, 2.923], $P = 0.7857$, $I^2 = 80.57\%$) or gastric cancer ($n = 2$, RR: 1.316, 95% CI: [0.679, 2.551], $P = 0.4160$, $I^2 = 0\%$) (**Supplementary Figure 5A**).

Correlation Between SIRT1 Expression and Clinicopathological Characteristics of Cancers in Different Countries

We performed analysis of correlation between SIRT1 expression and clinicopathological characteristics of cancers in different countries (**Supplementary Table 4**). The results showed that SIRT1 overexpression was associated with a higher TNM stage ($n = 17$, RR: 1.638, 95% CI: [1.404, 1.911], $P < 0.0001$, $I^2 = 41.16\%$) (**Supplementary Figure 4B**) and lymphatic metastasis in China ($n = 11$, RR: 1.411, 95% CI: [1.155, 1.724], $P = 0.0007$, $I^2 = 68.48\%$), and not with lymphatic metastasis in Japan ($n = 3$, RR: 0.964, 95% CI: [0.657, 1.415]), or Korea ($n = 12$, RR: 1.166, 95% CI: [0.898, 1.516]) (**Supplementary Figure 6A**).

Correlation Between SIRT1 Expression and Clinicopathological Characteristics of Cancers in Asian and Caucasian

We performed analysis of correlation between SIRT1 expression and clinicopathological characteristics of cancers in Asian and Caucasian (**Supplementary Table 4**). The results showed that SIRT1 overexpression predicted a significantly higher TNM stage in Asian population with cancers ($n = 30$, RR: 1.323, 95% CI: [1.124, 1.559], $P = 0.0008$, $I^2 = 78.76\%$) rather than that in Caucasian population ($n = 3$, RR: 0.919, 95% CI: [0.744, 1.136], $P = 0.4352$, $I^2 = 0\%$) (**Supplementary Figure 4C**). However, publication bias was suspected based on the Egger's test ($P = 0.0070$) rather than Begg's test ($P = 0.1827$).

Elevated SIRT1 expression predicted a significantly distant metastasis in Caucasian population with cancers ($n = 2$, RR:

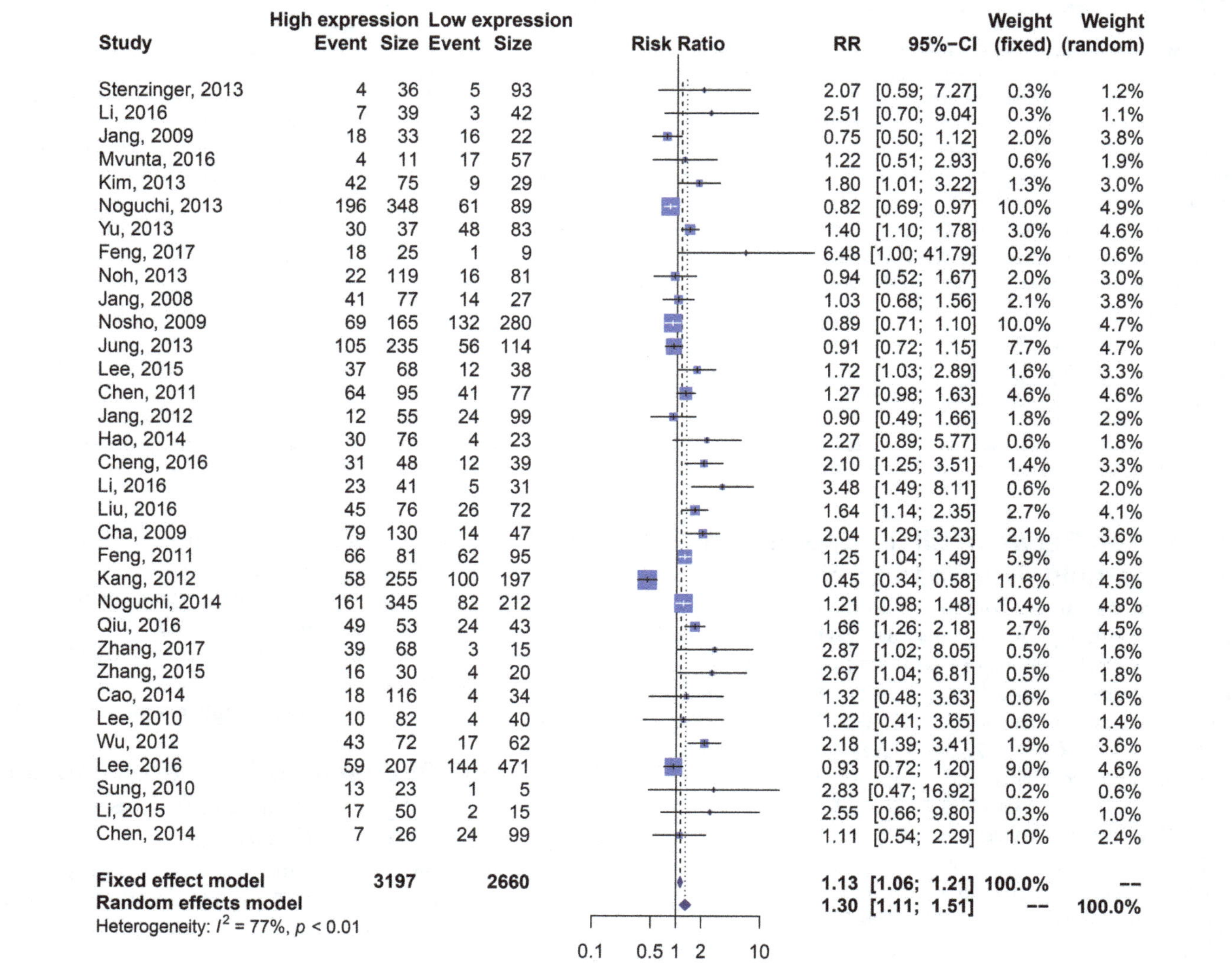

FIGURE 4 | Forest plots of tumor stage compared SIRT1 overexpression with underexpression.

3.830, 95% CI: [1.445, 10.154], $P = 0.0069$, $I^2 = 0\%$), but not in Asian population ($n = 12$, RR: 1.422, 95% CI: [0.913, 2.217], $P = 0.1198$, $I^2 = 72.85\%$) (**Supplementary Figure 5B**).

Elevated SIRT1 expression predicted a significantly higher lymphatic metastasis in Asian population with cancers ($n = 29$, RR: 1.239, 95% CI: [1.056, 1.453], $P = 0.0086$, $I^2 = 86.81\%$), but not correlated with lymphatic metastasis in Caucasian population ($n = 3$, RR: 0.777, 95% CI: [0.526, 1.147], $P = 0.2040$, $I^2 = 76.11\%$) (**Supplementary Figure 6B**).

Meta-Regression Analysis of Heterogeneity for Overall Survival and Publication Bias

We performed a meta-regression to explore the source of high heterogeneity for OS (**Table 4**). All potential factors could not significantly explain heterogeneity in the meta-analyses of the SIRT1 expression with survival outcomes in the *post-hoc* analysis, with the exception of ethnicity (**Supplementary Table 5**). Meta-regression analysis demonstrated a statistically significant correlation between ethnicity and OS ($P = 0.022$). From the meta-regression result, we conducted a subgroup analysis with groups of patients Asian or Caucasian (**Supplementary Figure 1C**). This subgroup analysis demonstrated a significantly lower heterogeneity value in Asian group ($n = 40$, RR: 1.708, 95% CI: [1.406, 2.076], $I^2 = 69.59\%$), which suggests that the high SIRT1 expression has stronger efficacy in the Asian population than the Caucasian population.

Meta-regression also used to explore the source of high heterogeneity for clinicopathological outcomes (Further details are provided in **Supplementary Table 6**). As to tumor stage, meta-regression analysis demonstrated a statistically significant correlation between tumor stage and country ($P < 0.05$), published year ($P = 0.0169$), and sample size ($P = 0.0004$). This subgroup analysis demonstrated a significantly lower heterogeneity value in China ($n = 17$, RR: 1.638, 95% CI: [1.404, 1.911], $I^2 = 41.16\%$), which suggests that the high SIRT1

Study	High expression Event	High expression Size	Low expression Event	Low expression Size	RR	95%-CI	Weight (fixed)	Weight (random)
Stenzinger, 2013	27	36	71	93	0.98	[0.79; 1.22]	2.9%	4.4%
Li, 2016	22	39	16	52	1.83	[1.12; 3.00]	1.0%	3.2%
Mvunta, 2016	2	11	10	57	1.04	[0.26; 4.10]	0.2%	0.9%
Kim, 2013	12	74	3	30	1.62	[0.49; 5.34]	0.3%	1.2%
Noguchi, 2013	156	348	52	89	0.77	[0.62; 0.95]	6.1%	4.5%
Yu, 2013	23	37	29	83	1.78	[1.21; 2.62]	1.3%	3.7%
He, 2015	34	54	13	32	1.55	[0.97; 2.47]	1.2%	3.3%
Noh, 2013	1	119	1	81	0.68	[0.04; 10.73]	0.1%	0.3%
Jang, 2012	103	208	178	289	0.80	[0.68; 0.95]	10.9%	4.6%
Jung, 2013	98	235	47	114	1.01	[0.78; 1.32]	4.6%	4.2%
Lv, 2014	23	32	41	88	1.54	[1.13; 2.11]	1.6%	4.0%
Cha, 2009	95	130	18	47	1.91	[1.31; 2.78]	1.9%	3.7%
Feng, 2011	67	81	61	95	1.29	[1.08; 1.54]	4.1%	4.6%
Kang, 2012	96	255	213	293	0.52	[0.44; 0.62]	14.5%	4.6%
Noguchi, 2014	172	255	173	302	1.18	[1.03; 1.34]	11.6%	4.7%
Qiu, 2016	50	53	22	43	1.84	[1.37; 2.49]	1.8%	4.1%
Zhang, 2017	46	68	5	15	2.03	[0.97; 4.23]	0.6%	2.2%
Zhang, 2015	13	30	6	20	1.44	[0.66; 3.17]	0.5%	2.1%
Cao, 2014	46	116	21	34	0.64	[0.45; 0.91]	2.4%	3.9%
Jin, 2015	39	87	63	232	1.65	[1.21; 2.26]	2.5%	4.0%
Kim, 2015	78	117	133	161	0.81	[0.70; 0.93]	8.2%	4.7%
Lee, 2010	36	82	16	20	0.55	[0.40; 0.76]	1.9%	4.0%
Chung, 2016	58	146	52	198	1.51	[1.11; 2.06]	3.2%	4.1%
Lee, 2016	120	206	237	470	1.16	[1.00; 1.34]	10.6%	4.7%
Sung, 2010	14	23	1	5	3.04	[0.51; 18.11]	0.1%	0.6%
Gharabaghi, 2016	16	27	9	13	0.86	[0.53; 1.38]	0.9%	3.3%
Lin, 2015	23	36	133	224	1.08	[0.82; 1.41]	2.7%	4.2%
Noh, 2013	58	96	12	48	2.42	[1.44; 4.05]	1.2%	3.1%
Chen, 2014	12	26	26	99	1.76	[1.03; 2.99]	0.8%	3.0%
Fixed effect model		**3027**		**3327**	**1.05**	**[1.00; 1.10]**	**100.0%**	**--**
Random effects model					**1.17**	**[1.01; 1.36]**	**--**	**100.0%**

Heterogeneity: $I^2 = 86\%$, $p < 0.01$

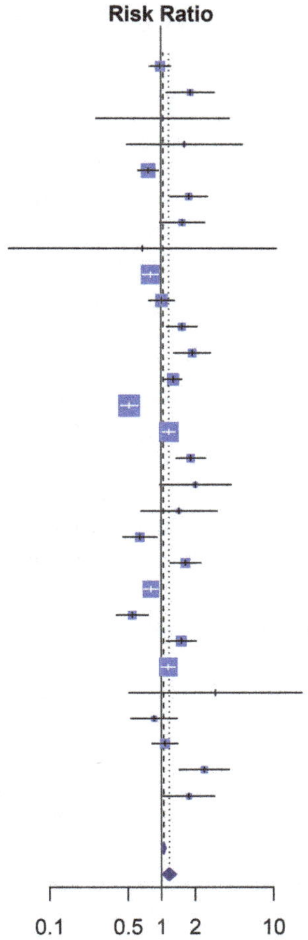

FIGURE 5 | Forest plots of lymphatic metastasis compared SIRT1 overexpression with underexpression.

Study	High expression Event	High expression Size	Low expression Event	Low expression Size	RR	95%-CI	Weight (fixed)	Weight (random)
Stenzinger, 2013	2	36	2	93	2.58	[0.38; 17.65]	0.9%	3.5%
Li, 2016	18	39	12	52	2.00	[1.10; 3.65]	8.8%	9.6%
Feng, 2016	39	49	17	40	1.87	[1.27; 2.76]	15.9%	10.8%
Kim, 2013	29	74	2	30	5.88	[1.50; 23.10]	2.4%	5.3%
Feng, 2017	8	25	7	9	0.41	[0.21; 0.80]	8.8%	9.2%
Jeh, 2017	2	16	22	86	0.49	[0.13; 1.88]	5.9%	5.4%
Jang, 2012	7	208	12	289	0.81	[0.32; 2.02]	8.5%	7.7%
Jung, 2013	23	235	17	114	0.66	[0.37; 1.18]	19.5%	9.7%
Lv, 2014	12	32	12	88	2.75	[1.38; 5.48]	5.4%	9.1%
Cha, 2009	3	130	1	47	1.08	[0.12; 10.17]	1.2%	2.8%
Noguchi, 2014	24	345	11	212	1.34	[0.67; 2.68]	11.6%	9.0%
Lee, 2010	27	82	3	40	4.39	[1.42; 13.61]	3.4%	6.5%
Wu, 2012	26	72	8	64	2.89	[1.41; 5.92]	7.2%	8.9%
Chen, 2014	2	26	1	99	7.62	[0.72; 80.76]	0.4%	2.5%
Fixed effect model		**1369**		**1263**	**1.61**	**[1.31; 1.97]**	**100.0%**	**--**
Random effects model					**1.56**	**[1.02; 2.39]**	**--**	**100.0%**

Heterogeneity: $I^2 = 71\%$, $p < 0.01$

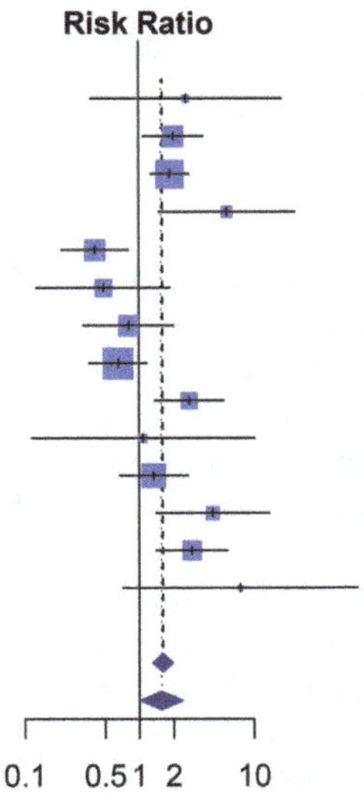

FIGURE 6 | Forest plots of distant metastasis compared SIRT1 overexpression with underexpression.

TABLE 4 | Meta-regression analysis of heterogeneity for overall survival.

Moderators	Variables of regression	$HR_{interaction}$ (95% CI)	*P*-value of regression	I^2	Cochrane Q (*P*-value)
Year	Year	1.001(0.990–1.012)	0.840	81.69%	<0.001
Sample size	Sample size	2.578(0.674–9.860)	0.166	43.18%	0.152
Follow up	Follow up	0.741(0.076–7.236)	0.796	72.89%	<0.001
Country	Intercept	1.648(1.291–2.104)	<0.001	71.56%	<0.001
	Germany	1.001(0.334–2.997)	0.999	71.56%	<0.001
	Hungary	0.388(0.143–1.051)	0.063	71.56%	<0.001
	Iran	1.523(0.380–6.105)	0.553	71.56%	<0.001
	Japan	1.134(0.463–2.775)	0.783	71.56%	<0.001
	Korea	1.079(0.695–1.675)	0.736	71.56%	<0.001
	Netherlands	0.600(0.285–1.263)	0.178	71.56%	<0.001
	Spain	1.330(0.405–4.374)	0.638	71.56%	<0.001
	USA	0.605(0.302–1.215)	0.158	71.56%	<0.001
Tumor type	Intercept	1.716(1.055–2.792)	0.030	75.22%	<0.001
	Colorectal cancer	0.543(0.293–1.008)	0.053	75.22%	<0.001
	Diffuse large B cell lymphoma	2.786(0.559–13.892)	0.211	75.22%	<0.001
	Endometrial carcinoma	0.629(0.082–4.849)	0.657	75.22%	<0.001
	Esophageal squamous cell carcinoma	1.044(0.412–2.640)	0.928	75.22%	<0.001
	Gastric Cancer	0.851(0.442–1.638)	0.630	75.22%	<0.001
	Hepatocellular Carcinoma	1.168(0.574–2.373)	0.668	75.22%	<0.001
	Laryngeal and hypopharyngeal carcinomas	0.326(0.078–1.370)	0.126	75.22%	<0.001
	NSCLC	1.071(0.521–2.204)	0.852	75.22%	<0.001
	Osteosarcoma	0.960(0.384–2.399)	0.930	75.22%	<0.001
	Ovarian cancer	1.135(0.478–2.692)	0.774	75.22%	<0.001
	Pancreatic ductal adenocarcinoma	0.961(0.294–3.144)	0.948	75.22%	<0.001
	Pelvis chondrosarcoma	0.711(0.080–6.345)	0.760	75.22%	<0.001
	Renal cell carcinoma	2.208(0.520–9.383)	0.283	75.22%	<0.001
	Soft tissue sarcoma	***5.863(1.115–30.823)***	***0.037***	75.22%	<0.001
	Uterine cervical cancer	0.880(0.208–3.727)	0.862	75.22%	<0.001
Race	Intercept	1.705(1.414–2.056)	<0.001	73.32%	<0.001
	Caucasian	***0.619(0.411–0.932)***	***0.022***	73.32%	<0.001
Sample type	Intercept	1.430(0.353–5.799)	0.617	81.72%	<0.001
	Tissue	1.097(0.267–4.510)	0.898	81.72%	<0.001

$HR_{interaction}$, interaction effect calculated by meta-regression; Positive direction indicates that possible moderators might strengthen OS in the SIRT1 overexpression relative to underexpression. Bold italics indicate statistically significant values (P < 0.05).

expression has stronger efficacy in the China population than the other countries. As to tumor size, meta-regression analysis demonstrated a statistically significant correlation between tumor size and published year ($P = 0.0260$). As to depth of tumor invasion, meta-regression analysis demonstrated a statistically significant correlation between depth of tumor invasion and sample size ($P = 0.0044$).

We used funnel plots and Egger's regression models to assess potential publication bias (**Tables 2**, **3**). The association between HRs (**Supplementary Figure 7**) or RRs (**Supplementary Figure 8**) and standard error for the SIRT1 expression was demonstrated in funnel plots, with each plot point representing a study. In regards to the OS, RFS, and TNM stage, we found that Egger's regression yielded potential publication bias (**Figure 7**).

DISCUSSION

In the current study, we conducted a meta-analysis of 13,138 subjects in 63 articles from PubMed, EMBASE and Cochrane library to evaluate prognostic and clinicopathological significance of SIRT1 expression in cancers. We found that elevated expression of SIRT1 was correlated with a poor OS of cancer patients, DFS, EFS, and PFS, but couldn't predict RFS or CCS. Elevated SIRT1 expression was associated with TNM stage, lymph node metastasis, and distant metastasis, but not with tumor size, depth of tumor invasion, differentiation, gender, or age. Our findings provide a clue to understanding prognostic and clinicopathological significance of SIRT1 expression in cancers.

Our current study indicates that overexpression of SIRT1 is correlated with poor OS, DFS, EFS, and PFS, but not with RFS or

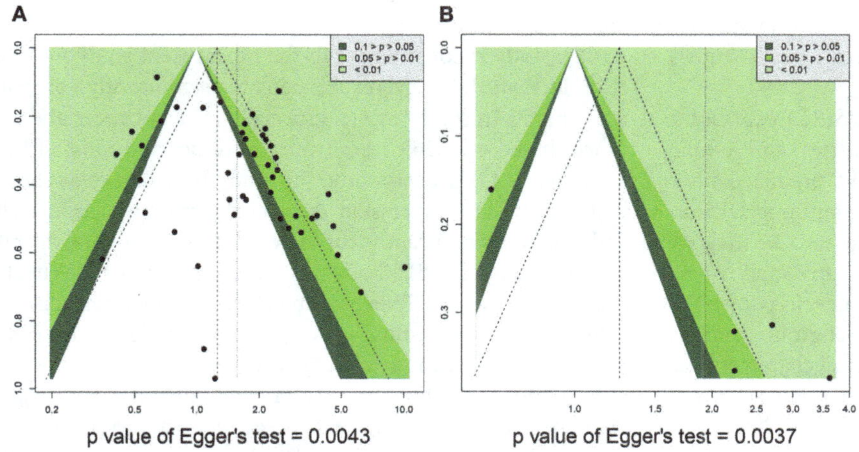

FIGURE 7 | Funnel plot for publication bias in overall survival, recurrence free survival, and TNM stage. **(A)** OS. **(B)** RFS. **(C)** TNM stage.

CCS, suggesting that SIRT1 expression is significantly correlated with poor prognosis as a global factor but not a restricted factor to tumor itself. It has been shown that SIRT1 is not a protein only found to a specific tissues or organs, instead, its expression can be found in almost all human tissues (1) and involved in a large variety of cellular processes, such as genomic stability, energy metabolism, senescence, gene transcription, and oxidative stress (5) by acting on a wide spectrum of proteins, including histones and transcription factors (2–4). This render SIRT1 plays multiple roles to regulate biological process in multi-systems. Melatonin is a pleiotropic molecule synthesized by pineal gland and many other organs and has important cytoprotective effects in many tissues including aging, neurodegenerative diseases, immunomodulation, and cancer and modulates DNA damage response (88, 89). Melatonin counteracts tumor metastases by modulating cell-cell and cell-matrix interaction, extracellular matrix remodeling, cytoskeleton reorganization, epithelial-mesenchymal transition, and angiogenesis (90). Recent studies showed that the upregulated SIRT1 signaling pathway is involved in protective effects of melatonin on vascular endothelium against aging-, oxidative stress-, lipopolysaccharide-, and ischemia-induced damage (91) and delays ovarian aging (92). SIRT1 is induced in normal cells and inhibited in tumor cells by melatonin (88, 89). SIRT1 may mediate the pleiotropic function of melatonin in cancer progression and metastasis. SIRT1 is an endocrine regulator of thyroid and parathyroid hormone function (93–95), and steroid hormone receptor activity (96, 97). SIRT1 is a regulator in immunity and autoimmunity, such as dendritic cell activation, T-regulatory cells (98–102). SIRT1 is also a regulator of lipid and carbohydrate metabolism (9, 103–105). In addition, SIRT1 regulates nervous system by inhibiting neuronal apoptosis and damage as well module nerve regeneration (103, 106, 107). Therefore, SIRT1 is a global factor for endocrine, immunity, metabolism, and nervous system, and affect poor OS, DFS, EFS, and PFS, but not with RFS or CCS in cancer patients.

In the current study, we found that SIRT1 overexpression was associated with TNM stage, lymph node metastasis, and distant metastasis, but not with tumor size, depth of tumor invasion, differentiation, gender, or age, suggesting that SIRT1 promotes metastasis but not growth, proliferation, and invasion of cancer tissues. Tumor is locally initiated and proliferated and may invade near tissues. Tumor size, depth of tumor invasion, and differentiation are terms used to characterize tumors which are locally confined in the early stage of malignancy (108, 109). Metastasis is the characteristics of advanced malignancy of cancer progression (110–113). Our data indicate that SIRT1 overexpression is associated with metastasis but not with tumor characteristics of early stage, suggesting that SIRT1 expression can predict advanced malignancy and is a potential therapeutic target for inhibiting metastasis of advanced cancer.

We performed subgroup analysis because of high heterogeneity in included studies. Correlation analysis between SIRT1 expression and prognosis of cancer types showed that SIRT1 overexpression predicted worse OS of osteosarcoma, esophageal squamous cell carcinoma, OS but not DFS of hepatocellular carcinoma, OS and DFS of breast carcinoma, OS and RFS of NSCLC, DFS but not OS or CCS in colorectal cancer, RFS and CCS but not OS of gastric cancer, RFS and CCS of renal cell carcinoma, CCS but not RFS in head and neck squamous cell carcinoma. SIRT1 overexpression cannot predict OS in ovarian cancer. Correlation analysis between SIRT1 expression and clinicopathological characteristics of cancers types showed that SIRT1 overexpression was associated with a higher TNM stage in hepatocellular carcinoma, but not in pancreatic ductal adenocarcinoma, ovarian cancer, colorectal cancer, gastric cancer, breast carcinoma, or NSCLC. SIRT1 overexpression was associated with distant metastasis in pancreatic ductal adenocarcinoma and breast carcinoma, but not in colorectal cancer or gastric cancer. From these results, we are unable to draw a unanimous conclusion, probably because there is a deficiency of studies that employ all prognostic indexes OS, DFS,

EFS, RFS, CCS, and PFS or a full range of clinicopathological characteristics to study the role of SIRT1 expression in survival of patients with a specific cancer type. More thorough studies are warranted.

Our subgroup correlation analysis between SIRT1 expression and prognosis of cancer in different countries and ethnic groups showed that high expression of SIRT1 predicted poor OS and DFS in China, poor OS and EFS but not DFS in Korea, poor OS in Japan, EFS in USA, but not OS in USA or Netherlands. Elevated SIRT1 expression predicted worse OS and DFS in Asian population with cancers, poor DFS but not OS in Caucasian population. Our subgroup analysis between SIRT1 expression and clinicopathological characteristics of cancers in different countries and ethnic groups showed that SIRT1 overexpression was associated with a higher TNM stage and lymphatic metastasis in China and Asian population except lymphatic metastasis in Japan or Korea, and not higher TNM stage and lymphatic metastasis in Caucasian population, We also found that SIRT1 overexpression predicted distant metastasis in Caucasian population, but not in Asians. These results indicate that ethnic background has influence on the role of SIRT1 expression in predicting the OS and clinicopathological characteristics of cancers. This is consistent with recent studies that showed SIRT1 expression is lower in NSCLC than the normal control group in a group of Chinese patients (15), and overexpressed in NSCLC in an Iran population (16). Our study showed that overexpression of SIRT1 predicted a worse OS in the Asian but not in the Caucasian, a higher TNM stage and lymphatic metastasis in Asian population especially in China but not in the Caucasian. This is consistent with the results of our meta-regression analysis. The effects of ethnic background on the role of SIRT1 expression in predicting the OS and clinicopathological characteristics of cancers need further collaborative investigation.

It has been established that there are significant differences between Asian and Caucasian populations in genetic and epigenetic background, dietary, environmental factors (114, 115). These factors are essential for not only initiation and progression, but also metastasis of cancers (116, 117). Mutations and extensive polymorphisms of SIRT1 were found in Chinese and Japanese (118–121) and 41 cancer lines (122). Although the data on mutations and polymorphisms of SIRT1 are very limited, we speculate that difference in SIRT1 mutations and polymorphisms may be one of accounts for difference in predicting OS and TNM stage and lymphatic metastasis of cancer by SIRT1 expression. This deserves further investigation (123).

It is known that metastasis is an independent predictor for poor prognosis of many cancer types (124–126). We find that elevated expression of SIRT1 was correlated with OS, DFS, EFS, and PFS. SIRT1 overexpression is also correlated with TNM stage, lymph node metastasis, and distant metastasis, but not with tumor size, depth of tumor invasion, differentiation, gender, or age. Overexpression of SIRT1 predicted a worse OS and higher TNM stage and lymphatic metastasis in Asian population especially in China. Therefore, overexpression of SIRT1 may promote lymphatic metastasis of cancers that lead to poor OS, DFS, EFS, and PFS. It is likely that SIRT1-mediated molecular events and biological processes could be an underlying mechanism for metastasis.

Our study is consistent with the most recent study by Wang et al. in that SIRT1 overexpression was significantly correlated with the OS in solid cancers, especially in liver cancer and lung cancer based on 7,369 cases from 37 studies and most of them are Asians (34). Consistently, the study by Hong et al showed that high SIRT1 expression correlated with vascular invasion and was not significantly correlated with overall survival rates in colon cancer (36). Study with 3024 patients by Wu et al showed that high SIRT1 expression predicts poor survival in non-colorectal gastrointestinal cancer, but not in colorectal cancer (35). SIRT1 expression was correlated with depth of invasion, lymph node metastasis and TNM stage and predicted a poor OS in colorectal cancer patients based on an analysis with seven studies (33). In an analysis of 1,650 patients in seven studies, high SIRT1 expression predicts a poor prognosis of gastric cancer patients and linked with patients' age, T stage, N stage, and tumor differentiation (32). Analysis by Cao et al. based on six studies involving 604 patients showed that SIRT1 expression was correlated with poor DFS and OS and high TNM stage and lymph node metastasis (31). However, we have performed study on survival and clinicopathological significance of SIRT1 expression in cancers more comprehensively. First, we included 63 eligible articles and a total of 13,138 participants in our study. These patients represented 9 countries and 16 cancer types as well as Asian and Caucasian ethnic groups. Second, we investigated both clinicopathological and prognostic significance of SIRT1 expression based on comprehensive clinical data and performed a series of subgroup analysis based on prognostic types, clinicopathological characteristics, cancer types, ethnic groups, countries. These stratifications provide more vehicles in understanding the survival and clinicopathological significance of SIRT1 expression in cancers.

There are also limitations in our study. Firstly, we found that heterogeneity existed in the meta-analysis as indicated by the I^2 values. It is predictable because of presence of inter-study differences in study design (prospective and retrospective), enrolled populations, treatment regimen, duration of follow-up, outcome measures, and other study and clinical characteristics (127). The heterogeneity among the studies remained, despite the usage of a random-effects model and subgroup analyses (128). Secondly, there is publication bias for SIRT1 expression and prognosis or clinicopathological characteristics as indicated by asymmetry of funnel plots for OS, DFS, EFS, RFS, CCS, PFS, and clinicopathological characteristics. Thirdly, we barely explored the correlation between SIRT1 overexpression and patient survival in terms of clinical parameters. Other elements that may contribute to the heterogeneity, such as therapeutic regimen, pathological grade, body mass index, and mean age, were not analyzed due to the lack of sufficient data (129). Fourthly, we performed a quantitative meta-analysis based mostly on secondary data, which could lead to inaccurate results because of a shortage of original individual patient data (130). Finally, we conducted our study based on the mRNA expression of SIRT1 or the protein levels, although the changes in the mRNA and protein levels of SIRT1 are consistent in several cancer types

(15, 16, 131, 132). The study by Hong et al who determined SIRT1 expression using immunohistochemistry showed similar results to ours study in relation with vascular invasion and overall survival rates in colon cancer (36). We should extensively investigate the prognostic and clinicopathological significance of SIRT1 expression at protein level in the future.

In conclusion, we have found that elevated expression of SIRT1 can predict poor OS, DFS, EFS, and PFS, but not with RFS or CCS, TNM stage, lymph node metastasis, and distant metastasis, but not tumor size, depth of tumor invasion, differentiation of cancers. Ethnic background has influence on the role of SIRT1 expression in predicting survival and clinicopathological characteristics of cancers. Overexpression of SIRT1 predicted a worse OS and higher TNM stage and lymphatic metastasis in Asian population especially in China. SIRT1-mediated molecular events and biological processes could be an underlying mechanism for metastasis and SIRT1 is a potential therapeutic target for inhibiting cancer metastasis. More studies that employ all prognostic indexes OS, DFS, EFS, RFS, CCS, and PFS or a full range of clinicopathological characteristics to study the role of SIRT1 expression in survival of patients with a specific cancer type, and mutations and polymorphisms of SIRT1 in cancers of different ethnic groups need to be further investigated in the future.

AUTHOR CONTRIBUTIONS

MS, DH, XGu, and HZ participated in research design. MS, WZ, MD, SX, XGo, PL, HL, and JZ performed data analysis. MS and XGu wrote or contributed to the writing of the manuscript.

SUPPLEMENTARY MATERIAL

Supplementary Table 1 | Databases searching terms. **(a)** Search criterion of Medline (via PubMed, from inception to April 1st, 2018) ($n = 2397$). **(b)** Search criterion of Embase (from 1966 to July 24, 2018) ($n = 2460$). **(c)** Search criterion of Cochrane Library (April 1st, 2018) ($n = 20$).

Supplementary Table 2 | Results of quality assessment using the Newcastle–Ottawa Scale for the included studies.

Supplementary Table 3 | Subgroup analysis for SIRT1 overexpression and the prognosis in cancers.

Supplementary Table 4 | Subgroup analysis for SIRT1 overexpression and clinicopathological parameters in cancers.

Supplementary Table 5 | Meta-regression analysis of heterogeneity for survival outcomes.

Supplementary Table 6 | Meta-regression analysis of heterogeneity for clinicopathological parameters in cancers.

Supplementary Figure 1 | Forest plot of subgroup analysis for SIRT1 overexpression and OS in cancers. **(A)** Cancer subgroup, **(B)** Country subgroup, **(C)** Ethnicity subgroup.

Supplementary Figure 2 | Forest plot of subgroup analysis for SIRT1 overexpression and DFS in cancers. **(A)** Cancer subgroup, **(B)** Country subgroup, **(C)** Ethnicity subgroup.

Supplementary Figure 3 | Forest plots of non-essential clinicopathological outcomes compared SIRT1 overexpression with underexpression. **(A)** Tumor size, **(B)** Depth of tumor invasion, **(C)** Differentiation, **(D)** Gender, **(E)** Age.

Supplementary Figure 4 | Forest plot of subgroup analysis for SIRT1 overexpression and TNM stage in cancers. **(A)** Cancer subgroup, **(B)** Country subgroup, **(C)** Ethnicity subgroup.

Supplementary Figure 5 | Forest plot of subgroup analysis for SIRT1 overexpression and distant metastasis in cancers. **(A)** Cancer subgroup, **(B)** Ethnicity subgroup.

Supplementary Figure 6 | Forest plot of subgroup analysis for SIRT1 overexpression and lymphatic metastasis in cancers. **(A)** Country subgroup, **(B)** Ethnicity subgroup.

Supplementary Figure 7 | Funnel plot for publication bias for SIRT1 expression and prognosis. **(A)** OS, **(B)** DFS, **(C)** EFS, **(D)** RFS, **(E)** CCS.

Supplementary Figure 8 | Funnel plot for publication bias for SIRT1 expression and clinicopathological characteristics. **(A)** Age, **(B)** Gender, **(C)** Tumor stage, **(D)** Distant metastasis, **(E)** Lymphatic invasion, **(F)** Tumor size, **(G)** Depth of tumor invasion, **(H)** Differentiation.

REFERENCES

1. Fagerberg L, Hallstrom BM, Oksvold P, Kampf C, Djureinovic D, Odeberg J, et al. Analysis of the human tissue-specific expression by genome-wide integration of transcriptomics and antibody-based proteomics. *Mol Cell Proteomics.* (2014) 13:397–406. doi: 10.1074/mcp.M113.035600
2. Jang SH, Min KW, Paik SS, Jang KS. Loss of SIRT1 histone deacetylase expression associates with tumour progression in colorectal adenocarcinoma. *J Clin Pathol.* (2012) 65:735–9. doi: 10.1136/jclinpath-2012-200685
3. Derr RS, van Hoesel AQ, Benard A, Goossens-Beumer IJ, Sajet A, Dekker-Ensink NG, et al. High nuclear expression levels of histone-modifying enzymes LSD1, HDAC2 and SIRT1 in tumor cells correlate with decreased survival and increased relapse in breast cancer patients. *BMC Cancer.* (2014) 14:604. doi: 10.1186/1471-2407-14-604
4. Xu Z, Yang Y, Li B, Li Y, Xia K, Li X, et al. Checkpoint suppressor 1 suppresses transcriptional activity of ERalpha and breast cancer cell proliferation via deacetylase SIRT1. *Cell Death Dis.* (2018) 9:559. doi: 10.1038/s41419-018-0629-3

5. Tran D, Bergholz J, Zhang H, He H, Wang Y, Zhang Y, et al. Insulin-like growth factor-1 regulates the SIRT1-p53 pathway in cellular senescence. *Aging Cell.* (2014) 13:669–78. doi: 10.1111/acel.12219
6. Imai S, Guarente L. Ten years of NAD-dependent SIR2 family deacetylases: implications for metabolic diseases. *Trends Pharmacol Sci.* (2010) 31:212–20. doi: 10.1016/j.tips.2010.02.003
7. Sebastian C, Satterstrom FK, Haigis MC, Mostoslavsky R. From sirtuin biology to human diseases: an update. *J Biol Chem.* (2012) 287:42444–52. doi: 10.1074/jbc.R112.402768
8. Carafa V, Rotili D, Forgione M, Cuomo F, Serretiello E, Hailu GS, et al. Sirtuin functions and modulation: from chemistry to the clinic. *Clin Epigenet.* (2016) 8:61. doi: 10.1186/s13148-016-0224-3
9. Zhu S, Dong Z, Ke X, Hou J, Zhao E, Zhang K, et al. The roles of sirtuins family in cell metabolism during tumor development. *Semin Cancer Biol.* (2018). doi: 10.1016/j.semcancer.2018.11.003. [Epub ahead of print].
10. Liu T, Liu PY, Marshall GM. The critical role of the class III histone deacetylase SIRT1 in cancer. *Cancer Res.* (2009) 69:1702–5. doi: 10.1158/0008-5472.CAN-08-3365
11. Fang Y, Nicholl MB. Sirtuin 1 in malignant transformation: friend or foe? *Cancer Lett.* (2011) 306:10–4. doi: 10.1016/j.canlet.2011.02.019
12. Fang Y, Nicholl MB. A dual role for sirtuin 1 in tumorigenesis. *Curr Pharm Des.* (2014) 20:2634–6.
13. Xu Y, Qin Q, Chen R, Wei C, Mo Q. SIRT1 promotes proliferation, migration, and invasion of breast cancer cell line MCF-7 by upregulating DNA polymerase delta1 (POLD1). *Biochem Biophys Res Commun.* (2018) 502:351–7. doi: 10.1016/j.bbrc.2018.05.164
14. Xia X, Zhou X. Knockdown of SIRT1 inhibits proliferation and promotes apoptosis of paclitaxel-resistant human cervical cancer cells. *Cell Mol Biol.* (2018) 64:36–41.
15. Yang F. The expression and mechanism of Sirt1 and AMPK in nonsmall cell lung cancer. *J BUON.* (2018) 23:106–10.
16. Gharabaghi MA. Diagnostic investigation of BIRC6 and SIRT1 protein expression level as potential prognostic biomarkers in patients with non-small cell lung cancer. *Clin Respir J.* (2018) 12:633–8. doi: 10.1111/crj.12572
17. Tan J, Liu Y, Maimaiti Y, Wang C, Yan Y, Zhou J, et al. Combination of SIRT1 and Src overexpression suggests poor prognosis in luminal breast cancer. *Onco Targets Ther.* (2018) 11:2051–61. doi: 10.2147/OTT.S162503
18. Shuang T, Wang M, Zhou Y, Shi C. Over-expression of Sirt1 contributes to chemoresistance and indicates poor prognosis in serous epithelial ovarian cancer (EOC). *Med Oncol.* (2015) 32:260. doi: 10.1007/s12032-015-0706-8
19. Noguchi A, Kikuchi K, Zheng H, Takahashi H, Miyagi Y, Aoki I, et al. SIRT1 expression is associated with a poor prognosis, whereas DBC1 is associated with favorable outcomes in gastric cancer. *Cancer Med.* (2014) 3:1553–61. doi: 10.1002/cam4.310
20. Li C, Wang L, Zheng L, Zhan X, Xu B, Jiang J, et al. SIRT1 expression is associated with poor prognosis of lung adenocarcinoma. *Onco Targets Ther.* (2015) 8:977–84. doi: 10.2147/ott.s82378
21. Lee H, Kim KR, Noh SJ, Park HS, Kwon KS, Park BH, et al. Expression of DBC1 and SIRT1 is associated with poor prognosis for breast carcinoma. *Hum Pathol.* (2011) 42:204–13. doi: 10.1016/j.humpath.2010.05.023
22. Chen X, Sun K, Jiao S, Cai N, Zhao X, Zou H, et al. High levels of SIRT1 expression enhance tumorigenesis and associate with a poor prognosis of colorectal carcinoma patients. *Sci Rep.* (2014) 4:7481. doi: 10.1038/srep07481
23. Chen X, Hokka D, Maniwa Y, Ohbayashi C, Itoh T, Hayashi Y. Sirt1 is a tumor promoter in lung adenocarcinoma. *Oncol Lett.* (2014) 8:387–93. doi: 10.3892/ol.2014.2057
24. Kim JR, Moon YJ, Kwon KS, Bae JS, Wagle S, Yu TK, et al. Expression of SIRT1 and DBC1 is associated with poor prognosis of soft tissue sarcomas. *PLoS ONE.* (2013) 8:e74738. doi: 10.1371/journal.pone.0074738
25. Wu M, Wei W, Xiao X, Guo J, Xie X, Li L, et al. Expression of SIRT1 is associated with lymph node metastasis and poor prognosis in both operable triple-negative and non-triple-negative breast cancer. *Med Oncol.* (2012) 29:3240–9. doi: 10.1007/s12032-012-0260-6
26. Chen HC, Jeng YM, Yuan RH, Hsu HC, Chen YL. SIRT1 promotes tumorigenesis and resistance to chemotherapy in hepatocellular carcinoma and its expression predicts poor prognosis. *Ann Surg Oncol.* (2012) 19:2011–9. doi: 10.1245/s10434-011-2159-4
27. Cha EJ, Noh SJ, Kwon KS, Kim CY, Park BH, Park HS, et al. Expression of DBC1 and SIRT1 is associated with poor prognosis of gastric carcinoma. *Clin Cancer Res.* (2009) 15:4453–9. doi: 10.1158/1078-0432.ccr-08-3329
28. Jang KY, Hwang SH, Kwon KS, Kim KR, Choi HN, Lee NR, et al. SIRT1 expression is associated with poor prognosis of diffuse large B-cell lymphoma. *Am J Surg Pathol.* (2008) 32:1523–31. doi: 10.1097/PAS.0b013e31816b6478
29. Noguchi A, Li X, Kubota A, Kikuchi K, Kameda Y, Zheng H, et al. SIRT1 expression is associated with good prognosis for head and neck squamous cell carcinoma patients. *Oral Surg Oral Med Oral Pathol Oral Radiol.* (2013) 115:385–92. doi: 10.1016/j.oooo.2012.12.013
30. Jung W, Hong KD, Jung WY, Lee E, Shin BK, Kim HK, et al. SIRT1 expression is associated with good prognosis in colorectal cancer. *Korean J Pathol.* (2013) 47:332–9. doi: 10.4132/KoreanJPathol.2013.47.4.332
31. Cao YW, Li YC, Wan GX, Du XM, Li F. Clinicopathological and prognostic role of SIRT1 in breast cancer patients: a meta-analysis. *Int J Clin Exp Med.* (2015) 8:616–24.
32. Jiang B, Chen JH, Yuan WZ, Ji JT, Liu ZY, Wu L, et al. Prognostic and clinical value of Sirt1 expression in gastric cancer: A systematic meta-analysis. *J Huazhong Univ Sci Technolog Med Sci.* (2016) 36:278–84. doi: 10.1007/s11596-016-1580-0
33. Zu G, Ji A, Zhou T, Che N. Clinicopathological significance of SIRT1 expression in colorectal cancer: a systematic review and meta analysis. *Int J Surg.* (2016) 26:32–7. doi: 10.1016/j.ijsu.2016.01.002
34. Wang C, Yang W, Dong F, Guo Y, Tan J, Ruan S, et al. The prognostic role of Sirt1 expression in solid malignancies: a meta-analysis. *Oncotarget.* (2017) 8:66343–51. doi: 10.18632/oncotarget.18494
35. Wu S, Jiang J, Liu J, Wang X, Gan Y, Tang Y. Meta-analysis of SIRT1 expression as a prognostic marker for overall survival in gastrointestinal cancer. *Oncotarget.* (2017) 8:62589–99. doi: 10.18632/oncotarget.19880
36. Hong WG, Pyo JS. The clinicopathological significance of SIRT1 expression in colon cancer: an immunohistochemical study and meta-analysis. *Pathol Res Pract.* (2018) 214:1550–5. doi: 10.1016/j.prp.2018.07.022
37. Parmar MK, Torri V, Stewart L. Extracting summary statistics to perform meta-analyses of the published literature for survival endpoints. *Stat Med.* (1998) 17:2815–34.
38. Tierney JF, Stewart LA, Ghersi D, Burdett S, Sydes MR. Practical methods for incorporating summary time-to-event data into meta-analysis. *Trials.* (2007) 8:16. doi: 10.1186/1745-6215-8-16
39. Stuck AE, Rubenstein LZ, Wieland D. Bias in meta-analysis detected by a simple, graphical test. Asymmetry detected in funnel plot was probably due to true heterogeneity. *BMJ.* (1998) 316: 469; author reply 470–461.
40. Stenzinger A, Endris V, Klauschen F, Sinn B, Lorenz K, Warth A, et al. High SIRT1 expression is a negative prognosticator in pancreatic ductal adenocarcinoma. *BMC Cancer.* (2013) 13:450. doi: 10.1186/1471-2407-13-450
41. Li S, Hong H, Lv H, Wu G, Wang Z. SIRT 1 overexpression is associated with metastasis of Pancreatic Ductal Adenocarcinoma (PDAC) and promotes migration and growth of PDAC cells. *Med Sci Monit.* (2016) 22:1593–600. doi: 10.12659/MSM.896697
42. Teramae M, Fukuda T, Wada T, Kawanishi M, Imai K, Yamauchi M, et al. Sirtuin1 expression predicts the efficacy of neoadjuvant chemotherapy for locally advanced uterine cervical cancer. *Mol Clin Oncol.* (2015) 3:73–8. doi: 10.3892/mco.2014.427
43. Asaka R, Miyamoto T. Sirtuin 1 promotes the growth and cisplatin resistance of endometrial carcinoma cells: a novel therapeutic target. *Lab Invest.* (2015) 95:1363–73. doi: 10.1038/labinvest.2015.119
44. Jang KY, Kim KS, Hwang SH, Kwon KS, Kim KR, Park HS, et al. Expression and prognostic significance of SIRT1 in ovarian epithelial tumours. *Pathology.* (2009) 41:366–71. doi: 10.1080/00313020902884451
45. Mvunta DH, Miyamoto T, Asaka R, Yamada Y, Ando H, Higuchi S, et al. Overexpression of SIRT1 is associated with poor outcomes in patients with ovarian carcinoma. *Appl Immunohistochem Mol Morphol.* (2017) 25:415–21. doi: 10.1097/pai.0000000000000316
46. Zhang N, Xie T, Xian M, Wang YJ, Li HY, Ying MD, et al. SIRT1 promotes metastasis of human osteosarcoma cells. *Oncotarget.* (2016) 7:79654–69. doi: 10.18632/oncotarget.12916

47. Feng H, Guo P, Wang J, Xu J, Xie C, Gao F. Expression of Leptin and Sirtuin-1 is associated with poor prognosis in patients with osteosarcoma. *Pathol Res Pract.* (2016) 212:319–24. doi: 10.1016/j.prp.2016.02.002
48. Yu XM, Liu Y, Jin T, Liu J, Wang J, Ma C, et al. The expression of SIRT1 and DBC1 in laryngeal and hypopharyngeal carcinomas. *PLoS ONE.* (2013) 8:e66975. doi: 10.1371/journal.pone.0066975
49. Batra A, Kashyap S, Singh L, Bakhshi S. Sirtuin1 expression and correlation with histopathological features in retinoblastoma. *Ocul Oncol Pathol.* (2015) 2:86–90. doi: 10.1159/000439594
50. Chen GQ, Tian H, Yue WM, Li L, Li SH, Qi L, et al. SIRT1 expression is associated with lymphangiogenesis, lymphovascular invasion and prognosis in pN0 esophageal squamous cell carcinoma. *Cell Biosci.* (2014) 4:48. doi: 10.1186/2045-3701-4-48
51. He Z, Yi J, Jin L, Pan B, Chen L, Song H. Overexpression of Sirtuin-1 is associated with poor clinical outcome in esophageal squamous cell carcinoma. *Tumour Biol.* (2016) 37:7139–48. doi: 10.1007/s13277-015-4459-y
52. Feng H, Wang J, Xu J, Xie C, Gao F, Li Z. The expression of SIRT1 regulates the metastaticplasticity of chondrosarcoma cells by inducing epithelial-mesenchymal transition. *Sci Rep.* (2017) 7:41203. doi: 10.1038/srep41203
53. Noh SJ, Kang MJ, Kim KM, Bae JS, Park HS, Moon WS, et al. Acetylation status of P53 and the expression of DBC1, SIRT1, and androgen receptor are associated with survival in clear cell renal cell carcinoma patients. *Pathology.* (2013) 45:574–80. doi: 10.1097/PAT.0b013e3283652c7a
54. Jeh SU, Park JJ, Lee JS, Kim DC, Do J, Lee SW, et al. Differential expression of the sirtuin family in renal cell carcinoma: aspects of carcinogenesis and prognostic significance. *Urol Oncol.* (2017) 35:675.e9–675.e15. doi: 10.1016/j.urolonc.2017.08.016
55. Ren Y, Gu Y, Wang W, Wang J, Li X, Wang Y, et al. Expression of the significance of silent information regulator type-1 in Angioimmunoblastic T-cell lymphoma is greater association with tumorigenesis and has strong implications for adverse prognosis. *Cell Cycle.* (2016) 15:1545–51. doi: 10.1080/15384101.2016.1172157
56. Nosho K, Shima K, Irahara N, Kure S, Firestein R, Baba Y, et al. SIRT1 histone deacetylase expression is associated with microsatellite instability and CpG island methylator phenotype in colorectal cancer. *Mod Pathol.* (2009) 22:922–32. doi: 10.1038/modpathol.2009.49
57. Benard A, Goossens-Beumer IJ, van Hoesel AQ, Horati H, de Graaf W, Putter H, et al. Nuclear expression of histone deacetylases and their histone modifications predicts clinical outcome in colorectal cancer. *Histopathology.* (2015) 66:270–82. doi: 10.1111/his.12534
58. Lv L, Shen Z, Zhang J, Zhang H, Dong J, Yan Y, et al. Clinicopathological significance of SIRT1 expression in colorectal adenocarcinoma. *Med Oncol.* (2014) 31:965. doi: 10.1007/s12032-014-0965-9
59. Lee WY, Lee WT, Cheng CH, Chen KC, Chou CM, Chung CH, et al. Repositioning antipsychotic chlorpromazine for treating colorectal cancer by inhibiting sirtuin 1. *Oncotarget.* (2015) 6:27580–95. doi: 10.18632/oncotarget.4768
60. Cheng F, Su L, Yao C, Liu L, Shen J, Liu C, et al. SIRT1 promotes epithelial-mesenchymal transition and metastasis in colorectal cancer by regulating Fra-1 expression. *Cancer Lett.* (2016) 375:274–83. doi: 10.1016/j.canlet.2016.03.010
61. Chen J, Zhang B, Wong N, Lo AW, To KF, Chan AW, et al. Sirtuin 1 is upregulated in a subset of hepatocellular carcinomas where it is essential for telomere maintenance and tumor cell growth. *Cancer Res.* (2011) 71:4138–49. doi: 10.1158/0008-5472.can-10-4274
62. Jang KY, Noh SJ, Lehwald N, Tao GZ, Bellovin DI, Park HS, et al. SIRT1 and c-Myc promote liver tumor cell survival and predict poor survival of human hepatocellular carcinomas. *PLoS ONE.* (2012) 7:e45119. doi: 10.1371/journal.pone.0045119
63. Hao C, Zhu PX, Yang X, Han ZP, Jiang JH, Zong C, et al. Overexpression of SIRT1 promotes metastasis through epithelial-mesenchymal transition in hepatocellular carcinoma. *BMC Cancer.* (2014) 14:978. doi: 10.1186/1471-2407-14-978
64. Cheng J, Liu C, Liu L, Chen X, Shan J, Shen J, et al. MEK1 signaling promotes self-renewal and tumorigenicity of liver cancer stem cells via maintaining SIRT1 protein stabilization. *Oncotarget.* (2016) 7:20597–611. doi: 10.18632/oncotarget.7972
65. Li Y, Xu S, Li J, Zheng L, Feng M, Wang X, et al. SIRT1 facilitates hepatocellular carcinoma metastasis by promoting PGC-1alpha-mediated mitochondrial biogenesis. *Oncotarget.* (2016) 7:29255–74. doi: 10.18632/oncotarget.8711
66. Liu L, Liu C, Zhang Q, Shen J, Zhang H, Shan J, et al. SIRT1-mediated transcriptional regulation of SOX2 is important for self-renewal of liver cancer stem cells. *Hepatology.* (2016) 64:814–27. doi: 10.1002/hep.28690
67. Feng AN, Zhang LH, Fan XS, Huang Q, Ye Q, Wu HY, et al. Expression of SIRT1 in gastric cardiac cancer and its clinicopathologic significance. *Int J Surg Pathol.* (2011) 19:743–50. doi: 10.1177/1066896911412181
68. Kang Y, Jung WY, Lee H, Lee E, Kim A, Kim BH. Expression of SIRT1 and DBC1 in gastric adenocarcinoma. *Korean J Pathol.* (2012) 46:523–31. doi: 10.4132/KoreanJPathol.2012.46.6.523
69. Qiu G, Li X. The prognostic role of SIRT1-autophagy axis in gastric cancer. *Evid Based Complement Alternat Med.* (2016) 2016:6869415. doi: 10.1155/2016/5989681
70. Szasz AM, Lanczky A, Nagy A, Forster S, Hark K, Green JE, et al. Cross-validation of survival associated biomarkers in gastric cancer using transcriptomic data of 1,065 patients. *Oncotarget.* (2016) 7:49322–33. doi: 10.18632/oncotarget.10337
71. Zhang S, Huang S, Deng C, Cao Y, Yang J, Chen G, et al. Co-ordinated overexpression of SIRT1 and STAT3 is associated with poor survival outcome in gastric cancer patients. *Oncotarget.* (2017) 8:18848–60. doi: 10.1016/j.nut.2016.09.008
72. Zhang LH, Huang Q, Fan XS, Wu HY, Yang J, Feng AN. Clinicopathological significance of SIRT1 and p300/CBP expression in gastroesophageal junction (GEJ) cancer and the correlation with E-cadherin and MLH1. *Pathol Res Pract.* (2013) 209:611–7. doi: 10.1016/j.prp.2013.03.012
73. Ren NS, Ji M, Tokar EJ, Busch EL, Xu X, Lewis D, et al. Haploinsufficiency of SIRT1 enhances glutamine metabolism and promotes cancer development. *Curr Biol.* (2017) 27:483–94. doi: 10.1016/j.cub.2016.12.047
74. Shin DH, Choi YJ, Jin P, Yoon H, Chun YS, Shin HW, et al. Distinct effects of SIRT1 in cancer and stromal cells on tumor promotion. *Oncotarget.* (2016) 7:23975–87. doi: 10.18632/oncotarget.8073
75. Zhang XZ, Chen SQ, Cheng ML, Cao FL, Cheng YF. The expression and correlation of SIRT1 and Phospho-SIRT1 in colorectal cancer. *Int J Clin Exp Med.* (2015) 8:809–17.
76. Cao YW, Li WQ, Wan GX, Li YX, Du XM, Li YC, et al. Correlation and prognostic value of SIRT1 and Notch1 signaling in breast cancer. *J Exp Clin Cancer Res.* (2014) 33:97. doi: 10.1186/s13046-014-0097-2
77. Jin MS, Hyun CL, Park IA, Kim JY, Chung YR, Im SA, et al. SIRT1 induces tumor invasion by targeting epithelial mesenchymal transition-related pathway and is a prognostic marker in triple negative breast cancer. *Tumour Biol.* (2016) 37:4743–53. doi: 10.1007/s13277-015-4231-3
78. Kim H, Lee KH, Park IA, Chung YR, Im SA, Noh DY, et al. Expression of SIRT1 and apoptosis-related proteins is predictive for lymph node metastasis and disease-free survival in luminal A breast cancer. *Virchows Arch.* (2015) 467:563–70. doi: 10.1007/s00428-015-1815-7
79. Chung SY, Jung YY, Park IA, Kim H, Chung YR, Kim JY, et al. Oncogenic role of SIRT1 associated with tumor invasion, lymph node metastasis, and poor disease-free survival in triple negative breast cancer. *Clin Exp Metastasis.* (2016) 33:179–85. doi: 10.1007/s10585-015-9767-5
80. Lee JJ, Lee HJ, Son BH, Kim SB, Ahn JH, Ahn SD, et al. Expression of FOXM1 and related proteins in breast cancer molecular subtypes. *Int J Exp Pathol.* (2016) 97:170–7. doi: 10.1111/iep.12187
81. Chung YR, Kim H, Park SY, Park IA, Jang JJ, Choe JY, et al. Distinctive role of SIRT1 expression on tumor invasion and metastasis in breast cancer by molecular subtype. *Hum Pathol.* (2015) 46:1027–35. doi: 10.1016/j.humpath.2015.03.015
82. Zhang W, Luo J, Yang F, Wang Y, Yin Y, Strom A, et al. BRCA1 inhibits AR-mediated proliferation of breast cancer cells through the activation of SIRT1. *Sci Rep.* (2016) 6:22034. doi: 10.1038/srep22034
83. Sung JY, Kim R, Kim JE, Lee J. Balance between SIRT1 and DBC1 expression is lost in breast cancer. *Cancer Sci.* (2010) 101:1738–44. doi: 10.1111/j.1349-7006.2010.01573.x

84. Lin SY, Peng F. Association of SIRT1 and HMGA1 expression in non-small cell lung cancer. *Oncol Lett.* (2016) 11:782–8. doi: 10.3892/ol.2015.3914
85. Noh SJ, Baek HA, Park HS, Jang KY, Moon WS, Kang MJ, et al. Expression of SIRT1 and cortactin is associated with progression of non-small cell lung cancer. *Pathol Res Pract.* (2013) 209:365–70. doi: 10.1016/j.prp.2013.03.011
86. Zhang T, Rong N, Chen J, Zou C, Jing H, Zhu X, et al. SIRT1 expression is associated with the chemotherapy response and prognosis of patients with advanced NSCLC. *PLoS ONE.* (2013) 8:e79162. doi: 10.1371/journal.pone.0079162
87. Grbesa I, Pajares MJ, Martinez-Terroba E, Agorreta J, Mikecin AM, Larrayoz M, et al. Expression of sirtuin 1 and 2 is associated with poor prognosis in non-small cell lung cancer patients. *PLoS ONE.* (2015) 10:e0124670. doi: 10.1371/journal.pone.0124670
88. Majidinia M, Sadeghpour A, Mehrzadi S, Reiter RJ, Khatami N, Yousefi B. Melatonin: a pleiotropic molecule that modulates DNA damage response and repair pathways. *J Pineal Res.* (2017) 63:e12416. doi: 10.1111/jpi.12416
89. Mayo JC, Sainz RM, Gonzalez Menendez P, Cepas V, Tan DX, Reiter RJ. Melatonin and sirtuins: a "not-so unexpected" relationship. *J Pineal Res.* (2017) 62:e12391. doi: 10.1111/jpi.12391
90. Su SC, Hsieh MJ, Yang WE, Chung WH, Reiter RJ, Yang SF. Cancer metastasis: mechanisms of inhibition by melatonin. *J Pineal Res.* (2017) 62:e12370. doi: 10.1111/jpi.12370
91. Lee FY, Sun CK, Sung PH, Chen KH, Chua S, Sheu JJ, et al. Daily melatonin protects the endothelial lineage and functional integrity against the aging process, oxidative stress, and toxic environment and restores blood flow in critical limb ischemia area in mice. *J Pineal Res.* (2018) 65:e12489. doi: 10.1111/jpi.12489
92. Tamura H, Kawamoto M, Sato S, Tamura I, Maekawa R, Taketani T, et al. Long-term melatonin treatment delays ovarian aging. *J Pineal Res.* (2017) 62:e12381. doi: 10.1111/jpi.12381
93. Cordeiro A, de Souza LL, Oliveira LS, Faustino LC, Santiago LA, Bloise FF, et al. Thyroid hormone regulation of Sirtuin 1 expression and implications to integrated responses in fasted mice. *J Endocrinol.* (2013) 216:181–93. doi: 10.1530/JOE-12-0420
94. Thakran S, Sharma P, Attia RR, Hori RT, Deng X, Elam MB, et al. Role of sirtuin 1 in the regulation of hepatic gene expression by thyroid hormone. *J Biol Chem.* (2013) 288:807–18. doi: 10.1074/jbc.M112.437970
95. Fei Y, Shimizu E, McBurney MW, Partridge NC. Sirtuin 1 is a negative regulator of parathyroid hormone stimulation of matrix metalloproteinase 13 expression in osteoblastic cells: role of sirtuin 1 in the action of PTH on osteoblasts. *J Biol Chem.* (2015) 290:8373–82. doi: 10.1074/jbc.M114.602763
96. Dai Y, Ngo D, Forman LW, Qin DC, Jacob J, Faller DV. Sirtuin 1 is required for antagonist-induced transcriptional repression of androgen-responsive genes by the androgen receptor. *Mol Endocrinol.* (2007) 21:1807–21. doi: 10.1210/me.2006-0467
97. Moore RL, Dai Y, Faller DV. Sirtuin 1 (SIRT1) and steroid hormone receptor activity in cancer. *J Endocrinol.* (2012) 213:37–48. doi: 10.1530/JOE-11-0217
98. Kong S, McBurney MW, Fang D. Sirtuin 1 in immune regulation and autoimmunity. *Immunol Cell Biol.* (2012) 90:6–13. doi: 10.1038/icb.2011.102
99. Yang H, Lee SM, Gao B, Zhang J, Fang D. Histone deacetylase sirtuin 1 deacetylates IRF1 protein and programs dendritic cells to control Th17 protein differentiation during autoimmune inflammation. *J Biol Chem.* (2013) 288:37256–66. doi: 10.1074/jbc.M113.527531
100. Akimova T, Xiao H, Liu Y, Bhatti TR, Jiao J, Eruslanov E, et al. Targeting sirtuin-1 alleviates experimental autoimmune colitis by induction of Foxp3+ T-regulatory cells. *Mucosal Immunol.* (2014) 7:1209–20. doi: 10.1038/mi.2014.10
101. Luciano JA, Kautza B, Darwiche S, Martinez S, Stratimirovic S, Waltz P, et al. Sirtuin 1 agonist minimizes injury and improves the immune response following traumatic shock. *Shock.* (2015) 44(Suppl. 1):149–55. doi: 10.1097/SHK.0000000000000412
102. Owczarczyk AB, Schaller MA, Reed M, Rasky AJ, Lombard DB, Lukacs NW. Sirtuin 1 regulates dendritic cell activation and autophagy during respiratory syncytial virus-induced immune responses. *J Immunol.* (2015) 195:1637–46. doi: 10.4049/jimmunol.1500326
103. Zhang Y, Li H, Cao Y, Zhang M, Wei S. Sirtuin 1 regulates lipid metabolism associated with optic nerve regeneration. *Mol Med Rep.* (2015) 12:6962–8. doi: 10.3892/mmr.2015.4286
104. Alayon AN, Ortega Avila JG, Echeverri Jimenez I. Carbohydrate metabolism and gene expression of sirtuin 1 in healthy subjects after Sacha inchi oil supplementation: a randomized trial. *Food Funct.* (2018) 9:1570–7. doi: 10.1039/c7fo01956d
105. Cao MM, Lu X, Liu GD, Su Y, Li YB, Zhou J. Resveratrol attenuates type 2 diabetes mellitus by mediating mitochondrial biogenesis and lipid metabolism via Sirtuin type 1. *Exp Ther Med.* (2018) 15:576–84. doi: 10.3892/etm.2017.5400
106. Yan P, Bai L, Lu W, Gao Y, Bi Y, Lv G. Regulation of autophagy by AMP-activated protein kinase/sirtuin 1 pathway reduces spinal cord neurons damage. *Iran J Basic Med Sci.* (2017) 20:1029–36. doi: 10.22038/IJBMS.2017.9272
107. Shi X, Pi L, Zhou S, Li X, Min F, Wang S, et al. Activation of Sirtuin 1 Attenuates High Glucose-Induced Neuronal Apoptosis by Deacetylating p53. *Front Endocrinol.* (2018) 9:274. doi: 10.3389/fendo.2018.00274
108. Knudsen BS, Vasioukhin V. Mechanisms of prostate cancer initiation and progression. *Adv Cancer Res.* (2010) 109:1–50. doi: 10.1016/B978-0-12-380890-5.00001-6
109. Leong SP, Aktipis A, Maley C. Cancer initiation and progression within the cancer microenvironment. *Clin Exp Metastasis.* (2018). doi: 10.1007/s10585-018-9921-y. [Epub ahead of print].
110. Patel LR, Camacho DF, Shiozawa Y, Pienta KJ, Taichman RS. Mechanisms of cancer cell metastasis to the bone: a multistep process. *Future Oncol.* (2011) 7:1285–97. doi: 10.2217/fon.11.112
111. Farnsworth RH, Achen MG, Stacker SA. The evolving role of lymphatics in cancer metastasis. *Curr Opin Immunol.* (2018) 53:64–73. doi: 10.1016/j.coi.2018.04.008
112. Franchino F, Ruda R, Soffietti R. Mechanisms and Therapy for Cancer Metastasis to the Brain. *Front Oncol.* (2018) 8:161. doi: 10.3389/fonc.2018.00161
113. Hamidi H, Ivaska J. Every step of the way: integrins in cancer progression and metastasis. *Nat Rev Cancer.* (2018) 18:533–48. doi: 10.1038/s41568-018-0038-z
114. Hur YM, Kaprio J, Iacono WG, Boomsma DI, McGue M, Silventoinen K, et al. Genetic influences on the difference in variability of height, weight and body mass index between Caucasian and East Asian adolescent twins. *Int J Obes.* (2008) 32:1455–67. doi: 10.1038/ijo.2008.144
115. Tarabay M, Elshazli R, Settin A. African vs. Caucasian and Asian difference for the association of interleukin-10 promotor polymorphisms with type 2 diabetes mellitus (a meta-analysis study). *Meta Gene.* (2016) 9:10–7. doi: 10.1016/j.mgene.2016.02.006
116. Chatterjee A, Rodger EJ, Eccles MR. Epigenetic drivers of tumourigenesis and cancer metastasis. *Semin Cancer Biol.* (2018) 51:149–59. S1044-579X(17)30053-6
117. Pavlidis ET, Pavlidis TE. Current molecular and genetic aspects of pancreatic cancer, the role of Metastasis Associated Proteins (MTA): a review. *J Invest Surg.* (2018) 31:54–66. doi: 10.1080/08941939.2016.1269854
118. Shimoyama Y, Suzuki K, Hamajima N, Niwa T. Sirtuin 1 gene polymorphisms are associated with body fat and blood pressure in Japanese. *Transl Res.* (2011) 157:339–47. doi: 10.1016/j.trsl.2011.02.004
119. Shimoyama Y, Mitsuda Y, Tsuruta Y, Suzuki K, Hamajima N, Niwa T. SIRTUIN 1 gene polymorphisms are associated with cholesterol metabolism and coronary artery calcification in Japanese hemodialysis patients. *J Ren Nutr.* (2012) 22:114–9. doi: 10.1053/j.jrn.2011.10.025
120. Chen Z, Zhai Y, Zhang W, Teng Y, Yao K. Single Nucleotide Polymorphisms of the Sirtuin 1 (SIRT1) gene are associated with age-related macular degeneration in chinese han individuals: a case-control pilot study. *Medicine.* (2015) 94:e2238. doi: 10.1097/MD.0000000000002238
121. Lv Y, Lin S, Peng F. SIRT1 gene polymorphisms and risk of lung cancer. *Cancer Manag Res.* (2017) 9:381–6. doi: 10.1016/j.canlet.2017.09.001
122. Han J, Hubbard BP, Lee J, Montagna C, Lee HW, Sinclair DA, et al. Analysis of 41 cancer cell lines reveals excessive allelic loss and novel mutations in the SIRT1 gene. *Cell Cycle.* (2013) 12:263–70. doi: 10.4161/cc.23056
123. Mei ZB, Duan CY, Li CB, Cui L, Ogino S. Prognostic role of tumor PIK3CA mutation in colorectal cancer: a systematic review and meta-analysis. *Ann Oncol.* (2016) 27:1836–48. doi: 10.1093/annonc/mdw264

124. Tsutsumi S, Watanabe R, Tabe Y, Fujii T, Morita H, Kigure W, et al. Extranodal metastasis predicts poor survival in advanced colorectal cancer. *Hepatogastroenterology.* (2012) 59:372–4. doi: 10.5754/hge10139
125. Funazo T, Nomizo T, Kim YH. Liver metastasis is associated with poor progression-free survival in patients with non-small cell lung cancer treated with nivolumab. *J Thorac Oncol.* (2017) 12:e140–1. doi: 10.1016/j.jtho.2017.04.027
126. Ambe PC, Godde D, Storkel S, Zirngibl H, Bonicke L. Extra nodular metastasis is a poor prognostic factor for overall survival in node-positive patients with colorectal cancer. *Int J Colorectal Dis.* (2018) 33:403–9. doi: 10.1007/s00384-018-2991-0
127. Mei Z, Shi L, Wang B, Yang J, Xiao Z, Du P, et al. Prognostic role of pretreatment blood neutrophil-to-lymphocyte ratio in advanced cancer survivors: a systematic review and meta-analysis of 66 cohort studies. *Cancer Treat Rev.* (2017) 58:1–13. doi: 10.1016/j.ctrv.2017.05.005
128. Mei Z, Liang M, Li L, Zhang Y, Wang Q, Yang W. Effects of statins on cancer mortality and progression: a systematic review and meta-analysis of 95 cohorts including 1,111,407 individuals. *Int J Cancer.* (2017) 140:1068–81. doi: 10.1002/ijc.30526
129. Xiao Y, Zheng L, Mei Z, Xu C, Liu C, Chu X, et al. The impact of metformin use on survival in prostate cancer: a systematic review and meta-analysis. *Oncotarget.* (2017) 8:100449–58. doi: 10.18632/oncotarget.22117
130. Mei ZB, Zhang ZJ, Liu CY, Liu Y, Cui A, Liang ZL, et al. Survival benefits of metformin for colorectal cancer patients with diabetes: a systematic review and meta-analysis. *PLoS ONE.* (2014) 9:e91818. doi: 10.1371/journal.pone.0091818
131. Rifai K, Judes G, Idrissou M, Daures M, Bignon YJ, Penault-Llorca F, et al. Dual SIRT1 expression patterns strongly suggests its bivalent role in human breast cancer. *Oncotarget.* (2017) 8:110922–30. doi: 10.18632/oncotarget.23006
132. Subramaniyan B, Kumar V, Mathan G. Effect of sodium salt of Butrin, a novel compound isolated from Butea monosperma flowers on suppressing the expression of SIRT1 and Aurora B kinase-mediated apoptosis in colorectal cancer cells. *Biomed Pharmacother.* (2017) 90:402–13. doi: 10.1016/j.biopha.2017.03.086

13

SIRT1 and Estrogen Signaling Cooperation for Breast Cancer Onset and Progression

Sergio Liarte [1], José Luis Alonso-Romero [2] and Francisco José Nicolás [1]**

[1] *Laboratorio de Oncología Molecular y TGFβ, Instituto Murciano de Investigaciones Biosanitarias Arrixaca, Murcia, Spain,*
[2] *Servicio de Oncología, Hospital Clínico Universitario Virgen de la Arrixaca, Murcia, Spain*

***Correspondence:**
Sergio Liarte
sdll1@um.es
Francisco José Nicolás
franciscoj.nicolas2@carm.es

Breast cancer remains a significant female mortality cause. It constitutes a multifactorial disease for which research on environmental factors offers little help in predicting onset or progression. The pursuit for its foundations by analyzing hormonal changes as a motive for disease development, indicates that increased exposure to estrogens associates with increased risk. A prevalent number of breast cancer cases show dependence on the increased activity of the classic nuclear estrogen receptor (ER) for cell proliferation and survival. SIRT1 is a Type III histone deacetylase which is receiving increasing attention due to its ability to perform activities over relevant non-histone proteins and transcription factors. Interestingly, concomitant SIRT1 overexpression is commonly found in ER-positive breast cancer cases. Both proteins had been shown to directly interact, in a process related to altered intracellular signaling and aberrant transcription, then promoting tumor progression. Moreover, SIRT1 activities had been also linked to estrogenic effects through interaction with the G-protein coupled membrane bound estrogen receptor (GPER). This work aims to summarize present knowledge on the interplay between SIRT1 and ER/GPER for breast cancer onset and progression. Lastly, evidences on the ability of SIRT1 to interact with TGFß signaling, a concurrent pathway significantly involved in breast cancer progression, are reported. The potential of this research field for the development of innovative strategies in the assessment of orphan breast cancer subtypes, such as triple negative breast cancer (TNBC), is discussed.

Keywords: SIRT1, sex steroids, estrogen receptor, GPER, breast cancer, TNBC

INTRODUCTION

Breast cancer (BC) is the most frequent tumor in women and a prevailing cause for female cancer mortality (1). It constitutes a multifactorial disease for which epidemiologic studies over environmental determinants offer little help in predicting disease onset or progression, thus, gender, aging, diagnosed first-degree relatives or previous history of BC remain dominant risk factors (2, 3). The pursuit for BC causes over molecular biology techniques led to the establishment of few genetic markers, such as *BRCA1, BRCA2, or DBC-1,* which driver mutation predispose for disease while also explaining cases of familiar clustering; still, the majority of mutations detected account for genes of low penetrance and frequently altered across genomes (4). Whilst, concurrent research efforts tried to find a predictable BC marker or cause based on hormonal changes.Although for most of hormonal hypothesis proposed data is still inconclusive (2, 5), it is accepted that increased exposure to estrogens associates with higher risk, while reducing exposure is believed to result in protection (6). Therefore, factors such as early menarche, nulliparity or late menopause are associated with enhanced BC likelihood.

Observations on BC incidence are thought to be significantly contributed by the activities of classic nuclear hormone receptors for estrogens and progesterone (ER, PR). This is supported by tumor characterization using microarray techniques, which allowed to discriminate BC subtypes on the expression of key molecular markers including classic receptors. Applying such methods, BC is classified in ascending order indicating for aggressiveness: luminal-A; luminal-B (HER2−); luminal-B (HER2+); HER2-enriched; and basal-like. The first three subtypes share positivity for the expression of ER and/or PR along with the presence or absence of the human epidermal growth factor receptor 2 (Erb-B2; HER2), member of the epidermal growth factor receptor (HER/EGFR/ERBB) family. At last, the basal-like, which displays worsened prognosis and develops predominantly in pre-menopausal women, is characterized for the expression of specific basal-epithelium markers such as keratins (7). However, in clinical practice, cost-effective immunohistochemical methods are preferred to determine receptor presence, as such sub-typing, while providing prognostic information, also allow setting therapies to target specific oncogenic markers (**Table 1**). The anatomopathological absence of ER, PR, and HER2 led to the expression "triple negative" (TNBC), discerning cases devoid for all three markers (15). Worth noting, TNBC is somewhat regarded a surrogate for basal-like, as 70–80% overlap has been described between classifications (8, 16). In any case, while BC triage usually allows for adapted treatments improving prognosis in receptor-positive categories, that does not apply for TNBC cases, for which the lack of targeted approaches frequently restrict options to chemotherapy, with obvious consequences for the prognosis and lethality of the disease (17).

Interest on histone deacetylases (HDACs) is expanding as accumulated findings highlight their impact on regular physiology and pathological condition, staying SIRT1 the most studied (18). Sirtuins comprise a family of proteins (SIRT1–7) described as type III HDACs relying on NAD+ availability to perform a gatekeeping role in the configuration of the cell transcriptome, function that appears highly dependent on the cellular context and has been involved in a variety of biological processes, from modulating energy metabolism to development and cellular senescence (19–21). Intriguingly, Sirtuins in general and SIRT1 in particular display a paradoxical role in cancer, with histological studies showing increased or decreased expression patterns upon cancer origin and/or stage (22–24). In that sense, numerous contributions support the notion that SIRT1 activities influence hormone receptors (HR) actions, expressly those mediating long-term estrogenic effects in the mammary gland, namely the classic ERs, for which a relevant degree of interdependence between these factors has been described with apparent importance for BC onset and development. Moreover, interaction between the anew membrane-bound G-protein coupled estrogen receptor (GPER), which ubiquitously mediates short-term estrogenic effects, and SIRT1 has been also proposed, an interplay which could help fostering BC survivability and progression. Altogether, the conjoint actions of SIRT1 and HRs pose deep implications for BC onset and progression, which turn significantly relevant for the case of drug-resistant cases and conceivably HER2-enriched and TNBC. From that scope, this review synthetizes current knowledge on this emerging field.

KNOWN IMPLICATIONS OF SIRT1 FOR CANCER ONSET AND PROGRESSION

Initially described to deacetylate histones H1, H2, and H4 (18), SIRT1 is supposed to contribute to chromatin remodeling beneficial for tumor progression. However, despite obvious epigenetic capabilities, HDACs and SIRT1 current relevance for cancer strive on their now known ability to act on different substrates. SIRT1 is regarded an established modulator of significant non-histone nuclear proteins, such as p53, E2F1, or NF-kB (25, 26). SIRT1 overexpression has been related to tumor cell survival through the deacetylation and subsequent degradation of the p53 tumor suppressor (27, 28). Additionally, SIRT1 is known to deacetylate the FOXO family of transcription factors, resulting in repression of pro-apoptotic elements (29–31). In this line, using both hormone-responsive and TNBC models, MCF-7 and MDA-MB-231 cell lines respectively, SIRT1 has been found to localize to the promoters of silenced tumor suppressor genes, state reverted upon SIRT1 activity inhibition (32). Additionally, there is open debate on the ability of SIRT1 to act over cytosolic targets, with proposed tumorigenic implications related to PI3K/IGF-1R signaling (33, 34).

Moreover, SIRT1 shows a convoluted role in the regulation of the epithelial-mesenchymal transition (EMT) process, with apparent relevance in the case of reproductive tumors such as prostate and BC (35, 36). Notably, SIRT1 has been found to upregulate the expression of matrix-metalloproteinases in BC cells, condition known to promote invasiveness (37, 38). Moreover, SIRT1 activities seem to coordinate cancer stem cell-EMT changeover through deacetylation of a complex circuitry of transcription factors (39). To this regard, SIRT1 has been recently found to interact with Smad proteins, TGFß signaling canonical transducers (40). Interestingly, TGFß deregulation is regarded a cornerstone for EMT and tumor dispersion, among others markers, affecting the expression of matrix-metalloproteinases (4). While having a demonstrated role on the degradation of the inhibitory-Smad Smad7, SIRT1 has been also shown to relate with receptor-regulated Smads (Smad2 and Smad3), possibly coactivator-Smad Smad4 as well, in a process linked to altered transcriptional output (36, 40–42). Consequently, such interplay prompts for wide implications on cell transformation and tumor progression/dispersion.

ESTROGEN SIGNALING AND BREAST CANCER: THE ER PATHWAY

Among steroids, estrogens comprise a set of hormones involved in the development and maintenance of the female reproductive system, the main representative of which is 17ß-estradiol (E2),

TABLE 1 | Breast cancer anatomopathological surrogate definitions based on immunohistochemical subtyping methods.

Definition marker	Luminal A-like	Luminal B-like (HER2 negative)	Luminal B-like (HER2 positive)	HER2 positive (non-luminal)	Triple negative (ductal)
Erb-B2	–*	–*	+*	+*	–*
ER	+	+	+	–	–
PR	+	–/↓	+	–	–
Other relevant	Ki-67↓	Ki-67↑	Ki-67		Cytokeratins**
Prevalence	30∼70%	10∼20%		10∼20%	15∼25%
Main treatment strategy	Endocrine therapy	Endocrine therapy Cytotoxic		anti-HER2 Cytotoxic	Cytotoxic
Recurrence Risk	↓	↑		↓	↑↑
SIRT1		∼74%		∼55%	∼42%

*Concurrent marker detection is achieved for establishing subtypes. Not mentioned minor special histological types may respond to targeted therapies. Erb-B2, human epidermal growth factor receptor 2 (HER2); *overexpressed or amplified; ER, Estrogen Receptor; PR, Progesterone Receptor; Ki-67, proliferation marker; Cytokeratins, basal-like marker (8–14). **highly overexpressed; ↓low expression/risk; ↑high expression/risk; ↑↑very high expression/risk.*

constituting a major hormonal input along the monthly cycle. For its synthesis, androgens are converted into estrogens on the action of CYP19A1, known as Aromatase, an enzyme being mainly expressed in the ovaries but found in other tissues including the mammary gland (43). ERα and ERß correspond with the classic HRs responsible for E2 long-term effects (44). Both receptors, along with PR, integrate into the nuclear receptor family, which include sex steroids receptors as well as receptors for corticosteroids (45). Its members mostly localize to the nucleoplasm, but a minority of isoforms which help fine-modulating the overall response may also appear at alternate locations, involving a cytoplasmic-nuclear shuttling mechanism (46, 47). Although ERα and ERß share significant sequence homology, both receptors display unique expression patterns depending on either tissue or organ. ERα signaling comes crucial for the regulation of mammary gland development and function (44), also contributing to cancer onset and progression. Elevated ERα levels expressed in benign breast epithelium correlate with enhanced BC risk, whereas estrogen-dependent cancers require of E2 for cell survival and growth (44). Worth noting, PR positivity can be usually regarded a surrogate of ER positivity, as PR expression requires proper ER functioning to occur (48).

The principal ER activation mechanism requires E2 binding, which allows conformational changes promoting receptor dimerization and nuclear translocation to interact with estrogen response elements (ERE) present in the DNA to regulate transcription (44). Additionally, alternate mechanisms for ER activation and modulation had been described through cross-linking with signaling pathways like EGFR/PI3K/ERK, based on changes of ER phosphorylation status (49, 50). Upon landing on EREs, E2-ER complexes further recruit several co-activator proteins such as p300, PPARγ, and PGCα, which leads to histone acetylation and chromatin remodeling necessary for the regulation of transcription (51). Moreover, active ERα also recruit members of the FOXO family into transcriptomic complexes, interplay that has been characterized to greatly influence transcriptomic outcomes, with implications for mammary morphogenesis, BC onset and progression to drug resistant states (52–56).

At the clinic, hormone-responsive BC is usually managed in a straightforward manner due to the multiplicity of pharmacological approaches based in the use of Aromatase inhibitors along with selective ER modulators and downregulators, like Tamoxifen or Fulvestrant, which diminish ER-mediated E2-responses at the breast (57). Consequently, these cases are mostly associated with favorable prognosis. Still, hormone-responsive tumors frequently transform over time into an estrogen-independence status, gaining the ability to proliferate in the absence of hormonal input. This conversion usually becomes a critical step for BC clinical progression, as it is related to increased aggressiveness. In that sense, ER-negative cases at diagnosis are believed to have lost ERα expression over time due to gene silencing, thus reducing therapeutic options targeting HRs and thus associating with less favorable prognosis (58).

ESTROGEN SIGNALING AND BREAST CANCER: THE GPER PATHWAY

Despite the fact that classical HRs may be missing for some BC cases, however, it is now acknowledged that estrogen stimulation would still play a powerful role for the evolution of the disease through the actions of membrane-coupled ERs. Turning into the XXI century, the existence of a membrane-coupled ER was revealed, that would be responsible for most of E2 rapid physiological responses which at the time lacked of proper molecular explanation. This marker corresponded with a G-protein coupled receptor which could be located both at the endoplasmic reticulum and the plasmatic membranes (59, 60). Initial reports indicated that through its binding to E2, GPER actions resulted in cAMP and inositol triphosphate production, triggering intracellular calcium mobilization. However, it was rapidly established that its actions also resulted in the transactivation of diverse intracellular signaling cascades including MAP-Kinases, PI3K, or eNOS (61–63). In this line, further research also found GPER able to attune E2-mediated transcription regulation. This was established on co-expression experiments showing the existence of a functional cooperation between canonical-ERα-mediated and short-time-GPER-mediated signaling through a mechanism relying on the activation MAP-Kinases, capable of promoting post-translational modifications such as altering ERα phosphorylation status (64). Moreover, additional studies established GPER to be ubiquitously expressed through both reproductive and non-reproductive tissues (65), thus posing new challenges for the understanding of estrogen physiology. In that sense, it was not long before GPER was proposed to contribute for cancer development (61). Still, GPER's specific role for both neoplastic transformation and cancer progression remains unclear, as its actions seem to be highly depend on tissue origin (66). Yet, although anatomopathological studies on GPER expression are not included in routine clinical practices, in the case of estrogen-dependent tumors and especially BC, several works show that its altered expression can be associated with cancer progression, supporting a potential prognostic value (67–69).

At the molecular level, diverse studies advocate for GPER's ability to affect cancer cell survivability and proliferation, by influencing a myriad of signaling pathways responsible for cell cycle regulation or apoptosis control. They also play a role in the regulation of angiogenesis required for tumor nourishment and development [reviewed at (66)]. Moreover, GPER signaling has been proposed to distinctly affect cell migration and cancer invasiveness. Calpains are non-lysosomal proteases that are implicated in the regulation of cell adherence to the extracellular matrix and motility (70). Interestingly, it was reported that incubation of ER-negative BC cells with GPER agonists G-1 promoted Calpain-1 activity and altered adhesion to matrigel (71). Also in this line, GPER has been described to adjust EGFR/PI3K/ERK intracellular signaling, favoring expression changes of migration markers such as SNAIL or ß1-integrin, as well as altering plasticity of cellular adhesions by the activation of the focal adhesion kinase (FAK) (72). Conjointly, these abilities of GPER to promote viability and motility provide a molecular framework for estrogen stimulation of cancer cells despite ER-negativity. Notably, epidemiologic studies would deem clinical functionality to these capacities, as prevalence for GPER overexpression is found in HER2-enriched, basal-like and TNBC cases, also associated with both distant metastasis and recurrence (67, 73).

ESTROGEN SIGNALING AND BREAST CANCER: NOTED SIRT1 INFLUENCE

Numerous contributions support the notion that SIRT1 activities decisively impact HRs actions in relation to disease. With regard to classic ERs, in cellular models, E2 stimulation has been found to promote SIRT1 expression under direct influence of ERα transcriptomic complexes, observation matched by the prevalent detection of elevated levels for SIRT1 manifested for most of ERα-positive BC samples (74, 75). Interestingly, the ability of SIRT1 to interact with p300, PPARγ, and PGCα, ERα transcriptomic co-activators, has been proved to affect chromatin remodeling, disturbing developmental processes (76–78). Following studies found SIRT1 inhibition resulted in suppressed ERα expression, interfering with E2-dependent cell growth in healthy as well as malignant mammary epithelial cells (79, 80). In this line, inhibition of SIRT1 has been found to lessen ERα mediated repression of NRF2-dependent detoxifying enzymes in MCF-7 cells (81).

Simultaneously, significant efforts had been put to apprehend the effects of a less subtle SIRT1-ER interaction mechanism. Interestingly, ERα has been found to relate to and be a target for SIRT1. Upon E2-ERα activation, p300 stabilizes receptor complexes through acetylation in a process that can be reversed by SIRT1 (82). These findings initially suggested a SIRT1 inhibitory role over estrogen signaling. Still, changes in ERα acetylation status are considered to have limited effects (83). On the other hand, as previously mentioned, active ERα recruits FOXO family members into transcriptomic complexes, factors which also fall under SIRT1 spectrum of actions. Within the BC context, a recent report showed FOXN3 to be able to recruit SIRT1 into ERE-dependent transcriptomic complexes, promoting reduced transcriptomic output (84). Interestingly, alterations of FOXM1 and FOXO3a levels had been previously linked to SIRT1 aberrant activity, especially in TNBC (85).

Regarding the interaction between SIRT1 and GPER, knowledge is scarce. Nonetheless, using ER-negative HER2-enriched BC cells, it was recently described that E2 actions via GPER can result in SIRT1 overexpression through activation of the EGFR/ERK/c-fos/AP-1 transduction pathway (86). Interestingly, such induction contributed specifically to enhanced cancer cell survival and proliferation, as it was reversed by the use of SIRT1 inhibitors or GPER silencing as well. Notably, these effects were also observed in cancer associated fibroblast obtained from BC patients (86), posing challenging questions for this interplay in BC progression.

PRESENT AND FUTURE CLINICAL VALUE OF THE ESTROGEN SIGNALING/SIRT1 INTERPLAY

Finding ways to better screen and characterize BC, especially drug-resistant cases and TNBC, constitutes a standing challenge of cancer research. Efforts to establish a SIRT1 prognostic value for BC are increasing, as its overexpression can be commonly detected (9). Recent meta-analysis gathering non-connected data sources, while finding association with higher tumor stage, failed to detect correlation between SIRT1 expression levels and BC overall survival; however, these works addressed statistics letting out BC subtyping (87). Notwithstanding, a single retrospective study incorporating 822 BC patients found SIRT1 expression to correlate with tumor aggressiveness and reduced disease-free-survival (DFS) (88). Interestingly, when BC subtyping is considered, SIRT1 overexpression associates with ER-positivity and likely shortened DFS (9). Moreover, while not associated with HER2-enriched or TNBC status, concomitant SIRT1 overexpression successfully dictates for lymph-node metastasis likelihood (9), observation which has been linked to the ability of SIRT1 to promote an altered expression of key EMT markers such as E-Cadherin, Vimentin, and SNAIL-1 (89). Hence, although data so far may be considered insufficient or poorly curated,

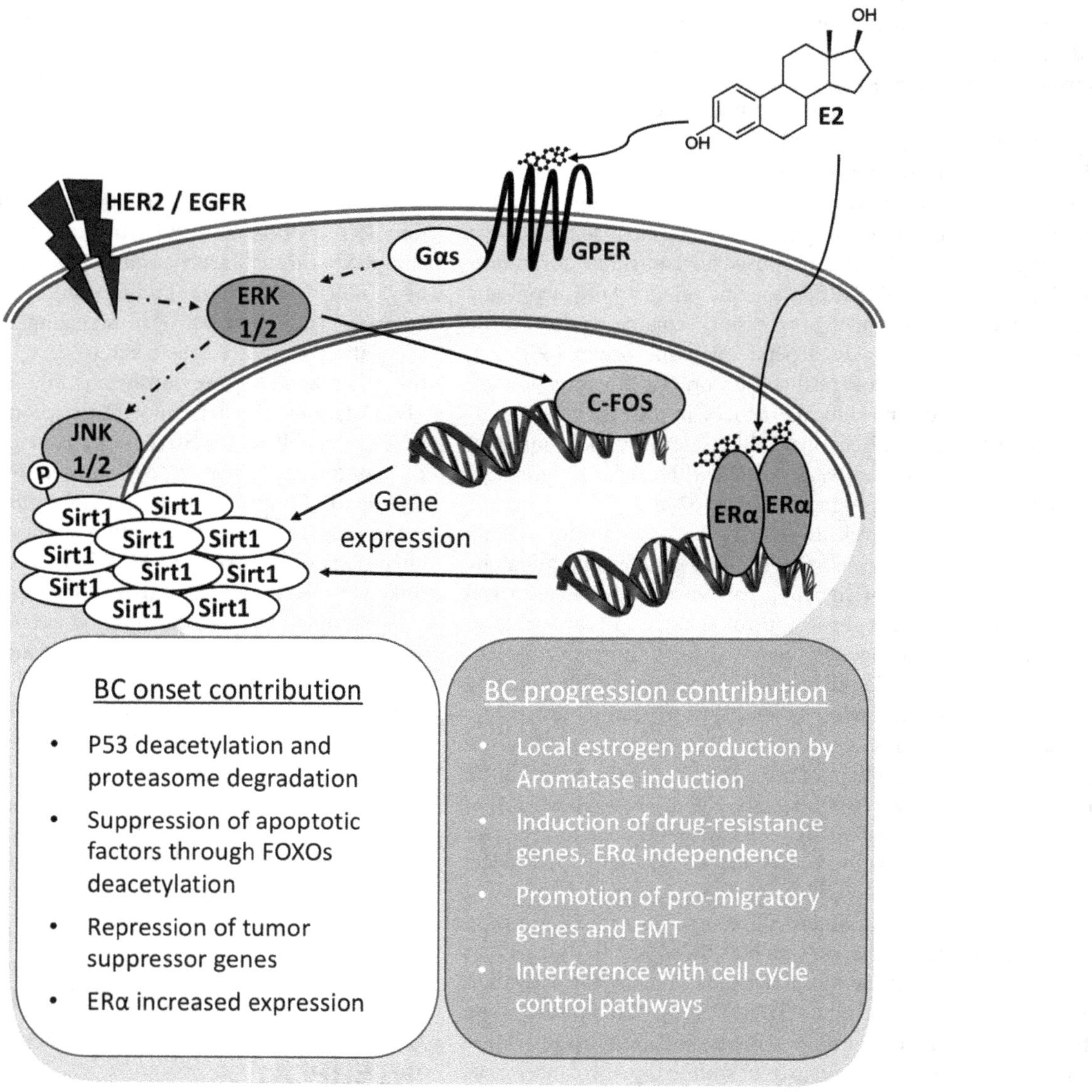

FIGURE 1 | Sirt1 overexpression contributes to Breast Cancer onset and progression. In breast cancer cells Sirt1 overexpression can be achieved independently through either nuclear (ERα) or membrane bound G-protein coupled estrogen receptor (GPER) signaling. Total activity is also modulated by phosphorylation status. Increased Sirt1 activities and interaction with diverse factors result in pleiotropic effects supporting cell survival and transformation for cancer onset. Continued activity contributes to cell de-differentiation and epithelium to mesenchyme transition (EMT).

the accumulated evidence allows to consider SIRT1 histological detection as a valuable marker for assessing BC status, also providing hints on metastasis and relapse odds.

Per BC tumor progression, it is speculated whether SIRT1 has a role in determining tumor conversion to a drug-refractory phenotype. It has been reported that SIRT1 activity helps increasing expression of drug-resistance genes (90), in a process that involves FOXO1 deacetylation and reverts upon SIRT1 suppression (91, 92). Noteworthy, SIRT1 activity is mainly regulated by upholding absolute protein levels with little variation overtime (35), although modulation of its actions depending on MAPK-mediated phosphorylation has been also described (93). To this extent, two considerations should be made. Firstly, it ought to be reminded that estrogen signaling via either HR can augment SIRT1 levels (74, 86). Interestingly, elevated SIRT1 levels has been reported to promote increased Aromatase activity both in ER-positive and TNBC cell lines (94), thereby allowing for local E2 production. Secondly, it should be noted that MAP-kinases signaling can be activated by overexpressed HER2 subunits dimerizing with EGFR and triggering the PI3K/ERK pathway (95). Consequently, a SIRT1 potential role assisting evolution to ER-independence turns reasonable, as deleterious abilities, including aberrant modulation of p53 and FOXO or expression of drug-resistance genes, could be maintained via SIRT1 overexpression depending on GPER signaling, perhaps also through MAP-kinases dependent activation. In that sense, recent reports showing linkage between SIRT1 overexpression and enhanced SRC and AKT activities in different TNBC cell lines would support the latter notion (96, 97). Worth considering as well, classic ERs and GPER display dissimilar behavior upon exposure to pharmaceutical modulators like Tamoxifen and Fulvestrant, which in the case of GPER appear to have an agonistic function (66). Moreover, in cellular models, GPER activation has been described to negatively affect ERα protein levels (71), perhaps fostering the transition. Hence, considering that solid tumors are composed by a clones plethora subject to selective pressure, it is tempting to propose the monitoring of SIRT1 expression/activity as source of information on the efficiency of treatments related to tumor evolution at the cellular scale. To this regard, procedures based on liquid-biopsy techniques would offer an appropriate framework for such approach (98).

On the aspect of treatments, many efforts had tried to assess the potential of suppressing SIRT1 activities. However, after several years, effects described on the many inhibitors discovered and interference studies do not agree with each other. This is regarded as the result of dissimilar mechanistic involved in knocking-out or knocking-down the enzymatic activity and also on the specificity of inhibitors used (99). Yet, modulators of SIRT1 activity may still retain potential as co-adjuvant treatments, due to sensitizing capabilities useful at specific BC environments (100). In this sense, sirtuins in general, and SIRT1 in particular, have been shown to interact with numerous signaling pathways which decisively affect different aspects of the cell physiology. That is the case with the recently described interaction of SIRT1 with TGFß canonical-signaling-transducers, the Smad proteins. SIRT1 has been found incorporated into Smad-mediated transcriptomic complexes, its activity linked to reduced Smad acetylation and decreased nuclear half-life (36, 40–42). Lack of proper TGFß response is considered a major mechanism for EMT through regulating the expression of key cell adherence and migration markers (4). Interestingly, this TGFß dependent regulation involves the participation of FOXO factors (101, 102). Hence, the overexpression of SIRT1 in BC cells has the potential to facilitate aberrant regulation through these system, thus contributing for the EMT process and cancer progression. Moreover, as signaling via GPER and HER2 are known to trigger MAP-Kinases activation, and activated MAP-Kinases had been related to SIRT1 augmented activity, this interplay provides an additional framework for the promotion of both tumor ER-independence and EMT progression, potentially offering opportunity to develop tailored strategies, which would come particularly useful for the case of TNBC. Perhaps, next-generation inhibitors, with better specificity and increased potency, may provide advancements in this field.

Finally, a brief but necessary mention should be made on non-coding RNAs. Increasing efforts attempt to discriminate the relevance of both long-non-coding and micro-RNAs in BC pathogenesis and progression, due to their dual role as an additional prognostic information source and potential therapeutic targets (103, 104). Not surprisingly, distinct signatures could be found in BC depending ER status (105). In that sense, exposure to either estrogens or selective ER modulators had been shown extensively affect through classic ERs the microRNA profile of different mammary cell lines (106). Interestingly, within the BC context, SIRT1 activity appears to be highly conditioned by the non-coding-RNA environment, with several long- and microRNA species affected by endocrine signaling being able to promote or downregulate its expression 107, 108). Further research in this area may again probe helpful for the development of strategies targeting intrinsic BC subtypes.

CONCLUDING REMARKS

The accumulated evidence prompts to consider SIRT1 as an integrated player into the transduction network activated by estrogens, both through ERs and GPER, in the mammary tissue (**Figure 1**). This tight cooperation conceptualizes and supports a SIRT1 promoting role in mammary tumorigenesis, with meaning for both disease onset and progression. These implications are to be considered both in the case of signaling triggered upon endogenous estrogens exposure, also in the case of exposure to environmental pollutants like xenoestrogens, phytoestrogens, and other synthetic compounds; let aside for the response to BC treatments based on estrogen modulators. Consequently, SIRT1 detection has potential to become a powerful prognostic indicator for tumor evolution and response to chemotherapeutics. Moreover, a better understanding at the molecular level of its cooperation and impact in the signaling through connected pathways may provide opportunity for the development of innovative therapy approaches in the assessment of BC and particularly TNBC cases.

AUTHOR CONTRIBUTIONS

SL conceptualized the work, performed searches in literature databases and prepared, reviewed and edited the original draft of the manuscript. JA-R contributed with formal analysis and the incorporation of clinical aspects, also reviewed the original draft. FN supervised the project, was responsible for funding acquisition and reviewed and edited the original draft. All authors read and approved the final manuscript.

ACKNOWLEDGMENTS

We are indebted to the Hospital Clínico Universitario Virgen de la Arrixaca that strongly supported this research.

REFERENCES

1. Jemal A, Bray F, Center MM, Ferlay J, Ward E, Forman D. Global cancer statistics. *CA Cancer J Clin.* (2011) 61:69–90. doi: 10.3322/caac.20107
2. Hindle WH. Hormone alterations in breast cancer: examining the hypotheses. *Medscape Womens Health.* (1999) 4:4.
3. Narod SA. Early-onset breast cancer: what do we know about the risk factors?: a countercurrents series. *Curr Oncol.* (2011) 18, 204–205. doi: 10.3747/co.v18i5.938
4. Velloso FJ, Bianco AF, Farias JO, Torres NE, Ferruzo PY, Anschau V, et al. The crossroads of breast cancer progression: insights into the modulation of major signaling pathways. *Onco Targets Ther.* (2017) 10:5491–524. doi: 10.2147/OTT.S142154
5. Folkerd E, Dowsett M. Sex hormones and breast cancer risk and prognosis. *Breast* (2013) 22 (Suppl. 2):S38–43. doi: 10.1016/j.breast.2013.07.007
6. Martin AM, Weber BL. Genetic and hormonal risk factors in breast cancer. *J Natl Cancer Inst.* (2000) 92:1126–35. doi: 10.1093/jnci/92.14.1126
7. Sorlie T, Perou CM, Tibshirani R, Aas T, Geisler S, Johnsen H, et al. Gene expression patterns of breast carcinomas distinguish tumor subclasses with clinical implications. *Proc Natl Acad Sci USA.* (2001) 98:10869–74. doi: 10.1073/pnas.191367098
8. Goldhirsch A, Winer EP, Coates AS, Gelber RD, Piccart-Gebhart M, Thurlimann B, et al. Personalizing the treatment of women with early breast cancer: highlights of the St Gallen International Expert Consensus on the Primary Therapy of Early Breast Cancer 2013. *Ann Oncol.* (2013) 24:2206–23. doi: 10.1093/annonc/mdt303
9. Chung YR, Kim H, Park SY, Park IA, Jang JJ, Choe JY, et al. Distinctive role of SIRT1 expression on tumor invasion and metastasis in breast cancer by molecular subtype. *Hum Pathol.* (2015) 46:1027–35. doi: 10.1016/j.humpath.2015.03.015
10. Voduc KD, Cheang MC, Tyldesley S, Gelmon K, Nielsen TO, Kennecke H. Breast cancer subtypes and the risk of local and regional relapse. *J Clin Oncol.* (2010) 28:1684–91. doi: 10.1200/JCO.2009.24.9284
11. Kumar N, Patni P, Agarwal A, Khan MA, Parashar N. Prevalence of molecular subtypes of invasive breast cancer: A retrospective study. *Med J Armed Forces India* (2015) 71:254–8. doi: 10.1016/j.mjafi.2015.04.006
12. Howlader N, Altekruse SF, Li CI, Chen VW, Clarke CA, Ries LA, et al. US incidence of breast cancer subtypes defined by joint hormone receptor and HER2 status. *J Natl Cancer Inst.* (2014) 106. doi: 10.1093/jnci/dju055
13. Cadoo KA, Fornier MN, Morris PG. Biological subtypes of breast cancer: current concepts and implications for recurrence patterns. *Q J Nucl Med Mol Imaging* (2013) 57:312–21.
14. Metzger-Filho O, Sun Z, Viale G, Price KN, Crivellari D, Snyder RD, et al. Patterns of Recurrence and outcome according to breast cancer subtypes in lymph node-negative disease: results from international breast cancer study group trials VIII and IX. *J Clin Oncol.* (2013) 31:3083–90. doi: 10.1200/JCO.2012.46.1574
15. Brenton JD, Carey LA, Ahmed AA, Caldas C. Molecular classification and molecular forecasting of breast cancer: ready for clinical application? *J Clin Oncol.* (2005) 23:7350–60. doi: 10.1200/JCO.2005.03.3845
16. Prat A, Adamo B, Cheang MC, Anders CK, Carey LA, Perou CM. Molecular characterization of basal-like and non-basal-like triple-negative breast cancer. *Oncologist* (2013) 18:123–33. doi: 10.1634/theoncologist.2012-0397
17. Venkitaraman R. Triple-negative/basal-like breast cancer: clinical, pathologic and molecular features. *Expert Rev Anticancer Ther.* (2010) 10:199–207. doi: 10.1586/era.09.189
18. Buler M, Andersson U, Hakkola J. Who watches the watchmen? Regulation of the expression and activity of sirtuins. *FASEB J.* (2016) 30:3942–60. doi: 10.1096/fj.201600410RR
19. Haigis MC, Sinclair DA. Mammalian sirtuins: biological insights and disease relevance. *Annu Rev Pathol.* (2010) 5:253–95. doi: 10.1146/annurev.pathol.4.110807.092250
20. Stunkel W, Campbell RM. Sirtuin 1 (SIRT1): the misunderstood HDAC. *J Biomol Screen* (2011) 16:1153–69. doi: 10.1177/1087057111422103
21. Martinez-Redondo P, Vaquero A. The diversity of histone versus nonhistone sirtuin substrates. *Genes Cancer* (2013) 4:148–63. doi: 10.1177/1947601913483767
22. Bosch-Presegue L, Vaquero A. The dual role of sirtuins in cancer. *Genes Cancer* (2011) 2:648–62. doi: 10.1177/1947601911417862
23. Nakagawa T, Guarente L. Sirtuins at a glance. *J Cell Sci.* (2011) 124:833–8. doi: 10.1242/jcs.081067
24. Simmons GE Jr, Pruitt WM, Pruitt K. Diverse roles of SIRT1 in cancer biology and lipid metabolism. *Int J Mol Sci.* (2015) 16:950–65. doi: 10.3390/ijms16010950
25. Michan S, Sinclair D. Sirtuins in mammals: insights into their biological function. *Biochem J.* (2007) 404:1–13. doi: 10.1042/BJ20070140
26. Yamamoto H, Schoonjans K, Auwerx J. Sirtuin functions in health and disease. *Mol Endocrinol.* (2007) 21:1745–55. doi: 10.1210/me.2007-0079
27. Luo J, Nikolaev AY, Imai S, Chen D, Su F, Shiloh A, et al. Negative control of p53 by Sir2alpha promotes cell survival under stress. *Cell* (2001) 107:137–48. doi: 10.1016/S0092-8674(01)00524-4
28. Ford J, Jiang M, Milner J. Cancer-specific functions of SIRT1 enable human epithelial cancer cell growth and survival. *Cancer Res.* (2005) 65:10457–63. doi: 10.1158/0008-5472.CAN-05-1923
29. Brunet A, Sweeney LB, Sturgill JF, Chua KF, Greer PL, Lin Y, et al. Stress-dependent regulation of FOXO transcription factors by the SIRT1 deacetylase. *Science* (2004) 303:2011–5. doi: 10.1126/science.1094637
30. Motta MC, Divecha N, Lemieux M, Kamel C, Chen D, Gu W, et al. Mammalian SIRT1 represses forkhead transcription factors. *Cell* (2004) 116:551–63. doi: 10.1016/S0092-8674(04)00126-6
31. Jiang S, Yang Z, Di S, Hu W, Ma Z, Chen F, et al. Novel role of forkhead box O 4 transcription factor in cancer: bringing out the good or the bad. *Semin Cancer Biol.* (2018) 50:1–12. doi: 10.1016/j.semcancer.2018.04.007
32. Pruitt K, Zinn RL, Ohm JE, Mcgarvey KM, Kang SH, Watkins DN, et al. Inhibition of SIRT1 reactivates silenced cancer genes without loss of promoter DNA hypermethylation. *PLoS Genet.* (2006) 2:e40. doi: 10.1371/journal.pgen.0020040
33. Byles V, Chmilewski LK, Wang J, Zhu L, Forman LW, Faller DV, et al. Aberrant cytoplasm localization and protein stability of SIRT1 is regulated by PI3K/IGF-1R signaling in human cancer cells. *Int J Biol Sci.* (2010) 6:599–612. doi: 10.7150/ijbs.6.599
34. Bai W, Zhang X. Nucleus or cytoplasm? The mysterious case of SIRT1's subcellular localization. *Cell Cycle* (2016) 15:3337–8. doi: 10.1080/15384101.2016.1237170
35. Byles V, Zhu L, Lovaas JD, Chmilewski LK, Wang J, Faller DV, et al. SIRT1 induces EMT by cooperating with EMT transcription factors and enhances prostate cancer cell migration and metastasis. *Oncogene* (2012) 31:4619–29. doi: 10.1038/onc.2011.612
36. Simic P, Williams EO, Bell EL, Gong JJ, Bonkowski M, Guarente L. SIRT1 suppresses the epithelial-to-mesenchymal transition in cancer metastasis and organ fibrosis. *Cell Rep.* (2013) 3:1175–86. doi: 10.1016/j.celrep.2013.03.019
37. Nakopoulou L, Tsirmpa I, Alexandrou P, Louvrou A, Ampela C, Markaki S, et al. MMP-2 protein in invasive breast cancer and the impact of MMP-2/TIMP-2 phenotype on overall survival. *Breast Cancer Res Treat.* (2003) 77:145–55. doi: 10.1023/A:1021371028777
38. Abdelmawgoud H, El Awady RR. Effect of Sirtuin 1 inhibition on matrix metalloproteinase 2 and Forkhead box O3a expression in breast cancer cells. *Genes Dis.* (2017) 4:240–6. doi: 10.1016/j.gendis.2017.11.001
39. Shi L, Tang X, Qian M, Liu Z, Meng F, Fu L, et al. A SIRT1-centered circuitry regulates breast cancer stemness and metastasis. *Oncogene* (2018). doi: 10.1038/s41388-018-0370-5
40. Garcia-Vizcaino EM, Liarte S, Alonso-Romero JL, Nicolas FJ. Sirt1 interaction with active Smad2 modulates transforming growth factor-beta regulated transcription. *Cell Commun Signal.* (2017) 15:50. doi: 10.1186/s12964-017-0205-y
41. Kume S, Haneda M, Kanasaki K, Sugimoto T, Araki SI, Isshiki K, et al. SIRT1 inhibits transforming growth factor beta-induced apoptosis in glomerular mesangial cells via Smad7 deacetylation. *J Biol Chem.* (2007) 282:151–8. doi: 10.1074/jbc.M605904200
42. Li J, Qu X, Ricardo SD, Bertram JF, Nikolic-Paterson DJ. Resveratrol inhibits renal fibrosis in the obstructed kidney: potential role in deacetylation of Smad3. *Am J Pathol.* (2010) 177:1065–71. doi: 10.2353/ajpath.2010.090923
43. Hilborn E, Stal O, Jansson A. Estrogen and androgen-converting enzymes 17beta-hydroxysteroid dehydrogenase and their involvement in cancer: with

a special focus on 17beta-hydroxysteroid dehydrogenase type 1, 2, and breast cancer. *Oncotarget* (2017) 8:30552–62. doi: 10.18632/oncotarget.15547
44. Burns KA, Korach KS. Estrogen receptors and human disease: an update. *Arch Toxicol.* (2012) 86:1491–504. doi: 10.1007/s00204-012-0868-5
45. Mangelsdorf DJ, Thummel C, Beato M, Herrlich P, Schutz G, Umesono K, et al. The nuclear receptor superfamily: the second decade. *Cell* (1995) 83:835–9. doi: 10.1016/0092-8674(95)90199-X
46. Levin ER, Hammes SR. Nuclear receptors outside the nucleus: extranuclear signalling by steroid receptors. *Nat Rev Mol Cell Biol.* (2016) 17:783–97. doi: 10.1038/nrm.2016.122
47. Schreihofer DA, Duong P, Cunningham RL. N-terminal truncations in sex steroid receptors and rapid steroid actions. *Steroids* (2018) 133:15–20. doi: 10.1016/j.steroids.2017.10.018
48. Nadji M, Gomez-Fernandez C, Ganjei-Azar P, Morales AR. Immunohistochemistry of estrogen and progesterone receptors reconsidered: experience with 5,993 breast cancers. *Am J Clin Pathol.* (2005) 123:21–7. doi: 10.1309/4WV79N2GHJ3X1841
49. Weigel NL, Zhang Y. Ligand-independent activation of steroid hormone receptors. *J Mol Med.* (1998) 76:469–79. doi: 10.1007/s0010900 50241
50. Cenni B, Picard D. Ligand-independent activation of steroid receptors: new roles for old players. *Trends Endocrinol Metab.* (1999) 10:41–6. doi: 10.1016/S1043-2760(98)00121-0
51. Sanchez R, Nguyen D, Rocha W, White JH, Mader S. Diversity in the mechanisms of gene regulation by estrogen receptors. *Bioessays* (2002) 24:244–54. doi: 10.1002/bies.10066
52. Bernardo GM, Lozada KL, Miedler JD, Harburg G, Hewitt SC, Mosley JD, et al. FOXA1 is an essential determinant of ERalpha expression and mammary ductal morphogenesis. *Development* (2010) 137:2045–54. doi: 10.1242/dev.043299
53. Millour J, Constantinidou D, Stavropoulou AV, Wilson MS, Myatt SS, Kwok JM, et al. FOXM1 is a transcriptional target of ERalpha and has a critical role in breast cancer endocrine sensitivity and resistance. *Oncogene* (2010) 29:2983–95. doi: 10.1038/onc.2010.47
54. Ross-Innes CS, Stark R, Teschendorff AE, Holmes KA, Ali HR, Dunning MJ, et al. Differential oestrogen receptor binding is associated with clinical outcome in breast cancer. *Nature* (2012) 481:389–93. doi: 10.1038/nature10730
55. Sanders DA, Ross-Innes CS, Beraldi D, Carroll JS, Balasubramanian S. Genome-wide mapping of FOXM1 binding reveals co-binding with estrogen receptor alpha in breast cancer cells. *Genome Biol.* (2013) 14:R6. doi: 10.1186/gb-2013-14-1-r6
56. Bergamaschi A, Madak-Erdogan Z, Kim YJ, Choi YL, Lu H, Katzenellenbogen BS. The forkhead transcription factor FOXM1 promotes endocrine resistance and invasiveness in estrogen receptor-positive breast cancer by expansion of stem-like cancer cells. *Breast Cancer Res.* (2014) 16:436. doi: 10.1186/s13058-014-0436-4
57. Early Breast Cancer Trialists' Collaborative Group, Davies C, Godwin J, Gray R, Clarke M, Cutter D, et al. Relevance of breast cancer hormone receptors and other factors to the efficacy of adjuvant tamoxifen: patient-level meta-analysis of randomised trials. *Lancet* (2011) 378:771–84. doi: 10.1016/S0140-6736(11)60993-8
58. Cleator S, Heller W, Coombes RC. Triple-negative breast cancer: therapeutic options. *Lancet Oncol.* (2007) 8:235–44. doi: 10.1016/S1470-2045(07)70074-8
59. Carmeci C, Thompson DA, Ring HZ, Francke U, Weigel RJ. Identification of a gene (GPR30) with homology to the G-protein-coupled receptor superfamily associated with estrogen receptor expression in breast cancer. *Genomics* (1997) 45:607–17. doi: 10.1006/geno.1997.4972
60. Filardo EJ, Quinn JA, Bland KI, Frackelton AR Jr. Estrogen-induced activation of Erk-1 and Erk-2 requires the G protein-coupled receptor homolog, GPR30, and occurs via trans-activation of the epidermal growth factor receptor through release of HB-EGF. *Mol Endocrinol.* (2000) 14:1649–60. doi: 10.1210/mend.14.10.0532
61. Filardo EJ. Epidermal growth factor receptor (EGFR) transactivation by estrogen via the G-protein-coupled receptor, GPR30: a novel signaling pathway with potential significance for breast cancer. *J Steroid Biochem Mol Biol.* (2002) 80:231–8. doi: 10.1016/S0960-0760(01)00190-X
62. Revankar CM, Cimino DF, Sklar LA, Arterburn JB, Prossnitz ER. A transmembrane intracellular estrogen receptor mediates rapid cell signaling. *Science* (2005) 307:1625–30. doi: 10.1126/science.1 106943
63. Bologa CG, Revankar CM, Young SM, Edwards BS, Arterburn JB, Kiselyov AS, et al. Virtual and biomolecular screening converge on a selective agonist for GPR30. *Nat Chem Biol.* (2006) 2:207–12. doi: 10.1038/nchembio775
64. Gao F, Ma X, Ostmann AB, Das SK. GPR30 activation opposes estrogen-dependent uterine growth via inhibition of stromal ERK1/2 and estrogen receptor alpha (ERalpha) phosphorylation signals. *Endocrinology* (2011) 152:1434–47. doi: 10.1210/en.2010-1368
65. Olde B, Leeb-Lundberg LM. GPR30/GPER1: searching for a role in estrogen physiology. *Trends Endocrinol Metab.* (2009) 20:409–16. doi: 10.1016/j.tem.2009.04.006
66. Jacenik D, Cygankiewicz AI, Krajewska WM. The G protein-coupled estrogen receptor as a modulator of neoplastic transformation. *Mol Cell Endocrinol.* (2016) 429:10–8. doi: 10.1016/j.mce.2016.04.011
67. Filardo EJ, Graeber CT, Quinn JA, Resnick MB, Giri D, Delellis RA, et al. Distribution of GPR30, a seven membrane-spanning estrogen receptor, in primary breast cancer and its association with clinicopathologic determinants of tumor progression. *Clin Cancer Res.* (2006) 12:6359–66. doi: 10.1158/1078-0432.CCR-06-0860
68. Ignatov T, Weissenborn C, Poehlmann A, Lemke A, Semczuk A, Roessner A, et al. GPER-1 expression decreases during breast cancer tumorigenesis. *Cancer Invest.* (2013) 31:309–15. doi: 10.3109/07357907.2013.789901
69. Aiad HA, Wahed MM, Asaad NY, El-Tahmody M, Elhosary E. Immunohistochemical expression of GPR30 in breast carcinoma of Egyptian patients: an association with immunohistochemical subtypes. *APMIS* (2014) 122:976–84. doi: 10.1111/apm.12241
70. Franco SJ, Huttenlocher A. Regulating cell migration: calpains make the cut. *J Cell Sci.* (2005) 118:3829–38. doi: 10.1242/jcs.02562
71. Chen Y, Li Z, He Y, Shang D, Pan J, Wang H, et al. Estrogen and pure antiestrogen fulvestrant (ICI 182 780) augment cell-matrigel adhesion of MCF-7 breast cancer cells through a novel G protein coupled estrogen receptor (GPR30)-to-calpain signaling axis. *Toxicol Appl Pharmacol.* (2014) 275:176–81. doi: 10.1016/j.taap.2014.01.005
72. Yuan J, Liu M, Yang L, Tu G, Zhu Q, Chen M, et al. Acquisition of epithelial-mesenchymal transition phenotype in the tamoxifen-resistant breast cancer cell: a new role for G protein-coupled estrogen receptor in mediating tamoxifen resistance through cancer-associated fibroblast-derived fibronectin and beta1-integrin signaling pathway in tumor cells. *Breast Cancer Res.* (2015) 17:69. doi: 10.1186/s13058-015-0579-y
73. Steiman J, Peralta EA, Louis S, Kamel O. Biology of the estrogen receptor, GPR30, in triple negative breast cancer. *Am J Surg.* (2013) 206:698–703. doi: 10.1016/j.amjsurg.2013.07.014
74. Elangovan S, Ramachandran S, Venkatesan N, Ananth S, Gnana-Prakasam JP, Martin PM, et al. SIRT1 is essential for oncogenic signaling by estrogen/estrogen receptor alpha in breast cancer. *Cancer Res.* (2011) 71:6654–64. doi: 10.1158/0008-5472.CAN-11-1446
75. Lee H, Kim KR, Noh SJ, Park HS, Kwon KS, Park BH, et al. Expression of DBC1 and SIRT1 is associated with poor prognosis for breast carcinoma. *Hum Pathol.* (2011) 42:204–13. doi: 10.1016/j.humpath.2010.05.023
76. Fulco M, Schiltz RL, Iezzi S, King MT, Zhao P, Kashiwaya Y, et al. Sir2 regulates skeletal muscle differentiation as a potential sensor of the redox state. *Mol Cell* (2003) 12:51–62. doi: 10.1016/S1097-2765(03)00226-0
77. Picard F, Kurtev M, Chung N, Topark-Ngarm A, Senawong T, Machado De Oliveira R, et al. Sirt1 promotes fat mobilization in white adipocytes by repressing PPAR-gamma. *Nature* (2004) 429:771–6. doi: 10.1038/nature02583
78. Rodgers JT, Lerin C, Haas W, Gygi SP, Spiegelman BM, Puigserver P. Nutrient control of glucose homeostasis through a complex of PGC-1alpha and SIRT1. *Nature* (2005) 434:113–8. doi: 10.1038/nature 03354
79. Yao Y, Li H, Gu Y, Davidson NE, Zhou Q. Inhibition of SIRT1 deacetylase suppresses estrogen receptor signaling. *Carcinogenesis* (2010) 31:382–7. doi: 10.1093/carcin/bgp308
80. Li H, Rajendran GK, Liu N, Ware C, Rubin BP, Gu Y. SirT1 modulates the estrogen-insulin-like growth factor-1 signaling for postnatal

development of mammary gland in mice. *Breast Cancer Res.* (2007) 9:R1. doi: 10.1186/bcr1632
81. Yao Y, Brodie AM, Davidson NE, Kensler TW, Zhou Q. Inhibition of estrogen signaling activates the NRF2 pathway in breast cancer. *Breast Cancer Res Treat* (2010) 124:585–91. doi: 10.1007/s10549-010-1023-8
82. Kim MY, Woo EM, Chong YT, Homenko DR, Kraus WL. Acetylation of estrogen receptor alpha by p300 at lysines 266 and 268 enhances the deoxyribonucleic acid binding and transactivation activities of the receptor. *Mol Endocrinol.* (2006) 20:1479–93. doi: 10.1210/me.2005-0531
83. Popov VM, Wang C, Shirley LA, Rosenberg A, Li S, Nevalainen M, et al. The functional significance of nuclear receptor acetylation. *Steroids* (2007) 72:221–30. doi: 10.1016/j.steroids.2006.12.001
84. Xu Z, Yang Y, Li B, Li Y, Xia K, Yang Y, et al. Checkpoint suppressor 1 suppresses transcriptional activity of ERalpha and breast cancer cell proliferation via deacetylase SIRT1. *Cell Death Dis.* (2018) 9:559. doi: 10.1038/s41419-018-0629-3
85. Lee JJ, Lee HJ, Son BH, Kim SB, Ahn JH, Ahn SD, et al. Expression of FOXM1 and related proteins in breast cancer molecular subtypes. *Int J Exp Pathol.* (2016) 97:170–7. doi: 10.1111/iep.12187
86. Santolla MF, Avino S, Pellegrino M, De Francesco EM, De Marco P, Lappano R, et al. SIRT1 is involved in oncogenic signaling mediated by GPER in breast cancer. *Cell Death Dis.* (2015) 6:e1834. doi: 10.1038/cddis.2015.201
87. Wang C, Yang W, Dong F, Guo Y, Tan J, Ruan S, et al. The prognostic role of Sirt1 expression in solid malignancies: a meta-analysis. *Oncotarget* (2017) 8:66343–51. doi: 10.18632/oncotarget.18494
88. Derr RS, Van Hoesel AQ, Benard A, Goossens-Beumer IJ, Sajet A, Dekker-Ensink NG, et al. High nuclear expression levels of histone-modifying enzymes LSD1, HDAC2 and SIRT1 in tumor cells correlate with decreased survival and increased relapse in breast cancer patients. *BMC Cancer* (2014) 14:604. doi: 10.1186/1471-2407-14-604
89. Jin MS, Hyun CL, Park IA, Kim JY, Chung YR, Im SA, et al. SIRT1 induces tumor invasion by targeting epithelial mesenchymal transition-related pathway and is a prognostic marker in triple negative breast cancer. *Tumour Biol.* (2016) 37:4743–53. doi: 10.1007/s13277-015-4231-3
90. Wang Z, Chen W. Emerging roles of SIRT1 in cancer drug resistance. *Genes Cancer* (2013) 4:82–90. doi: 10.1177/1947601912473826
91. Choi HK, Cho KB, Phuong NT, Han CY, Han HK, Hien TT, et al. SIRT1-mediated FoxO1 deacetylation is essential for multidrug resistance-associated protein 2 expression in tamoxifen-resistant breast cancer cells. *Mol Pharm.* (2013) 10:2517–27. doi: 10.1021/mp400287p
92. Jiang S, Li T, Yang Z, Hu W, Yang Y. Deciphering the roles of FOXO1 in human neoplasms. *Int J Cancer.* (2018). doi: 10.1002/ijc.31338
93. Sasaki T, Maier B, Koclega KD, Chruszcz M, Gluba W, Stukenberg PT, et al. Phosphorylation regulates SIRT1 function. *PLoS ONE* (2008) 3:e4020. doi: 10.1371/journal.pone.0004020
94. Holloway KR, Barbieri A, Malyarchuk S, Saxena M, Nedeljkovic-Kurepa A, Cameron Mehl M, et al. SIRT1 positively regulates breast cancer associated human aromatase (CYP19A1) expression. *Mol Endocrinol.* (2013) 27:480–90. doi: 10.1210/me.2012-1347
95. Harari D, Yarden Y. Molecular mechanisms underlying ErbB2/HER2 action in breast cancer. *Oncogene* (2000) 19:6102–14. doi: 10.1038/sj.onc.1203973
96. Tan J, Liu Y, Maimaiti Y, Wang C, Yan Y, Zhou J, et al. Combination of SIRT1 and Src overexpression suggests poor prognosis in luminal breast cancer. *Onco Targets Ther.* (2018) 11:2051–61. doi: 10.2147/OTT.S162503
97. Jin X, Wei Y, Xu F, Zhao M, Dai K, Shen R, et al. SIRT1 promotes formation of breast cancer through modulating Akt activity. *J Cancer* (2018) 9:2012–23. doi: 10.7150/jca.24275
98. Forte VA, Barrak DK, Elhodaky M, Tung L, Snow A, Lang JE. The potential for liquid biopsies in the precision medical treatment of breast cancer. *Cancer Biol Med.* (2016) 13:19–40. doi: 10.20892/j.issn.2095-3941.2016.0007
99. Hu J, Jing H, Lin H. Sirtuin inhibitors as anticancer agents. *Future Med Chem.* (2014) 6:945–66. doi: 10.4155/fmc.14.44
100. Fatehi D, Soltani A, Ghatrehsamani M. SRT1720, a potential sensitizer for radiotherapy and cytotoxicity effects of NVB-BEZ235 in metastatic breast cancer cells. *Pathol Res Pract.* (2018) 214:889–95. doi: 10.1016/j.prp.2018.04.001
101. Yang Z, Jiang S, Cheng Y, Li T, Hu W, Ma Z, et al. FOXC1 in cancer development and therapy: deciphering its emerging and divergent roles. *Ther Adv Med Oncol.* (2017) 9:797–816. doi: 10.1177/1758834017742576
102. Ma Z, Xin Z, Hu W, Jiang S, Yang Z, Yan X, et al. Forkhead box O proteins: crucial regulators of cancer EMT. *Semin Cancer Biol.* (2018)50: 21–31. doi: 10.1016/j.semcancer.2018.02.004
103. Graveel CR, Calderone HM, Westerhuis JJ, Winn ME, Sempere LF. Critical analysis of the potential for microRNA biomarkers in breast cancer management. *Breast Cancer* (2015) 7:59–79. doi: 10.2147/BCTT.S43799
104. Luqmani YA, Alam-Eldin N. Overcoming resistance to endocrine therapy in breast cancer: new approaches to a nagging problem. *Med Princ Pract.* (2016) 25(Suppl. 2):28–40. doi: 10.1159/000444451
105. Xiao B, Zhang W, Chen L, Hang J, Wang L, Zhang R, et al. Analysis of the miRNA-mRNA-lncRNA network in human estrogen receptor-positive and estrogen receptor-negative breast cancer based on TCGA data. *Gene* (2018) 658:28–35. doi: 10.1016/j.gene.2018.03.011
106. Klinge, C. M. miRNAs regulated by estrogens, tamoxifen, and endocrine disruptors and their downstream gene targets. *Mol Cell Endocrinol.* (2015) 418(Pt 3):273–97. doi: 10.1016/j.mce.2015.01.035
107. Liang Y, Song X, Li Y, Sang Y, Zhang N, Zhang H, et al. A novel long non-coding RNA-PRLB acts as a tumor promoter through regulating miR-4766-5p/SIRT1 axis in breast cancer. *Cell Death Dis.* (2018) 9:563. doi: 10.1038/s41419-018-0582-1
108. Karbasforooshan H, Roohbakhsh A, Karimi G. SIRT1 and microRNAs: the role in breast, lung and prostate cancers. *Exp Cell Res.* (2018) 367:1–6. doi: 10.1016/j.yexcr.2018.03.023

14

Insulin/IGF-1R, SIRT1 and FOXOs Pathways—An Intriguing Interaction Platform for Bone and Osteosarcoma

Consolato Sergi[1,2,3*†], Fan Shen[2†] and Song-Mei Liu[4†]

[1] Department of Orthopedics, Tianyou Hospital, Wuhan University of Science and Technology, Wuhan, China, [2] Department of Laboratory Medicine and Pathology, University of Alberta, Edmonton, AB, Canada, [3] Department of Pediatrics, Stollery Children's Hospital, Edmonton, AB, Canada, [4] Center for Gene Diagnosis, Zhongnan Hospital of Wuhan University, Wuhan, China

***Correspondence:**
Consolato Sergi
sergi@ualberta.ca
orcid.org/0000-0002-2779-7879

†Fan Shen
orcid.org/0000-0001-7432-8891
Song-Mei Liu
orcid.org/0000-0001-9276-6078

Aging is a substantial risk factor for the development of osteoarthritis (OA) and, probably, an essential substrate for the development of neoplastic disease of the bone, such as osteosarcoma, which is the most common malignant mesenchymal primary bone tumor. Genetic studies have established that the insulin/insulin-like growth factor 1 (IGF-1)/phosphatidylinositol-3 kinase (PI3K)/AKT (Protein Kinase B) signal transduction pathway is involved across species, including nematodes, fruit flies, and mammals. SIRT1, a phylogenetically-conserved family of deacetylases, seems to play pleiotropic effects in epithelial malignancies of the liver and interact with the IGF-1/PI3K/AKT signal transduction pathway. Some of the most critical processes in degenerative conditions may indeed include the insulin/IGF1R and SIRT1 signaling pathways as well as some specific transcription factors. The Forkhead box O (FOXO) transcription factors (FOXOs) control diverse cellular functions, such as metabolism, longevity, and cell death. FOXOs play a critical role in the IGF-1/PI3K/AKT signal transduction pathway. FOXOs can indeed be modulated to reduce age-related diseases. FOXOs have advantageous inhibitory effects on fibroblast and myofibroblast activation, which are accompanied by a subsequent excessive production of extracellular matrix. FOXOs can block or decrease the fibrosis levels in numerous organs. Previously, we observed a correlation between nuclear FOXO3 and high caspase-8 expression, which induces cellular apoptosis in response to harmful external stimuli. In this perspective, we emphasize the current advances and interactions involving the insulin/IGF1R, SIRT1, and FOXOs pathways in the bone and osteosarcoma for a better understanding of the mechanisms potentially underpinning tissue degeneration and tumorigenesis.

Keywords: IGF1, FOXO, SIRT1, signaling pathways, bone, osteosarcoma

INTRODUCTION

Aging is a substantial risk factor for the development of inflammatory conditions, such as osteoarthritis (OA) and, probably, other degenerative, and neoplastic diseases of the bone, such as Paget disease of the bone and osteosarcoma (1, 2). Some growth factors linked to cartilage repair following damage in animal models have been considered to increase the risk of neoplasia (3–7). In this paper, we review the insulin/IGF1R, SIRT1, and FOXOs signaling pathways and emphasize the interaction involving these crucial factors in the bone physiology and oncogenesis, with regard to osteosarcoma, which is considered the most common mesenchymal malignant primary tumor of the skeletal system.

INSULIN/IGF1R SIGNALING PATHWAY

The insulin/IGF-1 signaling system (IIS) is the route that regulates not only the organism's metabolism, but also the growth, development, and longevity concerning the availability status of nutrients. It is an ancient system. In fact, it is highly conserved across species. In invertebrates, e.g., in the worm *C. elegans*, the IIS system begins with the secretion of numerous, insulin-like peptides in reply to food or, ultimately, to the sensory perception of food. These insulin-like ligands can connect to a single (common) receptor, called the insulin/IGF-1 like tyrosine kinase receptor or *dauer* formation 2 (DAF-2). In the 1990s, two DAF genes, DAF-2, and DAF-16, were discovered after isolating *dauer-constitutive* (DAF-c) mutants and *dauer-defective* mutants (DAF-d). The worm *C. elegans*, under conditions of high population density and low food, forms an alternative 3rd larval stage, called the *dauer* stage. This stage is resistant to dehydration and harsh environments (8). The *C. elegans* genome encodes AGE-1 adaptor protein (AAP-1), a single PI3K adaptor subunit, and a putative IRS homolog, i.e., the adaptor protein or insulin receptor substrate (IST-1) homolog (9). After the ligand binds, the signal is progressively transduced from the activated receptor to AGE-1, which is a phosphatidylinositol 3-kinase either directly or using the adaptor protein called IST-1 (9). The phosphatidylinositol 3-kinase AGE-1 changes the phospholipid PIP2 into the second messenger PIP3. Subsequently, the increased level of PIP3 initiates the 3-phosphoinositide-dependent protein kinase 1 (PDK1) and the protein kinases B1 and B2 (PKB1 and PKB2). Ultimately, it leads to the phosphorylation of the DAF-16 molecule, which causes its extrusion from the nucleus to the cytoplasm (10). DAF-18, a homolog of the mammalian phosphatase and tensin homolog (PTEN), can dephosphorylate PIP3 to PIP2. Gene mutations in daf-2 and kinase components of the IIS pathway harboring reduction of functional significance can extend the life span of the worm. Conversely, mutations harboring the same meaning but in daf-18 abolish the life-span extension of daf-2 and age-1 mutants. The downstream targets of DAF-16 include metabolic genes, cellular stress response genes, and genes encoding antimicrobial peptides (11, 12). The fruit fly (*Drosophila melanogaster*) shows powerful similarities to *C. elegans* about the IIS pathway. In the fruit fly, multiple extracellular ligands are binding to a single tyrosine kinase receptor, which is a transmembrane protein, the insulin/IGF-1 common receptor. The binding of the ligands to the common receptor promotes some intracellular phosphorylation events that end in the phosphorylation and nuclear extrusion of dFOXO. In the fruit fly, several indirect losses of function gene mutations have been linked to an enhancement of the life span, such as the insulin receptor and its substrate. These events are particularly pronounced in the female fruit fly. In mammals, the core of the insulin/IGF-1 signaling path is preserved, but there is an increase in complexity moving from invertebrates to vertebrates. Specifically, there are three different ligand molecules of insulin/IFG-1 receptor in mammals. They include insulin, IGF-1, and IGF-2. Also, there are three diverse mammalian insulin/IGF tyrosine kinase receptors, including insulin receptor (IR), IGF-1 receptor (IGF-1R), and the so-called orphan IR related receptor (IRR). An orphan receptor is a protein that harbors a structure similar to other identified receptors but whose endogenous ligand has not yet been discovered. Following the ligand binding, the activated IGF-1 or insulin receptor starts the phosphorylation of numerous intracellular substrates. The phosphorylated substrates give precise docking sites for intracellular effectors. These sites include the growth-factor-receptor-bound protein-2 (Grb2) and the p85 regulatory subunit of PI-3K. Eventually, it leads to the activation of two major signaling pathways, which are the Ras-MAPK pathway and the PI-3K-PKB/AKT pathway. The former path (PI-3K-PKB/AKT) has been shown to regulate most of the metabolic effects of insulin/IGF-1 signaling (13). The latter pathway (Ras-MAPK) gave evidence of the regulation of most of the effects (mitogenic) of insulin/IGF-1 signaling. Also, most of the crucial components of the insulin/IGF-1 signaling cascade show some further complexity in mammals, because different forms have been revealed that are encoded by several genes and/or isoforms determined by a single gene.

SIRT1 SIGNALING PATHWAY

In mammals, Sirtuins constitute a family of NAD+-dependent deacetylases (14–19). Seven members (SIRT1–SIRT7) are included in this family. All of them share the conserved Sirtuin domain conferring NAD+-dependent deacetylase activity (20). However, they also have different amino- and carboxy-terminal extensions. Also, they display distinct subcellular localization and biological functions. Although SIRT1 is predominantly located in the nucleus, it transfers between the nucleus and the cytoplasm during the ontogenesis and in response to physiological stress and pathological conditions. If SIRT1 is located in the nucleus, different is the situation for SIRT2, SIRT3, SIRT4, and SIRT5. The proteins SIRT3 through SIRT5 are located in the mitochondria, while SIRT2 is mostly identified in the cytoplasm. Like SIRT1, SIRT6, and SIRT7 are localized in the nucleus. The former is a chromatin-associated protein, while the latter is found in the nucleolus. In mammals, deacetylase activity was reported as conserved, but the acyl group preference is different according to the Sirtuins with SIRT4-7 harboring a weak or, probably, undetectable deacetylase activity *in vitro* (21–23). An efficient demyristoylase activity is found in SIRT2, while SIRT5 has a demalonylase and lysine desuccinylase activities associated with an adequate and efficient NAD+-dependent protein. SIRT4 and SIRT6 harbor ADP-ribosyltransferase activity. In mammals, Sirtuins are crucial in regulating a broad variety of cellular processes, including metabolism, oxidative/anti-oxidative balance, mitochondrial homeostasis, autophagy, and apoptosis as well as pathological conditions, such as inflammation. SIRT1 has been proved to repress inflammation in multiple cells and tissues (24–26). Moreover, there is an important contribution of Sirtuins in aging and aging-related diseases, such as obesity, type 2 diabetes mellitus (T2DM), cardiovascular disease, neurodegenerative diseases, and cancer (16, 17). Most probably, SIRT1 (and SIRT6 for certain aspects) is the most extensively characterized proteins of this class. In several species and across species, the nuclear factor kappa-light-chain-enhancer of activated B cells (NF-κB) remains a chief transcriptional factor in cellular physiology. NF-κB is a complex that panels the transcription of DNA, production of several cytokines, and, ultimately, cell survival. In the cell, NF-κB is tangled in responses to stimuli such as stress, free radicals, cytokines, but also bacterial or viral antigens as well as heavy metals, ultraviolet irradiation, oxidized lipoproteins. NF-κB mediates the expression of multiple inflammatory factors, including IL-1β, IL-6, and TNF-α. The nuclear translocation and activation of NF-κB rely on its acetylation. SIRT1 deacetylates NF-κB (p65 subunit) at lysine 310 (K310). It inhibits the transcriptional activity of NF-κB. A co-repressive action has also been identified with transducing-like enhancer of split 1 (TLE1). SIRT1 interacts with TLE1 to inhibit NF-κB-mediated transcription and suppress inflammation (27, 28). Other two actions of the SIRT1 are well-known and include (1) the deacetylation of activator protein-1 (AP-1) able to decrease the expression of cyclooxygenase 2 (COX-2) in macrophages and (2) the deacetylation of TP53 to repress macrophage activation. Sirtuins significantly contribute to their functions on insulin resistance. The activation of SIRT1 leads to the repression of c-Jun N-terminal kinases (JNKs) and inhibitor of NF-κB kinase subunit beta (IKK-β) inflammatory pathways substantially. JNKs were initially discovered as kinases that bind and phosphorylate c-Jun on Ser-63 and Ser-73 (two serine amino acid residues) within its transcriptional activation domain (29, 30). They are a member of the mitogen-activated protein kinase (MAPK) family and are responsive to stress stimuli. IKK- β is a protein that in humans is encoded by the gene labeled inhibitor of kappa light polypeptide and gene enhancer in B-cells, kinase beta (IKBKB). SIRT1 improves glucose tolerance, reduced hyperinsulinemia, and enhanced systemic insulin sensitivity and Sirtl controls specifically the inflammatory status of macrophages and T lymphocytes regulating the metabolism and that of adipose tissues in obese mice (31, 32). Besides, SIRT1 promotes mitochondrial biogenesis by deacetylating the peroxisome proliferator-activated receptor and gamma coactivator 1-alpha (PGC-1α), which is a transcriptional coactivator that regulates mitochondrial biogenesis and respiration. SIRT1 activator resveratrol induces PGC-1α increasing the number of mitochondria, and this may have a beneficial effect in T2DM patients, who have fewer mitochondria in the muscle than insulin-sensitive individuals. SIRT1 activator resveratrol inducing PGC-1α activity protects mice against diet-induced obesity and insulin resistance (33–35). Mitochondria biogenesis is found in a balance with the clearance of damaged mitochondria (mitophagy or mitochondria autophagy). SIRT1 binds to and deacetylates autophagy (ATG) regulators (e.g., ATG5, ATG7, and ATG8) to promote mitophagy (29, 36–39). SIRT1 also deacetylates Forkhead box protein O1 (FoxO1) and Forkhead box protein O3a (FoxO3a). Both deacetylations induce the expression of elements of the autophagy machinery. The deacetylation and activation of FoxO3a upregulate the expression of MnSOD and catalase, which is an enzyme detected in almost all living organisms exposed to O_2. Catalase catalyzes the decomposition of hydrogen peroxide (H_2O_2) to water and O_2. Calatase plays a major role in protecting the cell from oxidative damage by reactive oxygen species (ROS). Finally, SIRT1 promotes the transcriptional activity of Nuclear factor (erythroid-derived 2)-like 2 (NRF2). SIRT1 acts in this way by deacetylating it. SIRT1 upregulates the expression of NRF2 target antioxidant genes, including mitochondrial antioxidant manganese superoxide dismutase (MnSOD), catalase, heme oxygenase-1 (HO-1), and glutathione (29, 40, 41). Overall, Sirtuins are histone deacetylases that are crucial in regulating organismal lifespan as well as oxidative stress and DNA damage.

FOXOS SIGNALING PATHWAY—GENERAL REMARKS

An impressive class of transcription factors for cancer therapeutic modulation is represented by the forkhead box transcription factors (FOXO) family. FOXOs or FOXO proteins are growth factors and stress-related factors. These transcription factors naturally reside in the nucleus of cells and function as regulators of gene transcription. FOXO proteins may be transferred to the cytoplasm and go through degradation of the ubiquitin-proteasome pathway (UPP), which is the chief mechanism for protein catabolism in the mammalian cell. Following translation of the mRNA into proteins, and no cellular survival initiative of growth factors, FOXOs translocate to the nucleus upregulating a series of target genes of the cell cycle, stress resistance, and longevity. FOXOs regulate numerous cellular functions, and these functions include cellular differentiation, cellular proliferation, DNA damage, apoptosis, DNA repair, and oxidative stress modulation (42–45). These very delicate functions indicate how dysregulation of the FOXOs may implicate abnormal cellular and tissue physiology, tumorigenesis, and neoplastic progression. Different from most common transcription regulators, such as extracellular signal-regulated kinase (ERK), which are located in the cytoplasm where kinases are phosphorylated and translocated into the nucleus, FOXOs are transcription factors with a nuclear location. Growth factor pathways endorse the nuclear exclusion and translocation of phosphorylated FOXO to the cytoplasm. In the cytosol, the phosphorylated FOXO is subjected to degradation via the UPP. The founding member of the FOX family is the forkhead transcription factor of the forkhead box (FOX) family in the fruit fly *Drosophila melanogaster*, of which a mutation in Foxo genes results in defective head shrinkage. The forkhead box is a conserved domain, which has been described due to a butterfly-like appearance on nuclear magnetic resonance and X-ray crystallography. This domain consists of three α-helices and three β-sheets that are accompanied with two loops usually referred to like the wings. In invertebrates, there is only one FOXO gene, termed dFOXO in the fruit fly and daf-16 in the worm. Conversely, there are four FOXO genes, FOXO1, 3, 4, and 6 in mammals. In the mammals, forkhead transcription factors of the O class, i.e., FOXO1, FOXO3, FOXO4, and FOXO6 proteins, play a paramount role in the usual functional complexity of the cell, its proliferation, differentiation, and death as well as in the progression of several diseases. FOXO1 is a transcription factor that plays crucial roles in the regulation of gluconeogenesis and glycogenolysis by insulin signaling and is also vital to the decision for a preadipocyte to commit to adipogenesis. In mammals, FOXO localization at the subcellular level is exquisitely controlled by post-translational modifications, including ubiquitination, phosphorylation, and acetylation (29, 44–52). During development and tumorigenesis, the protein kinase B (AKT) path plays a significant role in cell growth and survival. AKT is activated by AKT kinase PDK1/2. AKT kinase PDK1/2 is considered to be a downstream target kinase of phospholipid kinase phosphatidylinositol 3-kinase (PI3K). In mammals, there are three isoforms which are determined by distinct loci. FOXOs are proteins active in growth factor signaling. In the pathway, they are positioned downstream of AKT. In addition to AKT, there are negative regulators of FOXOs, including the casein kinase 1 (CK1), dual-specificity tyrosine-phosphorylation-regulated kinase 1A (DYRK1A), serum and glucocorticoid-regulated kinase (SGK), IκB kinase (IKK), and the ubiquitous ERK. Other kinases, which control FOXOs are c-Jun N-terminal kinase (JNK) and mammalian ste20-like kinase (MST1) which act under circumstances of elevated oxidative stress. In the last few years, it has been suggested how FOXO regulation may contribute to fibrosis of several organs (42). In particular, FOXO1/3 have been demonstrated to have promising inhibitory effects on fibroblast activation and extracellular matrix production improving the degree of fibrosis levels in several organs, including the heart, kidney, liver, and lung (42). FOXOs have been cataloged to be tumor suppressors due to their antiproliferative and pro-apoptotic actions, despite some data revealed unpredicted functions of FOXOs in the advancement of cancer and in modifying responses to cancer treatment (49). A complex array of posttranslational modifications regulates FOXO transcriptional activity. These posttranslational modifications can be either activating or inactivating. These modifications alter modify the DNA binding affinity, nuclear import and export, and alter the pattern of transcriptional activity for specific target (53). FOXO factors play a crucial role in cell fate decision.

FOXO AND BONE

In a concerted fashion, bone is continuously degraded and replaced by the action of operating cells toward growth and operating cells toward remodeling. The builder cells are the osteoblasts, while the refining cells are the osteoclasts. This process of regeneration is active throughout the entire life of a vertebrate organism and is also present during tumorigenesis. Neoplasm is intrinsically linked to inflammation, and this aspect is not only relevant to the liver, where parasitic cholangitis can evolve to cancer, but it is a phenomenon across several organs and structures, including the skeletal system (54). Osteoclasts, which are short-lived giant multinucleated cells, arise from the fusion of myeloid lineage progenitor cells. They are under the influence of macrophage colony-stimulating factor (M-CSF) and the receptor activator of nuclear κ-B ligand (RANKL) and their respective receptors (55). The action of proteolytic enzymes and hydrogen ions (H^+) on the mineralized bone matrix evolves along all life of an individual. The "podosome belt" that tightly adheres to the bone area targeted for removal relies on a polarized secretion of proteolytic enzymes and H^+ ions (56–58). In the skeleton of an adult individual, bone mass is maintained, but the process is more complicated than thought initially. The maintenance of the bone mass requires the activity of both the re-absorption process and the re-apposition process. Thus, the resorption process is regulated by the osteoclast, while the deposition of new bone relies on osteoblasts. Human pathology and aging determine an imbalance between bone deposition and resorption. Conversely, osteoblasts are short-lived mesenchymal cells derived from bone progenitor cells that express the osteoblast identifying transcriptions factors RUNX2 and OSTERIX1 (59–62). FOXOs repress proliferation of OSTERIX1+ committed osteoblast precursors by inhibiting the canonical Wnt/β-catenin signaling (59). The osteoblasts are responsible for the deposition of osseous matrix (osteoid) in the bony tissue spaces emptied by the osteoclasts. One of the critical aspects of bone remodeling is played by the Wnt signaling (63). The WNT proteins present in the extracellular space bind to receptor frizzled and coreceptor lipoprotein-like receptor protein (LRP) 5/6 present on the cell surface of mesenchymal progenitors. The Wnt-frizzled and Wnt-LRP 5/6 binding triggers an intracellular set of events, which culminates in the release of β-catenin from a proteasomal degradation complex, its translocation into the nucleus, and subsequent binding T-cell factor/lymphoid enhancer factor (TCF/LEF) transcription factors. This bond β-catenin—TCF/LEF can activate or suppress the expression of Wnt target genes (64). Although most of the osteoblasts once finished their function die by apoptosis, a subgroup of them will incorporate in the bone matrix becoming long-lived dendritic cells called osteocytes. The osteocytes are a strong pillar in bone remodeling by producing RANKL and sclerostin, which are essential for both bone resorption and deposition, respectively (65).

The FOXO1, 3, and 4 proteins are critical for bone development, and the control of bone mass in both physiology and pathology (**Figure 1**). FOXOs are essential regulators of osteoclast differentiation and bone resorption by decreasing the ROS (66). The loss of all FOXO1, 3, and 4 in osteoclast progenitors does increase proliferation, osteoclast formation, and bone resorption, which lead to reduced trabecular and cortical bone mass. Contrarywise, gain-of-function of FOXO3 inhibits bone resorption by osteoclast differentiation. This aspect results by an increase of the expression of catalase, as an example of antioxidant enzymes able to impede H_2O_2 (66). The accumulation of ROS is due to RANKL, which decrease the levels and activity of FOXO1, 3, and 4 via AKT-mediated phosphorylation and proteasomal degradation (66–69). FOXOs also excite heme oxygenase-1 (HO-1) to be expressed in osteoclast progenitors. Furthermore, macrophages are the site where HO-1 catabolizes heme and attenuates oxidative phosphorylation and ATP production in mitochondria

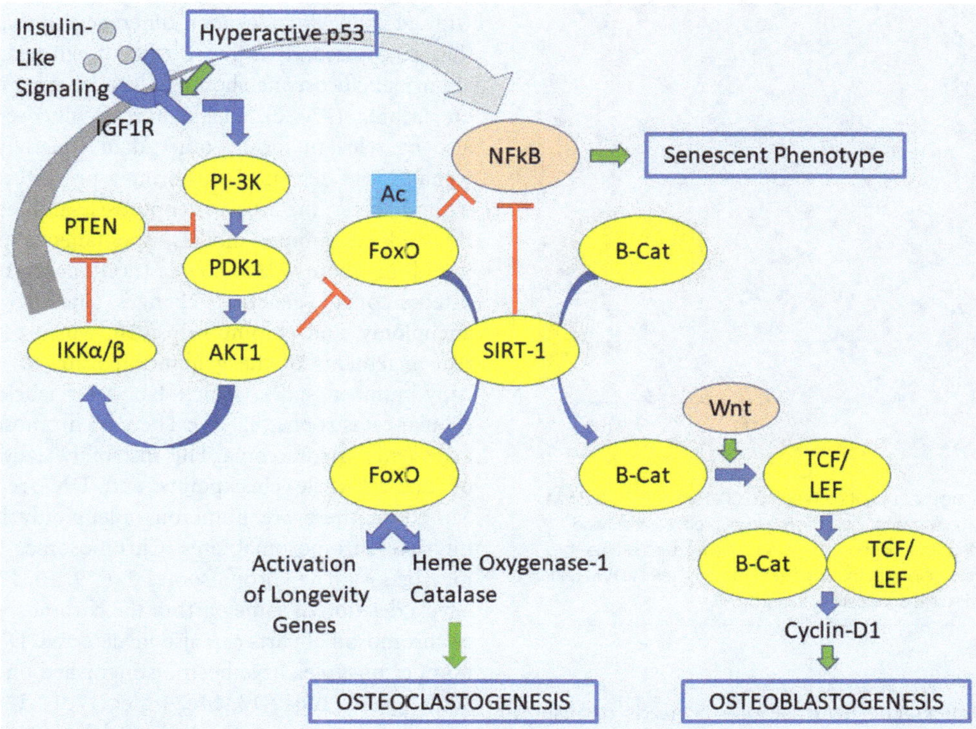

FIGURE 1 | Signaling pathways contemplating insulin-like signaling/IGFR1, FOXOs, and SIRT1 for the osteoclastogenesis and osteoblastogenesis. In this original picture is also depicted the occurrence of a hyperactive p53. A hyperactive p53 would be a condition leading to osteosarcoma-genesis. The abbreviations of this figure are shown in the text and please see the text for details.

(70). Overall, HO-1 contributes to the anti-osteoclastogenic effects of FOXOs. Further, FOXOs act directly to reduce the osteoblastogenesis by restraining Wnt signaling in which FOXOs bind to and sidetrack β-catenin away from TCF/LEF-mediated transcription. Consequently, there is a decrease in cyclin D1 and cell proliferation, and finally bone mass (59). However, FOXOs seems also to promote survival of osteoblasts by increasing the expression of catalase and superoxide dismutase, two major antioxidant enzymes, preventing oxidative cellular stress (71, 72). Also, FOXO1 promotes the accumulation of glutathione, a peptide that reduces ROS due to its redox-active sulfhydryl moieties. There is also a paracrine mechanism, but details of this process are still missing. The anti-osteoclastogenic actions of FOXOs are probably due to stimulation of osteoprotegerin (OPG), which is the decoy receptor for RANKL (59, 73).

MOLECULAR INTERACTION BETWEEN IGF-1, SIRT1, AND FOXOS

The PI3K-PKB/AKT pathway is the canonical pathway regulating the transcriptional activity of FOXOs. While FOXOs and SIRT1 add conceptually to the longevity of the bone through an equilibrated balance of bone formation and bone remodeling, the action related to IGF1 and IGF-R1 may act in the opposite direction. SIRT1 mediates posttranslational modifications of FOXOs and seems to prevent bone resorption and stimulate bone formation. Multiple kinases can modulate FOXOs through phosphorylation, and post-translational changes may work influencing FOXO activity. These modifications include methylation, ubiquitination, acetylation, PARylation, glycosylation, and hydroxylation. Poly ADP-ribosylation (PARylation) is a highly dynamic post-translation protein modification at DNA lesions, which is catalyzed by poly (ADP-ribose) polymerases (74). The accumulation of FOXOs in the nucleus determines its binding to various transcription-cofactors regulating the transcription of genes involved in the cell cycle, apoptosis, metabolism, redox homeostasis, angiogenesis, and GFR signaling. As seen that insulin-like signaling leads to PI(3)K activation, this tie induces AKT to inhibit FOXO by phosphorylation. Also, the human tumor suppressor PTEN inhibits AKT activity, conceivably by phosphorylation of PIP3. In the setting of oxidative stress, cells with high AMP/ATP ratios determine an increase of JNK and AMPK. Both kinases activate FOXOs by phosphorylation, and the active form of FOXOs relocates to the nucleus. Once in the nucleus, it promotes the expression of genes that promote longevity (75). Oxidative stress activates JNK with the consequence to increase the FOXOs activity. Subsequently, FOXOs reduces both WNT signaling and insulin-like signaling (ILS). The decreased Wnt signaling leads to protein aggregation, which involves the early cell degeneration with the formation of abnormal exocellular bodies,

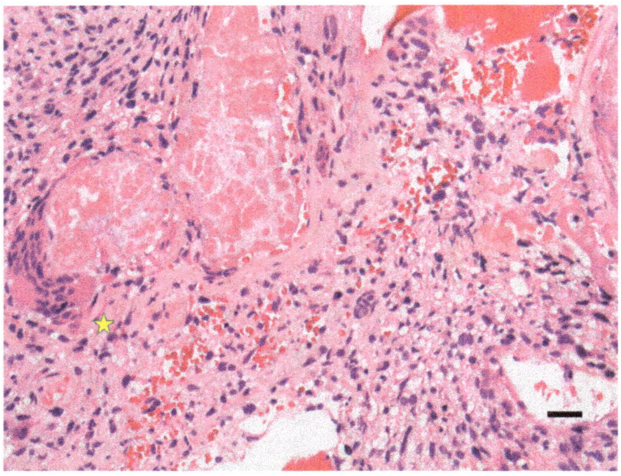

FIGURE 2 | This is an original microphotograph (X200, Hematoxylin & Eosin staining) of osteosarcoma showing osteoclastogenesis (left, asterisk) and osteoblastogenesis (right). The diagnosis of osteosarcoma relies on the identification of anaplastic cells with the osteoid formation (Hematoxylin and Eosin staining, X100 original magnification, bar: 20 μm).

e.g., β-amyloid plaques. The decrease of ILS heads to insulin resistance, hyperglycemia, and development of T2DM (30, 76).

OSTEOSARCOMA: THE MOST FREQUENT MALIGNANT MESENCHYMAL TUMOR OF BONE

The osteogenic sarcoma of the skeletal system or bone osteosarcoma is a malignant mesenchymal tumor of bone. It is the most common primary bony malignancy with both active osteoclastogenesis and osteoblastogenesis (**Figure 2**). The osteosarcoma derives from primitive bone-forming mesenchymal cells. The incidence rates of osteosarcoma per year per million of persons are about 4.0% for the range of 0–14 years and 5.0% for children aged 0–19 years, being eighth (2.4%) in the pediatric cancer incidence after leukemia (30%), brain tumors (22.3%), neuroblastoma (7.3%), nephroblastoma (5.6%), lymphoma of non-Hodgkin type (4.5%), rhabdomyosarcoma (3.1%), and retinoblastoma (2.8%) (1). Similar to other neoplasms, osteosarcoma has a bimodal age distribution, having the first peak during adolescence and the second peak in the elderly. Since the first peak is in the 10-14-year-old age group, there is an essential endocrinologic coincidence to be considered. This time corresponds to the pubertal growth spurt and may indicate a close relationship between the endocrinologic changes occurring during the adolescent growth spurt and the endocrinologic platforms of the bone metabolism. In the elderly osteosarcoma, there is a strong link with Paget disease of the bone. That there is a connection with the pubertal growth spurt, it may also be supported from the most frequent site of osteosarcoma. Indeed, it occurs near the metaphyseal growth plates of the long bones of the extremities (1). Although death rates for osteosarcoma have been declining by about 1% per year, the global 5 year survival rate for this tumor is 68%, without substantial gender difference. It has been suggested that osteosarcoma is more often identified in patients with abnormal glucose metabolism, although clear epidemiology data are lacking (77–80). The abnormal glucose metabolism may also be relevant locally other than generally. Interestingly, a teenager was described harboring a premature aging syndrome with diabetes mellitus, osteoporosis, and osteosarcoma (81). By studying animal models, spontaneous osteosarcoma was found in about 7% diabetic (non-obese) mice (79, 80). In osteosarcoma, genetics changes include point-mutations, aneuploidy, and chromothripsis, in which there are numerous rearrangements of the genome. It leads to oscillations of the copy number states, which has been labeled as a dramatic cellular catastrophe (82, 83). There is chromosomal instability in osteogenic osteosarcoma. This instability leads to the breakdown of the cell-cycle checkpoints and DNA-repair mechanisms. Moreover, there are numerous aneuploidy losses or gains at multiple chromosomal sites. Chromosomes 9, 10, 13, and 17 may be lost. The chromosomes 3, 6, 9, 10, 13, 17, and 18 may have a deletion of some parts of the chromosome. Amplification of chromosomal parts can also be detected. DNA sequence copy number upsurges have been distinguished on the regions 1q21, 3q26, 6p, 8q, 12q12-13, 14q24-qter, 17p11-12 of the autosomes and on the regions Xp11.2-21, and Xq12 of the allosomes. In most of the regions harboring chromosomal changes, there are sites of tumor suppressors and oncogenes. Apart of tumor suppressor and oncogenic sites, there are regions involved in the transcription procedure of the genetic information, including c-MYC and c-FOS that seem to play substantial roles in the etiology and/or pathogenesis (84, 85). In listing the other oncogenes connected with amplifications in osteosarcoma, we need to mention Cell Division Cycle five-Like (*CDC5L*), Mitogen-Activated Protein Kinase 7 (*MAPK7*), Mesenchymal to Epithelial Transition (*MET*), *PIM1*, peripheral myelin protein 22 (*PMP22*), DNA Primase Subunit 1 (*PRIM1*) other than Runt Related Transcription Factor 2 (*RUNX2*), and Vascular endothelial growth factor A (*VEGFA*) (86). Of these genes, *MAPK7*, *MET*, *PIM1*, *PMP22*, *RUNX2*, and *VEGFA* have been described to be associated with diabetes (87–91). Finally, epigenetic changes have also been demonstrated to play a role in osteosarcoma. Epigenetic modifications are specific changes in gene expression that are not due to direct changes in the DNA sequence. In osteosarcoma, there are epigenetic changes, which include methylation of DNA and modification of histones, nucleosome remodeling, and RNA-facilitated events (84, 92–94). Among others, p16 is a tumor-suppressor protein that plays a central role in osteosarcoma. The tumor suppressor p16 is a cell-cycle regulation factor, which acts by decelerating cells progression. The methylation of the cytosine residue within a gene can alter its expression. This event occurs in cytosine-phosphate-guanine (CpG) islands, i.e., DNA sites of 200 bp or more, GC rate >50%, and a detected-to-expected CpG ratio >60%. Gene silencing is the consequence of the methylation of CpG islands in promoter regions. The hypermethylation, when it occurs, reduces the genetic expression at the p16INK4 locus (84). Moreover, lysine-specific demethylase 1 (LSD1), a histone demethylase of the cell, is overexpressed in osteosarcoma. Cell lines treated with the inhibitor of LSD1 exhibit reduced cell growth (84, 95). Likewise, demethylation of the promoter regions of TSSC3, which is a proapoptotic gene, caused in overexpression of the gene with the consequence of suppression of the osteosarcoma cells (96). The demethylation of tumor-suppressor genes in osteosarcoma seems to alter the metastatic capability of the tumor (97, 98). Some microRNAs have also been identified and suggested to be markers of prognosis influencing the genetic expression of osteosarcoma (99). Transcription factors, which enable the process of transcribing coding information from the DNA to single-stranded RNA by binding to promoter sequences on the genome, are carefully supervised in cells at different levels. Osteosarcoma cells show that such regulatory mechanism is disturbed. The study of both FOS and JUN has evidenced that their oncogenes are upregulated in osteosarcoma. Both FOS and JUN are components of the activator protein one complex, which is a transcription factor that controls cell proliferation, differentiation, and metabolism in the bone. The activator protein one complex has also been concerned in the tendency of these tumors to invade and metastasize (100–102). Intranuclear MYC, which is a transcription factor and endorses cellular growth and proliferation, is also overexpressed in osteosarcoma. It is also linked with struggle to conventional chemotherapy protocols (85, 103, 104). That transcription factors play an important role in osteosarcoma may be underlined by the discovery that niclosamide, a traditional anti-helminthic drug, is successful in some osteosarcomas by inducing apoptosis and inhibiting cell-cycle progression in osteosarcoma cells. Niclosamide inhibits the transcription factors E2F1, AP1, and c-MYC-responsive reporters strongly (105, 106). Melatonin, which is a hormone, produced mainly by the pineal gland, regulates wakefulness, and protects mesenchymal stem cells of the bone marrow against iron overload-induced aberrant differentiation and cellular senescence, has also been seen influencing the progression of osteosarcoma *in vitro*. Melatonin weakens osteosarcoma cell invasion by inhibition of the c-Jun N-terminal kinase pathway (107, 108). Melatonin increased and decreased the activation of ERK 1/2 and JNK 1/2, respectively, in a dose-dependent manner in U2OS and HOS osteosarcoma cells (108). This occurred while exerting no apparent influence on the level and activation of P38, AKT, PTK2 protein tyrosine kinase 2 (PTK2), also known as focal adhesion kinase or FAK, steroid receptor coactivator, or Rapidly accelerated fibrosarcoma (RAF).

IGF-1, SIRT1, AND FOXO1 IN OSTEOSARCOMA

In osteosarcoma, increased levels of IGF-1 and IGF-1R have been found that seem to lead to tumor progression through transformation, proliferation, decreased susceptibility to apoptosis, and a phenotype prone to metastasis, including increase cell motility, invasion, and angiogenesis (109–111). Also, an over-expression of IGF-1/IGF-1R signaling also contributes to tumor cell survival, metastasis, and resistance to chemotherapy protocols. Some worrisome data for patients harboring osteosarcoma regard the interaction of IGF-1 signaling and osteosarcoma suggesting that supplementation of osteosarcoma cell lines with IGF-1 increases their growth (112, 113). IGF-1 stimulates cell growth, and proliferation exceeds cell death. In fact, the IGF-1 signaling pathway is activated in osteosarcoma promoting proliferation and chemotherapy resistance by activating the AKT signaling pathway. Jentzsch et al.'s study suggest that local IGF-1 expression is associated with more aggressive tumor types. Although relatively rare in human, the osteosarcoma is 27 times more frequent in dogs (114). In the canine osteosarcoma, IGF-1R mRNA and protein expression are strictly associated with surgical stage and distant metastasis (115). MacEwen et al. have indeed demonstrated that IGF-1R expression is correlated with a poor prognosis of both human and canine osteosarcoma (116).

The role of SIRT1 in cancer is controversially discussed. SIRT1 promotes osteosarcoma metastasis by regulating the expression of genes that are associated with a metastatic phenotype. Zhang et al. found that SIRT1 was upregulated in most primary osteosarcoma tumors when compared with normal tissues (117). In this investigation, Zhang et al. hypothesize that SIRT1 might be coupled with a metastatic phenotype in human osteosarcoma. Cell migration and wound-healing assays supported the invasive activity of osteosarcoma cells and downregulating SIRT1 with shRNA inhibition determined that the migration ability of osteosarcoma cells *in vitro* decreased. It blocked tumor lung metastasis in mice (117). Other groups have challenged this data. In other investigations, SIRT1 inhibits tumor progression, deacetylates β-catenin, drives cell proliferation, and inhibits carcinogenesis in patients harboring colon cancer (118, 119). These incongruencies have been explained considering the different features of various tumors.

FOXO1 is generally low or absent in osteosarcoma, and the FOXO1 locus has been associated with copy number variation (CNV) and loss of heterozygosity (LOH) in osteosarcoma confirming that chromosomal aberrations may be (at least partially) responsible for the low FOXO1 expression in some cases of osteosarcoma (120). In osteosarcoma cell lines, the activation of FOXO1 promotes the pathway leading to cell cycle arrest and apoptosis that has been associated with repressed Wnt/β-catenin signaling. The inhibition of FOXO1 induced cell proliferation and decreased the osteogenic differentiation of osteosarcoma cells. By rebuilding the FOXO1 activity, there was impaired proliferation and apoptosis. Both the retinoblastoma-1 gene (RB1) and FOXO1 are situated in 13q14. This locus is often associated with recurrent losses in osteosarcoma (121–123). Interestingly, patients that harbor a loss of 13q14 show lower event-free survival. Other tumors, including cellular angiofibroma, spindle cell lipoma, as well as mammary and vaginal myofibroblastomas, may share a monoallelic loss of RB1 and FOXO1, although none of them is a malignant tumor (124). Guan et al. (120) identified no point mutations in the coding sequence or DNA hypermethylation in the promoter region of FOXO1, which is similar to what has been published in previous studies, i.e., FOXO1 might be involved in the genomic loss, but rarely engaged in mutation or DNA hypermethylation in tumorigenesis. The same authors found five gains, six losses, and 15 cases of LOH of the FOXO1 locus in 34 cases of osteosarcoma by analysis of whole-genome sequencing (120). Guan et al. found that FOXO1 represses the survival of osteosarcoma cells by inhibition of the Wnt/β-catenin signaling, showing that the inhibition of Wnt/β-catenin signaling by FOXOs is conserved during the development of bone and osseous tumorigenesis. FOXO1 does not seem to have any significant influence on the subcellular localization of β-catenin, but FOXO1 inhibits expression of β-catenin. FOXO1 activation induces cell cycle arrest and its inhibition by impairing osteogenic differentiation of osteosarcoma cell lines considering that FOXO1 is a positive promoter of osteoblastogenesis *in vitro* (125). FOXO1 loss might contribute to the disturbed terminal differentiation observed in osteosarcoma. The rebuilding of FOXO1 activity could be a potential therapeutic strategy for therapy of osteosarcoma.

CONCLUSIONS

There is an intricate relationship that does occur in the interaction of IGF1, SIRT1, and FOXOs in the skeletal system. This relationship is particularly essential not only for altered bone metabolism, i.e., deposition and absorption of osteoid but also putatively for the inflammatory status that may trigger osteosarcoma to develop. A research platform in metabolomics of bone tumors is growing, and the mole of data will shape the treatment of osteosarcoma of the 21st century.

AUTHOR CONTRIBUTIONS

CS conceived the study and wrote the manuscript. FS critically reviewed the signaling pathways. S-ML critically reviewed the manuscript. All authors approved the final manuscript.

REFERENCES

1. Ottaviani G, Jaffe N. The epidemiology of osteosarcoma. *Cancer Treat Res.* (2009) 152:3–13. doi: 10.1007/978-1-4419-0284-9_1
2. Ogura K, Higashi T, Kawai A. Statistics of bone sarcoma in Japan: report from the Bone and soft tissue tumor registry in Japan. *J Orthop Sci.* (2017) 22:133–43. doi: 10.1016/j.jos.2016.10.006
3. Jung M, Tuischer JS, Sergi C, Gotterbarm T, Pohl J, Richter W, et al. Local application of a collagen type I/hyaluronate matrix and growth and differentiation factor 5 influences the closure of osteochondral defects in a minipig model by enchondral ossification. *Growth Factors.* (2006) 24:225–32. doi: 10.1080/08977190600926969
4. Simank HG, Sergi C, Jung M, Adolf S, Eckhardt C, Ehemann V, et al. Effects of local application of growth and differentiation factor-5 (GDF-5) in a full-thickness cartilage defect model. *Growth Factors.* (2004) 22:35–43.doi: 10.1080/08977190310001645207
5. Simank HG, Herold F, Schneider M, Maedler U, Ries R, Sergi C. Growth and differentiation factor 5 (GDF-5) composite improves the healing of necrosis of the femoral head in a sheep model. Analysis of an animal model. *Orthopade.* (2004) 33:68–75. doi: 10.1007/s00132-003-0541-z
6. Manggold J, Sergi C, Becker K, Lukoschek M, Simank HG. A new animal model of femoral head necrosis induced by intraosseous injection of ethanol. *Lab Anim.* (2002) 36:173–80. doi: 10.1258/0023677021912460
7. Simank HG, Manggold J, Sebald W, Ries R, Richter W, Ewerbeck V, et al. Bone morphogenetic protein-2 and growth and differentiation factor-5 enhance the healing of necrotic bone in a sheep model. *Growth Factors.* (2001) 19:247–57. doi: 10.3109/08977190109001090
8. Gottlieb S, Ruvkun G. daf-2, daf-16 and daf-23: genetically interacting genes controlling Dauer formation in Caenorhabditis elegans. *Genetics.* (1994) 137:107–20.
9. Wolkow CA, Munoz MJ, Riddle DL, Ruvkun G. Insulin receptor substrate and p55 orthologous adaptor proteins function in the Caenorhabditis elegans daf-2/insulin-like signaling pathway. *J Biol Chem.* (2002) 277:49591–7. doi: 10.1074/jbc.M207866200
10. Weinkove D, Halstead JR, Gems D, Divecha N. Long-term starvation and ageing induce AGE-1/PI 3-kinase-dependent translocation of DAF-16/FOXO to the cytoplasm. *BMC Biol.* (2006) 4:1. doi: 10.1186/1741-7007-4-1
11. Tissenbaum HA. DAF-16: FOXO in the Context of *C. elegans*. *Curr Top Dev Biol.* (2018) 127:1–21. doi: 10.1016/bs.ctdb.2017.11.007
12. Sun X, Chen WD, Wang YD. DAF-16/FOXO transcription factor in aging and longevity. *Front Pharmacol.* (2017) 8:548. doi: 10.3389/fphar.2017.00548
13. Giatti S, Mastrangelo R, D'Antonio M, Pesaresi M, Romano S, Diviccaro S, et al. Neuroactive steroids and diabetic complications in the nervous system. *Front Neuroendocrinol.* (2018) 48:58–69. doi: 10.1016/j.yfrne.2017.07.006
14. Gabay O, Sanchez C. Epigenetics, sirtuins and osteoarthritis. *Joint Bone Spine.* (2012) 79:570–3. doi: 10.1016/j.jbspin.2012.04.005
15. Gabay O, Clouse KA. Epigenetics of cartilage diseases. *Joint Bone Spine.* (2016) 83:491–4. doi: 10.1016/j.jbspin.2015.10.004
16. Wang Y, He J, Liao M, Hu M, Li W, Ouyang H, et al. An overview of Sirtuins as potential therapeutic target: structure, function and modulators. *Eur J Med Chem.* (2019) 161:48–77. doi: 10.1016/j.ejmech.2018.10.028
17. Zhou S, Tang X, Chen HZ. Sirtuins and insulin resistance. *Front Endocrinol.* (2018) 9:748. doi: 10.3389/fendo.2018.00748
18. Song J, Yang B, Jia X, Li M, Tan W, Ma S, et al. Distinctive roles of Sirtuins on diabetes, protective or detrimental? *Front Endocrinol.* (2018) 9:724. doi: 10.3389/fendo.2018.00724
19. Zhu S, Dong Z, Ke X, Hou J, Zhao E, Zhang K, et al. The roles of sirtuins family in cell metabolism during tumor development. *Semin Cancer Biol.* (2018). doi: 10.1016/j.semcancer.2018.11.003. [Epub ahead of print].
20. Strømland Ø, Niere M, Nikiforov AA, VanLinden MR, Heiland I, Ziegler M. Keeping the balance in NAD metabolism. *Biochem Soc Trans.* (2019). doi: 10.1042/BST20180417. [Epub ahead of print].
21. Morigi M, Perico L, Benigni A. Sirtuins in renal health and disease. *J Am Soc Nephrol.* (2018) 29:1799–809. doi: 10.1681/ASN.2017111218
22. Yamagata K, Yoshizawa T. Transcriptional regulation of metabolism by SIRT1 and SIRT7. *Int Rev Cell Mol Biol.* (2018) 335:143–66. doi: 10.1016/bs.ircmb.2017.07.009
23. Chen R, Xu M, Hogg RT, Li J, Little B, Gerard RD, et al. The acetylase/deacetylase couple CREB-binding protein/Sirtuin 1 controls hypoxia-inducible factor 2 signaling. *J Biol Chem.* (2012) 287:30800–11. doi: 10.1074/jbc.M111.244780
24. Abed E, Delalandre A, Lajeunesse D. Beneficial effect of resveratrol on phenotypic features and activity of osteoarthritic osteoblasts. *Arthritis Res Ther.* (2017) 19:151. doi: 10.1186/s13075-017-1365-2
25. Tamaki N, Cristina Orihuela-Campos R, Inagaki Y, Fukui M, Nagata T, Ito HO. Resveratrol improves oxidative stress and prevents the progression of periodontitis via the activation of the Sirtl/AMPK and the Nrf2/antioxidant defense pathways in a rat periodontitis model. *Free Radic Biol Med.* (2014) 75:222–9. doi: 10.1016/j.freeradbiomed.2014.07.034
26. Huang W, Shang WL, Wang HD, Wu WW, Hou SX. Sirtl overexpression protects murine osteoblasts against TNF-alpha-induced injury in vitro by suppressing the NF-kappaB signaling pathway. *Acta Pharmacol Sin.* (2012) 33:668–74. doi: 10.1038/aps.2011.189

27. Jeong WY, Kim JB, Kim HJ, Kim CW. Extremely low-frequency electromagnetic field promotes astrocytic differentiation of human bone marrow mesenchymal stem cells by modulating SIRT1 expression. *Biosci Biotechnol Biochem.* (2017) 81:1356–62. doi: 10.1080/09168451.2017.1308243
28. Magni M, Buscemi G, Zannini L. Cell cycle and apoptosis regulator 2 at the interface between DNA damage response and cell physiology. *Mutat Res.* (2018) 776:1–9. doi: 10.1016/j.mrrev.2018.03.004
29. Beyfuss K, Hood DA. A systematic review of p53 regulation of oxidative stress in skeletal muscle. *Redox Rep.* (2018) 23:100–17. doi: 10.1080/13510002.2017.1416773
30. Erol A. Insulin resistance is an evolutionarily conserved physiological mechanism at the cellular level for protection against increased oxidative stress. *Bioessays.* (2007) 29:811–8. doi: 10.1002/bies.20618
31. Liu G, Bi Y, Xue L, Zhang Y, Yang H, Chen X, et al. Dendritic cell SIRT1-HIF1alpha axis programs the differentiation of CD4+ T cells through IL-12 and TGF-beta1. *Proc Natl Acad Sci USA.* (2015) 112:E957–65. doi: 10.1073/pnas.1420419112
32. Lo Sasso G, Menzies KJ, Mottis A, Piersigilli A, Perino A, Yamamoto H, et al. SIRT2 deficiency modulates macrophage polarization and susceptibility to experimental colitis. *PLoS ONE.* (2014) 9:e103573. doi: 10.1371/journal.pone.0103573
33. Ning Z, Li Y, Liu D, Owoicho Orgah J, Zhu J, Wang Y, et al. Tetrahydroxystilbene glucoside delayed senile symptoms in old mice via regulation of the AMPK/SIRT1/PGC-1alpha signaling cascade. *Gerontology.* (2018) 64:457–65. doi: 10.1159/000487360
34. Fujita Y, Yamashita T. Sirtuins in neuroendocrine regulation and neurological diseases. *Front Neurosci.* (2018) 12:778. doi: 10.3389/fnins.2018.00778
35. Hsu YC, Wu YT, Tsai CL, Wei YH. Current understanding and future perspectives of the roles of sirtuins in the reprogramming and differentiation of pluripotent stem cells. *Exp Biol Med.* (2018) 243:563–75. doi: 10.1177/1535370218759636
36. Karbasforooshan H, Roohbakhsh A, Karimi G. SIRT1 and microRNAs: the role in breast, lung and prostate cancers. *Exp Cell Res.* (2018) 367:1–6. doi: 10.1016/j.yexcr.2018.03.023
37. Jiang W, Zhang X, Hao J, Shen J, Fang J, Dong W, et al. SIRT1 protects against apoptosis by promoting autophagy in degenerative human disc nucleus pulposus cells. *Sci Rep.* (2014) 4:7456. doi: 10. 1038/srep07456
38. Girardelli M, Basaldella F, Paolera SD, Vuch J, Tommasini A, Martelossi S, et al. Genetic profile of patients with early onset inflammatory bowel disease. *Gene.* (2018) 645:18–29. doi: 10.1016/j.gene.2017.12.029
39. Chiu B, Jantuan E, Shen F, Chiu B, Sergi C. Autophagy-inflammasome interplay in heart failure: a systematic review on basics, pathways, and therapeutic perspectives. *Ann Clin Lab Sci.* (2017) 47:243–52.
40. Truong VL, Jun M, Jeong WS. Role of resveratrol in regulation of cellular defense systems against oxidative stress. *Biofactors.* (2018) 44:36–49. doi: 10.1002/biof.1399
41. Yoon DS, Choi Y, Lee JW. Cellular localization of NRF2 determines the self-renewal and osteogenic differentiation potential of human MSCs via the P53-SIRT1 axis. *Cell Death Dis.* (2016) 7:e2093. doi: 10.1038/cddis.2016.3
42. Xin Z, Ma Z, Hu W, Jiang S, Yang Z, Li T, et al. FOXO1/3: Potential suppressors of fibrosis. *Ageing Res Rev.* (2018) 41:42–52. doi: 10.1016/j.arr.2017.11.002
43. Luo CT, Li MO. Foxo transcription factors in T cell biology and tumor immunity. *Semin Cancer Biol.* (2018) 50:13–20. doi: 10.1016/j.semcancer.2018.04.006
44. Tia N, Singh AK, Pandey P, Azad CS, Chaudhary P, Gambhir IS. Role of Forkhead Box O (FOXO) transcription factor in aging and diseases. *Gene.* (2018) 648:97–105. doi: 10.1016/j.gene.2018.01.051
45. Ma J, Matkar S, He X, Hua X. FOXO family in regulating cancer and metabolism. *Semin Cancer Biol.* (2018) 50:32–41. doi: 10.1016/j.semcancer.2018.01.018
46. Monsalve M, Prieto I, de Bem AF, Olmos Y. Methodological Approach for the Evaluation of FOXO as a positive regulator of antioxidant genes. *Methods Mol Biol.* (2019) 1890:61–76. doi: 10.1007/978-1-4939-8900-3_6
47. Mukherjee A, Hollern DP, Williams OG, Rayburn TS, Byrd WA, Yates C, et al. A Review of FOXI3 regulation of development and possible roles in cancer progression and metastasis. *Front Cell Dev Biol.* (2018) 6:69. doi: 10.3389/fcell.2018.00069
48. Kim HN, Iyer S, Ring R, Almeida M. The role of FoxOs in bone health and disease. *Curr Top Dev Biol.* (2018) 127:149–63. doi: 10.1016/bs.ctdb.2017.10.004
49. Jiang S, Li T, Yang Z, Hu W, Yang Y. Deciphering the roles of FOXO1 in human neoplasms. *Int J Cancer.* (2018) 143:1560–8. doi: 10.1002/ijc.31338
50. Miao C, Li Y, Zhang X. The functions of FoxO transcription factors in epithelial wound healing. *Australas J Dermatol.* (2018). doi: 10.1111/ajd.12952. [Epub ahead of print].
51. Yadav RK, Chauhan AS, Zhuang L, Gan B. FoxO transcription factors in cancer metabolism. *Semin Cancer Biol.* (2018) 50:65–76. doi: 10.1016/j.semcancer.2018.01.004
52. Hou T, Li Z, Zhao Y, Zhu WG. Mechanisms controlling the anti-neoplastic functions of FoxO proteins. *Semin Cancer Biol.* (2018) 50:101–14. doi: 10.1016/j.semcancer.2017.11.007
53. Wang Y, Zhou Y, Graves DT. FOXO transcription factors: their clinical significance and regulation. *Biomed Res Int.* (2014) 2014:925350. doi: 10.1155/2014/925350
54. Al-Bahrani R, Abuetabh Y, Zeitouni N, Sergi C. Cholangiocarcinoma: risk factors, environmental influences and oncogenesis. *Ann Clin Lab Sci.* (2013) 43:195–210.
55. Teitelbaum SL, Ross FP. Genetic regulation of osteoclast development and function. *Nat Rev Genet.* (2003) 4:638–49. doi: 10.1038/nrg1122
56. Baruzzi A, Berton G. The tyrosine kinase Abl is a component of macrophage podosomes and is required for podosome formation and function. *Eur J Immunol.* (2012) 42:2720–6. doi: 10.1002/eji.201142270
57. Ray BJ, Thomas K, Huang CS, Gutknecht MF, Botchwey EA, Bouton AH. Regulation of osteoclast structure and function by FAK family kinases. *J Leukoc Biol.* (2012) 92:1021–8. doi: 10.1189/jlb.0512259
58. Smith H, Whittall C, Weksler B, Middleton J. Chemokines stimulate bidirectional migration of human mesenchymal stem cells across bone marrow endothelial cells. *Stem Cells Dev.* (2012) 21:476–86. doi: 10.1089/scd.2011.0025
59. Iyer S, Ambrogini E, Bartell SM, Han L, Roberson PK, de Cabo R, et al. FOXOs attenuate bone formation by suppressing Wnt signaling. *J Clin Invest.* (2013) 123:3409–19. doi: 10.1172/JCI68049
60. Iyer S, Han L, Bartell SM, Kim HN, Gubrij I, de Cabo R, et al. Sirtuin1 (Sirt1) promotes cortical bone formation by preventing beta-catenin sequestration by FoxO transcription factors in osteoblast progenitors. *J Biol Chem.* (2014) 289:24069–78. doi: 10.1074/jbc.M114.561803
61. Lee YM, Shin SI, Shin KS, Lee YR, Park BH, Kim EC. The role of sirtuin 1 in osteoblastic differentiation in human periodontal ligament cells. *J Periodontal Res.* (2011) 46:712–21. doi: 10.1111/j.1600-0765.2011. 01394.x
62. Piemontese M, Onal M, Xiong J, Han L, Thostenson JD, Almeida M, et al. Low bone mass and changes in the osteocyte network in mice lacking autophagy in the osteoblast lineage. *Sci Rep.* (2016) 6:24262. doi: 10.1038/srep24262
63. Baron R, Kneissel M. WNT signaling in bone homeostasis and disease: from human mutations to treatments. *Nat Med.* (2013) 19:179–92. doi: 10.1038/nm.3074
64. Clevers H, Nusse R. Wnt/beta-catenin signaling and disease. *Cell.* (2012) 149:1192–205. doi: 10.1016/j.cell.2012.05.012
65. Jilka RL, O'Brien CA. The role of osteocytes in age-related bone loss. *Curr Osteoporos Rep.* (2016) 14:16–25. doi: 10.1007/s11914-016-0297-0
66. Bartell SM, Kim HN, Ambrogini E, Han L, Iyer S, Serra Ucer S, et al. FoxO proteins restrain osteoclastogenesis and bone resorption by attenuating H2O2 accumulation. *Nat Commun.* (2014) 5:3773. doi: 10.1038/ncomms4773
67. Liu W, Wang S, Wei S, Sun L, Feng X. Receptor activator of NF-kappaB (RANK) cytoplasmic motif, 369PFQEP373, plays a predominant role in osteoclast survival in part by activating Akt/PKB and its downstream effector AFX/FOXO4. *J Biol Chem.* (2005) 280:43064–72. doi: 10.1074/jbc.M509006200
68. Tan P, Guan H, Xie L, Mi B, Fang Z, Li J, et al. FOXO1 inhibits

osteoclastogenesis partially by antagnozing MYC. *Sci Rep.* (2015) 5:16835. doi: 10.1038/srep16835
69. Tan T, Wang L, Wang B. Collagen and prostaglandin E(2) regulate aromatase expression through the PI3K/AKT/IKK and the MAP kinase pathways in adipose stromal cells. *Mol Med Rep.* (2015) 12:4766–72. doi: 10.3892/mmr.2015.3901
70. Jais A, Einwallner E, Sharif O, Gossens K, Lu TT, Soyal SM, et al. Heme oxygenase-1 drives metaflammation and insulin resistance in mouse and man. *Cell.* (2014) 158:25–40. doi: 10.1016/j.cell.2014.04.043
71. Ambrogini E, Almeida M, Martin-Millan M, Paik JH, Depinho RA, Han L, et al. FoxO-mediated defense against oxidative stress in osteoblasts is indispensable for skeletal homeostasis in mice. *Cell Metab.* (2010) 11:136–46. doi: 10.1016/j.cmet.2009.12.009
72. Rached MT, Kode A, Xu L, Yoshikawa Y, Paik JH, Depinho RA, et al. FoxO1 is a positive regulator of bone formation by favoring protein synthesis and resistance to oxidative stress in osteoblasts. *Cell Metab.* (2010) 11:147–60. doi: 10.1016/j.cmet.2010.01.001
73. Ferron M, Wei J, Yoshizawa T, Del Fattore A, DePinho RA, Teti A, et al. Insulin signaling in osteoblasts integrates bone remodeling and energy metabolism. *Cell.* (2010) 142:296–308. doi: 10.1016/j.cell.2010.06.003
74. Wei H, Yu X. Functions of PARylation in DNA Damage Repair Pathways. *Genomics Proteomics Bioinformatics.* (2016) 14:131–9. doi: 10.1016/j.gpb.2016.05.001
75. Henderson ST, Johnson TE. daf-16 integrates developmental and environmental inputs to mediate aging in the nematode Caenorhabditis elegans. *Curr Biol.* (2001) 11:1975–80. doi: 10.1016/S0960-9822(01)00594-2
76. Manolopoulos KN, Klotz LO, Korsten P, Bornstein SR, Barthel A. Linking Alzheimer's disease to insulin resistance: the FoxO response to oxidative stress. *Mol Psychiatry.* (2010) 15:1046–52. doi: 10.1038/mp.2010.17
77. Mishra PJ. MicroRNAs as promising biomarkers in cancer diagnostics. *Biomark Res.* (2014) 2:19. doi: 10.1186/2050-7771-2-19
78. Schmid C, Ghirlanda-Keller C, Zapf J. Effects of IGF-I and -II, IGF binding protein-3 (IGFBP-3), and transforming growth factor-beta (TGF-beta) on growth and apoptosis of human osteosarcoma Saos-2/B-10 cells: lack of IGF-independent IGFBP-3 effects. *Eur J Endocrinol.* (2001) 145:213–21.
79. Gilbert MP, Pratley RE. The impact of diabetes and diabetes medications on bone health. *Endocr Rev.* (2015) 36:194–213. doi: 10.1210/er.2012-1042
80. Kavirayani AM, Foreman O. Retrospective study of spontaneous osteosarcomas in the nonobese diabetic strain and nonobese diabetic-derived substrains of mice. *Vet Pathol.* (2010) 47:482–7. doi: 10.1177/0300985810363699
81. Okamoto N, Satomura K, Hatsukawa Y, Hayashida M, Saijo K, Ohno T, et al. Premature aging syndrome with osteosarcoma, cataracts, diabetes mellitus, osteoporosis, erythroid macrocytosis, severe growth and developmental deficiency. *Am J Med Genet.* (1997) 69:169–70.
82. Stephens PJ, Greenman CD, Fu B, Yang F, Bignell GR, Mudie LJ, et al. Massive genomic rearrangement acquired in a single catastrophic event during cancer development. *Cell.* (2011) 144:27–40. doi: 10.1016/j.cell.2010.11.055
83. Maher CA, Wilson RK. Chromothripsis and human disease: piecing together the shattering process. *Cell.* (2012) 148:29–32. doi: 10.1016/j.cell.2012.01.006
84. Morrow JJ, Khanna C. Osteosarcoma genetics and epigenetics: emerging biology and candidate therapies. *Crit Rev Oncogenesis.* (2015) 20:173–97. doi: 10.1615/CritRevOncog.2015013713
85. Gamberi G, Benassi MS, Bohling T, Ragazzini P, Molendini L, Sollazzo MR, et al. C-myc and c-fos in human osteosarcoma: prognostic value of mRNA and protein expression. *Oncology.* (1998) 55:556–63.
86. Mutsaers AJ, Walkley CR. Cells of origin in osteosarcoma: mesenchymal stem cells or osteoblast committed cells? *Bone.* (2014) 62:56–63. doi: 10.1016/j.bone.2014.02.003
87. Zhu Y, Ma WQ, Han XQ, Wang Y, Wang X, Liu NF. Advanced glycation end products accelerate calcification in VSMCs through HIF-1alpha/PDK4 activation and suppress glucose metabolism. *Sci Rep.* (2018) 8:13730. doi: 10.1038/s41598-018-31877-6
88. Zhang YY, Li C, Yao GF, Du LJ, Liu Y, Zheng XJ, et al. Deletion of macrophage mineralocorticoid receptor protects hepatic steatosis and insulin resistance through ERalpha/HGF/Met pathway. *Diabetes.* (2017) 66:1535–47. doi: 10.2337/db16-1354
89. Katare R, Caporali A, Zentilin L, Avolio E, Sala-Newby G, Oikawa A, et al. Intravenous gene therapy with PIM-1 via a cardiotropic viral vector halts the progression of diabetic cardiomyopathy through promotion of prosurvival signaling. *Circ Res.* (2011) 108:1238–51. doi: 10.1161/CIRCRESAHA.110.239111
90. Lomas-Soria C, Perez-Ramirez IF, Caballero-Perez J, Guevara-Gonzalez RG, Guevara-Olvera L, Loarca-Pina G, et al. Cooked common beans (Phaseolus vulgaris L.) modulate renal genes in streptozotocin-induced diabetic rats. *J Nutr Biochem.* (2015) 26:761–8. doi: 10.1016/j.jnutbio.2015.02.006
91. Sun AP, Tang L, Liao Q, Zhang H, Zhang YS, Zhang J. Coexistent charcot-marie-tooth type 1A and type 2 diabetes mellitus neuropathies in a Chinese family. *Neural Regen Res.* (2015) 10:1696–9. doi: 10.4103/1673-5374.167771
92. Li B, Ye Z. Epigenetic alterations in osteosarcoma: promising targets. *Mol Biol Rep.* (2014) 41:3303–15. doi: 10.1007/s11033-014-3193-7
93. Roberts SB, Wootton E, De Ferrari L, Albagha OM, Salter DM. Epigenetics of osteoarticular diseases: recent developments. *Rheumatol Int.* (2015) 35:1293–305. doi: 10.1007/s00296-015-3260-y
94. Cui J, Wang W, Li Z, Zhang Z, Wu B, Zeng L. Epigenetic changes in osteosarcoma. *Bull Cancer.* (2011) 98:E62–8. doi: 10.1684/bdc.2011.1400
95. Bennani-Baiti IM, Machado I, Llombart-Bosch A, Kovar H. Lysine-specific demethylase 1 (LSD1/KDM1A/AOF2/BHC110) is expressed and is an epigenetic drug target in chondrosarcoma, Ewing's sarcoma, osteosarcoma, and rhabdomyosarcoma. *Hum Pathol.* (2012) 43:1300–7. doi: 10.1016/j.humpath.2011.10.010
96. Li Y, Huang Y, Lv Y, Meng G, Guo QN. Epigenetic regulation of the pro-apoptosis gene TSSC3 in human osteosarcoma cells. *Biomed Pharmacother.* (2014) 68:45–50. doi: 10.1016/j.biopha.2013.10.006
97. Mu X, Sultankulov B, Agarwal R, Mahjoub A, Schott T, Greco N, et al. Chick embryo extract demethylates tumor suppressor genes in osteosarcoma cells. *Clin Orthopaedics Relat Res.* (2014) 472:865–73. doi: 10.1007/s11999-013-3104-6
98. Zhou C, Tan W, Lv H, Gao F, Sun J. Hypoxia-inducible microRNA-488 regulates apoptosis by targeting Bim in osteosarcoma. *Cell Oncol.* (2016) 39:463–71. doi: 10.1007/s13402-016-0288-2
99. Dong J, Liu Y, Liao W, Liu R, Shi P, Wang L. miRNA-223 is a potential diagnostic and prognostic marker for osteosarcoma. *J Bone Oncol.* (2016) 5:74–9. doi: 10.1016/j.jbo.2016.05.001
100. Broadhead ML, Clark JC, Myers DE, Dass CR, Choong PF. The molecular pathogenesis of osteosarcoma: a review. *Sarcoma.* (2011) 2011:959248. doi: 10.1155/2011/959248
101. Wu JX, Carpenter PM, Gresens C, Keh R, Niman H, Morris JW, et al. The proto-oncogene c-fos is over-expressed in the majority of human osteosarcomas. *Oncogene.* (1990) 5:989–1000.
102. Franchi A, Calzolari A, Zampi G. Immunohistochemical detection of c-fos and c-jun expression in osseous and cartilaginous tumours of the skeleton. *Virchows Archiv Int J Pathol.* (1998) 432:515–9.
103. Shimizu T, Ishikawa T, Sugihara E, Kuninaka S, Miyamoto T, Mabuchi Y, et al. c-MYC overexpression with loss of Ink4a/Arf transforms bone marrow stromal cells into osteosarcoma accompanied by loss of adipogenesis. *Oncogene.* (2010) 29:5687–99. doi: 10.1038/onc.2010.312
104. Scionti I, Michelacci F, Pasello M, Hattinger CM, Alberghini M, Manara MC, et al. Clinical impact of the methotrexate resistance-associated genes C-MYC and dihydrofolate reductase (DHFR) in high-grade osteosarcoma. *Ann Oncol.* (2008) 19:1500–8. doi: 10.1093/annonc/mdn148
105. Liao Z, Nan G, Yan Z, Zeng L, Deng Y, Ye J, et al. The anthelmintic drug niclosamide inhibits the proliferative activity of human osteosarcoma cells by targeting multiple signal pathways. *Curr Cancer Drug Targets.* (2015) 15:726–38. doi: 10.2174/1568009615666150629132157
106. Osasan S, Zhang M, Shen F, Paul PJ, Persad S, Sergi C. Osteogenic

Sarcoma: A 21st century review. *Anticancer Res.* (2016) 36:4391–8. doi: 10.21873/anticanres.10982

107. Yang F, Yang L, Li Y, Yan G, Feng C, Liu T, et al. Melatonin protects bone marrow mesenchymal stem cells against iron overload-induced aberrant differentiation and senescence. *J Pineal Res.* (2017) 63:e12422. doi: 10.1111/jpi.12422
108. Lu KH, Su SC, Lin CW, Hsieh YH, Lin YC, Chien MH, et al. Melatonin attenuates osteosarcoma cell invasion by suppression of C-C motif chemokine ligand 24 through inhibition of the c-Jun N-terminal kinase pathway. *J Pineal Res.* (2018) 65:e12507. doi: 10.1111/jpi.12507
109. Hong SH, Briggs J, Newman R, Hoffman K, Mendoza A, LeRoith D, et al. Murine osteosarcoma primary tumour growth and metastatic progression is maintained after marked suppression of serum insulin-like growth factor I. *Int J Cancer.* (2009) 124:2042–9. doi: 10.1002/ijc.24169
110. Jentzsch T, Robl B, Husmann M, Bode-Lesniewska B, Fuchs B. Worse prognosis of osteosarcoma patients expressing IGF-1 on a tissue microarray. *Anticancer Res.* (2014) 34:3881–9.
111. Viereck V, Siggelkow H, Pannem R, Braulke T, Scharf JG, Kubler B. Alteration of the insulin-like growth factor axis during *in vitro* differentiation of the human osteosarcoma cell line HOS 58. *J Cell Biochem.* (2007) 102:28–40. doi: 10.1002/jcb.21274
112. Wang YH, Han XD, Qiu Y, Xiong J, Yu Y, Wang B, et al. Increased expression of insulin-like growth factor-1 receptor is correlated with tumor metastasis and prognosis in patients with osteosarcoma. *J Surg Oncol.* (2012) 105:235–43. doi: 10.1002/jso.22077
113. Borinstein SC, Barkauskas DA, Bernstein M, Goorin A, Gorlick R, Krailo M, et al. Analysis of serum insulin growth factor-1 concentrations in localized osteosarcoma: a children's oncology group study. *Pediatr Blood Cancer.* (2014) 61:749–52. doi: 10.1002/pbc.24778
114. Simpson S, Dunning MD, de Brot S, Grau-Roma L, Mongan NP, Rutland CS. Comparative review of human and canine osteosarcoma: morphology, epidemiology, prognosis, treatment and genetics. *Acta Vet Scand.* (2017) 59:71. doi: 10.1186/s13028-017-0341-9
115. Maniscalco L, Iussich S, Morello E, Martano M, Gattino F, Miretti S, et al. Increased expression of insulin-like growth factor-1 receptor is correlated with worse survival in canine appendicular osteosarcoma. *Vet J.* (2015) 205:272–80. doi: 10.1016/j.tvjl.2014.09.005
116. MacEwen EG, Pastor J, Kutzke J, Tsan R, Kurzman ID, Thamm DH, et al. IGF-1 receptor contributes to the malignant phenotype in human and canine osteosarcoma. *J Cell Biochem.* (2004) 92:77-91. doi: 10.1002/jcb.20046
117. Zhang N, Xie T, Xian M, Wang YJ, Li HY, Ying MD, et al. SIRT1 promotes metastasis of human osteosarcoma cells. *Oncotarget.* (2016) 7:79654–69. doi: 10.18632/oncotarget.12916
118. Firestein R, Blander G, Michan S, Oberdoerffer P, Ogino S, Campbell J, et al. The SIRT1 deacetylase suppresses intestinal tumorigenesis and colon cancer growth. *PLoS ONE.* (2008) 3:e2020. doi: 10.1371/journal.pone.0002020
119. Kabra N, Li Z, Chen L, Li B, Zhang X, Wang C, et al. SirT1 is an inhibitor of proliferation and tumor formation in colon cancer. *J Biol Chem.* (2009) 284:18210–7. doi: 10.1074/jbc.M109.000034
120. Guan H, Tan P, Xie L, Mi B, Fang Z, Li J, et al. FOXO1 inhibits osteosarcoma oncogenesis via Wnt/beta-catenin pathway suppression. *Oncogenesis.* (2015) 4:e166. doi: 10.1038/oncsis.2015.25
121. Kresse SH, Ohnstad HO, Paulsen EB, Bjerkehagen B, Szuhai K, Serra M, et al. LSAMP, a novel candidate tumor suppressor gene in human osteosarcomas, identified by array comparative genomic hybridization. *Genes Chromosomes Cancer.* (2009) 48:679–93. doi: 10.1002/gcc.20675
122. Blattmann C, Thiemann M, Stenzinger A, Roth EK, Dittmar A, Witt H, et al. Establishment of a patient-derived orthotopic osteosarcoma mouse model. *J Transl Med.* (2015) 13:136. doi: 10.1186/s12967-015-0497-x
123. Sadikovic B, Park PC, Selvarajah S, Zielenska M. Array comparative genomic hybridization in osteosarcoma. *Methods Mol Biol.* (2013) 973:227–47. doi: 10.1007/978-1-62703-281-0_15
124. Magro G, Righi A, Casorzo L, Antonietta T, Salvatorelli L, Kacerovska D, et al. Mammary and vaginal myofibroblastomas are genetically related lesions: fluorescence in situ hybridization analysis shows deletion of 13q14 region. *Hum Pathol.* (2012) 43:1887–93. doi: 10.1016/j.humpath.2012.01.015
125. Siqueira MF, Flowers S, Bhattacharya R, Faibish D, Behl Y, Kotton DN, et al. FOXO1 modulates osteoblast differentiation. *Bone.* (2011) 48:1043–51. doi: 10.1016/j.bone.2011.01.019

15

Sirtuins and Insulin Resistance

Shuang Zhou [1]*, Xiaoqiang Tang* [2*] *and Hou-Zao Chen* [3*]

[1] Internal Medicine, Peking Union Medical College Hospital, Beijing, China, [2] Key Laboratory of Birth Defects and Related Diseases of Women and Children of MOE, State Key Laboratory of Biotherapy, West China Second University Hospital, Sichuan University, Chengdu, China, [3] State Key Laboratory of Medical Molecular Biology, Department of Biochemistry and Molecular Biology, Institute of Basic Medical Sciences, Chinese Academy of Medical Sciences & Peking Union Medical College, Beijing, China

***Correspondence:**
Xiaoqiang Tang
tangxiaoqiang@scu.edu.cn
Hou-Zao Chen
chenhouzao@ibms.cams.cn;
houzao@gmail.com

The mammalian Sirtuins (SIRT1-7) are an evolutionarily conserved family of NAD$^+$-dependent deacylase and mono-ADP-ribosyltransferase. Sirtuins display distinct subcellular localizations and functions and are involved in cell survival, senescence, metabolism and genome stability. Among the mammalian Sirtuins, SIRT1 and SIRT6 have been thoroughly investigated and have prominent metabolic regulatory roles. Moreover, SIRT1 and SIRT6 have been implicated in obesity, insulin resistance, type 2 diabetes mellitus (T2DM), fatty liver disease and cardiovascular diseases. However, the roles of other Sirtuins are not fully understood. Recent studies have shown that these Sirtuins also play important roles in inflammation, mitochondrial dysfunction, and energy metabolism. Insulin resistance is the critical pathological trait of obesity and metabolic syndrome as well as the core defect in T2DM. Accumulating clinical and experimental animal evidence suggests the potential roles of the remaining Sirtuins in the regulation of insulin resistance through diverse biological mechanisms. In this review, we summarize recent advances in the understanding of the functions of Sirtuins in various insulin resistance-associated physiological processes, including inflammation, mitochondrial dysfunction, the insulin signaling pathway, glucose, and lipid metabolism. In addition, we highlight the important gaps that must be addressed in this field.

Keywords: sirtuins, insulin resistance, senescaging, inflammation, mitochondrial dysfunction

INTRODUCTION

The increasing prevalence of obesity and associated metabolic syndrome (including type 2 diabetes mellitus [T2DM], nonalcoholic fatty liver disease [NAFLD], atherosclerosis and atherosclerotic heart disease) is an increasingly severe challenge in public health (1). Insulin resistance is the critical, universal pathological feature of these diseases, especially T2DM. Insulin is a major hormone secreted by pancreatic β cells after nutrient stimulation and plays a critical role in reducing blood glucose concentration by facilitating glucose uptake by skeletal muscle and adipose tissue and inhibiting endogenous glucose production in the liver (2–4). Insulin resistance occurs when cells are incapable of efficiently responding to a normal dose of insulin (2–4). The development of insulin resistance is a multistep, complex process influenced by genetics and environments (3). Although the precise pathogenesis of insulin resistance remains incompletely understood, several mechanisms are proposed to be involved, including defects in the insulin signaling pathway, ectopic lipid accumulation, systemic inflammation, mitochondrial dysfunction, oxidative stress, and endoplasmic reticulum (ER) stress, as reviewed elsewhere (1, 5, 6).

The mammalian Sirtuins are a family of NAD^+-dependent deacetylases (7). This family consists of seven members (SIRT1-SIRT7), which share the conserved Sirtuin domain conferring NAD^+-dependent deacetylase activity but have variable amino- and carboxy-terminal extensions and display distinct subcellular localization and biological functions (8, 9). SIRT1 is mainly localized to the nucleus (10), but it shuttles between the nucleus and cytoplasm during development and in response to physiological and pathological stress (11). In contrast to SIRT1, mammalian SIRT2 is mainly localized to the cytoplasm (10, 12) but is also found in the nucleus (13). SIRT3, SIRT4, and SIRT5 are localized to mitochondria (10, 14), whereas SIRT6 and SIRT7 are found in the nucleus (10). SIRT6 is a chromatin-associated protein, and SIRT7 resides in the nucleolus (15, 16). Deacetylase activity was initially reported as conserved in mammalian Sirtuins, but different Sirtuins exhibit different acyl group preferences (17). Among the seven Sirtuins, SIRT4-7 exhibit weak or undetectable deacetylation activity *in vitro* (10, 18). SIRT2 reportedly possesses efficient demyristoylase activity (18). SIRT5 is reportedly an efficient NAD^+-dependent protein, lysine desuccinylase and demalonylase (19), while SIRT4 and SIRT6 reportedly possess ADP-ribosyltransferase activity (20, 21).

Mammalian Sirtuins regulate a wide variety of cellular processes, including metabolism, mitochondrial homeostasis, oxidative stress, inflammation, autophagy and apoptosis (22). Sirtuins also play important roles in aging and aging-related diseases, such as obesity, T2DM, cardiovascular disease, cancer, neurodegenerative diseases (23). SIRT1 and SIRT6 are the most extensively characterized Sirtuins. A large body of literature indicates that these two Sirtuins play an important role in metabolism, and they have also recently attracted increased attention with regard to their protective roles in maintaining insulin sensitivity, as reviewed elsewhere (24–26). Compared to the metabolic roles of SIRT1 and SIRT6, the metabolic roles of other Sirtuins remain poorly understood. Here, we review the recent advances in the understanding of the roles of Sirtuins in inflammation, mitochondrial dysfunction, and oxidative stress and discuss their possible roles in insulin resistance.

SIRTUINS IN INFLAMMATION

Obesity-induced chronic, low-grade inflammation is one of the most important contributors to the pathogenesis of insulin resistance (27–29). Adipose tissue is not only an insulin-targeting organ for lipid metabolism but also an endocrine organ that secretes hormones, cytokines, and chemokines to influence insulin sensitivity. For instance, adipocytes secrete adipokines, such as leptin and adiponectin, to promote insulin sensitivity (30, 31), and resistin and retinol-binding protein 4 (RBP4) to impair insulin sensitivity (32, 33). Importantly, adipose tissue is a critical initiator of the inflammatory response to obesity (28). In obesity, metabolism and gene expression of adipocytes change, resulting in increased lipolysis of adipocytes, the release of free fatty acids and proinflammatory cytokines and activation of M1 macrophages (27–29). M1 macrophages produce a large number of proinflammatory mediators, such as TNF-α, IL-1β, and resistin, that act on adipocytes to induce an insulin-resistant state and activate inflammatory pathways in insulin-targeting cells. Ultimately, ectopic lipid deposition and increased expression of inflammatory mediators in the liver and skeletal muscle lead to impaired insulin signaling and exacerbate systemic insulin resistance (29). Signals from all the proinflammatory mediators converge on inflammatory signaling pathways, including jun-n-terminal kinase (JNK) and inhibitor of nuclear factor κB (NF-κB) kinase (IKK) (27, 34, 35). Inhibition of insulin receptor downstream signaling is the primary mechanism for inflammation-induced insulin resistance (27). Activated JNK or IKK can phosphorylate the insulin receptor (IR) and insulin receptor substrate (IRS) proteins and decrease their tyrosine phosphorylation, thus leading to decreased activation of PI3-kinase and Akt and resistance to the metabolic actions of insulin (34, 36). In addition, activation of the JNK and IKK pathways can induce the production of inflammatory mediators, while the Sirtuin family plays essential roles in inflammation, which comprehensively contributes to insulin resistance.

Inflammatory Transcriptional Factor

NF-κB is a key transcriptional factor that mediates the expression of multiple inflammatory factors, including TNF-α, IL-1β, and IL-6. The acetylation of NF-κB promotes its nuclear translocation and activation. SIRT1 has been demonstrated to repress inflammation in multiple tissues and cells (37–40). In particular, SIRT1 suppresses inflammation in both adipocytes (39, 41) and macrophages (42), which leads to a reduction of adipose tissue inflammation. SIRT1 deacetylates p65 subunit of NF-κB at lysine 310 (K310) and inhibits the transcriptional activity of NF-κB (43). Moreover, SIRT1 interacts with transducing-like enhancer of split 1 (TLE1), a co-repressor of NF-κB, to inhibit NF-κB-mediated transcription (44). In addition, SIRT1 deacetylates activator protein-1 (AP-1) to reduce the expression of COX-2 in macrophages and deacetylates p53 to repress macrophage activation (45, 46). Similar to SIRT1, SIRT2 also binds to NF-κB and mediates the deacetylation of NF-κB subunit p65 at K310, which leads to the inhibition of the expression of NF-κB target inflammatory genes in fibroblasts, macrophages and microglial cells (47–49). SIRT2-mediated inhibition of NF-κB and inflammation contributes to its anti-inflammatory function in an experimental colitis mouse model (49), neuroinflammation (48, 50, 51), collagen-induced arthritis (52), and microvascular inflammation in *ob/ob* septic mice (53). In addition to SIRT2, SIRT4 can regulate the activation of NF-κB. SIRT4 has been shown to negatively regulate cigarette smoke extract (CSE)-induced NF-κB activation by inhibiting the degradation of IκBα and inhibiting NF-κB target gene expression, including the proinflammatory cytokines IL-1β, TNF-α, and IL-6, resulting in inhibition of CSE-induced mononuclear cell adhesion to human pulmonary microvascular endothelial cells (54). SIRT4 can prevent NF-κB nuclear translocation as well as the transcriptional activity of NF-κB, thereby suppressing inflammation in human umbilical vein endothelial cells (55). Interestingly, the role of SIRT5 in inflammation is controversial.

Recently, Qin and colleagues showed that SIRT5 deficiency decreased toll-like receptor (TLR)-triggered inflammation in both acute and immunosuppressive phases of sepsis (56). Mechanistically, SIRT5 competes with SIRT2 to interact with NF-κB p65 in a deacetylase activity-independent manner and thus blocks the deacetylation of p65 by SIRT2, which consequently leads to the activation of the NF-κB pathway and induction of its downstream cytokines in macrophages (56). However, Wang and colleagues found that SIRT5 desuccinylates and actives pyruvate kinase isoform M2 (PKM2) by promoting its dimerization and nuclear accumulation, thereby decreasing proinflammatory cytokine IL-1β production in LPS-activated macrophages (57). As hyperproduction of IL-1β contributes to increased susceptibility to inflammatory bowel disease, *Sirt5*-deficient mice are more susceptible to dextran sulfate sodium (DSS)-induced colitis (57). Interestingly, *Sirt6* deficient mice display increased expression of NF-κB-dependent genes in multiple tissues (58). *Sirt6* deletion increases inflammation in the mice adipose tissue and promotes HFD-induced insulin resistance (59, 60). Mechanistically, SIRT6 binds to the NF-κB subunit RelA and deacetylates histone H3 lysine 9 (H3K9) at NF-κB target gene promoters, which leads to a reduction of NF-κB target gene expression (58). These findings suggest that the Sirtuins target inflammatory transcriptional factors (e.g., NF-κB and AP1) directly or indirectly to contribute to insulin resistance comprehensively.

Inflammasome

The anti-inflammatory role of Sirtuins involves other mechanisms. The Nod-like receptor family, pyrin domain-containing 3 (NLRP3) inflammasome is a multiprotein complex that orchestrates the innate immune responses of macrophages by controlling the activation of caspase-1 and the release of the proinflammatory cytokines IL-1β and IL-18 (61–63). Obesity-related inflammation is partly mediated by the NLRP3 inflammasome, and NLRP3 activation exacerbates obesity-linked diseases (64, 65). Resveratrol, a SIRT1 activator, inhibits ionizing irradiation-induced inflammation in mesenchymal stem cells *via* suppressing NLRP3 inflammasome activation (66). In a murine model of sepsis, *Sirt1* deletion results in increasing lung inflammasome activation and inflammatory lung injury (67). A recent study demonstrated that silybin prevents NLRP3 inflammasome activation during NAFLD through SIRT2 (68). However, further studies are needed to clarify the mechanism underlying SIRT2-mediated regulation of NLRP3 inflammasome activity. In a human fasting/refeeding study, Traba and colleagues observed that fasting leads to a reduction in NLRP3 inflammasome activation (69). SIRT3 deletion in a human macrophage line increases NLRP3 inflammasome activation, accompanied by excessive mitochondrial ROS production (69). Pharmacologic and genetic SIRT3 activation enhances mitochondrial function and suppresses NLRP3 activity in THP-1 monocyte cells and in leukocytes extracted from healthy volunteers and from refeeding individuals (69). The authors concluded that nutrient levels regulate the NLRP3 inflammasome partly through SIRT3-mediated mitochondrial homeostatic control. Similarly, Chen *et al.* reported that trimethylamine-N-oxide (TMAO) increases ROS production by inhibiting the SIRT3-SOD2-mitochondrial signaling pathway, which leads to NLRP3 inflammasome activation and consequently promotes vascular inflammation (70). Defective autophagy in monocytes or macrophages might result in NLRP3 inflammasome activation and cause vascular metabolic inflammation (71–73). Acetylation of ATG5, an autophagy-related protein, inhibits autophagosome maturation and induces NLRP3 inflammasome activation (74). Recently, Liu and colleagues demonstrated that SIRT3 binds with ATG5 and deacetylates it, while SIRT3-deficient macrophages display impaired autophagy, leading to accelerated NLRP3 inflammasome activation and endothelial dysfunction (73). These studies suggest that SIRT3 may inhibit NLRP3 inflammasome activation by regulating mitochondrial function, ROS production, and autophagy. As SIRT2 has also been shown to regulate NLRP3 inflammasome activation (68), the potential synergistic effect on regulation of NLRP3 inflammasome activation between SIRT3 and SIRT2 needs further study. Previous studies have highlighted the anti-inflammatory role of SIRT3 in obesity-related diseases, including insulin resistance. The function of SIRT3 in inflammasome regulation largely depends on SIRT3-mediated activation of MnSOD and suppression of oxidative stress. These findings implicate that the SIRT1-SIRT3 indirectly regulate the activation of the NLRP3 inflammasome, which may be involved in the modulation of insulin resistance. However, whether Sirtuins directly regulate inflammasome remains unknown.

Sirtuins, Inflammation and Insulin Resistance

The roles of Sirtuins in inflammation significantly contribute to their functions during insulin resistance. For instance, activation of SIRT1 leads to the repression of JNK and IKK inflammatory pathways greatly and subsequently improves glucose tolerance, reduced hyperinsulinemia, and enhanced systemic insulin sensitivity (40). SIRT1 also controls the inflammatory status of macrophages and T lymphocytes to regulate the metabolism (insulin sensitivity) and inflammation of adipose tissues in obese mice (41, 75–77). In addition, SIRT6 is important for macrophage activation and TNFα production (78). Myeloid *Sirt6* deficiency causes insulin resistance in HFD–fed mice by eliciting macrophage polarization toward an M1 phenotype (79), and facilitates the development of HFD-induced atherosclerosis (80). Deletion of *Sirt6* in T cells or myeloid-derived cells is sufficient to induce liver inflammation and fibrosis (81). Interestingly, SIRT1 and SIRT6 can coordinate a switch from glucose to fatty acid oxidation during the acute inflammatory response (82). Therefore, Sirtuins not only regulate the inflammatory pathways within the target cells (e.g., hepatocytes, skeletal muscle cells, adipocytes) to affect their insulin sensitivity but also regulate inflammatory cells infiltrated in the organs, where the Sirtuins respond to inflammatory and metabolic insults and subsequently regulate insulin sensitivity and disease by targeting inflammatory cell activation and differentiation. Notably, the Sirtuins may also cooperate in diverse types of cells or within the same type of cell during inflammation-associated insulin resistance.

SIRTUINS IN MITOCHONDRIAL DYSFUNCTION

Mitochondria are the primary site for ATP generation and ROS production. Mitochondrial dysfunction results in decreased ATP production, increased ROS production and accumulated mitochondrial DNA damage, which contribute to insulin resistance (5). Cells eliminate ROS by expressing endogenous antioxidant enzymes, including manganese superoxide dismutase (MnSOD), catalase, glutathione peroxidase (GPX) and glutathione reductase (GRx) (83, 84). An imbalance between the production of ROS and antioxidant enzymes leads to oxidative stress, which has been implicated in the pathogenesis of insulin resistance, obesity, and diabetes (1, 85).

SIRT1

There are fewer mitochondria in muscles of T2DM patients than those of insulin-sensitive individuals (86). Marked reduction of oxidative phosphorylation in the mitochondria can be detected in the liver and skeletal muscle of T2DM patients and insulin-resistant individuals (87, 88). Peroxisome proliferator-activated receptor gamma coactivator 1-alpha (PGC-1α) is a transcriptional coactivator that regulates mitochondrial biogenesis and respiration (89, 90). SIRT1 has been shown to deacetylate PGC-1α at several lysine residues and regulates PGC-1α activity, which activates the transcription of genes involved in mitochondrial biogenesis (91). SIRT1 activator resveratrol promotes PGC-1α activity and increases the number of mitochondria in muscle cells, which improves mitochondrial function and protects mice against diet-induced obesity and insulin resistance (92). In addition to mitochondria biogenesis, SIRT1 regulates mitochondrial function through clearance of damaged mitochondria (93). Mechanistically, SIRT1 binds to and deacetylates autophagy regulators (including ATG5, ATG7, and ATG8) to induce mitochondria autophagy or mitophagy (93). SIRT1-mediated deacetylation of FoxO1 and FoxO3a is also known to induce the expression of autophagy pathway components (94, 95). Accumulating evidence has shown that SIRT1 safeguards cells from oxidative stress. SIRT1 reduces ros production by deacetylating and activating FoxO3a to upregulate expression of MnSOD and catalase (95, 96). SIRT1 promotes the transcriptional activity of Nuclear factor (erythroid-derived 2)-like 2 (NRF2) by deacetylating it and upregulates the expression of NRF2 target antioxidant genes, including *MnSOD*, *catalase*, *glutathione*, and *heme oxygenase-1* (*HO-1*) (97).

SIRT2

Oxidative stress increases SIRT2 expression *in vivo* and *in vitro* (98, 99). SIRT2 can bind to FoxO3a and deacetylate it, leading to an increase in FoxO3a transcriptional activity, upregulation of the expression of FoxO target genes such as *MnSOD*, *Bim*, and $p27^{Kip1}$, and a consequent decrease in ROS generation (98). Nicotinamide adenine dinucleotide phosphate (NADPH) is a functionally important metabolite that is required to generate the reduced form of glutathione (GSH) to maintain cellular redox potential. In response to oxidative stimuli, SIRT2 deacetylates and activates glucose 6-phosphate dehydrogenase (G6PD), a key enzyme in the pentose phosphate pathway (PPP), resulting in increased cytosolic NADPH to attenuate oxidative damage (100). Similarly, oxidative stress increases the glycolytic enzyme phosphoglycerate mutase (PGAM)-SIRT2 interaction, leading to deacetylation and activation of PGAM, which increases the cellular NADPH level to counteract oxidative damage (101). Lysine 4-oxononanoylation (4-ONylation) is a newly discovered histone posttranslational modification that disrupts the interaction between histone H3 and DNA, thereby preventing nucleosome assembly under oxidative stress (102). SIRT2 was reported to remove the 4-oxononanoyl (4-ONyl) lysine groups on histones and attenuate the negative impact of protein 4-ONylation caused by oxidative stress (103). This study provides novel evidence that SIRT2 may exert antioxidation effects through epigenetic modification. Oxidative stress is not completely caused by mitochondria, and whether SIRT2 can influence oxidative stress by regulating mitochondrial function is unclear.

Interestingly, a recent work by Liu and colleagues observed that SIRT2 can localize to the inner mitochondrial membrane of mouse central nervous system cells and that the acetylation of several metabolic mitochondrial proteins is altered in *Sirt2*-deficient mice. In mice, deletion of *Sirt2* causes mitochondrial morphological changes, increases oxidative stress and decreases ATP production in MEFs and brain tissues (104), indicating that SIRT2 may deacetylate antioxidant enzymes in the mitochondria directly.

SIRT3

SIRT3, a central mitochondrial deacetylase, deacetylates, and activates mitochondrial enzymes to regulate mitochondrial metabolism, oxidative stress, cell survival, and longevity (105). SIRT3 has been shown to play a pivotal role in maintaining mitochondrial function and ROS homeostasis. For example, SIRT3 deacetylates complex I and complex II of the electron transport chain to promote electron transport and regulate energy homeostasis (106, 107). SIRT3 deacetylates cyclophilin D (CypD), the regulatory component of the mitochondrial permeability transition pore (mPTP), preventing opening of the mPTP and mitochondrial dysfunction (108). SIRT3 binds to and deacetylates 8-oxoguanine-DNA glycosylase 1 (OGG1), a DNA repair enzyme that excises 7,8-dihydro-8-oxoguanine from the damaged genome, resulting in the repair of mitochondrial DNA (mtDNA) damage, protection of mitochondrial integrity, defense against mitochondrial dysfunction and prevention of stress-induced cellular apoptosis (109). In contrast, *Sirt3* deficiency has been linked to increased ROS production (110, 111). The antioxidant action of SIRT3 involves MnSOD and mitochondrial isocitrate dehydrogenase 2 (IDH2). SIRT3 has been shown to block cardiac hypertrophy by deacetylating FOXO3a and upregulating the expression of FOXO3a target genes such as *MnSOD* and *catalase*, decreasing ROS generation (112). Notably, the antioxidative action of SIRT3 may also be attributed to its direct deacetylation and promotion of the enzyme activity of

MnSOD. SIRT3 deacetylates two critical lysine residues (K53 and K89) of MnSOD that promote MnSOD antioxidation activity, thereby reducing cellular ROS (113). Direct deacetylation of lysine residues, including K68 and K122 by SIRT3, also increases the enzyme activity of MnSOD and decreases ROS production (114, 115). In addition to MnSOD, SIRT3 directly deacetylates and activates mitochondrial IDH2, which results in increased NADPH levels and an increased ratio of reduced to oxidized GSH in mitochondria, thus protecting cells from oxidative stress-induced damage (110, 116). These studies suggest that SIRT3 activity is necessary to prevent mitochondrial dysfunction and reduce oxidative stress.

SIRT4

SIRT4 functions as an efficient mitochondrial ADP-ribosyl transferase that negatively impacts gene expression and various metabolic processes in mitochondria. Our previous work demonstrated that SIRT4 promotes angiotensin II-induced development of cardiac hypertrophy by inhibiting the interaction of SIRT3 and MnSOD, which increases MnSOD acetylation levels, decreases its activity and leads to elevated ROS accumulation (117). SIRT4 may play a role different from that of SIRT3 in regulating mitochondrial function and oxidative stress. *Sirt4* deficiency *in vivo* and *in vitro* increases the expression of genes involved in fatty acid β-oxidation and oxidative phosphorylation, thus enhancing fatty acid oxidation and mitochondrial respiration in liver and muscle (118, 119). SIRT4 increases stress-induced mitochondrial ROS production and interacts with the long form of GTPase optic atrophy 1 (L-OPA1) to promote mitochondrial fusion, thereby inhibiting mitophagy and decreasing the removal of dysfunctional mitochondria (120).

SIRT5

SIRT5 functions to deacetylate, demalonylate, and desuccinylate multiple proteins in mitochondria (19). SIRT5 is involved in the regulation of mitochondrial fatty acid β-oxidation, the urea cycle, and cellular respiration (84, 121). SIRT5 binds to, desuccinylates and activates copper-zinc superoxide dismutase 1 (SOD1) to eliminate ROS (122). Moreover, SIRT5 desuccinylates IDH2 and deglutarylates G6PD, thus activating both NADPH-producing enzymes to scavenge ROS (123). SIRT5 also binds, desuccinylates and inhibits the activity of the glycolysis enzyme PKM2, which facilitates the diversion of glucose metabolites into the pentose phosphate shunt and then produces sufficient NADPH to eliminate ROS (123). Interestingly, a very recent study showed that SIRT5 is present in peroxisomes and can bind, desuccinylate and inhibit ACOX1, the first and rate-limiting enzyme in fatty acid β-oxidation and a major producer of H_2O_2, attenuating peroxisome-induced oxidative stress (124).

SIRT6

SIRT6 plays an important role in DNA repair, genomic stability, and cellular senescence, however, the role of SIRT6 in oxidative stress has not been well clarified. According to recent studies, SIRT6 is believed to protect cells against oxidative stress. Pan et al. (125) found that SIRT6 serves as an NRF2 coactivator by interacting with NRF2 and RNA polymerase II to transactivate NRF2-regulated antioxidant genes, including HO-1. SIRT6 activates AMPK-FoxO3a axis to initiate expression of *MnSOD* and *catalase* and protects cardiomyocytes against ischemia/reperfusion-induced injury (126).

SIRT7

Sirt7 deficiency in mice induces multisystemic mitochondrial dysfunction (127). SIRT7 deacetylates GABPβ1, a master regulator of nuclear-encoded mitochondrial genes, enables it to form the transcriptionally active GABPa/GABPβ heterotetramer, and promotes mitochondria function (127). Additionally, the mitochondrial unfolded protein response [UPR(mt)] is mediated by the interplay of SIRT7 and NRF1 and is coupled to cellular energy metabolism and proliferation (128).

SIRTUINS IN INSULIN SIGNALING PATHWAYS

Insulin Secretion

Under the condition of insulin resistance, normal pancreatic β cells increase the production of insulin to maintain blood glucose levels. However, this compensatory response fails, and relative insulin insufficiency develops. Then, glucose tolerance is impaired, and T2DM eventually occurs. SIRT1, SIRT4, and SIRT6 reportedly regulate pancreatic β cell function (**Figure 1**) (24, 129, 130). According to accumulating evidence, SIRT1 and SIRT6 repress pancreatic β cell dysfunction, attenuating the development of T2DM. β cell-specific SIRT1 transgenic mice exhibit enhanced insulin secretion and improved glucose tolerance to high glucose stimulation (131). Mechanistically, through repressing UCP2 expression, SIRT1 enhances ATP production in pancreatic β cells, to shut down the potassium channel, resulting in the influx of calcium and finally the secretion of insulin (131, 132). SIRT1 can induce *NeuroD* and *MafA* expression *via* deacetylating and activating FoxO1, which protects pancreatic β cells against oxidative damage and preserves pancreatic β cells function (133). In contrast to SIRT1 and SIRT6, SIRT4 functions as a negative regulator of insulin secretion in β cells. Glutamate dehydrogenase (GDH) promotes the metabolism of glutamate and glutamine, generating ATP to further promote insulin secretion. In pancreatic β cells, SIRT4 represses the activity of GDH by ADP-ribosylation, thereby downregulating insulin secretion in response to amino acids under calorie-sufficient conditions (20). SIRT4 also controls leucine oxidation to regulate insulin secretion (134). Given that SIRT3 deacetylases GDH and increases its activity in hepatocytes (135), SIRT3 may function in β cell mitochondria to promote insulin secretion. Recent studies have provided evidence to support this notion. Caton *et al.* observed that SIRT3 expression markedly decreases in islets isolated from T2DM patients, as well as in mouse islets or INS1 cells (136). *Sirt3* knockdown in INS1 cells results in increased production of cellular ROS and IL-1β, increased β cell apoptosis and reduced insulin secretion (136). SIRT3 deficiency predisposes pancreatic β cells to oxidative stress-induced dysfunction and reduces glucose-induced insulin secretion (137). By contrast, SIRT3 overexpression inhibits ER stress and attenuates palmitate-induced pancreatic β cell

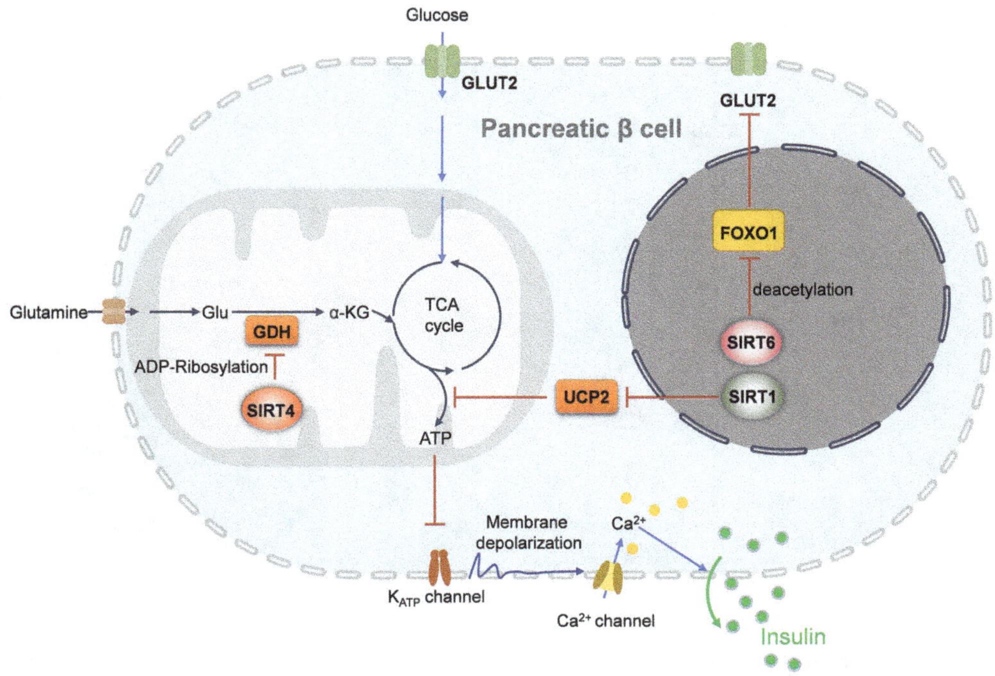

FIGURE 1 | Sirtuins regulates insulin secretion of pancreatic beta cells. In the nucleus, SIRT1 induces insulin secretion through the reduction of UCP2 expression and the enhancement of depolarization in pancreatic β cells, while SIRT6 deacetylates FOXO1 and promotes the expression of GLUT2, which facilitates glucose uptake and insulin secretion. In the mitochondria, SIRT4 promotes the ADP-ribosylation and inactivation of GDH, leading the repression of ATP generation and inhibition of insulin secretion. UCP2, uncoupling protein 2; Glu, glutamate; GDH, glutamate dehydrogenase; GLUT2, glucose transporter 2; α-KG, alpha-ketoglutarate.

dysfunction (138, 139). Therefore, SIRT3 and SIRT4 play opposing roles in regulating insulin secretion in pancreatic β cells. In addition, insulin secretion impairment is observed in *Sirt6* knockout pancreatic β cells, which is mediated by suppression of the FoxO1-Pdx1-Glut2 pathway (140). *Sirt6* deletion in pancreatic β cells also reduces ATP production and increases mitochondrial damage which induces cell apoptosis and impairs glucose-stimulated insulin secretion (129, 141). β cell-specific *Sirt6*-ko mice are glucose intolerance and are defective in glucose-stimulated insulin secretion, in spite do not show abnormality in endocrine morphology, pancreatic β cell mass or insulin production (130). *Sirt6* deficiency also results in aberrant upregulation of thioredoxin-interacting protein (TXNIP) in pancreatic β cells, which inhibits insulin secretion (130).

Insulin Signaling Pathway

Insulin resistance, the inability of cells to efficiently respond to a normal dose of insulin, is caused by impaired insulin signaling and postreceptor intracellular defects (4). Insulin binding to its receptor results in IR phosphorylating itself and several intracellular substrates. The phosphorylated substrates interact with intracellular effectors, leading to the activation of the PI3K-Akt pathway, which is responsible for most of the metabolic actions of insulin, and the Ras-MAPK pathway, which controls cell growth and differentiation (4, 142). Impaired Akt activation is a key factor in metabolic disorders involving insulin resistance. Accumulating evidence suggests that Sirtuins participate in insulin signaling in target cells (**Figure 2**).

SIRT1 positively regulates insulin signaling and Akt activation at multiple levels. SIRT1 represses transcription of *PTPN1*, a negative regulator of the insulin signal transduction cascade, at the chromatin level and improves insulin sensitivity (3). Knockdown of *Sirt1* in 3T3-L1 adipocytes increases phosphorylation of JNK, as well as serine phosphorylation of insulin receptor substrate 1 (IRS-1), which leads to decrease tyrosine phosphorylation of IRS-1, and then inhibit phosphorylation of Akt (39). Inhibition of SIRT1 activity reduces insulin-induced IRS-2 deacetylation, which prevents insulin-induced IRS-2 tyrosine phosphorylation (143). SIRT1 mediates deacetylation of Akt regulates binding of Akt to phosphatidylinositol 3,4,5-trisphosphate (PIP3) which is necessary for Akt membrane localization and activation (144).

SIRT2 can directly regulate the insulin signaling pathway, but its role is controversial. SIRT2 can deacetylate and activate Akt through the Akt/glycogen synthase kinase-3β (GSK3β)/β-catenin signaling pathway, finally resulting in aberrant proliferation and survival of myeloid leukemia cells and epithelial-mesenchymal transition of HCC (145, 146). Interestingly, Ramakrishnan and colleagues showed that SIRT2 is a novel Akt interactor and is required for optimal Akt activation under normal conditions (147). Pharmacological or genetic inhibition of SIRT2 decreases Akt activation in 3T3-L1 preadipocytes and HeLa cells, whereas SIRT2 overexpression enhances the activation of Akt and its

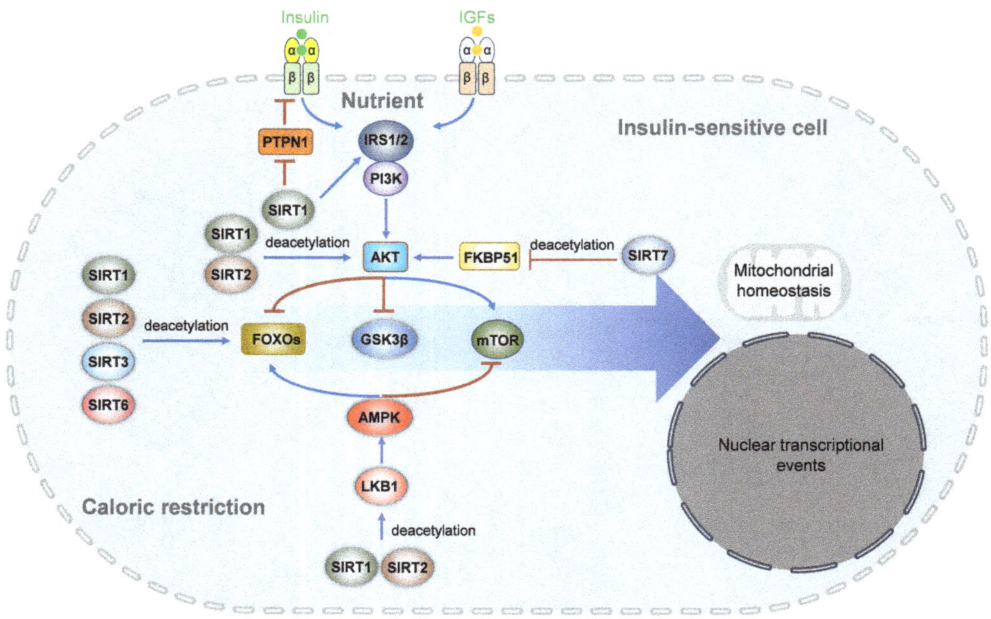

FIGURE 2 | Sirtuins regulates insulin signaling pathways. In nutrient enough conditions, insulin and insulin-like growth factors activate the IRS-PI3K-AKT signaling and downstream FOXO and mTOR signaling to regulate multiple aspects of metabolism, survival, mitochondrial homeostasis, nuclear transcriptional events, and other cellular behaviors. The insulin receptor activation is inhibited by PTPN1, which is repressed by SIRT1. SIRT1 also deacetylates IRS2 and represses IRS1 phosphorylation and PI3K-AKT activation. SIRT1 and SIRT2 also deacetylate AKT to activate its activation directly, while SIRT7 indirectly inhibits AKT activation by deacetylating FKBP51. Under energetic stress or caloric restriction, multiple members of the Sirtuins family are activated. SIRT1, SIRT2, SIRT3, and SIRT6 can directly deacetylate FOXOs (FOXO1 and FOXO3a), while SIRT1 and SIRT2 activate the LKB1-AMPK signaling to activate FOXO and inhibit mTOR signaling. IGF, insulin-like growth factor; IRS, insulin receptor substrate; PTPN1, tyrosine-protein phosphatase non-receptor type 1; PI3K, phosphatidylinositol-4,5-bisphosphate 3-kinase; mTOR, mammalian target of rapamycin; AMPK, AMP-activated protein kinase; LKB1, liver kinase B1; FKBP51, FK506-binding protein 51; GSK3β, glycogen synthase kinase-3 beta.

downstream targets, such as GSK3 and p70-S6-kinase (147). Insulin-induced Akt activation requires Akt binding to inositol 1,4,5-trisphosphate, which leads to Akt conformational changes and facilitates its phosphorylation by PDK1 and mTORC1 (147). Acetylation at Lys20 blocks Akt activation by restricting the binding of Akt to inositol 1,4,5-trisphosphate (144). However, the authors were unable to detect Akt acetylation in the experiment, and they could not determine whether the effects of SIRT2 on Akt are dependent on changing the acetylation level of Akt (147). However, the opposite results have also been reported. Arora et al. reported that SIRT2 is upregulated in insulin-resistant skeletal muscle cells, and inhibition of SIRT2 by pharmacological or genetic means improves phosphorylation of Akt and GSK3β and increases insulin-stimulated glucose uptake (148). Similarly, in insulin-resistant neuro-2a cells, inhibition of SIRT2 by pharmacological or genetic means also enhances the activity of Akt and increases insulin-stimulated glucose uptake (149). Therefore, SIRT2 may regulate Akt in both direct (activity-dependent) and indirect (activity-independent) manners, which may largely rely on the metabolic status of the cells. SIRT2 can deacetylate and regulate the function of FOxO transcription factors, which are direct Akt targets (98, 150). Interestingly, the Akt-independent pathway also contributes to the function of SIRT2 in the regulation of insulin sensitivity. TUG acetylation modulates its interaction with Golgi matrix proteins and enhances its function to trap GLUT4 storage vesicles in intracellular (151). Insulin mobilizes the exocytic translocation of GLUT4 glucose transporters by triggering TUG proteolysis to accelerate glucose uptake in fat and muscle. SIRT2-mediated TUG deacetylation controls insulin sensitivity *in vivo* and *in vitro* (151).

The role of SIRT6 in the insulin signaling pathway is controversial. *Sirt6*-deficient mice die about 4 weeks of age, exhibiting severe metabolic defects, including low insulin and hypoglycemia (15). Xiao et al. found that *Sirt6* deficiency increases Akt phosphorylation through modulating insulin signaling upstream of Akt, including insulin receptor, IRS1, IRS2, and enhances insulin signaling, leading to hypoglycemia (152). On the contrary, *Sirt6* transgenic mice show increased insulin sensitivity in skeletal muscle and liver and exhibit enhanced insulin-induced Akt activation in gastrocnemius (153).

In addition, SIRT7 can regulate Akt signaling. SIRT7 regulates the acetylation of FKBP51, which then regulates Akt activation. Acetylated FKBP51 enhances Akt activity by blocking its interaction with PHLPP-Akt. SIRT7 deacetylates FKBP51 at two major lysine residues. SIRT7 suppresses Akt activation and modulates cell sensitivity to genotoxic agents (154). The inhibitory effects of SIRT7 on Akt activation were also observed in murine hearts.

SIRTUINS IN INSULIN-SENSITIVE ORGANS

Adipose tissue, liver, and muscle are the primary insulin-responsive organs. Insulin regulates blood glucose concentrations by suppressing hepatic glucose output and stimulating glucose uptake by muscle and adipose tissue. In addition, insulin promotes energy storage in adipose tissue, liver, and muscle by stimulating lipogenesis, glycogen, and protein synthesis but inhibiting lipolysis, glycogenolysis and protein catabolism (155).

The impaired lipogenic/adipogenic capacity of adipose tissue leads to increased body fat mass and adverse metabolic consequences (4, 156). Adipose tissue is not only an excessive energy storage pot but also a highly active endocrine organ that secretes proteins, adipokines, cytokines and chemokines to influence insulin sensitivity. Circulating FFAs derived from adipocytes are involved in the accumulation of triglycerides and fatty acid-derived metabolites in muscle and liver, which is a contributing factor to insulin resistance (155). In addition, adipose tissue is an important initiator of the inflammatory response to obesity (28), and FFAs from adipose tissue are important ER stress-triggering factors (28).

The liver, as the central organ responsible for maintaining lipid and glucose hemostasis in the body, plays a crucial role in insulin sensitivity and metabolic diseases. During prolonged fasting or starvation, the liver converts lipids to available energy through fatty acid oxidation and provides glucose to maintain normal blood glucose, initially by glycogenolysis and then by switching to gluconeogenesis (157, 158). Under energy abundance conditions, the liver promotes glycogenesis and lipogenesis to store energy. Insulin stimulates glycogen accumulation and blocks gluconeogenesis and glycogenolysis in the liver to suppress hepatic glucose output (155, 158, 159). In the condition of insulin resistance, suppression of hepatic glucose output is impaired, while increased FFA from adipocytes leads to ectopic lipid accumulation in the liver, which exacerbates insulin resistance (29).

Skeletal muscle is the major site for insulin-stimulated glucose disposal *in vivo* as well as the main energy consumer of lipid catabolism that strongly influences whole-body lipid metabolism (155, 160). The ability to switch between glucose and lipid oxidation is crucial for skeletal muscle to maintain physiological function and metabolic hemostasis (161). Intramuscular fatty acid metabolite accumulation may cause insulin resistance (162).

The functions of Sirtuins in regulating glucose and lipid metabolism as well as insulin sensitivity have been widely investigated in adipose tissue, liver and skeletal muscles (**Figure 3**).

SIRT1 and Insulin-Sensitive Organs

SIRT1 Regulates Fatty Acid and Glucose Metabolism in the Liver

The role of SIRT1 in regulating hepatic gluconeogenesis is controversial under the condition of calorie restriction. Resveratrol has been shown to improve glucose homeostasis in insulin-resistant mice by reducing hepatic gluconeogenesis and increase insulin sensitivity in adipose tissue, skeletal muscle and liver (163). On the contrary, resveratrol causes nuclear translocation of FoxO1 in hepatocytes *via* SIRT1-dependent deacetylation, which leads to activation of gluconeogenesis and increased hepatic glucose output (164). Pyruvate induces SIRT1 protein in the liver during fasting, and once SIRT1 is induced, which can increase gluconeogenic genes expression and promote hepatic glucose output through interacting and deacetylating PGC-1α (165). Conversely, during prolonged fasting, SIRT1 deacetylates CREB regulated transcription coactivator 2 (CRTC2) and promotes its ubiquitin-dependent degradation to inhibit gluconeogenic gene expression, leading to decreased hepatic glucose output (166). On the other hand, upregulation of FOXO1 and PGC-1α activity by SIRT1 leads to activation of gluconeogenic gene expression in hepatic cells and increase hepatic glucose production (157, 166). In addition, SIRT1 regulates the activity of PGC-1α, and glycolytic enzyme phosphoglycerate mutase-1 (PGAM1), inducing repression of glycolytic genes in response to fasting (165, 167). These studies suggest an important role of SIRT1 in maintaining energy balance under fasting. Liver-specific *Sirt1* ko mice develop hepatic steatosis when underwent fasting and obesity when fed with HFD in insulin-dependent and independent manners (38, 168). *Sirt1* transgenic mice show better glucose tolerance and insulin sensitivity and are almost entirely protected from hepatic steatosis with HFD treatment (37, 169). On one hand, SIRT1 deacetylates and activates PGC-1α, increasing fatty acid β-oxidation in the liver (38). On the other hand, SIRT1 plays an important role in inhibiting lipogenesis in the liver. For example, resveratrol can increase the levels of sterol regulatory element-binding protein (SREBP), a critical regulator of lipid and sterol homeostasis in eukaryotes, in livers of alcohol-treated mice and alleviate alcoholic fatty liver (170). SRT1720, a SIRT1 activator, ameliorates fatty liver through suppressing the expression of lipogenic enzymes, including SREBP-1c, acetyl-CoA carboxylase, and fatty acid synthase, in obesity and insulin resistant mice (171). SIRT1 can directly deacetylate SREBP, and control SREBP protein stability *via* SREBP ubiquitination, leading to attenuating SREBP target lipogenic gene expression and inhibiting lipid synthesis and fat storage (172). Otherwise, SIRT1 activation by polyphenols acts as an upstream regulator in the LKB1/AMPK signaling axis, resulting in repression expression of acetyl-CoA carboxylase and fatty acid synthase and reduction of lipid accumulation in hepatocytes (173).

SIRT1 Regulates Adipocyte Differentiation and Adipogenesis

PPARγ and CCAAT/enhancer-binding protein α (C/EBPα) are master regulators of adipogenesis (156, 174). SIRT1 overexpression inhibits the expression of PPARγ and C/EBPα in 3T3-L1 adipocytes (175). SIRT1 represses PPARγ by docking with its cofactors nuclear receptor co-repressor (NCoR) and silencing mediator of retinoid and thyroid hormone receptors (SMRT) and suppresses adipogenesis (175). In differentiated fat cells, upregulation of SIRT1 by resveratrol triggers lipolysis and loss of fat, but SIRT1 inhibitor nicotinamide reduces the release of free fatty acid (175).

	Liver				Adipose tissue				Skeletal Muscle	
	Fatty acid oxidation	Lipogenesis	Glycolysis	Gluconeogenesis	Thermogenesis	Browning	Adipogenesis	Fatty acid oxidation	Glycolysis	Fatty acid oxidation
SIRT1	FOXO1(+), PGC1α(+), CRTC2(-), PPARα(+)	SREBP1c(-), AMPK(+)	HIF1α(-), FOXO1(+), PGC1α(+), PGAM-1(-)	FOXO1(+), PGC1α(+), PPARα(+), CRTC2(-)		PPARγ(-), Prdm16(+)	FOXO1(+), PPARγ(-)		PGC1α(+)	PGC1α(+), AMPK(+), PPARα(+)
SIRT2	PGC1α(+)	ACLY(-)	GKRP(+)	PEPCK1(+)			FOXO1(+)	PGC1α(+)		
SIRT3	LCAD(+)		PDH(+), IDH2(+), NDUFA9(+)		PGC1α(+)	PGC1α(+), SDH(+)			PDH(+), HK2(+)	
SIRT4	PPARα(+), AMPK(+)		PDH(-)				MCD(-)			MCD(-)
SIRT5	ECHA(+), HCDH(+)		GAPDH(+)	GAPDH(+)						
SIRT6	CPT1(+), AOX(+)	SREBP-2(-), ACC(-), SCD(-), FAS(-)	GK(-)	GCN5(+)	PGC1α(+)	PGC1α(+)	KIF5C(-)		AMPK(+)	AMPK(+)
SIRT7	GABPβ1(+)	DCAF1/DDB1/CUL4B (-)	PGK1(-)	G6PC(+)			SIRT1(-), PPARγ(+)			

FIGURE 3 | Sirtuins regulates metabolism in insulin-target organs. The functions of Sirtuins in the regulation of glucose and fatty acid metabolism in the liver, adipose tissue, and skeletal muscle. The (–) indicates Sirtuin represses the activation/expression of this target, whereas (+) indicates Sirtuin promotes the activation/expression of the target. The green background indicates Sirtuin promotes the biological process whereas the pink background indicates the Sirtuin represses the biological process. PGC-1α, peroxisome proliferator-activated receptor gamma coactivator 1-alpha; TORC2, CREB regulated transcription coactivator 2; PPARα, peroxisome proliferator-activated receptor alpha; SREBP1c, Sterol response element-binding protein 1c; AMPK, AMP-activated protein kinase; HIF1α, hypoxia-inducible factor 1 alpha; PGAM-1, phosphoglycerate mutase 1; CRTC2, CREB regulated transcription coactivator 2; PPARγ, peroxisome proliferator-activated receptor gamma; Prdm16, PR domain containing 16; PEPCK1, phosphoenolpyruvate carboxykinase 1; LCAD, long-chain acyl-CoA dehydrogenase; PDH, pyruvate dehydrogenase; IDH2, isocitrate dehydrogenase; NDUFA9, NADH dehydrogenase [ubiquinone] 1 alpha subcomplex subunit 9; SDH, succinate dehydrogenase; HK2, hexokinase 2; MCD, malonyl-CoA decarboxylase; ECHA, trifunctional enzyme subunit alpha; HCDH, hydroxyacyl-Coenzyme A dehydrogenase; GAPDH, Glyceraldehyde 3-phosphate dehydrogenase; SREBP-2, sterol regulatory element-binding protein 2; ACC, acetyl-CoA carboxylase; SCD, stearoyl-CoA desaturase; FAS, fatty acid synthase; GK, glucokinase; GCN5, general control non-repressed protein 5; KIF5C, kinesin heavy chain isoform 5C; GABPβ1, GA binding protein β1; DCAF1/DDB1/GUL4B, DDB1-CUL4-associated factor 1 (DCAF1)/damage-specific DNA binding protein 1 (DDB1)/cullin 4B (CUL4B) complex; PGK1, phosphoglycerate kinase 1; G6PC, glucose-6-phosphatase, catalytic subunit; GKRP, glucokinase regulatory protein.

SIRT1 Regulates Lipid Metabolism in Skeletal Muscle

There is a strong correlation between the presence of intramyocellular lipid in skeletal muscle and liver and progression of T2DM (176, 177). Fasting induces PGC-1α deacetylation by SIRT1 in skeletal muscle, and that is required for activation of mitochondrial fatty acid oxidation genes (178). SIRT1 overexpression protects C2C12 myotubes against fatty acid-induced insulin resistance through transcriptional repression of PTP1B (3). In skeletal muscle, SIRT1 acts downstream of AMPK signaling, deacetylates and modulates the activity of PGC-1α, FOXO1, and FOXO3a to inhibit lipogenesis and promote energy consumption (179). SIRT1 overexpression or resveratrol treatment increases insulin-induced Akt phosphorylation and activation *via* interacting with the PI3K adapter subunit p85 (180). These studies suggest SIRT1 plays a positive role in ameliorating insulin sensitivity in skeletal muscle. However, several studies have demonstrated that skeletal muscle-specific overexpression of SIRT1 does not enhance whole-body energy expenditure or skeletal muscle insulin sensitivity under normal or overfeeding conditions (181, 182). These controversial results suggest SIRT1 in other metabolic tissues, such as adipose tissue, liver or intestinal tissue, may play a role in the metabolic benefits of SIRT1 activation (183). Notably, high-intensity interval training increases SIRT1 activity in human skeletal muscle and mice with muscle-specific inactivation of the SIRT1 deacetylase domain displayed reduced myofiber size, impaired muscle regeneration, and derepression of muscle developmental genes (184, 185). Therefore, SIRT1-mediated metabolic balance is important for skeletal muscle homeostasis and regeneration.

SIRT2 and Insulin-Sensitive Organs

SIRT2 Regulates Adipocyte Differentiation and Adipogenesis

SIRT2 is widely distributed and has been detected in a wide range of metabolic tissues, including the brain, muscle, liver, pancreas and adipose tissue. SIRT2 expression is regulated by metabolic status. For instance, the expression of SIRT2 is elevated in the white adipose tissue (WAT) of cr mice (98). SIRT2 gene expression increased in the peripheral blood mononuclear cells of obese subjects following an 8-week hypocaloric diet (186). By contrast, SIRT2 protein expression in visceral WAT from human obese subjects and a mouse model of diet-induced obesity is downregulated compared with that in WAT from lean controls

(187). SIRT2 gene expression is significantly lower in peripheral blood mononuclear cells of obese children with insulin resistance than in those without insulin resistance (188). A growing body of literature has indicated that SIRT2 is involved in regulating various metabolic processes, including adipocyte differentiation, hepatic gluconeogenesis, and insulin action. SIRT2 mRNA is more abundant than other Sirtuins in adipose tissue *in vivo* and preadipocytes in culture (150), implicating the possible important role of SIRT2 in adipose tissue. FOXO1 acts as an adipogenesis inhibitor (189). In adipose tissue, FOXO1 can interact with PPARγ and negatively regulate its transcriptional activity (190) or bind to the PPARγ promoter region and suppress its expression (191). In mouse 3T3-L1 preadipocytes, SIRT2 interacts with and deacetylates FOXO1, which antagonizes FOXO1 phosphorylation and promotes nuclear retention of FOXO1, leading to repression of the expression of *PPARγ* and *C/EBPα* as well as genes marking terminal adipocyte differentiation, such as *Glut4*, *aP2*, and *fatty acid synthase* (150). SIRT2 also suppresses adipogenesis by deacetylating FOXO1 to promote the binding of FOXO1 to PPARγ and subsequent repression of PPARγ transcriptional activity (192). Increased *de novo* lipogenesis is an important contributor to increased adipose mass (193). ATP-citrate lyase (ACLY) is the building block for *de novo* lipid synthesis, which converts glucose-derived citrate into acetyl-CoA (194). ACLY is acetylated on multiple lysine residues in response to high glucose and promotes lipogenesis, while SIRT2 deacetylates and destabilizes ACLY, leading to reduced lipogenesis (195). Transcriptional regulators such as PPARs and the coactivator PGC-1α play key roles in the process of fatty acid β-oxidation, which determines whole-body energy expenditure (196). Through transcriptional repression of SIRT2, hypoxia-inducible factor 1α (HIF1α) decreases deacetylation of PGC-1α and further diminishes fatty acid β-oxidation in WAT. Adipocyte-specific HIF1α inactivation leads to increased expression of SIRT2 and attenuates dietary-driven obesity in mice (187). These studies suggest that SIRT2 contributes to the control of adipose tissue mass by inhibiting adipogenesis and lipogenesis but promoting fatty acid β-oxidation.

SIRT2 Participates in Gluconeogenesis in the Liver

SIRT2 deacetylates and subsequently increases the stability of PEPCK1, the gluconeogenic rate-limiting enzyme under conditions of glucose deprivation, leading to increased gluconeogenesis (197, 198). FOXO1 and PGC-1α reportedly activate the process of gluconeogenesis in the liver by increasing the transcription of gluconeogenic enzyme genes and are considered negative regulators of insulin sensitivity in the liver (199–201). Insulin suppresses gluconeogenesis by regulating the FOXO1-PGC-1α interaction (199). SIRT2 deacetylates and activates FOXO1/PGC-1α in adipocytes (150, 187, 192), which implies that SIRT2 may enhance gluconeogenesis through the FOXO1-PGC-1α pathway. However, whether the role of SIRT2 in gluconeogenesis depends on different nutrient conditions must be elucidated. In addition, the roles of SIRT2 in metabolic diseases are largely unknown.

SIRT3

Human SIRT3 is expressed in a variety of metabolically active tissues, including muscle, liver, kidney, heart, brain, and BAT (202–204). The expression of SIRT3 in the liver and adipose tissue of mice increases during cr (205–208). A single nucleotide polymorphism in the human *SIRT3* gene has been correlated with the reduced enzymatic efficiency of SIRT3 and the development of metabolic syndrome (209). Compared with WT mice, *Sirt3*-KO mice fed an HFD show accelerated obesity, insulin resistance, hyperlipidemia, and hepatic steatosis (209).

SIRT3 Participates in WAT/BAT Metabolism and Thermogenesis

High levels of SIRT3 occur in the BAT. Cold exposure upregulates SIRT3 expression in the BAT. Increasing the expression of PGC-1α and uncoupling protein 1 (UCP1) by sustained expression of SIRT3 in brown adipocytes leads to increased thermogenesis (7, 206). Fatty acid β-oxidation in the BAT of *Sirt3*-KO mice is significantly reduced (210). Although SIRT3 maintains a low level in WAT (206), several studies refer to the role of SIRT3 in regulating WAT lipid metabolism. cr activates SIRT3 expression in both white and brown adipose tissue; SIRT3 expression decreases in the BAT of several lines of genetically obese mice (206). In a human study, SIRT3 gene expression was decreased in VAT from morbid subjects (211) and WAT from children with obesity (212). Although the role of SIRT3 in WAT lipid metabolism is intricate and unclear, these studies suggest that SIRT3 may play a protective role in obesity.

SIRT3 Regulates Fatty Acid Oxidation in the Liver

Sirt3-deficient mice show higher levels of fatty acid β-oxidation intermediate products and triglycerides in the liver during fasting and develop hepatic steatosis (210). Metabolomic analyses of fasted *Sirt3*-deficient mice revealed that SIRT3 is involved in fatty acid β-oxidation and modulates fatty acid β-oxidation at multiple points, such as short-chain L-3-hydroxy acyl-CoA dehydrogenase (SCHAD), very-long-chain acyl-CoA dehydrogenase (VLCAD) and 3-ketoacyl-CoA thiolase, in addition to LCAD (208). LCAD is a key enzyme in mitochondrial fatty acid β-oxidation, and LCAD deficiency causes hepatic steatosis and hepatic insulin resistance (213, 214). SIRT3 promotes hepatic fatty acid β-oxidation through deacetylation and activation of LCAD (210). However, hepatocyte-specific *Sirt3*-KO mice do not show any obvious metabolic phenotype under either chow or HFD conditions, despite a marked global hyperacetylation of mitochondrial proteins (215). These conflicting findings from global *Sirt3*-KO mice and tissue-specific KO mice suggest that the roles of SIRT3 in other cell types may be important for SIRT3-mediated metabolic effects in the liver.

SIRT3 Regulates Glucose Metabolism in Skeletal Muscle

SIRT3 expression decreases in the skeletal muscle of diabetic and HFD-fed mice (36, 216). CR and exercise upregulate SIRT3 expression in mouse skeletal muscle (162). These findings suggest that SIRT3 is involved in skeletal muscle metabolism. Although muscle-specific *Sirt3* KO in mice shows no obvious effects on global metabolic hemostasis under normal conditions (215), striking results have been shown in global *Sirt3*-KO mice. Global *Sirt3*-KO mice exhibit decreased oxygen consumption and enhanced oxidative stress in skeletal muscle that leads to impaired insulin signaling (36). The deletion of *Sirt3 in vivo* and *in vitro* induces hyperacetylation of the pyruvate dehydrogenase (PDH) E1α subunit and leads to decreased PDH enzymatic activity (161). Inhibition of PDH activity reduces glucose oxidation and results in a switch to fatty acid β-oxidation, thus leading to a loss of skeletal muscle metabolic flexibility (161). In addition, HFD-fed *Sirt3*-KO mice exhibit increased insulin resistance due to defects in skeletal muscle glucose uptake (217). These studies suggest that SIRT3 may protect insulin sensitivity in skeletal muscle.

SIRT4

SIRT4 Regulates Lipogenesis

The expression of SIRT4 is upregulated in the liver and adipose tissues in rodents fed an HFD (218, 219). SIRT4 deacetylates and inhibits malonyl CoA decarboxylase (MCD), an enzyme producing acetyl-CoA from malonyl CoA, consequently repressing fatty acid oxidation but promoting lipogenesis in WAT and skeletal muscle under nutrient abundance conditions. *Sirt4*-KO mice display increased exercise tolerance and protection against diet-induced obesity (220).

SIRT4 Regulates Fatty Acid Oxidation

SIRT4 inhibition in mouse primary hepatocytes increases fatty acid oxidation gene expression, leading to increased fat oxidative capacity in liver (118). The same result is obtained in muscle (118). Similarly, primary hepatocytes from *Sirt4*-KO mice exhibit higher rates of fatty acid oxidation. SIRT4 suppresses PPARα activity and inhibits hepatic fatty acid oxidation by modulating SIRT1 activity (221). Livers from NAFLD patients exhibit increased SIRT4 and lipogenic gene expression (222). These results support the notion that SIRT4 is likely to inhibit fatty acid oxidation and potentiate ectopic lipid storage in liver and skeletal muscle.

SIRT5

SIRT5 in the Regulation of Fatty Acid Metabolism

SIRT5 is highly expressed in metabolic tissues, including the heart, skeletal muscle, brain, liver, and kidney (121). Using a label-free quantitative proteomic approach, Rardin et al. characterized the lysine succinylome in liver mitochondria and revealed a major role for SIRT5 in regulating many metabolic pathways, including β-oxidation and ketogenesis (223). Park et al. revealed that SIRT5 desuccinylates a set of metabolic enzymes in mitochondria that are involved in amino acid degradation, the TCA cycle and fatty acid metabolism (224). In contrast to the other two mitochondrial Sirtuins, SIRT5 protein levels do not change during CR (121, 207). However, similar to *Sirt3*-KO and *Sirt4*-KO mice, *Sirt5*-KO mice do not show any overt metabolic abnormalities under either normal chow or HFD conditions (225). Sirt5 deficiency does not protect or sensitize mice to the development of HFD-induced obesity, hypertension, and insulin resistance (225). The results from *Sirt5*-KO mice suggest that SIRT5 is not dispensable for cellular metabolism, at least under normal conditions. Subsequent studies have shown promising results. In humans, *SIRT5* gene expression decreases in the liver of NAFLD patients (222), and the expression of *SIRT5* in adipose tissue is positively correlated with insulin sensitivity (226). Using affinity enrichment and label-free quantitative proteomics, Nishida *et al.* characterized the SIRT5-regulated lysine malonylome (227). Pathway analysis identified gluconeogenesis and glycolysis as the pathways most enriched in SIRT5-regulated malonylated proteins (227). SIRT5 regulates glyceraldehyde phosphate dehydrogenase (GAPDH), a glycolytic enzyme, through demalonylation of lysine 184 (227). According to these results, SIRT5 may play a critical role in regulating glucose and lipid metabolism and preserving insulin sensitivity. Mitochondria-specific Sirtuin knockout mice show no obvious metabolic abnormalities, indicating that mitochondrial Sirtuins serve as nutrient sensors to maintain energy homeostasis.

SIRT6 and Insulin-Sensitive Organs

SIRT6 Regulates Adipogenesis, Lipid Metabolism and Thermogenesis in Adipose Tissue

SIRT6 expression is decreased in adipose tissue of *db/db* mice but increased in adipose tissue of human individuals with weight loss (228, 229), suggesting that SIRT6 plays a role in adipose tissue. Chen et al. (230) demonstrated that SIRT6 is required for mitotic clonal expansion during adipogenesis by inhibiting expression of kinesin family member 5C (KIF5C) and subsequent increasing CK2 kinase activity. *Sirt6* transgenic mice exhibit resistance to HFD-induced obesity and insulin resistance (231). Conversely, fat-specific *Sirt6* knockout increases blood glucose levels and hepatic steatosis, and sensitizes mice to HFD-induced obesity and insulin resistance (59, 60, 232). SIRT6 overexpression downregulates a set of PPARγ target genes that are involved in lipid metabolism, lipid transport and adipogenesis (231). Especially, SIRT6 decreases expressions of ANGPTL4, a negative regulator of lipoprotein lipase, and diglyceride acyltransferase 1 (DGAT1), a key enzyme in triglycerides synthesis, leading to the increased serum triglyceride clearance and reducing triglyceride synthesis in adipose tissues (231). *Sirt6* deletion decreases FoxO1 transcriptional activity by increasing its acetylation and phosphorylation and reduces expression of adipose triglyceride lipase (ATGL), a key lipolytic enzyme, reducing lipolysis (59). Fat-specific *Sirt6* knockout not only induces obesity and insulin resistance but also impairs the thermogenic function of brown adipocytes (232). Yao et al. (232) found *Sirt6* deletion decreases ATF2 binding to the PGC-1α promoter, leading to reducing the expression of PGC-1α and PGC-1α target thermogenic genes.

SIRT6 Represses Gluconeogenesis and Lipid Accumulation in the Liver

The hepatic SIRT6 level is reduced in obese/diabetic mice and gluconeogenic genes were higher in *Sirt6*-deficient livers whereas ectopic re-expression of SIRT6 suppressed gluconeogenesis and normalizes glycemia (228, 233). Mechanistically, SIRT6 interacts with and increases the activity of general control non-repressed protein 5 (GCN5), an acetyltransferase, which, in turn, catalyzes the acetylation of PGC-1α, suppressing gluconeogenic gene expression such as *phosphoenolpyruvate carboxykinase C (PEPCK-C)* and *glucose 6-phosphatase*, and resulting in repression of hepatic glucose output (228). p53 directly activates expression of SIRT6, which subsequently interacts with and deacetylates FoxO1, leading to FoxO1 export to the cytoplasm, and finally, reduce the expression of gluconeogenetic genes such as *glucose 6-phosphatase alpha* and *phosphoenolpyruvate carboxykinase 1* (234). Human fatty liver samples exhibited significantly lower levels of SIRT6 than normal controls and liver-specific deletion of *Sirt6* in mice causes increased glycolysis, triglyceride synthesis, reduced β-oxidation, and leads to liver steatosis (235). Rosiglitazone, an agonist of PPARγ, increases the expression of SIRT6, PGC-1α, and FoxO1, and AMPK phosphorylation in rat liver and ameliorates hepatic lipid accumulation (236). *Sirt6* knockdown abolished the effects of rosiglitazone (236), suggesting *Sirt6* at least partly mediates the metabolic effects of rosiglitazone. Altogether, those evidence suggest that SIRT6 significantly participates in glucose and lipid metabolism in the liver.

SIRT6 Increases Insulin Sensitivity in the Skeletal Muscle

SIRT6 also regulates metabolic homeostasis in the skeletal muscle. *Sirt6* transgenic mice show enhanced insulin sensitivity in skeletal muscle and exhibit enhanced insulin-induced activation of Akt in the gastrocnemius (153). By contrast, skeletal muscle-specific *Sirt6* ko mice exhibit impaired glucose homeostasis and insulin sensitivity, attenuating whole-body energy expenditure (237). Mechanistically, *Sirt6* deletion decreases AMPK activity and subsequently decreases the expression of genes involved in glucose and lipid uptake, fatty acid oxidation, and mitochondrial oxidative phosphorylation (237). Further studies are needed to elucidate the direct mechanism underlying SIRT6 function in skeletal muscle.

SIRT7

SIRT7 Regulates Fatty Acid Metabolism in Adipose Tissues

SIRT7 is the least characterized Sirtuin of the seven mammalian Sirtuins. SIRT7 protein levels are high in the liver, spleen, and testis, whereas are low in the muscle, heart, and brain of mice (16). In human, *Sirt7* mRNA is expressed in various tissues (10). Recent reports clarify the important roles of SIRT7 in a variety of biological processes including DNA repair, chromatin assembly, and aging. However, the role of SIRT7 in metabolism remains largely unknown. The expression of *Sirt7* mRNA level is upregulated in adipose tissues of obese patients (238). In HFD-fed mice, *Sirt7* knockout decreased the expression of the fatty acid transporter CD36 in WAT (239). In addition, *Sirt7* knockout led to an increase of thermogenesis along with increased expression of UCP1 and DIO2 in BAT (239). These results suggest SIRT7 regulates lipid metabolism in adipocytes. Recently, Fang *al et.* found that SIRT7 restricts SIRT1 activity by preventing SIRT1 auto-deacetylation, and increasing SIRT1 activity in *Sirt7*-KO mice blocks PPARγ and adipocyte differentiation, thereby decreases the accumulation of white fat (240, 241). Together, these findings implicate the important role of SIRT7 in the regulation of fatty acid metabolism.

SIRT7 Regulates Fatty Acid and Glucose Metabolism in the Liver

Up to now, there are three studies linking SIRT7 to the liver lipid metabolism using independently generated mouse models. Shin et al. reported that *Sirt7*-KO mice developed steatosis resembling human fatty liver disease (242). Selectively overexpression of SIRT7 in the liver of *Sirt7*-KO mice *via* adeno-associated virus 8 (AAV8)-mediated gene transfer prevents the development of fatty liver (242). The authors found expressions of inflammatory markers and lipogenic genes are increased in *Sirt7*-deficient livers, and they clarified the underlying mechanism as SIRT7 repressing the expression of ribosomal proteins through decreasing Myc activity and further suppressing ER stress (242). Ryu et al. generated a different *Sirt7*-KO mouse by deleting exons 6-9, and observed more general metabolic defects including hepatic microvesicular steatosis, increased blood lactate levels, reduced exercise performance, cardiac dysfunction and age-related hearing loss induced by multisystemic mitochondrial dysfunction (127). Mechanistically, SIRT7 deacetylates GABPβ1, thereby enables it to form the transcriptionally active GABPα/GABPβ heterotetramer, and then promotes mitochondria function (127). Another study has the opposite result. Yoshizawa *et al.* reported that *Sirt7*-KO mice, deleting exons 4-9, are resistant to HFD induced fatty liver, obesity, and glucose intolerance (239). TR4 is a nuclear receptor involved in lipid metabolism and its target genes increase fatty acid uptake and triglyceride synthesis and storage (243). Hepatic SIRT7 was reported to increase TR4 expression through binding with DCAF1/DDB1/CUL4B E3 ubiquitin ligase complex and inhibiting TR4 degradation (239). It is difficult to explain the divergence of three *Sirt7*-KO mouse models with different genetic background. Liver-specific knockout or *Sirt7* transgene mouse model may be helpful to clarify the role of SIRT7 in liver lipid metabolism (239, 242). In addition to lipid metabolism, SIRT7 is involved in glucose metabolism. SIRT7 regulates acetylation at the K323 site of phosphoglycerate kinase 1 (PGK1), an important enzyme in glycolysis, decreases PGK1 enzyme activity and inhibits glycolysis in liver cancer cells (244). Yoshizawa *et al.* Found that *Sirt7*-KO mice show decreased expression of the hepatic glucose-6-phosphatase catalytic subunit (G6PC), a key gluconeogenic enzyme, and resistance to glucose intolerance (239). Mechanistically, glucose deprivation stimulates SIRT7 binding to the promoter of G6PC, and deacetylating H3K18 in the G6PC promoter, which results in elevated G6PC expression and promotion of hepatic gluconeogenesis (245).

SIRTUINS IN AGING-RELATED METABOLIC DEFECTS

Aging is a complex process accompanied by the declines in basal metabolic rate and physical activity. Aging is one of the major risk factors contributing to the development of insulin resistance, obesity, T2DM and metabolic syndrome (246). During the aging process, chronic inflammation and mitochondria dysfunction in pancreatic β cells and insulin-sensitive organs have been demonstrated to be major mechanisms linking aging and insulin resistance (247–250). As mentioned above, Sirtuins play important roles in regulating inflammation and mitochondria function. Sirtuins are critically involved in lifespan and healthspan. Deficiency of Sirtuins (SIRT1, SIRT6, and SIRT7) is associated with shortened lifespan and metabolic diseases (251). Our recent evidence also demonstrated that SIRT2 deficiency also facilitated the aging-related development of cardiac dysfunction, including hypertrophy and fibrosis (252). By contrast, germline or cell-specific overexpression of SIRT1 or SIRT6 were reported to expand lifespan and defense metabolic diseases in insulin-dependent and independent manners (253–255).

Sirtuin-targeted strategies show promising in repressing aging-related insulin resistance and metabolic diseases. For instance, the SIRT1 activator SRT1720 extends lifespan and improves the health of mice fed a standard diet (163, 256). It is well established that caloric restriction (CR), the Sirtuin activator, is an effective and reliable means to defense against aging and extend the lifespan and healthspan of mammals, including monkeys (257). Activation of vascular SIRT1 by CR leads to the repressing of aging-related metabolic vascular diseases, including atherosclerosis and aortic aneurysm (258–260). In human studies, CR also can reduce insulin resistance significantly and delay the onset of metabolic diseases (261, 262). Although the mechanisms by which CR extend lifespan are not fully understood, Sirtuins have been implicated to mediate beneficial effects of CR on aging (263). Notably, the CR mimetics (metformin, resveratrol, rapamycin) could expand lifespan and repress diseases related to insulin resistance in rodents partially through activation of Sirtuins (257, 264). Our data showed that SIRT2 contributes to the effects of metformin on aging-related diseases, including cardiac remodeling (252). Currently, clinical trials investigating the anti-aging effects of metformin is undergoing (ClinicalTrials.gov Identifier: NCT02432287).

Importantly, the Sirtuins do not function in individual metabolic organs or cell types alone during aging. Instead, the Sirtuins orchestrate the crosstalk between different organs or between different cell types within the local microenvironmental niche to maintain metabolic homeostasis and prevent against insulin resistance. The SIRT1 activator SRT3025 provides atheroprotection in *Apoe*$^{-/-}$ mice by reducing hepatic *Pcsk9* secretion and enhancing *Ldlr* expression (265). Resveratrol activates duodenal SIRT1 to initiate a gut-brain-liver neuronal axis that improves hypothalamic insulin sensitivity in rats (183). SIRT1 in intestinal stem cells also contributes to the protection roles of caloric restriction on aging (266). In addition, SIRT3 activation by nitrite and metformin improves insulin sensitivity in skeletal muscle and normalizes pulmonary hypertension associated with heart failure with preserved ejection fraction (267). Sirtuins also regulate inflammatory cells within the local microenvironmental niches to regulate insulin resistance in an autocrine or paracrine manner (41, 79, 80).

Therefore, targeting Sirtuins could be a promising strategy for improvement of insulin sensitivity and metabolic status of the whole body. However, activation of Sirtuins alone may not archive the biggest benefits because of the exhaustion of the endogenous NAD. Sirtuin activator in supplement with NAD precursor may represent a better therapeutic strategy for repressing aging-related insulin resistance and metabolic diseases.

CONCLUDING REMARKS

Insulin resistance is a critical pathological feature of obesity and metabolic syndrome and plays a key role in the pathogenesis of T2DM and attendant cardiovascular complications. Moreover, insulin resistance provides a therapeutic strategy to prevent, delay or treat T2DM, obesity, and metabolic syndrome by improving insulin sensitivity. Although insulin resistance is a complex metabolic disorder that has remained poorly understood, Sirtuin family members are involved in the potential cellular mechanisms of the pathogenesis of insulin resistance. According to accumulating evidence in the past decades, Sirtuin family members have emerged as a nutrient sensor to maintain energy homeostasis. Cellular and animal studies have demonstrated that Sirtuins play an important role in regulating glucose and lipids by modulating crucial enzymes in metabolic pathways and interfering with inflammation, oxidative stress, mitochondrial dysfunction, ER stress, and the insulin signaling pathway.

Sirtuins respond to environmental (diet and lifestyle) or metabolic (obesity, fasting, and diabetes) insults at mRNA and protein levels in insulin-sensing organs (268, 269). The roles of Sirtuins in regulating glucose and lipid metabolism as well as insulin resistance in liver, adipose tissue, and skeletal muscle make their importance in regulating metabolic diseases, including T2DM and diabetic complications (269).

Nevertheless, many additional studies are needed.

1. Different Sirtuins may have the same downstream targets, such as FoxO3a, FoxO1, PGC-1α, and GDH, and there is cross-talk among Sirtuin family members (56, 117, 270). How do different Sirtuin members coordinate to regulate the same downstream targets?
2. The Sirtuin family comprises NAD$^+$-dependent histone deacetylases; however, recent results have revealed that Sirtuin members can act in a deacetylase-independent manner (117). How can we determine the functions and activities of Sirtuins in addition to their deacetylation function in insulin resistance?
3. In addition to Sirtuins, there are other epigenetic modification enzymes, including SUV39H1 and EZH2 are involved in insulin resistance and T2DM (271–276). There is an interaction between SUV39H1 and Sirtuins, including SIRT1, SIRT3, and SIRT7 (277–281). EZH2 is reportedly the deacetylating substrate of SIRT1 (282, 283). SIRT2 negatively regulates JMJD2A expression in human non-small cell lung cancer tissues (284). Is JMJD2A involved in insulin resistance? In the condition of insulin resistance, how do these epigenetic modification enzymes influence each other and consequently act on insulin sensitivity?
4. Obesity, insulin resistance, and T2DM are aging-related abnormalities. Sirtuins, especially SIRT1, SIRT2, and SIRT6,

are characterized as protectors of aging and aging-related diseases. Whether the promotive effect of aging by the decline of Sirtuin activity is involved in insulin resistance deserves further investigation. In addition, cell senescence-induced organ dysfunction and aging (senescaging) are common during physiological and pathological aging processes (268). Selective elimination of senescent cells, or senolysis, was reported to delay aging and aging-related metabolic diseases including congestive decline, atherosclerosis, cardiac diseases, and osteoarthritis (285–291). However, it remains to elucidate that what are the physiological and pathological functions of cellular senescence in organs during aging and that whether Sirtuins regulate senescaging in insulin resistance and healthy conditions.

AUTHOR CONTRIBUTIONS

All authors listed have made a substantial, direct and intellectual contribution to the work. SZ is responsible for literature collection and article draft. XT designed the Figures and revised the manuscript. H-ZC is the leading principal investigator who directed the study and data analysis, and prepared the manuscript. All authors approved publication of this work.

ACKNOWLEDGMENTS

This work was supported by the National Natural Science Foundation of China (Grant Nos. 81600038, 31571193 and 81800273). H-ZC is also supported by the Youth Top-notch Talent Support Program and the Youth Yangtze River Scholar Program in China. XT is also supported by the Postdoctoral Innovative Talents Support Program (BX20180206), the China Postdoctoral Science Foundation (2018M631084) and Full-time Postdoctoral Research and Development Fund of Sichuan University (2018SCU12010). We apologize to those scientists whose work we could not highlight owing to space limitations. We thank Miss. Xiao-Feng Chen for reading the manuscript and helpful suggestions.

REFERENCES

1. Samuel VT, Shulman GI. Mechanisms for insulin resistance: common threads and missing links. *Cell* (2012) 148:852–71. doi: 10.1016/j.cell.2012.02.017
2. Saltiel AR. New perspectives into the molecular pathogenesis and treatment of type 2 diabetes. *Cell* (2001) 104:517–29. doi: 10.1016/S0092-8674(01)00239-2
3. Sun C, Zhang F, Ge X, Yan T, Chen X, Shi X, et al. SIRT1 improves insulin sensitivity under insulin-resistant conditions by repressing PTP1B. *Cell Metab.* (2007) 6:307–19. doi: 10.1016/j.cmet.2007.08.014
4. Gomes P, Fleming Outeiro T, Cavadas C. Emerging role of sirtuin 2 in the regulation of mammalian metabolism. *Trends Pharmacol Sci.* (2015) 36:756–68. doi: 10.1016/j.tips.2015.08.001
5. Kim JA, Wei Y, Sowers JR. Role of mitochondrial dysfunction in insulin resistance. *Circul Res.* (2008) 102:401–14. doi: 10.1161/CIRCRESAHA.107.165472
6. Muoio DM, Newgard CB. Mechanisms of disease: molecular and metabolic mechanisms of insulin resistance and beta-cell failure in type 2 diabetes. *Nat Rev.* (2008) 9:193–205. doi: 10.1038/nrm2327
7. Nogueiras R, Habegger KM, Chaudhary N, Finan B, Banks AS, Dietrich MO, et al. Sirtuin 1 and sirtuin 3: physiological modulators of metabolism. *Physiol Rev.* (2012) 92:1479–514. doi: 10.1152/physrev.00022.2011
8. Frye RA. Characterization of five human cDNAs with homology to the yeast SIR2 gene: Sir2-like proteins (sirtuins) metabolize NAD and may have protein ADP-ribosyltransferase activity. *Biochem Biophys Res Commun.* (1999) 260:273–9. doi: 10.1006/bbrc.1999.0897
9. North BJ, Verdin E. Sirtuins: Sir2-related NAD-dependent protein deacetylases. *Genome Biol.* (2004) 5:224. doi: 10.1186/gb-2004-5-5-224
10. Michishita E, Park JY, Burneskis JM, Barrett JC, Horikawa I. Evolutionarily conserved and nonconserved cellular localizations and functions of human SIRT proteins. *Mol Biol Cell* (2005) 16:4623–35. doi: 10.1091/mbc.e05-01-0033
11. Tanno M, Sakamoto J, Miura T, Shimamoto K, Horio Y. Nucleocytoplasmic shuttling of the NAD+-dependent histone deacetylase SIRT1. *J Biol Chem.* (2007) 282:6823–32. doi: 10.1074/jbc.M609554200
12. North BJ, Marshall BL, Borra MT, Denu JM, Verdin E. The human Sir2 ortholog, SIRT2, is an NAD+-dependent tubulin deacetylase. *Mol Cell* (2003) 11:437–44. doi: 10.1016/S1097-2765(03)00038-8
13. Vaquero A, Scher MB, Lee DH, Sutton A, Cheng HL, Alt FW, et al. SIRT2 is a histone deacetylase with preference for histone H4 Lys 16 during mitosis. *Genes Dev.* (2006) 20:1256–61. doi: 10.1101/gad.1412706
14. Huang JY, Hirschey MD, Shimazu T, Ho L, Verdin E. Mitochondrial sirtuins. *Biochim Biophys Acta* (2010) 1804:1645–51. doi: 10.1016/j.bbapap.2009.12.021
15. Mostoslavsky R, Chua KF, Lombard DB, Pang WW, Fischer MR, Gellon L, et al. Genomic instability and aging-like phenotype in the absence of mammalian SIRT6. *Cell* (2006) 124:315–29. doi: 10.1016/j.cell.2005.11.044
16. Ford E, Voit R, Liszt G, Magin C, Grummt I, Guarente L. Mammalian Sir2 homolog SIRT7 is an activator of RNA polymerase I transcription. *Genes Dev.* (2006) 20:1075–80. doi: 10.1101/gad.1399706
17. Rauh D, Fischer F, Gertz M, Lakshminarasimhan M, Bergbrede T, Aladini F, et al. An acetylome peptide microarray reveals specificities and deacetylation substrates for all human sirtuin isoforms. *Nat Commun.* (2013) 4:2327. doi: 10.1038/ncomms3327
18. Teng YB, Jing H, Aramsangtienchai P, He B, Khan S, Hu J, et al. Efficient demyristoylase activity of SIRT2 revealed by kinetic and structural studies. *Sci Rep.* (2015) 5:8529. doi: 10.1038/srep08529
19. Du J, Zhou Y, Su X, Yu JJ, Khan S, Jiang H, et al. SIRT5 is a NAD-dependent protein lysine demalonylase and desuccinylase. *Science* (2011) 334:806–9. doi: 10.1126/science.1207861
20. Haigis MC, Mostoslavsky R, Haigis KM, Fahie K, Christodoulou DC, Murphy AJ, et al. SIRT4 inhibits glutamate dehydrogenase and opposes the effects of calorie restriction in pancreatic beta cells. *Cell* (2006) 126:941–54. doi: 10.1016/j.cell.2006.06.057
21. Liszt G, Ford E, Kurtev M, Guarente L. Mouse Sir2 homolog SIRT6 is a nuclear ADP-ribosyltransferase. *J Biol Chem.* (2005) 280:21313–20. doi: 10.1074/jbc.M413296200
22. Guarente L, Franklin H. Epstein lecture: sirtuins, aging, and medicine. *N Engl J Med.* (2011) 364:2235–44. doi: 10.1056/NEJMra1100831
23. Morris BJ. Seven sirtuins for seven deadly diseases of aging. *Free Radic Biol Med.* (2013) 56:133–71. doi: 10.1016/j.freeradbiomed.2012.10.525
24. Liang F, Kume S, Koya D. SIRT1 and insulin resistance. *Nat Rev. Endocrinol.* (2009) 5:367–73. doi: 10.1038/nrendo.2009.101
25. Cao Y, Jiang X, Ma H, Wang Y, Xue P, Liu Y. SIRT1 and insulin resistance. *J Diabetes Compl.* (2016) 30:178–83. doi: 10.1016/j.jdiacomp.2015.08.022
26. Kuang J, Chen L, Tang Q, Zhang J, Li Y, He J. The role of SIRT6 in obesity and diabetes. *Front Physiol.* (2018) 9:135. doi: 10.3389/fphys.2018.00135
27. Wellen KE, Hotamisligil GS. Inflammation, stress, and diabetes. *J Clin Investig.* (2005) 115:1111–9. doi: 10.1172/JCI25102
28. Olefsky JM, Glass CK. Macrophages, inflammation, and insulin resistance. *Annu Rev Physiol.* (2010) 72:219–46. doi: 10.1146/annurev-physiol-021909-135846

29. Lumeng CN, Saltiel AR. Inflammatory links between obesity and metabolic disease. *J Clin Investig.* (2011) 121:2111–7. doi: 10.1172/JCI57132
30. Scherer PE. Adipose tissue: from lipid storage compartment to endocrine organ. *Diabetes* (2006) 55:1537–45. doi: 10.2337/db06-0263
31. Wang P, Mariman E, Renes J, Keijer J. The secretory function of adipocytes in the physiology of white adipose tissue. *J Cell Physiol.* (2008) 216:3–13. doi: 10.1002/jcp.21386
32. Steppan CM, Bailey ST, Bhat S, Brown EJ, Banerjee RR, Wright CM, et al. The hormone resistin links obesity to diabetes. *Nature* (2001) 409:307–12. doi: 10.1038/35053000
33. Yang Q, Graham TE, Mody N, Preitner F, Peroni OD, Zabolotny JM, et al. Serum retinol binding protein 4 contributes to insulin resistance in obesity and type 2 diabetes. *Nature* (2005) 436:356–62. doi: 10.1038/nature03711
34. Hirosumi J, Tuncman G, Chang L, Gorgun CZ, Uysal KT, Maeda K, et al. A central role for JNK in obesity and insulin resistance. *Nature* (2002) 420:333–6. doi: 10.1038/nature01137
35. Zick Y. Role of Ser/Thr kinases in the uncoupling of insulin signaling. *Int J Obes Related Metab Disord.* (2003) 27(Suppl. 3):S56–60. doi: 10.1038/sj.ijo.0802503
36. Jing E, Emanuelli B, Hirschey MD, Boucher J, Lee KY, Lombard D, et al. Sirtuin-3 (SIRT3) regulates skeletal muscle metabolism and insulin signaling via altered mitochondrial oxidation and reactive oxygen species production. *Proc Natl Acad Sci USA* (2011) 108:14608–13. doi: 10.1073/pnas.1111308108
37. Pfluger PT, Herranz D, Velasco-Miguel S, Serrano M, Tschop MH. SIRT1 protects against high-fat diet-induced metabolic damage. *Proc Natl Acad Sci USA* (2008) 105:9793–8. doi: 10.1073/pnas.0802917105
38. Purushotham A, Schug TT, Xu Q, Surapureddi S, Guo X, Li X. Hepatocyte-specific deletion of SIRT1 alters fatty acid metabolism and results in hepatic steatosis and inflammation. *Cell Metab.* (2009) 9:327–38. doi: 10.1016/j.cmet.2009.02.006
39. Yoshizaki T, Milne JC, Imamura T, Schenk S, Sonoda N, Babendure JL, et al. SIRT1 exerts anti-inflammatory effects and improves insulin sensitivity in adipocytes. *Mol Cell Biol.* (2009) 29:1363–74. doi: 10.1128/MCB.00705-08
40. Yoshizaki T, Schenk S, Imamura T, Babendure JL, Sonoda N, Bae EJ, et al. SIRT1 inhibits inflammatory pathways in macrophages and modulates insulin sensitivity. *Am J Physiol. Endocrinol Metab.* (2010) 298:E419–428. doi: 10.1152/ajpendo.00417.2009
41. Gillum MP, Kotas ME, Erion DM, Kursawe R, Chatterjee P, Nead KT, et al. SIRT1 regulates adipose tissue inflammation. *Diabetes* (2011) 60:3235–45. doi: 10.2337/db11-0616
42. Hui X, Zhang M, Gu P, Li K, Gao Y, Wu D, et al. Adipocyte SIRT1 controls systemic insulin sensitivity by modulating macrophages in adipose tissue. *EMBO Rep.* (2017) 18:645–57. doi: 10.15252/embr.201643184
43. Yeung F, Hoberg JE, Ramsey CS, Keller MD, Jones DR, Frye RA, et al. Modulation of NF-kappaB-dependent transcription and cell survival by the SIRT1 deacetylase. *EMBO J.* (2004) 23:2369–80. doi: 10.1038/sj.emboj.7600244
44. Ghosh HS, Spencer JV, Ng B, McBurney MW, Robbins PD. SIRT1 interacts with transducin-like enhancer of split-1 to inhibit nuclear factor kappaB-mediated transcription. *Biochem J.* (2007) 408:105–111. doi: 10.1042/BJ20070817
45. Zhang R, Chen HZ, Liu JJ, Jia YY, Zhang ZQ, Yang RF, et al. SIRT1 suppresses activator protein-1 transcriptional activity and cyclooxygenase-2 expression in macrophages. *J Biol Chem.* (2010) 285:7097–110. doi: 10.1074/jbc.M109.038604
46. Nakamura K, Zhang M, Kageyama S, Ke B, Fujii T, Sosa RA, et al. Macrophage heme oxygenase-1-SIRT1-p53 axis regulates sterile inflammation in liver ischemia-reperfusion injury. *J Hepatol.* (2017) 67:1232–42. doi: 10.1016/j.jhep.2017.08.010
47. Rothgiesser KM, Erener S, Waibel S, Luscher B, Hottiger MO. SIRT2 regulates NF-kappaB dependent gene expression through deacetylation of p65 Lys310. *J Cell Sci.* (2010) 123:4251–8. doi: 10.1242/jcs.073783
48. Pais TF, Szego EM, Marques O, Miller-Fleming L, Antas P, Guerreiro P, et al. The NAD-dependent deacetylase sirtuin 2 is a suppressor of microglial activation and brain inflammation. *EMBO J.* (2013) 32:2603–16. doi: 10.1038/emboj.2013.200
49. Lo Sasso G, Menzies KJ, Mottis A, Piersigilli A, Perino A, Yamamoto H, et al. SIRT2 deficiency modulates macrophage polarization and susceptibility to experimental colitis. *PLoS ONE* (2014) 9:e103573. doi: 10.1371/journal.pone.0103573
50. Zhang Y, Chi D. Overexpression of SIRT2 alleviates neuropathic pain and neuroinflammation through deacetylation of transcription factor nuclear factor-kappa B. *Inflammation* (2018) 41:569–78. doi: 10.1007/s10753-017-0713-3
51. Yuan F, Xu ZM, Lu LY, Nie H, Ding J, Ying WH et al. SIRT2 inhibition exacerbates neuroinflammation and blood–brain barrier disruption in experimental traumatic brain injury by enhancing NF-κB p65 acetylation and activation. *J Neurochem.* (2016) 136:581–93. doi: 10.1111/jnc.13423
52. Lin J, Sun B, Jiang C, Hong H, Zheng Y. SIRT2 suppresses inflammatory responses in collagen-induced arthritis. *Biochem Biophys Res Commun.* (2013) 441:897–903. doi: 10.1016/j.bbrc.2013.10.153
53. Wang X, Buechler NL, Martin A, Wells J, Yoza B, McCall CE, et al. Sirtuin-2 regulates sepsis inflammation in ob/ob mice. *PLoS ONE* (2016) 11:e0160431. doi: 10.1371/journal.pone.0160431
54. Chen Y, Wang H, Luo G, Dai X. SIRT4 inhibits cigarette smoke extracts-induced mononuclear cell adhesion to human pulmonary microvascular endothelial cells via regulating NF-kappaB activity. *Toxicol Lett.* (2014) 226:320–7. doi: 10.1016/j.toxlet.2014.02.022
55. Tao Y, Huang C, Huang Y, Hong L, Wang H, Zhou Z, et al. SIRT4 suppresses inflammatory responses in human umbilical vein endothelial cells. *Cardiovasc Toxicol.* (2015) 15:217–23. doi: 10.1007/s12012-014-9287-6
56. Qin K, Han C, Zhang H, Li T, Li N, Cao X. NAD(+) dependent deacetylase Sirtuin 5 rescues the innate inflammatory response of endotoxin tolerant macrophages by promoting acetylation of p65. *J Autoimmun.* (2017) 81:120–9. doi: 10.1016/j.jaut.2017.04.006
57. Wang F, Wang K, Xu W, Zhao S, Ye D, Wang Y, et al. SIRT5 desuccinylates and activates pyruvate kinase M2 to block macrophage IL-1beta production and to prevent DSS-induced colitis in mice. *Cell Rep.* (2017) 19:2331–44. doi: 10.1016/j.celrep.2017.05.065
58. Kawahara TL, Michishita E, Adler AS, Damian M, Berber E, Lin M, et al. SIRT6 links histone H3 lysine 9 deacetylation to NF-kappaB-dependent gene expression and organismal life span. *Cell* (2009) 136:62–74. doi: 10.1016/j.cell.2008.10.052
59. Kuang J, Zhang Y, Liu Q, Shen J, Pu S, Cheng S, et al. Fat-specific SIRT6 ablation sensitizes mice to high-fat diet-induced obesity and insulin resistance by inhibiting lipolysis. *Diabetes* (2017) 66:1159–71. doi: 10.2337/db16-1225
60. Xiong X, Zhang C, Zhang Y, Fan R, Qian X, Dong XC. Fabp4-Cre-mediated SIRT6 deletion impairs adipose tissue function and metabolic homeostasis in mice. *J Endocrinol.* (2017) 233:307–14. doi: 10.1530/JOE-17-0033
61. Franchi L, Eigenbrod T, Munoz-Planillo R, Nunez G. The inflammasome: a caspase-1-activation platform that regulates immune responses and disease pathogenesis. *Nat Immunol.* (2009) 10:241–7. doi: 10.1038/ni.1703
62. Lamkanfi M, Dixit VM. Mechanisms and functions of inflammasomes. *Cell* (2014) 157:1013–22. doi: 10.1016/j.cell.2014.04.007
63. Youm YH, Nguyen KY, Grant RW, Goldberg EL, Bodogai M, Kim D, et al. The ketone metabolite beta-hydroxybutyrate blocks NLRP3 inflammasome-mediated inflammatory disease. *Nat Med.* (2015) 21:263–9. doi: 10.1038/nm.3804
64. Vandanmagsar B, Youm YH, Ravussin A, Galgani JE, Stadler K, Mynatt RL, et al. The NLRP3 inflammasome instigates obesity-induced inflammation and insulin resistance. *Nat Med.* (2011) 17:179–88. doi: 10.1038/nm.2279
65. Lee HM, Kim JJ, Kim HJ, Shong M, Ku BJ, Jo EK. Upregulated NLRP3 inflammasome activation in patients with type 2 diabetes. *Diabetes* (2013) 62:194–204. doi: 10.2337/db12-0420
66. Fu Y, Wang Y, Du L, Xu C, Cao J, Fan T, et al. Resveratrol inhibits ionising irradiation-induced inflammation in MSCs by activating SIRT1 and limiting NLRP-3 inflammasome activation. *Int J Mol Sci.* (2013) 14:14105–18. doi: 10.3390/ijms140714105
67. Gao R, Ma Z, Hu Y, Chen J, Shetty S, Fu J. SIRT1 restrains lung inflammasome activation in a murine model of sepsis. *Am J Physiol.* (2015) 308:L847–853. doi: 10.1152/ajplung.00274.2014
68. Zhang B, Xu D, She L, Wang Z, Yang N, Sun R, et al. Silybin inhibits NLRP3 inflammasome assembly through the NAD(+)/SIRT2 pathway in

mice with nonalcoholic fatty liver disease. *FASEB J.* (2018) 32:757–67. doi: 10.1096/fj.201700602R

69. Traba J, Kwarteng-Siaw M, Okoli TC, Li J, Huffstutler RD, Bray A, et al. Fasting and refeeding differentially regulate NLRP3 inflammasome activation in human subjects. *J Clin Investig.* (2015) 125:4592–600. doi: 10.1172/JCI83260
70. Chen ML, Zhu XH, Lang HD, Mi MT. Trimethylamine-N-oxide induces vascular inflammation by activating the NLRP3 inflammasome through the SIRT3-SOD2-mtROS signaling pathway. *J Am Heart Assoc.* (2017) 6:e006347. doi: 10.1161/JAHA.117.006347
71. Harris J, Hartman M, Roche C, Zeng SG, O'Shea A, Sharp FA, et al. Autophagy controls IL-1beta secretion by targeting pro-IL-1beta for degradation. *J Biol Chem.* (2011) 286:9587–97. doi: 10.1074/jbc.M110.202911
72. Chen Y, Li X, Boini KM, Pitzer AL, Gulbins E, Zhang Y, et al. Endothelial Nlrp3 inflammasome activation associated with lysosomal destabilization during coronary arteritis. *Biochim Biophys Acta* (2015) 1853:396–408. doi: 10.1016/j.bbamcr.2014.11.012
73. Liu P, Huang G, Wei T, Gao J, Huang C, Sun M, et al. Sirtuin 3-induced macrophage autophagy in regulating NLRP3 inflammasome activation. *Biochim Biophys Acta* (2018) 1864:764–77. doi: 10.1016/j.bbadis.2017.12.027
74. Nakahira K, Haspel JA, Rathinam VA, Lee SJ, Dolinay T, Lam HC, et al. Autophagy proteins regulate innate immune responses by inhibiting the release of mitochondrial DNA mediated by the NALP3 inflammasome. *Nat Immunol.* (2011) 12:222–230. doi: 10.1038/ni.1980
75. Cho KW, Lumeng CN. SIRT1: a guardian at the gates of adipose tissue inflammation. *Diabetes* (2011) 60:3100–2. doi: 10.2337/db11-1308
76. Zhang J, Lee SM, Shannon S, Gao B, Chen W, Chen A, et al. The type III histone deacetylase SIRT1 is essential for maintenance of T cell tolerance in mice. *J Clin Invest.* (2009) 119:3048–58. doi: 10.1172/JCI38902
77. Liu Z, Gan L, Liu G, Chen Y, Wu T, Feng F, et al. SIRT1 decreased adipose inflammation by interacting with Akt2 and inhibiting mTOR/S6K1 pathway in mice. *J Lipid Res.* (2016) 57:1373–81. doi: 10.1194/jlr.M063537
78. Jiang H, Khan S, Wang Y, Charron G, He B, Sebastian C, et al. SIRT6 regulates TNF-alpha secretion through hydrolysis of long-chain fatty acyl lysine. *Nature* (2013) 496:110–3. doi: 10.1038/nature12038
79. Lee Y, Ka SO, Cha HN, Chae YN, Kim MK, Park SY, et al. Myeloid sirtuin 6 deficiency causes insulin resistance in high-fat diet–fed mice by eliciting macrophage polarization toward an m1 phenotype. *Diabetes* (2017) 66:2659–68. doi: 10.2337/db16-1446
80. Zhang ZQ, Ren SC, Tan Y, Li ZZ, Tang X, Wang TT et al. Epigenetic regulation of NKG2D ligands is involved in exacerbated atherosclerosis development in SIRT6 heterozygous mice. *Sci Rep.* (2016) 6:23912. doi: 10.1038/srep23912
81. Xiao C, Wang RH, Lahusen TJ, Park O, Bertola A, Maruyama T, et al. Progression of chronic liver inflammation and fibrosis driven by activation of c-JUN signaling in SIRT6 mutant mice. *J Biol Chem.* (2012) 287:41903–13. doi: 10.1074/jbc.M112.415182
82. Liu TF, Vachharajani VT, Yoza BK, McCall CE. NAD+-dependent sirtuin 1 and 6 proteins coordinate a switch from glucose to fatty acid oxidation during the acute inflammatory response. *J Biol Chem.* (2012) 287:25758–69. doi: 10.1074/jbc.M112.362343
83. Pham-Huy LA, He H, Pham-Huy C. Free radicals, antioxidants in disease and health. *Int J Biomed Sci.* (2008) 4:89–96.
84. Singh CK, Chhabra G, Ndiaye MA, Garcia-Peterson LM, Mack NJ, Ahmad N. The role of sirtuins in antioxidant and redox signaling. *Antiox Redox Signal.* (2018) 28:643–61. doi: 10.1089/ars.2017.7290
85. Maiese K. New insights for oxidative stress and diabetes mellitus. *Oxidat Med Cell Long.* (2015) 2015:875961. doi: 10.1155/2015/875961
86. Kelley DE, He J, Menshikova EV, Ritov VB. Dysfunction of mitochondria in human skeletal muscle in type 2 diabetes. *Diabetes* (2002) 51:2944–50. doi: 10.2337/diabetes.51.10.2944
87. Petersen KF, Dufour S, Befroy D, Garcia R, Shulman GI. Impaired mitochondrial activity in the insulin-resistant offspring of patients with type 2 diabetes. *N Engl J Med.* (2004) 350:664–71. doi: 10.1056/NEJMoa031314
88. Lowell BB, Shulman GI. Mitochondrial dysfunction and type 2 diabetes. *Science* (2005) 307:384–7. doi: 10.1126/science.1104343
89. Wu Z, Puigserver P, Andersson U, Zhang C, Adelmant G, Mootha V, et al. Mechanisms controlling mitochondrial biogenesis and respiration through the thermogenic coactivator PGC-1. *Cell* (1999) 98:115–24. doi: 10.1016/S0092-8674(00)80611-X
90. Finck BN, Kelly DP. PGC-1 coactivators: inducible regulators of energy metabolism in health and disease. *J Clin Investig.* (2006) 116:615–22. doi: 10.1172/JCI27794
91. Nemoto S, Fergusson MM, Finkel T. SIRT1 functionally interacts with the metabolic regulator and transcriptional coactivator PGC-1{alpha}. *J Biol Chem.* (2005) 280:16456–60. doi: 10.1074/jbc.M501485200
92. Lagouge M, Argmann C, Gerhart-Hines Z, Meziane H, Lerin C, Daussin F, et al. Resveratrol improves mitochondrial function and protects against metabolic disease by activating SIRT1 and PGC-1alpha. *Cell* (2006) 127:1109–22. doi: 10.1016/j.cell.2006.11.013
93. Lee IH, Cao L, Mostoslavsky R, Lombard DB, Liu J, Bruns NE, et al. A role for the NAD-dependent deacetylase SIRT1 in the regulation of autophagy. *Proc Natl Acad Sci USA* (2008) 105:3374–9. doi: 10.1073/pnas.0712145105
94. Hariharan N, Maejima Y, Nakae J, Paik J, Depinho RA, Sadoshima J. Deacetylation of FoxO by SIRT1 Plays an Essential Role in Mediating Starvation-Induced Autophagy in Cardiac Myocytes, *Circ Res.* (2010) 107:1470–82. doi: 10.1161/CIRCRESAHA.110.227371
95. Kume S, Uzu T, Horiike K, Chin-Kanasaki M, Isshiki K, Araki S, et al. Calorie restriction enhances cell adaptation to hypoxia through SIRT1-dependent mitochondrial autophagy in mouse aged kidney. *J Clin Investig.* (2010) 120:1043–55. doi: 10.1172/JCI41376
96. Brunet A, Sweeney LB, Sturgill JF, Chua KF, Greer PL, Lin Y, et al. Stress-dependent regulation of FOXO transcription factors by the SIRT1 deacetylase. *Science* (2004) 303:2011–15. doi: 10.1126/science.1094637
97. Zhang B, Zhai M, Li B, Liu Z, Li K, Jiang L, et al. Honokiol ameliorates myocardial ischemia/reperfusion injury in type 1 diabetic rats by reducing oxidative stress and apoptosis through activating the SIRT1-Nrf2 signaling pathway. *Oxidat Med Cell Long.* (2018) 2018:3159801. doi: 10.1155/2018/3159801
98. Wang F, Nguyen M, Qin FX, Tong Q. SIRT2 deacetylates FOXO3a in response to oxidative stress and caloric restriction. *Aging Cell* (2007) 6:505–14. doi: 10.1111/j.1474-9726.2007.00304.x
99. Lynn EG, McLeod CJ, Gordon JP, Bao J, Sack MN. SIRT2 is a negative regulator of anoxia-reoxygenation tolerance via regulation of 14-3-3 zeta and BAD in H9c2 cells. *FEBS Lett.* (2008) 582:2857–62. doi: 10.1016/j.febslet.2008.07.016
100. Wang YP, Zhou LS, Zhao YZ, Wang SW, Chen LL, Liu LX, et al. Regulation of G6PD acetylation by SIRT2 and KAT9 modulates NADPH homeostasis and cell survival during oxidative stress. *EMBO J.* (2014) 33:1304–20. doi: 10.1002/embj.201387224
101. Xu Y, Li F, Lv L, Li T, Zhou X, Deng CX, et al. Oxidative stress activates SIRT2 to deacetylate and stimulate phosphoglycerate mutase. *Cancer Res.* (2014) 74:3630–42. doi: 10.1158/0008-5472.CAN-13-3615
102. Galligan JJ, Rose KL, Beavers WN, Hill S, Tallman KA, Tansey WP, et al. Stable histone adduction by 4-oxo-2-nonenal: a potential link between oxidative stress and epigenetics. *J Am Chem Soc.* (2014) 136:11864–6. doi: 10.1021/ja503604t
103. Jin J, He B, Zhang X, Lin H, Wang Y. SIRT2 reverses 4-oxononanoyl lysine modification on histones. *J Am Chem Soc.* (2016) 138:12304–7. doi: 10.1021/jacs.6b04977
104. Liu G, Park SH, Imbesi M, Nathan WJ, Zou X, Zhu Y, et al. Loss of NAD-dependent protein deacetylase sirtuin-2 alters mitochondrial protein acetylation and dysregulates mitophagy. *Antioxid Redox Signal.* (2017) 26:849–63. doi: 10.1089/ars.2016.6662
105. Weir HJ, Lane JD, Balthasar N. SIRT3: a central regulator of mitochondrial adaptation in health and disease. *Genes Cancer* (2013) 4:118–24. doi: 10.1177/1947601913476949
106. Ahn BH, Kim HS, Song S, Lee IH, Liu J, Vassilopoulos A, et al. A role for the mitochondrial deacetylase SIRT3 in regulating energy homeostasis. *Proc Natl Acad Sci USA* (2008) 105:14447–52. doi: 10.1073/pnas.0803790105
107. Cimen H, Han MJ, Yang Y, Tong Q, Koc H, Koc EC. Regulation of succinate dehydrogenase activity by SIRT3 in mammalian mitochondria. *Biochemistry* (2010) 49:304–11. doi: 10.1021/bi901627u
108. Hafner AV, Dai J, Gomes AP, Xiao CY, Palmeira CM, Rosenzweig A, et al. Regulation of the mPTP by SIRT3-mediated deacetylation of CypD at lysine

166 suppresses age-related cardiac hypertrophy. *Aging* (2010) 2:914–23. doi: 10.18632/aging.100252
109. Cheng Y, Ren X, Gowda AS, Shan Y, Zhang L, Yuan YS, et al. Interaction of SIRT3 with OGG1 contributes to repair of mitochondrial DNA and protects from apoptotic cell death under oxidative stress. *Cell Death Dis.* (2013) 4:e731. doi: 10.1038/cddis.2013.254
110. Someya S, Yu W, Hallows WC, Xu J, Vann JM, Leeuwenburgh C, et al. SIRT3 mediates reduction of oxidative damage and prevention of age-related hearing loss under caloric restriction. *Cell* (2010) 143:802–12. doi: 10.1016/j.cell.2010.10.002
111. Finley LW, Carracedo A, Lee J, Souza A, Egia A, Zhang J, et al. SIRT3 opposes reprogramming of cancer cell metabolism through HIF1alpha destabilization. *Cancer Cell* (2011) 19:416–28. doi: 10.1016/j.ccr.2011.02.014
112. Sundaresan NR, Gupta M, Kim G, Rajamohan SB, Isbatan A, Gupta MP. SIRT3 blocks the cardiac hypertrophic response by augmenting Foxo3a-dependent antioxidant defense mechanisms in mice. *J Clin Investig.* (2009) 119:2758–71. doi: 10.1172/JCI39162
113. Qiu X, Brown K, Hirschey MD, Verdin E, Chen D. Calorie restriction reduces oxidative stress by SIRT3-mediated SOD2 activation. *Cell Metab.* (2010) 12:662–7. doi: 10.1016/j.cmet.2010.11.015
114. Chen Y, Zhang J, Lin Y, Lei Q, Guan KL, Zhao S, et al. Tumour suppressor SIRT3 deacetylates and activates manganese superoxide dismutase to scavenge ROS. *EMBO Rep.* (2011) 12:534–41. doi: 10.1038/embor.2011.65
115. Tao R, Coleman MC, Pennington JD, Ozden O, Park SH, Jiang H, et al. SIRT3-mediated deacetylation of evolutionarily conserved lysine 122 regulates MnSOD activity in response to stress. *Mol Cell* (2010) 40:893–904. doi: 10.1016/j.molcel.2010.12.013
116. Yu W, Dittenhafer-Reed KE, Denu JM. SIRT3 protein deacetylates isocitrate dehydrogenase 2 (IDH2) and regulates mitochondrial redox status. *J Biol Chem.* (2012) 287:14078–86. doi: 10.1074/jbc.M112.355206
117. Luo YX, Tang X, An XZ, Xie XM, Chen XF, Zhao X, et al. SIRT4 accelerates Ang II-induced pathological cardiac hypertrophy by inhibiting manganese superoxide dismutase activity. *Eur Heart J.* (2017) 38:1389–98. doi: 10.1093/eurheartj/ehw138
118. Nasrin N, Wu X, Fortier E, Feng Y, Bare OC, Chen S, et al. SIRT4 regulates fatty acid oxidation and mitochondrial gene expression in liver and muscle cells. *J Biol Chem.* (2010) 285:31995–2002. doi: 10.1074/jbc.M110.124164
119. Ho L, Titus AS, Banerjee KK, George S, Lin W, Deota S, et al. SIRT4 regulates ATP homeostasis and mediates a retrograde signaling via AMPK. *Aging* (2013) 5:835–49. doi: 10.18632/aging.100616
120. Lang A, Anand R, Altinoluk-Hambuchen S, Ezzahoini H, Stefanski A, Iram A, et al. SIRT4 interacts with OPA1 and regulates mitochondrial quality control and mitophagy. *Aging* (2017) 9:2163–89. doi: 10.18632/aging.101307
121. Nakagawa T, Lomb DJ, Haigis MC, Guarente L. SIRT5 Deacetylates carbamoyl phosphate synthetase 1 and regulates the urea cycle. *Cell* (2009) 137:560–70. doi: 10.1016/j.cell.2009.02.026
122. Lin ZF, Xu HB, Wang JY, Lin Q, Ruan Z, Liu FB, et al. SIRT5 desuccinylates and activates SOD1 to eliminate ROS. *Biochem Biophys Res Commun.* (2013) 441:191–5. doi: 10.1016/j.bbrc.2013.10.033
123. Zhou L, Wang F, Sun R, Chen X, Zhang M, Xu Q, et al. SIRT5 promotes IDH2 desuccinylation and G6PD deglutarylation to enhance cellular antioxidant defense. *EMBO Rep.* (2016) 17:811–22. doi: 10.15252/embr.201541643
124. Chen XF, Tian MX, Sun RQ, Zhang ML, Zhou LS, Jin L, et al. SIRT5 inhibits peroxisomal ACOX1 to prevent oxidative damage and is downregulated in liver cancer. *EMBO Rep.* (2018) 19:e45124. doi: 10.15252/embr.201745124
125. Pan H, Guan D, Liu X, Li J, Wang L, Wu J, et al. SIRT6 safeguards human mesenchymal stem cells from oxidative stress by coactivating NRF2. *Cell Res.* (2016) 26:190–205. doi: 10.1038/cr.2016.4
126. Wang XX, Wang XL, Tong MM, Gan L, Chen H, Wu SS, et al. SIRT6 protects cardiomyocytes against ischemia/reperfusion injury by augmenting FoxO3alpha-dependent antioxidant defense mechanisms. *Basic Res Cardiol.* (2016) 111:13. doi: 10.1007/s00395-016-0531-z
127. Ryu D, Jo YS, Lo Sasso G, Stein S, Zhang H, Perino A, et al. A SIRT7-dependent acetylation switch of GABPbeta1 controls mitochondrial function. *Cell Metab.* (2014) 20:856–69. doi: 10.1016/j.cmet.2014.08.001
128. Mohrin M, Shin J, Liu Y, Brown K, Luo H, Xi Y, et al. Stem cell aging. A mitochondrial UPR-mediated metabolic checkpoint regulates hematopoietic stem cell aging. *Science* (2015) 347:1374–7. doi: 10.1126/science.aaa2361
129. Xiong X, Sun X, Wang Q, Qian X, Zhang Y, Pan X, et al. SIRT6 protects against palmitate-induced pancreatic beta-cell dysfunction and apoptosis. *J Endocrinol.* (2016) 231:159–65. doi: 10.1530/JOE-16-0317
130. Qin K, Zhang N, Zhang Z, Nipper M, Zhu Z, Leighton J, et al. SIRT6-mediated transcriptional suppression of Txnip is critical for pancreatic beta cell function and survival in mice. *Diabetologia* (2018) 61:906–18. doi: 10.1007/s00125-017-4542-6
131. Moynihan KA, Grimm AA, Plueger MM, Bernal-Mizrachi E, Ford E, Cras-Meneur C, et al. Increased dosage of mammalian Sir2 in pancreatic beta cells enhances glucose-stimulated insulin secretion in mice. *Cell Metab.* (2005) 2:105–17. doi: 10.1016/j.cmet.2005.07.001
132. Bordone L, Motta MC, Picard F, Robinson A, Jhala US, Apfeld J, et al. SIRT1 regulates insulin secretion by repressing UCP2 in pancreatic beta cells. *PLoS Biol.* (2006) 4:e31. doi: 10.1371/journal.pbio.0040031
133. Kitamura YI, Kitamura T, Kruse JP, Raum JC, Stein R, Gu W, et al. FoxO1 protects against pancreatic beta cell failure through NeuroD and MafA induction. *Cell Metab.* (2005) 2:153–63. doi: 10.1016/j.cmet.2005.0 8.004
134. Anderson KA, Huynh FK, Fisher-Wellman K, Stuart JD, Peterson BS, Douros JD, et al. SIRT4 is a lysine deacylase that controls leucine metabolism and insulin secretion. *Cell Metab.* (2017) 25:838-855.e815. doi: 10.1016/j.cmet.2017.03.003
135. Lombard DB, Alt FW, Cheng HL, Bunkenborg J, Streeper RS, Mostoslavsky R, et al. Mammalian Sir2 homolog SIRT3 regulates global mitochondrial lysine acetylation. *Mol Cell Biol.* (2007) 27:8807–14. doi: 10.1128/MCB.01636-07
136. Caton PW, Richardson SJ, Kieswich J, Bugliani M, Holland ML, Marchetti P, et al. Sirtuin 3 regulates mouse pancreatic beta cell function and is suppressed in pancreatic islets isolated from human type 2 diabetic patients. *Diabetologia* (2013) 56:1068–77. doi: 10.1007/s00125-013-2851-y
137. Zhou Y, Chung ACK, Fan R, Lee HM, Xu G, Tomlinson B, et al. SIRT3 deficiency increased the vulnerability of pancreatic beta cells to oxidative stress-induced dysfunction. *Antiox Redox Signal.* (2017) 27:962–76. doi: 10.1089/ars.2016.6859
138. Kim M, Lee JS, Oh JE, Nan J, Lee H, Jung HS, et al. SIRT3 Overexpression attenuates palmitate-induced pancreatic beta-cell dysfunction. *PLoS ONE* (2015) 10:e0124744. doi: 10.1371/journal.pone.01 24744
139. Zhang HH, Ma XJ, Wu LN, Zhao YY, Zhang PY, Zhang YH, et al. Sirtuin-3 (SIRT3) protects pancreatic beta-cells from endoplasmic reticulum (ER) stress-induced apoptosis and dysfunction. *Mol Cell Biochem.* (2016) 420:95–106. doi: 10.1007/s11010-016-2771-5
140. Song MY, Wang J, Ka SO, Bae EJ, Park BH. Insulin secretion impairment in SIRT6 knockout pancreatic beta cells is mediated by suppression of the FoxO1-Pdx1-Glut2 pathway. *Sci Rep.* (2016) 6:30321. doi: 10.1038/srep30321
141. Xiong X, Wang G, Tao R, Wu P, Kono T, Li K, et al. Sirtuin 6 regulates glucose-stimulated insulin secretion in mouse pancreatic beta cells. *Diabetologia* (2016) 59:151–60. doi: 10.1007/s00125-015-3778-2
142. Taniguchi CM, Emanuelli B, Kahn CR. Critical nodes in signalling pathways: insights into insulin action. *Nat Rev Mol Cell Biol.* (2006) 7:85–96. doi: 10.1038/nrm1837
143. Zhang J. The direct involvement of SIRT1 in insulin-induced insulin receptor substrate-2 tyrosine phosphorylation. *J Biol Chem.* (2007) 282:34356–364. doi: 10.1074/jbc.M706644200
144. Sundaresan NR, Pillai VB, Wolfgeher D, Samant S, Vasudevan P, Parekh V, et al. The deacetylase SIRT1 promotes membrane localization and activation of Akt and PDK1 during tumorigenesis and cardiac hypertrophy. *Sci Signal.* (2011) 4:ra46. doi: 10.1126/scisignal.2001465
145. Dan L, Klimenkova O, Klimiankou M, Klusman JH, van den Heuvel-Eibrink MM, Reinhardt D, et al. The role of sirtuin 2 activation by nicotinamide phosphoribosyltransferase in the aberrant proliferation and survival of myeloid leukemia cells. *Haematologica* (2012) 97:551–9. doi: 10.3324/haematol.2011.055236
146. Chen J, Chan AW, To KF, Chen W, Zhang Z, Ren J, et al. SIRT2 overexpression in hepatocellular carcinoma mediates epithelial to mesenchymal transition by protein kinase B/glycogen synthase kinase-3beta/beta-catenin signaling. *Hepatology* (2013) 57:2287–98. doi: 10.1002/hep.26278

147. Ramakrishnan G, Davaakhuu G, Kaplun L, Chung WC, Rana A, Atfi A, et al. SIRT2 deacetylase is a novel AKT binding partner critical for AKT activation by insulin. *J Biol Chem.* (2014) 289:6054–66. doi: 10.1074/jbc.M113.537266
148. Arora A, Dey CS. SIRT2 negatively regulates insulin resistance in C2C12 skeletal muscle cells. *Biochim Biophys Acta* (2014) 1842:1372–8. doi: 10.1016/j.bbadis.2014.04.027
149. Arora A, Dey CS. SIRT2 regulates insulin sensitivity in insulin resistant neuronal cells. *Biochem Biophys Res Commun.* (2016) 474:747–52. doi: 10.1016/j.bbrc.2016.05.029
150. Jing E, Gesta S, Kahn CR. SIRT2 regulates adipocyte differentiation through FoxO1 acetylation/deacetylation. *Cell Metab.* (2007) 6:105–14. doi: 10.1016/j.cmet.2007.07.003
151. Belman JP, Bian RR, Habtemichael EN, Li DT, Jurczak MJ, Alcazar-Roman A, et al. Acetylation of TUG protein promotes the accumulation of GLUT4 glucose transporters in an insulin-responsive intracellular compartment. *J Biol Chem.* (2015) 290:4447–63. doi: 10.1074/jbc.M114.603977
152. Xiao C, Kim HS, Lahusen T, Wang RH, Xu X, Gavrilova O, et al. SIRT6 deficiency results in severe hypoglycemia by enhancing both basal and insulin-stimulated glucose uptake in mice. *J Biol Chem.* (2010) 285:36776–84. doi: 10.1074/jbc.M110.168039
153. Anderson JG, Ramadori G, Ioris RM, Galie M, Berglund ED, Coate KC, et al. Enhanced insulin sensitivity in skeletal muscle and liver by physiological overexpression of SIRT6. *Mol Metab* (2015) 4:846–56. doi: 10.1016/j.molmet.2015.09.003
154. Yu J, Qin B, Wu F, Qin S, Nowsheen S, Shan S, et al. Regulation of serine-threonine kinase Akt Activation by NAD$^+$-dependent deacetylase SIRT7. *Cell Rep.* (2017) 18:1229–40. doi: 10.1016/j.celrep.2017.01.009
155. Saltiel AR, Kahn CR. Insulin signalling and the regulation of glucose and lipid metabolism. *Nature* (2001) 414:799–806. doi: 10.1038/414799a
156. Farmer SR. Transcriptional control of adipocyte formation. *Cell Metab.* (2006) 4:263–273. doi: 10.1016/j.cmet.2006.07.001
157. Puigserver P, Rhee J, Donovan J, Walkey CJ, Yoon JC, Oriente F, et al. Insulin-regulated hepatic gluconeogenesis through FOXO1-PGC-1alpha interaction. *Nature* (2003) 423:550–5. doi: 10.1038/nature01667
158. Bouche C, Serdy S, Kahn CR, Goldfine AB. The cellular fate of glucose and its relevance in type 2 diabetes. *Endocrine Rev.* (2004) 25:807–30. doi: 10.1210/er.2003-0026
159. Weyer C, Bogardus C, Mott DM, Pratley RE. The natural history of insulin secretory dysfunction and insulin resistance in the pathogenesis of type 2 diabetes mellitus. *J Clin Investigat.* (1999) 104:787–94. doi: 10.1172/JCI7231
160. Smith AG, Muscat GE. Skeletal muscle and nuclear hormone receptors: implications for cardiovascular and metabolic disease. *Int J Biochem Cell Biol.* (2005) 37:2047–63. doi: 10.1016/j.biocel.2005.03.002
161. Jing E, O'Neill BT, Rardin MJ, Kleinridders A, Ilkeyeva OR, Ussar S, et al. SIRT3 regulates metabolic flexibility of skeletal muscle through reversible enzymatic deacetylation. *Diabetes* (2013) 62:3404–17. doi: 10.2337/db12-1650
162. Palacios OM, Carmona JJ, Michan S, Chen KY, Manabe Y, Ward JL, et al. Diet and exercise signals regulate SIRT3 and activate AMPK and PGC-1alpha in skeletal muscle. *Aging* (2009) 1:771–783. doi: 10.18632/aging.100075
163. Milne JC, Lambert PD, Schenk S, Carney DP, Smith JJ, Gagne DJ, et al. Small molecule activators of SIRT1 as therapeutics for the treatment of type 2 diabetes. *Nature* (2007) 450:712–6. doi: 10.1038/nature06261
164. Frescas D, Valenti L, Accili D. Nuclear trapping of the forkhead transcription factor FoxO1 via SIRT-dependent deacetylation promotes expression of glucogenetic genes. *J Biol Chem.* (2005) 280:20589–95. doi: 10.1074/jbc.M412357200
165. Rodgers JT, Lerin C, Haas W, Gygi SP, Spiegelman BM, Puigserver P. Nutrient control of glucose homeostasis through a complex of PGC-1alpha and SIRT1. *Nature* (2005) 434:113–8. doi: 10.1038/nature03354
166. Liu Y, Dentin R, Chen D, Hedrick S, Ravnskjaer K, Schenk S, et al. A fasting inducible switch modulates gluconeogenesis via activator/coactivator exchange. *Nature* (2008) 456:269–73. doi: 10.1038/nature07349
167. Hallows WC, Yu W, Denu JM. Regulation of glycolytic enzyme phosphoglycerate mutase-1 by SIRT1 protein-mediated deacetylation. *J Biol Chem.* (2012) 287:3850–8. doi: 10.1074/jbc.M111.317404
168. Li Y, Wong K, Giles A, Jiang J, Lee JW, Adams AC, et al. Hepatic SIRT1 attenuates hepatic steatosis and controls energy balance in mice by inducing fibroblast growth factor 21. *Gastroenterology* (2014) 146:539–549.e537. doi: 10.1053/j.gastro.2013.10.059
169. Li Y, Xu S, Giles A, Nakamura K, Lee JW, Hou X, et al. Hepatic overexpression of SIRT1 in mice attenuates endoplasmic reticulum stress and insulin resistance in the liver. *FASEB J.* (2011) 25:1664–79. doi: 10.1096/fj.10-173492
170. Ajmo JM, Liang X, Rogers CQ, Pennock B, You M. Resveratrol alleviates alcoholic fatty liver in mice. *Am J Physiol.* (2008) 295:G833–842. doi: 10.1152/ajpgi.90358.2008
171. Yamazaki Y, Usui I, Kanatani Y, Matsuya Y, Tsuneyama K, Fujisaka S, et al. Treatment with SRT1720, a SIRT1 activator, ameliorates fatty liver with reduced expression of lipogenic enzymes in MSG mice. *Am J Physiol.* (2009) 297:E1179–1186. doi: 10.1152/ajpendo.90997.2008
172. Walker AK, Yang F, Jiang K, Ji JY, Watts JL, Purushotham A, et al. Conserved role of SIRT1 orthologs in fasting-dependent inhibition of the lipid/cholesterol regulator SREBP. *Genes Dev.* (2010) 24:1403–17. doi: 10.1101/gad.1901210
173. Hou X, Xu S, Maitland-Toolan KA, Sato K, Jiang B, Ido Y, et al. SIRT1 regulates hepatocyte lipid metabolism through activating AMP-activated protein kinase. *J Biol Chem.* (2008) 283:20015–26. doi: 10.1074/jbc.M802187200
174. Gesta S, Tseng YH, Kahn CR. Developmental origin of fat: tracking obesity to its source. *Cell* (2007) 131:242–56. doi: 10.1016/j.cell.2007.10.004
175. Picard F, Kurtev M, Chung N, Topark-Ngarm A, Senawong T, Machado De Oliveira R, et al. SIRT1 promotes fat mobilization in white adipocytes by repressing PPAR-gamma. *Nature* (2004) 429:771–6. doi: 10.1038/nature02583
176. Guan HP, Li Y, Jensen MV, Newgard CB, Steppan CM, Lazar MA. A futile metabolic cycle activated in adipocytes by antidiabetic agents. *Nat Med.* (2002) 8:1122–8. doi: 10.1038/nm780
177. Kelley DE, Goodpaster BH, Storlien L. Muscle triglyceride and insulin resistance. *Annu Rev Nutr.* (2002) 22:325–46. doi: 10.1146/annurev.nutr.22.010402.102912
178. Gerhart-Hines Z, Rodgers JT, Bare O, Lerin C, Kim SH, Mostoslavsky R, et al. Metabolic control of muscle mitochondrial function and fatty acid oxidation through SIRT1/PGC-1alpha. *EMBO J.* (2007) 26:1913–23. doi: 10.1038/sj.emboj.7601633
179. Canto C, Gerhart-Hines Z, Feige JN, Lagouge M, Noriega L, Milne JC, et al. AMPK regulates energy expenditure by modulating NAD+ metabolism and SIRT1 activity. *Nature* (2009) 458:1056–60. doi: 10.1038/nature07813
180. Frojdo S, Durand C, Molin L, Carey AL, El-Osta A, Kingwell BA, et al. Phosphoinositide 3-kinase as a novel functional target for the regulation of the insulin signaling pathway by SIRT1. *Mol Cell Endocrinol.* (2011) 335:166–76. doi: 10.1016/j.mce.2011.01.008
181. White AT, McCurdy CE, Philp A, Hamilton DL, Johnson CD, Schenk S. Skeletal muscle-specific overexpression of SIRT1 does not enhance whole-body energy expenditure or insulin sensitivity in young mice. *Diabetologia* (2013) 56:1629–37. doi: 10.1007/s00125-013-2912-2
182. White AT, Philp A, Fridolfsson HN, Schilling JM, Murphy AN, Hamilton DL, et al. High-fat diet-induced impairment of skeletal muscle insulin sensitivity is not prevented by SIRT1 overexpression. *Am J Physiol.* (2014) 307:E764–772. doi: 10.1152/ajpendo.00001.2014
183. Côté CD, Rasmussen BA, Duca FA, Zadeh-Tahmasebi M, Baur JA, Daljeet M, et al. Resveratrol activates duodenal SIRT1 to reverse insulin resistance in rats through a neuronal network. *Nat Med.* (2015) 21:498. doi: 10.1038/nm.3821
184. James Ryall G, Dell'Orso S, Derfoul A, Juan A, Zare H, Feng X, et al. The NAD$^+$-dependent SIRT1 deacetylase translates a metabolic switch into regulatory epigenetics in skeletal muscle stem cells. *Cell Stem Cell* (2015) 16:171–83. doi: 10.1016/j.stem.2014.12.004
185. Gurd BJ, Perry CGR, Heigenhauser GJF, Spriet LL, Bonen A. High-intensity interval training increases SIRT1 activity in human skeletal muscle. *Appl Physiol Nutr Metab.* (2010) 35:350–7. doi: 10.1139/H10-030
186. Crujeiras AB, Parra D, Goyenechea E, Martinez JA. Sirtuin gene expression in human mononuclear cells is modulated by caloric restriction. *Eur J Clin Investig.* (2008) 38:672–8. doi: 10.1111/j.1365-2362.2008.01998.x
187. Krishnan J, Danzer C, Simka T, Ukropec J, Walter KM, Kumpf S, et al. Dietary obesity-associated Hif1alpha activation in adipocytes restricts fatty

acid oxidation and energy expenditure via suppression of the SIRT2-NAD+ system. *Genes Dev.* (2012) 26:259–70. doi: 10.1101/gad.180406.111

188. Arab Sadeghabadi Z, Nourbakhsh M, Pasalar P, Emamgholipour S, Golestani A, Larijani B, et al. Reduced gene expression of sirtuins and active AMPK levels in children and adolescents with obesity and insulin resistance. *Obes Res Clin Pract.* (2018) 12:167–73. doi: 10.1016/j.orcp.2017.10.004
189. Nakae J, Kitamura T, Kitamura Y, Biggs WH 3rd, Arden KC, Accili D. The forkhead transcription factor Foxol regulates adipocyte differentiation. *Dev Cell* (2003) 4:119–29. doi: 10.1016/S1534-5807(02)00401-X
190. Dowell P, Otto TC, Adi S, Lane MD. Convergence of peroxisome proliferator-activated receptor gamma and Foxol signaling pathways. *J Biol Chem.* (2003) 278:45485–91. doi: 10.1074/jbc.M309069200
191. Armoni M, Harel C, Karni S, Chen H, Bar-Yoseph F, Ver MR, et al. FOXO1 represses peroxisome proliferator-activated receptor-gamma1 and -gamma2 gene promoters in primary adipocytes. A novel paradigm to increase insulin sensitivity. *J Biol Chem.* (2006) 281:19881–91. doi: 10.1074/jbc.M600320200
192. Wang F, Tong Q. SIRT2 suppresses adipocyte differentiation by deacetylating FOXO1 and enhancing FOXO1's repressive interaction with PPARgamma. *Mol Biol Cell* (2009) 20:801–8. doi: 10.1091/mbc.e08-06-0647
193. Strable MS, Ntambi JM. Genetic control of *de novo* lipogenesis: role in diet-induced obesity. *Crit Rev Biochem Mol Biol.* (2010) 45:199–214. doi: 10.3109/10409231003667500
194. Wellen KE, Hatzivassiliou G, Sachdeva UM, Bui TV, Cross JR, Thompson CB. ATP-citrate lyase links cellular metabolism to histone acetylation. *Science* (2009) 324:1076–80. doi: 10.1126/science.1164097
195. Lin R, Tao R, Gao X, Li T, Zhou X, Guan KL, et al. Acetylation stabilizes ATP-citrate lyase to promote lipid biosynthesis and tumor growth. *Mol Cell* (2013) 51:506–18. doi: 10.1016/j.molcel.2013.07.002
196. Vega RB, Huss JM, Kelly DP. The coactivator PGC-1 cooperates with peroxisome proliferator-activated receptor alpha in transcriptional control of nuclear genes encoding mitochondrial fatty acid oxidation enzymes. *Mol Cell Biol.* (2000) 20:1868–76. doi: 10.1128/MCB.20.5.1868-1876.2000
197. Zhao S, Xu W, Jiang W, Yu W, Lin Y, Zhang T, et al. Regulation of cellular metabolism by protein lysine acetylation. *Science* (2010) 327:1000–4. doi: 10.1126/science.1179689
198. Jiang W, Wang S, Xiao M, Lin Y, Zhou L, Lei Q, et al. Acetylation regulates gluconeogenesis by promoting PEPCK1 degradation via recruiting the UBR5 ubiquitin ligase. *Mol Cell* (2011) 43:33–44. doi: 10.1016/j.molcel.2011.04.028
199. Herzig S, Long F, Jhala US, Hedrick S, Quinn R, Bauer A, et al. CREB regulates hepatic gluconeogenesis through the coactivator PGC-1. *Nature* (2001) 413:179–83. doi: 10.1038/35093131
200. Nakae J, Biggs WH 3rd, Kitamura T, Cavenee WK, Wright CV, Arden KC, et al. Regulation of insulin action and pancreatic beta-cell function by mutated alleles of the gene encoding forkhead transcription factor Foxol. *Nat Genet.* (2002) 32:245–53. doi: 10.1038/ng890
201. Yoon JC, Puigserver P, Chen G, Donovan J, Wu Z, Rhee J, et al. Control of hepatic gluconeogenesis through the transcriptional coactivator PGC-1. *Nature* (2001) 413:131–8. doi: 10.1038/35093050
202. Onyango P, Celic I, McCaffery JM, Boeke JD, Feinberg AP. SIRT3, a human SIR2 homologue, is an NAD-dependent deacetylase localized to mitochondria. *Proc Natl Acad Sci USA* (2002) 99:13653–8. doi: 10.1073/pnas.222538099
203. Su AI, Wiltshire T, Batalov S, Lapp H, Ching KA, Block D, et al. A gene atlas of the mouse and human protein-encoding transcriptomes. *Proc Natl Acad Sci USA* (2004) 101:6062–7. doi: 10.1073/pnas.0400782101
204. Wu C, Orozco C, Boyer J, Leglise M, Goodale J, Batalov S, et al. BioGPS: an extensible and customizable portal for querying and organizing gene annotation resources. *Genome Biol.* (2009) 10:R130. doi: 10.1186/gb-2009-10-11-r130
205. Han E, Hilsenbeck SG, Richardson A, Nelson JF. cDNA expression arrays reveal incomplete reversal of age-related changes in gene expression by calorie restriction. *Mech Ageing Dev.* (2000) 115:157–74. doi: 10.1016/S0047-6374(00)00119-6
206. Shi T, Wang F, Stieren E, Tong Q. SIRT3, a mitochondrial sirtuin deacetylase, regulates mitochondrial function and thermogenesis in brown adipocytes. *J Biol Chem.* (2005) 280:13560–7. doi: 10.1074/jbc.M414670200
207. Schwer B, Eckersdorff M, Li Y, Silva JC, Fermin D, Kurtev MV, et al. Calorie restriction alters mitochondrial protein acetylation. *Aging Cell* (2009) 8:604–6. doi: 10.1111/j.1474-9726.2009.00503.x
208. Hallows WC, Yu W, Smith BC, Devries MK, Ellinger JJ, Someya S, et al. SIRT3 promotes the urea cycle and fatty acid oxidation during dietary restriction. *Mol Cell* (2011) 41:139–49. doi: 10.1016/j.molcel.2011.01.002
209. Hirschey MD, Shimazu T, Jing E, Grueter CA, Collins AM, Aouizerat B, et al. SIRT3 deficiency and mitochondrial protein hyperacetylation accelerate the development of the metabolic syndrome. *Mol Cell* (2011) 44:177–90. doi: 10.1016/j.molcel.2011.07.019
210. Hirschey MD, Shimazu T, Goetzman E, Jing E, Schwer B, Lombard DB, et al. SIRT3 regulates mitochondrial fatty-acid oxidation by reversible enzyme deacetylation. *Nature* (2010) 464:121–5. doi: 10.1038/nature08778
211. Garcia-Fuentes E, Santiago-Fernandez C, Gutierrez-Repiso C, Mayas MD, Oliva-Olivera W, Coin-Araguez L, et al. Hypoxia is associated with a lower expression of genes involved in lipogenesis in visceral adipose tissue. *J Transl Med.* (2015) 13:373. doi: 10.1186/s12967-015-0732-5
212. Zamora-Mendoza R, Rosas-Vargas H, Ramos-Cervantes MT, Garcia-Zuniga P, Perez-Lorenzana H, Mendoza-Lorenzo P, et al. Dysregulation of mitochondrial function and biogenesis modulators in adipose tissue of obese children. *Int J Obes.* (2018) 42:618–24. doi: 10.1038/ijo.2017.274
213. Kurtz DM, Rinaldo P, Rhead WJ, Tian L, Millington DS, Vockley J, et al. Targeted disruption of mouse long-chain acyl-CoA dehydrogenase gene reveals crucial roles for fatty acid oxidation. *Proc Natl Acad Sci USA* (1998) 95:15592–7. doi: 10.1073/pnas.95.26.15592
214. Zhang D, Liu ZX, Choi CS, Tian L, Kibbey R, Dong J, et al. Shulman GI, Mitochondrial dysfunction due to long-chain Acyl-CoA dehydrogenase deficiency causes hepatic steatosis and hepatic insulin resistance. *Proc Natl Acad Sci USA* (2007) 104:17075–80. doi: 10.1073/pnas.0707060104
215. Fernandez-Marcos PJ, Jeninga EH, Canto C, Harach T, de Boer VC, Andreux P, et al. Muscle or liver-specific SIRT3 deficiency induces hyperacetylation of mitochondrial proteins without affecting global metabolic homeostasis. *Sci Rep.* (2012) 2:425. doi: 10.1038/srep00425
216. Yechoor VK, Patti ME, Ueki K, Laustsen PG, Saccone R, Rauniyar R, et al. Distinct pathways of insulin-regulated versus diabetes-regulated gene expression: an *in vivo* analysis in MIRKO mice. *Proc Natl Acad Sci USA* (2004) 101:16525–30. doi: 10.1073/pnas.0407574101
217. Lantier L, Williams AS, Williams IM, Yang KK, Bracy DP, Goelzer M, et al. SIRT3 is crucial for maintaining skeletal muscle insulin action and protects against severe insulin resistance in high-fat-fed mice. *Diabetes* (2015) 64:3081–92. doi: 10.2337/db14-1810
218. Chen YR, Fang SR, Fu YC, Zhou XH, Xu MY, Xu WC. Calorie restriction on insulin resistance and expression of SIRT1 and SIRT4 in rats. *Biochem Cell Biol.* (2010) 88:715–22. doi: 10.1139/O10-010
219. de Pinho L, Andrade JM, Paraiso A, Filho AB, Feltenberger JD, Guimaraes AL, et al. Diet composition modulates expression of sirtuins and renin-angiotensin system components in adipose tissue. *Obesity* (2013) 21:1830–5. doi: 10.1002/oby.20305
220. Laurent G, German NJ, Saha AK, de Boer VC, Davies M, Koves TR, et al. SIRT4 coordinates the balance between lipid synthesis and catabolism by repressing malonyl CoA decarboxylase. *Mol Cell* (2013) 50:686–98. doi: 10.1016/j.molcel.2013.05.012
221. Laurent G, de Boer VC, Finley LW, Sweeney M, Lu H, Schug TT, et al. SIRT4 represses peroxisome proliferator-activated receptor alpha activity to suppress hepatic fat oxidation. *Mol Cell Biol.* (2013) 33:4552–61. doi: 10.1128/MCB.00087-13
222. Wu T, Liu YH, Fu YC, Liu XM, Zhou XH. Direct evidence of sirtuin downregulation in the liver of non-alcoholic fatty liver disease patients. *Ann Clin Labor Sci.* (2014) 44:410–8.
223. Rardin MJ, He W, Nishida Y, Newman JC, Carrico C, Danielson SR, et al. SIRT5 regulates the mitochondrial lysine succinylome and metabolic networks. *Cell Metab.* (2013) 18:920–33. doi: 10.1016/j.cmet.2013.11.013
224. Park J, Chen Y, Tishkoff DX, Peng C, Tan M, Dai L, et al. SIRT5-mediated lysine desuccinylation impacts diverse metabolic pathways. *Mol Cell* (2013) 50:919–30. doi: 10.1016/j.molcel.2013.06.001
225. Yu J, Sadhukhan S, Noriega LG, Moullan N, He B, Weiss RS, et al. Metabolic characterization of a SIRT5 deficient mouse model. *Sci Rep.* (2013) 3:2806. doi: 10.1038/srep02806

226. Jukarainen S, Heinonen S, Ramo JT, Rinnankoski-Tuikka R, Rappou E, Tummers M, et al. Obesity is associated with low NAD(+)/SIRT pathway expression in adipose tissue of BMI-discordant monozygotic twins. *J Clin Endocrinol Metab.* (2016) 101:275–83. doi: 10.1210/jc.2015-3095
227. Nishida Y, Rardin MJ, Carrico C, He W, Sahu AK, Gut P, et al. SIRT5 Regulates both cytosolic and mitochondrial protein malonylation with glycolysis as a major target. *Mol Cell* (2015) 59:321–32. doi: 10.1016/j.molcel.2015.05.022
228. Dominy JE Jr, Lee Y, Jedrychowski MP, Chim H, Jurczak MJ, Camporez JP, et al. The deacetylase SIRT6 activates the acetyltransferase GCN5 and suppresses hepatic gluconeogenesis. *Mol Cell* (2012) 48:900–13. doi: 10.1016/j.molcel.2012.09.030
229. Moschen AR, Wieser V, Gerner RR, Bichler A, Enrich B, Moser P, et al. Adipose tissue and liver expression of SIRT1, 3, and 6 increase after extensive weight loss in morbid obesity. *J Hepatol.* (2013) 59:1315–22. doi: 10.1016/j.jhep.2013.07.027
230. Chen Q, Hao W, Xiao C, Wang R, Xu X, Lu H, et al. SIRT6 is essential for adipocyte differentiation by regulating mitotic clonal expansion. *Cell Rep.* (2017) 18:3155–66. doi: 10.1016/j.celrep.2017.03.006
231. Kanfi Y, Peshti V, Gil R, Naiman S, Nahum L, Levin E, et al. SIRT6 protects against pathological damage caused by diet-induced obesity. *Aging Cell* (2010) 9:162–73. doi: 10.1111/j.1474-9726.2009.00544.x
232. Yao L, Cui X, Chen Q, Yang X, Fang F, Zhang J, et al. Cold-inducible SIRT6 regulates thermogenesis of brown and beige fat. *Cell Rep.* (2017) 20:641–54. doi: 10.1016/j.celrep.2017.06.069
233. Zhong L, D'Urso A, Toiber D, Sebastian C, Henry RE, Vadysirisack DD, et al. The histone deacetylase SIRT6 regulates glucose homeostasis via Hif1alpha. *Cell* (2010) 140:280–93. doi: 10.1016/j.cell.2009.12.041
234. Zhang P, Tu B, Wang H, Cao Z, Tang M, Zhang C, et al. Tumor suppressor p53 cooperates with SIRT6 to regulate gluconeogenesis by promoting FoxO1 nuclear exclusion. *Proc Natl Acad Sci USA* (2014) 111:10684–9. doi: 10.1073/pnas.1411026111
235. Kim HS, Xiao C, Wang RH, Lahusen T, Xu X, Vassilopoulos A, et al. Hepatic-specific disruption of SIRT6 in mice results in fatty liver formation due to enhanced glycolysis and triglyceride synthesis. *Cell Metab.* (2010) 12:224–36. doi: 10.1016/j.cmet.2010.06.009
236. Yang SJ, Choi JM, Chae SW, Kim WJ, Park SE, Rhee EJ, et al. Activation of peroxisome proliferator-activated receptor gamma by rosiglitazone increases SIRT6 expression and ameliorates hepatic steatosis in rats. *PLoS ONE* (2011) 6:e17057. doi: 10.1371/journal.pone.0017057
237. Cui X, Yao L, Yang X, Gao Y, Fang F, Zhang J, et al. SIRT6 regulates metabolic homeostasis in skeletal muscle through activation of AMPK. *Am J Physiol Endocrinol Metab.* (2017) 313:E493–E505. doi: 10.1152/ajpendo.00122.2017
238. Kurylowicz A, Owczarz M, Polosak J, Jonas MI, Lisik W, Jonas M, et al. SIRT1 and SIRT7 expression in adipose tissues of obese and normal-weight individuals is regulated by microRNAs but not by methylation status. *Int J Obes.* (2016) 40:1635–42. doi: 10.1038/ijo.2016.131
239. Yoshizawa T, Karim MF, Sato Y, Senokuchi T, Miyata K, Fukuda T, et al. SIRT7 controls hepatic lipid metabolism by regulating the ubiquitin-proteasome pathway. *Cell Metab.* (2014) 19:712–21. doi: 10.1016/j.cmet.2014.03.006
240. Fang J, Ianni A, Smolka C, Vakhrusheva O, Nolte H, Kruger M, et al. SIRT7 promotes adipogenesis in the mouse by inhibiting autocatalytic activation of SIRT1. *Proc Natl Acad Sci USA* (2017) 114:E8352–E8361. doi: 10.1073/pnas.1706945114
241. Cioffi M, Vallespinos-Serrano M, Sara Trabulo M, Pablo Fernandez-Marcos J, Ashley Firment N, Berta Vazquez N, et al. MiR-93 Controls Adiposity via Inhibition of SIRT7 and Tbx3. *Cell Rep.* (2015) 12:1594–605. doi: 10.1016/j.celrep.2015.08.006
242. Shin J, He M, Liu Y, Paredes S, Villanova L, Brown K, et al. SIRT7 represses Myc activity to suppress ER stress and prevent fatty liver disease. *Cell Rep.* (2013) 5:654–65. doi: 10.1016/j.celrep.2013.10.007
243. Kang HS, Okamoto K, Kim YS, Takeda Y, Bortner CD, Dang H, et al. Nuclear orphan receptor TAK1/TR4-deficient mice are protected against obesity-linked inflammation, hepatic steatosis, and insulin resistance. *Diabetes* (2011) 60:177–88. doi: 10.2337/db10-0628
244. Hu H, Zhu W, Qin J, Chen M, Gong L, Li L, et al. Acetylation of PGK1 promotes liver cancer cell proliferation and tumorigenesis. *Hepatology* (2017) 65:515–28. doi: 10.1002/hep.28887
245. Jiang L, Xiong J, Zhan J, Yuan F, Tang M, Zhang C, et al. Ubiquitin-specific peptidase 7 (USP7)-mediated deubiquitination of the histone deacetylase SIRT7 regulates gluconeogenesis. *J Biol Chem.* (2017) 292:13296–311. doi: 10.1074/jbc.M117.780130
246. Hall JA, Dominy JE, Lee Y, Puigserver P. The sirtuin family's role in aging and age-associated pathologies. *J Clin Investig.* (2013) 123:973–9. doi: 10.1172/JCI64094
247. Petersen KF, Befroy D, Dufour S, Dziura J, Ariyan C, Rothman DL, et al. Mitochondrial dysfunction in the elderly: possible role in insulin resistance. *Science* (2003) 300:1140–2. doi: 10.1126/science.1082889
248. Park MH, Kim DH, Lee EK, Kim ND, Im DS, Lee J, et al. Age-related inflammation and insulin resistance: a review of their intricate interdependency. *Arch Pharm Res.* (2014) 37:1507–14. doi: 10.1007/s12272-014-0474-6
249. Fabbri E, Chia CW, Spencer RG, Fishbein KW, Reiter DA, Cameron D, et al. Insulin resistance is associated with reduced mitochondrial oxidative capacity measured by 31P-magnetic resonance spectroscopy in participants without diabetes from the baltimore longitudinal study of aging. *Diabetes* (2017) 66:170–6. doi: 10.2337/db16-0754
250. Wu H, Ballantyne CM. Skeletal muscle inflammation and insulin resistance in obesity. *J Clin Investig.* (2017) 127:43–54. doi: 10.1172/JCI88880
251. Finkel T, Deng CX. Mostoslavsky R, Recent progress in the biology and physiology of sirtuins. *Nature* (2009) 460:587–91. doi: 10.1038/nature08197
252. Tang X, Chen XF, Wang NY, Wang XM, Liang ST, Zheng W, et al. SIRT2 acts as a cardioprotective deacetylase in pathological cardiac hypertrophy. *Circulation* (2017) 136:2051–67. doi: 10.1161/CIRCULATIONAHA.117.028728
253. Kanfi Y, Naiman S, Amir G, Peshti V, Zinman G, Nahum L, et al. The sirtuin SIRT6 regulates lifespan in male mice. *Nature* (2012) 483:218. doi: 10.1038/nature10815
254. Sundaresan NR, Vasudevan P, Zhong L, Kim G, Samant S, Parekh V, et al. The sirtuin SIRT6 blocks IGF-Akt signaling and development of cardiac hypertrophy by targeting c-Jun. *Nat Med.* (2012) 18:1643. doi: 10.1038/nm.2961
255. Satoh A, Brace CS, Rensing N, Cliften P, Wozniak DF, Herzog ED, et al. SIRT1 extends life span and delays aging in mice through the regulation of Nk2 homeobox 1 in the DMH and LH. *Cell Metab.* (2013) 18:416–30. doi: 10.1016/j.cmet.2013.07.013
256. Sarah Mitchell J, Martin-Montalvo A, Evi Mercken M, Hector Palacios H, Theresa Ward M, Abulwerdi G, et al. The SIRT1 activator SRT1720 extends lifespan and improves health of mice fed a standard diet. *Cell Rep.* (2014) 6:836–43. doi: 10.1016/j.celrep.2014.01.031
257. Madeo F, Pietrocola F, Eisenberg T, Kroemer G. Caloric restriction mimetics: towards a molecular definition. *Nat Rev Drug Discov.* (2014) 13:727–40. doi: 10.1038/nrd4391
258. Chen HZ, Wang F, Gao P, Pei JF, Liu Y, Xu TT, et al. Age-associated sirtuin 1 reduction in vascular smooth muscle links vascular senescence and inflammation to abdominal aortic aneurysm. *Circ Res.* (2016) 119:1076–88. doi: 10.1161/CIRCRESAHA.116.308895
259. Liu Y, Wang TT, Zhang R, Fu WY, Wang X, Wang F, et al. Calorie restriction protects against experimental abdominal aortic aneurysms in mice. *J Exp Med.* (2016) 213:2473–88. doi: 10.1084/jem.20151794
260. Winnik S, Auwerx J, Sinclair DA, Matter CM. Protective effects of sirtuins in cardiovascular diseases: from bench to bedside. *Eur Heart J.* (2015) 36:3404–12. doi: 10.1093/eurheartj/ehv290
261. Weiss EP, Racette SB, Villareal DT, Fontana L, Steger-May K, Schechtman KB, et al. Washington University School of Medicine, Improvements in glucose tolerance and insulin action induced by increasing energy expenditure or decreasing energy intake: a randomized controlled trial. *Am J Clin Nutr.* (2006) 84:1033–42. doi: 10.1093/ajcn/84.5.1033
262. Meehan CA, Cochran E, Mattingly M, Gorden P, Brown RJ. Mild caloric restriction decreases insulin requirements in patients with type 2 diabetes and severe insulin resistance. *Medicine* (2015) 94:e1160. doi: 10.1097/MD.0000000000001160

263. Houtkooper RH, Pirinen E, Auwerx J. Sirtuins as regulators of metabolism and healthspan. *Nat Rev Mol Cell Biol.* (2012) 13:225–38. doi: 10.1038/nrm3293
264. Martin-Montalvo A, Mercken EM, Mitchell SJ, Palacios HH, Mote PL, Scheibye-Knudsen M, et al. improves healthspan and lifespan in mice. *Nat Commun.* (2013) 4:2192. doi: 10.1038/ncomms3192
265. Miranda MX, van Tits LJ, Lohmann C, Arsiwala T, Winnik S, Tailleux A, et al. The SIRT1 activator SRT3025 provides atheroprotection in Apoe-/- mice by reducing hepatic Pcsk9 secretion and enhancing Ldlr expression. *Eur Heart J.* (2015) 36:51–9. doi: 10.1093/eurheartj/ehu095
266. Igarashi M, Guarente L. mTORC1 and SIRT1 cooperate to foster expansion of gut adult stem cells during calorie restriction. *Cell* (2016) 166:436–50. doi: 10.1016/j.cell.2016.05.044
267. Lai YC, Tabima DM, Dube JJ, Hughan KS, Vanderpool RR, Goncharov DA, et al. SIRT3–AMP-activated protein kinase activation by nitrite and metformin improves hyperglycemia and normalizes pulmonary hypertension associated with heart failure with preserved ejection fraction. *Circulation* (2016) 133:717–31. doi: 10.1161/CIRCULATIONAHA.115.018935
268. Ding YN, Tang X, Chen HZ, Liu DP. Epigenetic regulation of vascular aging and age-related vascular diseases, In: Wang Z, editor. *Aging and Aging-Related Diseases: Mechanisms and Interventions*. Singapore: Springer (2018). p. 55–75. doi: 10.1007/978-981-13-1117-8_4
269. Bonkowski MS, Sinclair DA. Slowing ageing by design: the rise of NAD+ and sirtuin-activating compounds. *Nat Rev Mol Cell Biol.* (2016) 17:679. doi: 10.1038/nrm.2016.93
270. Masri S, Rigor P, Cervantes M, Ceglia N, Sebastian C, Xiao C, et al. Partitioning circadian transcription by SIRT6 leads to segregated control of cellular metabolism. *Cell* (2014) 158:659–72. doi: 10.1016/j.cell.2014.06.050
271. Villeneuve LM, Reddy MA, Lanting LL, Wang M, Meng L, Natarajan R. Epigenetic histone H3 lysine 9 methylation in metabolic memory and inflammatory phenotype of vascular smooth muscle cells in diabetes. *Proc Natl Acad Sci USA* (2008) 105:9047–52. doi: 10.1073/pnas.0803623105
272. Raychaudhuri N, Thamotharan S, Srinivasan M, Mahmood S, Patel MS, Devaskar SU. Postnatal exposure to a high-carbohydrate diet interferes epigenetically with thyroid hormone receptor induction of the adult male rat skeletal muscle glucose transporter isoform 4 expression. *J Nutr Biochem.* (2014) 25:1066–76. doi: 10.1016/j.jnutbio.2014.05.011
273. Yang B, Yang J, Bai J, Pu P, Liu J, Wang F, et al. SUV39H1 protects from myocardial ischemia-reperfusion injury in diabetic rats. *Cell Physiol Biochem.* (2014) 33:1176–85. doi: 10.1159/000358686
274. Jiang Z, Shi D, Tu Y, Tian J, Zhang W, Xing B, et al. Human proislet peptide promotes pancreatic progenitor cells to ameliorate diabetes through FOXO1/menin-mediated epigenetic regulation. *Diabetes* (2018) 67:1345–55. doi: 10.2337/db17-0885
275. Tian Y, Wong VW, Wong GL, Yang W, Sun H, Shen J, et al. Histone deacetylase HDAC8 promotes insulin resistance and beta-catenin activation in NAFLD-associated hepatocellular carcinoma. *Cancer Res.* (2015) 75:4803–16. doi: 10.1158/0008-5472.CAN-14-3786
276. Shi H, Munk A, Nielsen TS, Daughtry MR, Larsson L, Li S, et al. Skeletal muscle O-GlcNAc transferase is important for muscle energy homeostasis and whole-body insulin sensitivity. *Mol Metab.* (2018) 11:160–77. doi: 10.1016/j.molmet.2018.02.010
277. Vaquero A, Scher M, Erdjument-Bromage H, Tempst P, Serrano L, Reinberg D. SIRT1 regulates the histone methyl-transferase SUV39H1 during heterochromatin formation. *Nature* (2007) 450:440–4. doi: 10.1038/nature06268
278. Bosch-Presegue L, Raurell-Vila H, Marazuela-Duque A, Kane-Goldsmith N, Valle A, Oliver J, et al. Stabilization of SUV39H1 by SIRT1 is part of oxidative stress response and ensures genome protection. *Mol Cell* (2011) 42:210–23. doi: 10.1016/j.molcel.2011.02.034
279. Yang G, Zhang X, Weng X, Liang P, Dai X, Zeng S, et al. SUV39H1 mediated SIRT1 trans-repression contributes to cardiac ischemia-reperfusion injury. *Basic Res Cardiol.* (2017) 112:22. doi: 10.1007/s00395-017-0608-3
280. Ren JH, Hu JL, Cheng ST, Yu HB, Wong VKW, Law BYK, et al. SIRT3 restricts HBV transcription and replication via epigenetic regulation of cccDNA involving SUV39H1 and SETD1A histone methyltransferases. *Hepatology* (2018) 68:1260–76. doi: 10.1002/hep.29912
281. Kumari P, Popescu D, Yue S, Bober E, Ianni A, Braun T. SIRT7 inhibits SIRT1-mediated activation of SUV39H1. *Cell Cycle* (2018) 17:1403–12. doi: 10.1080/15384101.2018.1486166
282. Shu YN, Dong LH, Li H, Pei QQ, Miao SB, Zhang F, et al. CKII-SIRT1-SM22alpha loop evokes a self-limited inflammatory response in vascular smooth muscle cells. *Cardiovasc Res.* (2017) 113:1198–207. doi: 10.1093/cvr/cvx048
283. Li M, Hong W, Hao C, Li L, Wu D, Shen A, et al. SIRT1 antagonizes liver fibrosis by blocking hepatic stellate cell activation in mice. *FASEB J.* (2018) 32:500–11. doi: 10.1096/fj.201700612R
284. Xu W, Jiang K, Shen M, Qian Y, Peng Y. SIRT2 suppresses non-small cell lung cancer growth by targeting JMJD2A. *Biol Chem.* (2015) 396:929–36. doi: 10.1515/hsz-2014-0284
285. Baker DJ, Childs BG, Durik M, Wijers ME, Sieben CJ, Zhong J, et al. Naturally occurring p16 Ink4a-positive cells shorten healthy lifespan. *Nature* (2016) 530:184. doi: 10.1038/nature16932
286. Childs BG, Baker DJ, Wijshake T, Conover CA, Campisi J, van Deursen JM. Senescent intimal foam cells are deleterious at all stages of atherosclerosis. *Science* (2016) 354:472–7. doi: 10.1126/science.aaf6659
287. Childs BG, Li H, van Deursen JM. Senescent cells: a therapeutic target for cardiovascular disease. *J Clin Invest.* (2018) 128:1217–28. doi: 10.1172/JCI95146
288. Jeon OH, Kim C, Laberge RM, Demaria M, Rathod S, Vasserot AP, et al. Local clearance of senescent cells attenuates the development of post-traumatic osteoarthritis and creates a pro-regenerative environment. *Nat Med.* (2017) 23:775–81. doi: 10.1038/nm.4324
289. Jeon OH, David N, Campisi J, Elisseeff JH. Senescent cells and osteoarthritis: a painful connection. *J Clin Invest.* (2018) 128:1229–37. doi: 10.1172/JCI95147
290. Bussian TJ, Aziz A, Meyer CF, Swenson BL, van Deursen JM, Baker DJ. Clearance of senescent glial cells prevents tau-dependent pathology and cognitive decline. *Nature* (2018) 562:578–82. doi: 10.1038/s41586-018-0543-y
291. Baker DJ, Petersen RC. Cellular senescence in brain aging and neurodegenerative diseases: evidence and perspectives. *J Clin Invest.* (2018) 128:1208–16. doi: 10.1172/JCI95145

16

The Essential Role of SIRT1 in Hypothalamic-Pituitary Axis

Masaaki Yamamoto[1] *and Yutaka Takahashi*[2*]

[1] *Pituitary Center, Department of Medicine, Cedars-Sinai Medical Center, Los Angeles, CA, United States,* [2] *Division of Diabetes and Endocrinology, Department of Internal Medicine, Kobe University Graduate School of Medicine, Kobe, Japan*

Correspondence:
Yutaka Takahashi
takahash@med.kobe-u.ac.jp

The endocrine system plays an essential role in the physiological adaptation to malnutrition. The adaptive response of various hormones directs the energy utilization toward the survival functions and away from growth and reproduction. Particularly, the hypothalamic pituitary axis plays an integral and a central role in the regulation of endocrine organs. Sirtuin 1 (SIRT1) is a nicotinamide adenine dinucleotide (NAD)-dependent histone deacetylase that is activated in response to calorie restriction (CR). SIRT1 is involved in cellular processes via the deacetylation of histone as well as various transcription factors and signal transduction molecules and thereby modulates the endocrine/metabolic functions. There is much evidence to demonstrate clearly that SIRT1 in the hypothalamus, pituitary gland, and other target organs modifies the synthesis, secretion, and activities of hormones and in turn induces the adaptive responses. In this review, we discussed the role of SIRT1 in the hypothalamic pituitary axis and its pathophysiological significance.

Keywords: SIRT1, adaptation, calorie restriction, hypothalamus, pituitary

INTRODUCTION

The Physiological Role of Sirtuin 1 (SIRT1)

SIR2 is the first sirtuin protein to be discovered in *Saccharomyces cerevisae* (yeast) (1). SIR2 orthologs are highly conserved throughout various species including mammals, plants, bacteria, worms, flies, and fishes. In mammals, the seven SIR2 orthologs are termed SIRT1-7 and are presumed to be ubiquitously expressed in all the tissues (2). Sirtuins were initially reported as protein deacetylases and ADP ribosyltransferases (3, 4). However, subsequent analyses revealed that sirtuins exhibit various enzymatic activities. For instance, SIRT5 exhibits lysine-desuccinylase and -demalonylase activities (5, 6). These enzymatic activities of sirtuins are generally activated in response to CR by the utilization of nicotine adenine dinucleotide (NAD+) as the co-substrate.

Regarding the intracellular localization of sirtuins, SIRT1, SIRT6, and SIRT7 are localized in the nucleus and mostly regulates protein function by the post-translational modification via histone deacetylation (7). Moreover, SIRT1 localizes in the cytosol and directly deacetylates various transcription factors and cofactors. SIRT2 is localized in the cytosol and nucleus and is involved in the metabolic process and cell cycle regulation (8–11). SIRT3, SIRT4, and SIRT5 are localized in the mitochondria and regulate various metabolic enzyme activities and mitochondrial oxidative stress (9). Therefore, in the organisms, sirtuins coordinate the cellular responses to adapt to CR in their corresponding cellular compartments in which they occur.

Among the seven sirtuins, SIRT1 is the most studied and well-characterized sirtuin with respect to its physiological functions. SIRT1 is involved in the production of various hormones and maintenance of homeostasis by regulating the function of histones and transcription factors, to adapt to malnutrition in the endocrine and metabolic systems. For instance, SIRT1 modulates forkhead box protein O1 (FOXO1), peroxisome proliferator-activated receptor gamma coactivator 1-alpha (PGC-1α), signal transducer and activator of transcription (STAT3) (12–14). SIRT1 interacts with peroxisome proliferator-activated receptor (PPARγ) and represses its transcriptional activity to reduce adipogenesis in differentiated fat cells and mobilize free fatty acid from the white adipose tissues (15). Additionally, SIRT1 negatively regulates the mitochondrial uncoupling protein 2 (UCP2) expression and enhances the insulin secretion in response to glucose level elevation in the pancreas (16).

Recently, accumulating evidence suggests that SIRT1 plays important role in the homeostasis maintenance in the neuroendocrine system. Particularly, the hypothalamic pituitary axes play a central and an integral role in the neuroendocrine system.

PHYSIOLOGY OF THE HYPOTHALAMUS AND PITUITARY GLAND

The neuroendocrine system, especially the hypothalamus and pituitary gland play an essential role in the homeostasis maintenance via orchestrating the endocrine system as a regulatory machinery. The hypothalamus–pituitary complex connects the nervous system with the endocrine system that regulates the systemic hormone secretion in a direct or indirect manner. The neural signaling of central nervous system modifies the hypothalamus–pituitary axis and results in the regulation of corresponding target hormonal secretion (17).

The hypothalamus is responsible for the homeostasis maintenance by regulating the body temperature, appetite, thirst, energy expenditure, behavior, and circadian rhythm of the organisms (18). Moreover, the hypothalamus synthesizes and secretes various hypothalamic hormones that in turn stimulate or inhibit the secretion of pituitary hormones (19). The medial preoptic nucleus regulates the release of gonadotropic hormones and thermogenesis (20). The putative anterior paraventricular (aPV), the paraventricular nucleus (PVN), and the supraoptic nucleus (SON) consist of parvicellular neurons that release corticotropin-releasing hormone (CRH), thyrotropin-releasing hormone (TRH), growth hormone releasing hormone (GHRH), and somatostatin (SST), and magnocellular neurons that produce vasopressin (AVP) and oxytocin (OXT) (21–24).

The pituitary gland consists of anterior posterior lobes and the anterior lobe is functionally subdivided into six cell types based on the production of a specific hormone by each cell type (25). The growth hormone (GH), prolactin, adrenocorticotropic hormone (ACTH), thyroid stimulating hormone (TSH), and luteinizing hormone (LH) or follicular stimulating hormone (FSH) are secreted by the somatotroph, lactotroph, corticotroph, thyrotroph, and gonadotroph, respectively (26). The anterior pituitary hormones are mainly regulated by the release hormones or inhibitory hormones from the hypothalamus via the portal hypophyseal circulation into the anterior lobe and neural connection to the posterior lobe through the pituitary stalk (a physical and functional connection between the hypothalamus and pituitary gland) (27, 28). The hormones secreted by the pituitary gland circulate in the systemic blood flow and thereby stimulate the hormone secretion by each of their respective target organ. Generally, these pathways initiating from the hypothalamus to target organ via the pituitary gland are mainly classified into four axes depending on the target organ, namely, hypothalamus-pituitary-adrenal (HPA), hypothalamus-pituitary-thyroid (HPT), hypothalamus-pituitary-gonadal (HPG), and somatotropic axes. In this review, we described the SIRT1 involvement in each of the aforementioned axes in the subsequent subsections.

SIRT1 in Hypothalamus

In the hypothalamus, SIRT1 is expressed in the SF1 neuron in the ventromedial hypothalamic nucleus (VMH) and in the POMC and AgRP neuron in the arcuate nucleus (ARH), respectively (29–31). POMC neuron specific SIRT1 knockout mice exhibited energy imbalance due to the altered sympathetic activity (30). Also, deletion of SIRT1 in SF1 neurons caused insulin resistance in skeletal muscle. On the contrary, SIRT1 overexpression in SF1 neurons prevented from diet-induced obesity and insulin resistance (29). Both targeted overexpression of SIRT1 in POMC or AgRP neurons prevented age-associated weight gain. However, SIRT1 overexpression in POMC neurons enhanced the energy expenditure mediated by increment of sympathetic activity in adipose tissue while SIRT1 overexpression in AgRP neurons suppressed food intake, indicating a presence of nuclear specific mechanisms (31). Also, food restriction increases SIRT1 protein levels in the dorsomedial (DMH) and lateral hypothalamic nuclei (LH) (32). Brain specific SIRT1 overexpressing mice exhibited extended life span mediated by enhanced neural activity in DMH and LH, through increased orexin type 2 receptor (Ox2r) expression (32). These data indicate that region specific expression of SIRT1 plays an important role in the regulation of appetite, energy expenditure, general metabolism, and life span.

The HPA Axis

The HPA axis is an important neuroendocrine system that plays an essential role in the survival, stress response, metabolism, appetite, immunoreaction, mood, and behavior of the organisms. Corticotrophin releasing hormone (CRH) secreted by the PVN in the hypothalamus initiates stress response in the HPA axis via the production of proopiomelanocortin (POMC) by the pituitary corticotroph. POMC is a precursor polypeptide of ACTH and alpha-melanocyte stimulating hormone (αMSH) that are cleaved by prohormone convertases 1 and 2 (PC1 and PC2), respectively. ACTH induced by corticotroph stimulates the glucocorticoid production by the adrenal cortex.

The SIRT1 expression in the hypothalamic POMC neuron is enhanced by fasting and is associated with the reduced αMSH levels, although the significance to the HPA axis is unknown (33). On the other hand, another group reported that POMC neuron specific ablation of SIRT1 did not alter POMC, ACTH, and αMSH levels (30). The precursor pro-CRH is post-translationally processed by the PC1 and PC2. SIRT1 increases the PC2 levels in the PVN that in turn increases the active-CRH production and results in the HPA axis activation (34). In mouse corticotroph cell line (AtT20 cells), treatment with resveratrol (a SIRT1 activating compound) increased the PC1 and PC2 levels. In accordance with this, Ex-527 (a SIRT1 specific inhibitor) treatment decreased the PC1 and PC2 levels in AtT20 cells (33). Although there have been no reports demonstrating the expression of SIRT1 in the corticotrophs, these data suggest that SIRT1 may indirectly modulates the HPA axis by regulating the PC1 and PC2 levels. Additionally, resveratrol increased the expression and prolonged the half-life of P450 side chain cleavage enzyme (P450scc) in the adrenal gland that results in an increase in glucocorticoid secretion by the adrenal cortex (35). Moreover, the hypothalamic SIRT1 plays an important role in the energy homeostasis maintenance associated with the HPA axis. These data clearly indicate that SIRT1 in the hypothalamus, pituitary, and adrenal gland regulates the HPA axis activation that acts as an adaptive response to starvation (**Table 1**A).

The HPT Axis

The HPT axis is activated by the thyrotropin-releasing hormone (TRH) secretion by the hypothalamus when the hypothalamus senses low levels of circulating thyroid hormone. The TRH induces thyroid-stimulating hormone (TSH) secretion by thyrotroph cells in the pituitary that in turn stimulates the thyroid hormone (TH) secretion by the thyroid to maintain normal TH levels (36). SIRT1 is expressed in thyrotroph cells and enhances TSH endocytosis via the deacetylation of phosphatidylinositol-4-phosphate 5-kinase type 1γ (PIP5K1γ), which is a main enzyme that synthesizes phosphatidylinositol 4,5-bisphosphate in thyrotroph cells (37). Tyrotroph-specific SIRT1 knockout mice showed decreased TSH secretion resulting in decreased metabolic rate (37). Additionally, SIRT1 knockout in whole body exhibited hypermetabolism caused by an increased oxygen consumption in the hepatic mitochondria leading to the decreased body weight while the mice manifested hyperphagia, reduced serum thyroxin level, and decreased nocturnal physical activity (38). Interestingly, thyroxin treatment suppressed the fasting-induced SIRT1 expression as thyroxin negatively regulates the SIRT1 level and activity in the liver via TH receptor-β (39). These data indicate that the HPT axis and SIRT1 interact with each other and adaptively regulate metabolism (**Table 1**B).

The HPG Axis

The HPG axis is responsible for the reproduction, life cycle, and sexual dimorphism in the organisms. Gonadotropin-releasing hormone (GnRH) is secreted by GnRH neurons that diffusely localize and form a network named pulse-generator in the hypothalamus. The pulsatile secretion of GnRH stimulates the luteinizing hormone (LH) and follicle-stimulating hormone (FSH) secretion by pituitary gonadotroph cells and subsequently the gonads produce estrogen or testosterone (36, 40).

Although secondary effect of the general condition including body weight loss cannot be ruled out, SIRT1 knockout mice exhibited a diminished hypothalamic GnRH expression and in turn reduced serum LH and FSH levels and spermatogenesis arrest, suggesting an important role of SIRT1 in the HPG axis (41). Additionally, GnRH treatment decreases SIRT1 level via the miR-132/212 induction in the pituitary. This results in the downregulation of SIRT1-dependent FOXO1 deacetylation and a decrease in the FOXO1-mediated inhibition of Fshβ transcription that ultimately increases the Fshβ expression in rat primary pituitary cells and LβT2 cell line (42) (**Table 1**C).

The Somatotropic Axis

In the somatotropic axis, GH releasing hormone (GHRH) that is secreted by the hypothalamus induces the GH secretion by pituitary somatotroph cells. Circulating GH binds to GH receptor on hepatocytes and results in the increased serum insulin like growth factor-I (IGF-I) level (36). Moreover, GH induces local IGF-I production in various tissues including bone, muscle, and fat tissue. In various species, numerous evidences demonstrated that the reduced function of somatotropic axis extends lifespan in

TABLE 1 | The role of SIRT1 in hypothalamic-pituitary axis.

	A HPA axis		B HPT axis		C HPG axis		D Somatotrophic axis	
SIRT1	↑	↓	↑	↓	↑	↓	↑	↓
Hypothalamus	PC2 ↓ CRH ↓	POMC ↓				GnRH ↓		
Pituitary	a-MSH ↓ PC1/ PC2 ↓	PC1/ PC2 ↓	TSH ↑			LH ↓ FSH ↑	GH ↓	GH ↓
Periphery	Adrenal GC ↑			Thyroid T4 ↓		Testis Testosterone ↑	IGF-I ↓	IGF-I ↓

(A) HPA axis, (B) HPT axis, (C) HPG axis, (D) somatotrophic axis.

SIRT1↑, Overexpression/activation of SIRT1. SIRT1↓, Knockout/inhibition of SIRT1. GC, Glucocorticoid, T4, Thyroxine.

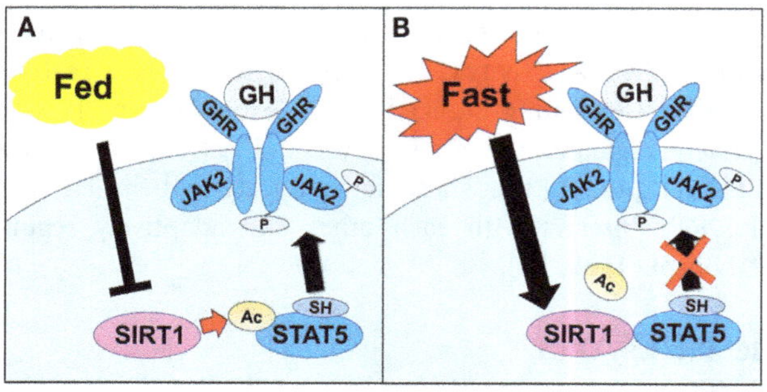

FIGURE 1 | The mechanisms through which SIRT1 regulates STAT5 activation by GH. **(A)** In the fed condition, the SH2 domain of STAT5 recognizes and binds to Tyr-phosphorylated GHR, causing JAK2 to phosphorylate and activate STAT5. **(B)** In the fasting condition, SIRT1 is activated and interacts with STAT5, thereby deacetylating Lys residues adjacent to the SH2 domain of STAT5. This results in an impaired ability to bind Tyr-phosphorylated GHR, which inhibits activation of STAT5. Excerpt from, Yamamoto et al. (60).

animal models (43–48). Regarding the underlying mechanisms, among the species which evolved from C. elegans to mouse, an evolutionarily conserved interplay between SIR2/SIRT1 and the somatotropic axis was reported in which SIR2/SIRT1 modulates the signaling molecules of somatotropic pathway (49–54).

SIRT1 brain-specific knockout (BSKO) mice exhibited dwarfism with small pituitary and reduced GH-IGF-I levels while the other pituitary hormonal levels were unaltered (55). Interestingly, SIRT6 BSKO manifested similar phenotype as that of SIRT1 BSKO. Despite the significant reduction in the number of somatotroph cells and GH content in the pituitary gland of SIRT6 BSKO, the hypothalamic GHRH and somatotropin release–inhibiting factor (SRIF) levels remained unaltered (56). Although the precise mechanism remains unclear in these models, it is speculated that aberrations during the pituitary somatotroph development and GH synthesis were presumably caused by the hypothalamic dysfunction or feedback dysregulation between the hypothalamus and pituitary gland.

Moreover, the direct role of SIRT1 in pituitary somatotroph cells was reported (57). The SIRT1 activation in somatotroph cells suppressed the GHRH-induced GH secretion in *in vivo* and *in vitro* studies. SIRT1 deacetylates glycogen synthase kinase 3 beta (GSK3β) and cAMP response element-binding protein (CREB). Deacetylated-GSK3β gets activated and inactivates CREB via protein phosphatase-1. Deacetylated-CREB exhibits a decrease in its activity and is unable to activate the transcription of POU domain, class 1, transcription factor 1 that results in the GH synthesis impairment (57). These data demonstrate that SIRT1 regulates the somatotropic axis in the hypothalamus and pituitary gland.

During starvation condition, it is well-known that the reduced serum IGF-I level is observed despite the elevated GH level. Moreover, it is reported that exogenous GH treatment did not increase the serum IGF-I level in starving individuals (58). This is considered as GH resistance status in the liver (59). In the organisms, it is considered that GH resistance is an adaptive response to survive during starvation and malnutrition conditions. These responses include the decreased IGF-I level inhibits growth and the elevated GH level causes insulin resistance and free fatty acid mobilization to avoid hypoglycemia. Therefore, we hypothesized that SIRT1 might negatively regulate the GH-dependent IGF-I production during starved condition in the liver. We demonstrated that hepatic SIRT1 directly deacetylates STAT5 and suppresses the tyrosine phosphorylation of STAT5 via GH that results in the impairment of GH signaling during fasting condition (60) (**Figure 1**).

Considering that the somatotropic axis utilizes energy to promote body growth, SIRT1 signaling basically utilizes energy to improve the survival of organisms during CR. Conclusively, SIRT1 plays an important role in switching from growth to survival mode in order to adapt to malnutrition by modulating the somatotropic axis at various steps (**Table 1**D).

CONCLUSION

These studies clearly demonstrated that SIRT1 is involved in the regulatory mechanism of hypothalamus-pituitary axis with respect to the homeostasis maintenance. The determination of a crosstalk between the neuroendocrine system and SIRT1 function is crucial as both of them play an important role in the homeostasis maintenance as well as the regulation of lifespan.

AUTHOR CONTRIBUTIONS

MY drafted the manuscript and MY and YT were responsible for the conception and design of this review.

REFERENCES

1. Klar AJ, Fogel S, Macleod K. MAR1-a Regulator of the HMa and HMalpha Loci in *Saccharomyces cerevisiae. Genetics* (1979) 93:37–50.
2. Baur JA, Ungvari Z, Minor RK, Le Couteur DG, de Cabo R. Are sirtuins viable targets for improving healthspan and lifespan? *Nat Rev Drug Discovery* (2012) 11:443–61. doi: 10.1038/nrd3738
3. Imai S, Armstrong CM, Kaeberlein M, Guarente L. Transcriptional silencing and longevity protein Sir2 is an NAD-dependent histone deacetylase. *Nature* (2000) 403:795–800. doi: 10.1038/35001622
4. Faraone-Mennella MR. A new facet of ADP-ribosylation reactions: SIRTs and PARPs interplay. *Front Biosci.* (2015) 20:458–73. doi: 10.2741/4319

5. Du J, Zhou Y, Su X, Yu JJ, Khan S, Jiang H, et al. Sirt5 is a NAD-dependent protein lysine demalonylase and desuccinylase. *Science* (2011) 334:806–9. doi: 10.1126/science.1207861
6. Peng C, Lu Z, Xie Z, Cheng Z, Chen Y, Tan M, et al. The first identification of lysine malonylation substrates and its regulatory enzyme. *Mol Cell Proteomics* (2011) 10:M111.012658. doi: 10.1074/mcp.M111.012658
7. Guarente L. Calorie restriction and sirtuins revisited. *Genes Dev.* (2013) 27:2072–85. doi: 10.1101/gad.227439.113
8. Serrano L, Martinez-Redondo P, Marazuela-Duque A, Vazquez BN, Dooley SJ, Voigt P, et al. The tumor suppressor SirT2 regulates cell cycle progression and genome stability by modulating the mitotic deposition of H4K20 methylation. *Genes Dev.* (2013) 27:639–53. doi: 10.1101/gad.211342.112
9. Watanabe H, Inaba Y, Kimura K, Matsumoto M, Kaneko S, Kasuga M, et al. Sirt2 facilitates hepatic glucose uptake by deacetylating glucokinase regulatory protein. *Nat Commun.* (2018) 9:30. doi: 10.1038/s41467-017-02537-6
10. Vaquero A, Scher MB, Lee DH, Sutton A, Cheng HL, Alt FW, et al. SirT2 is a histone deacetylase with preference for histone H4 Lys 16 during mitosis. *Genes Dev.* (2006) 20:1256–61. doi: 10.1101/gad.1412706
11. Dryden SC, Nahhas FA, Nowak JE, Goustin AS, Tainsky MA. Role for human SIRT2 NAD-dependent deacetylase activity in control of mitotic exit in the cell cycle. *Mol Cell Biol.* (2003) 23:3173–85. doi: 10.1128/MCB.23.9.3173-3185.2003
12. Liu Y, Dentin R, Chen D, Hedrick S, Ravnskjaer K, Schenk S, et al. A fasting inducible switch modulates gluconeogenesis via activator/coactivator exchange. *Nature* (2008) 456:269–73. doi: 10.1038/nature07349
13. Rodgers JT, Lerin C, Haas W, Gygi SP, Spiegelman BM, Puigserver P. Nutrient control of glucose homeostasis through a complex of PGC 1alpha and SIRT1. *Nature* (2005) 434:113–8. doi: 10.1038/nature03354
14. Nie Y, Erion DM, Yuan Z, Dietrich M, Shulman GI, Horvath TL, et al. STAT3 inhibition of gluconeogenesis is downregulated by SirT1. *Nat Cell Biol.* (2009) 11:492–500. doi: 10.1038/ncb1857
15. Picard F, Kurtev M, Chung N, Topark-Ngarm A, Senawong T, Machado De Oliveira R, et al. Sirt1 promotes fat mobilization in white adipocytes by repressing PPAR-gamma. *Nature* (2004) 429:771–6. doi: 10.1038/nature02583
16. Moynihan KA, Grimm AA, Plueger MM, Bernal-Mizrachi E, Ford E, Cras-Meneur C, et al. Increased dosage of mammalian Sir2 in pancreatic beta cells enhances glucose-stimulated insulin secretion in mice. *Cell Metabol.* (2005) 2:105–17. doi: 10.1016/j.cmet.2005.07.001
17. Suga H. Recapitulating Hypothalamus and Pituitary Development Using Embryonic Stem/Induced Pluripotent Stem Cells. In: Pfaff D, Christen Y, editors. *Stem Cells in Neuroendocrinology.* Cham (CH): Springer. (2016). p. 35–50.
18. Burbridge S, Stewart I, Placzek M. Development of the neuroendocrine hypothalamus. *Comprehens Physiol.* (2016) 6:623–43. doi: 10.1002/cphy.c150023
19. Xie Y, Dorsky RI. Development of the hypothalamus: conservation, modification and innovation. *Development* (2017) 144:1588–99. doi: 10.1242/dev.139055
20. Panzica GC, Viglietti-Panzica C, Balthazart J. The sexually dimorphic medial preoptic nucleus of quail: a key brain area mediating steroid action on male sexual behavior. *Front Neuroendocrinol.* (1996) 17:51–125. doi: 10.1006/frne.1996.0002
21. Morales-Delgado N, Castro-Robles B, Ferran JL, Martinez-de-la-Torre M, Puelles L, Diaz C. Regionalized differentiation of CRH, TRH, and GHRH peptidergic neurons in the mouse hypothalamus. *Brain Struc Funct.* (2014) 219:1083–111. doi: 10.1007/s00429-013-0554-2
22. Morales-Delgado N, Merchan P, Bardet SM, Ferran JL, Puelles L, Diaz C. Topography of somatostatin gene expression relative to molecular progenitor domains during ontogeny of the mouse hypothalamus. *Front Neuroanat.* (2011) 5:10. doi: 10.3389/fnana.2011.00010
23. Swanson LW, Sawchenko PE. Hypothalamic integration: organization of the paraventricular and supraoptic nuclei. *Annu Rev Neurosci.* (1983) 6:269–324. doi: 10.1146/annurev.ne.06.030183.001413
24. Gao Y, Sun T. Molecular regulation of hypothalamic development and physiological functions. *Mol Neurobiol.* (2016) 53:4275–85. doi: 10.1007/s12035-015-9367-z
25. Treier M, Rosenfeld MG. The hypothalamic-pituitary axis: co-development of two organs. *Curr Opin Cell Biol.* (1996) 8:833–43. doi: 10.1016/S0955-0674(96)80085-8
26. Scully KM, Rosenfeld MG. Pituitary development: regulatory codes in mammalian organogenesis. *Science* (2002) 295:2231–5. doi: 10.1126/science.1062736
27. Spanner R. [Physiology of the pituitary portal veins; blood supply of pituitary gland and hypothalamus by the pituitary circulation]. *Klinische Wochenschrift* (1952) 30:721–5. doi: 10.1007/BF01471289
28. Page RB. Pituitary blood flow. *Am J Physiol.* (1982) 243:E427–42.
29. Ramadori G, Fujikawa T, Anderson J, Berglund ED, Frazao R, Michan S, et al. SIRT1 deacetylase in SF1 neurons protects against metabolic imbalance. *Cell Metabol.* (2011) 14:301–12. doi: 10.1016/j.cmet.2011.06.014
30. Ramadori G, Fujikawa T, Fukuda M, Anderson J, Morgan DA, Mostoslavsky R, et al. SIRT1 deacetylase in POMC neurons is required for homeostatic defenses against diet-induced obesity. *Cell Metabol.* (2010) 12:78–87. doi: 10.1016/j.cmet.2010.05.010
31. Sasaki T, Kikuchi O, Shimpuku M, Susanti VY, Yokota-Hashimoto H, Taguchi R, et al. Hypothalamic SIRT1 prevents age-associated weight gain by improving leptin sensitivity in mice. *Diabetologia* (2014) 57:819–31. doi: 10.1007/s00125-013-3140-5
32. Satoh A, Brace CS, Rensing N, Cliften P, Wozniak DF, Herzog ED, et al. Sirt1 extends life span and delays aging in mice through the regulation of Nk2 homeobox 1 in the DMH and LH. *Cell Metabol.* (2013) 18:416–30. doi: 10.1016/j.cmet.2013.07.013
33. Toorie AM, Nillni EA. Minireview: Central Sirt1 regulates energy balance via the melanocortin system and alternate pathways. *Mol Endocrinol.* (2014) 28:1423–34. doi: 10.1210/me.2014-1115
34. Toorie AM, Cyr NE, Steger JS, Beckman R, Farah G, Nillni EA. The nutrient and energy sensor sirt1 regulates the hypothalamic-pituitary-adrenal (HPA) axis by altering the production of the prohormone convertase 2 (PC2) essential in the maturation of Corticotropin-releasing Hormone (CRH) from its prohormone in male rats. *J Biol Chem.* (2016) 291:5844–59. doi: 10.1074/jbc.M115.675264
35. Li D, Dammer EB, Sewer MB. Resveratrol stimulates cortisol biosynthesis by activating SIRT-dependent deacetylation of P450scc. *Endocrinology* (2012) 153:3258–68. doi: 10.1210/en.2011-2088
36. Sam S, Frohman LA. Normal physiology of hypothalamic pituitary regulation. *Endocrinol Metabol Clin North Am.* (2008) 37:1–22, vii. doi: 10.1016/j.ecl.2007.10.007
37. Akieda-Asai S, Zaima N, Ikegami K, Kahyo T, Yao I, Hatanaka T, et al. SIRT1 Regulates thyroid-stimulating hormone release by enhancing PIP5Kgamma activity through deacetylation of specific lysine residues in mammals. *PloS ONE* (2010) 5:e11755. doi: 10.1371/journal.pone.0011755
38. Boily G, Seifert EL, Bevilacqua L, He XH, Sabourin G, Estey C, et al. SirT1 regulates energy metabolism and response to caloric restriction in mice. *PloS ONE* (2008) 3:e1759. doi: 10.1371/journal.pone.0001759
39. Cordeiro A, de Souza LL, Oliveira LS, Faustino LC, Santiago LA, Bloise FF, et al. Thyroid hormone regulation of Sirtuin 1 expression and implications to integrated responses in fasted mice. *J Endocrinol.* (2013) 216:181–93. doi: 10.1530/JOE-12-0420
40. Veldhuis JD, Keenan DM, Liu PY, Iranmanesh A, Takahashi PY, Nehra AX. The aging male hypothalamic-pituitary-gonadal axis: pulsatility and feedback. *Mol Cell Endocrinol.* (2009) 299:14–22. doi: 10.1016/j.mce.2008.09.005
41. Kolthur-Seetharam U, Teerds K, de Rooij DG, Wendling O, McBurney M, Sassone-Corsi P, et al. The histone deacetylase SIRT1 controls male fertility in mice through regulation of hypothalamic-pituitary gonadotropin signaling. *Biol Rep.* (2009) 80:384–91. doi: 10.1095/biolreprod.108.070193
42. Lannes J, L'Hote D, Garrel G, Laverriere JN, Cohen-Tannoudji J, Querat B. Rapid communication: A microRNA-132/212 pathway mediates GnRH activation of FSH expression. *Mol Endocrinol.* (2015) 29:364–72. doi: 10.1210/me.2014-1390
43. Bartke A, Brown-Borg H. Life extension in the dwarf mouse. *Curr Topics Dev Biol.* (2004) 63:189–225. doi: 10.1016/S0070-2153(04)63006-7
44. Holzenberger M, Kappeler L, De Magalhaes Filho C. IGF-1 signaling and aging. *Exp Gerontol.* (2004) 39:1761–4. doi: 10.1016/j.exger.2004.08.017

45. Bartke A, Brown-Borg HM, Bode AM, Carlson J, Hunter WS, Bronson RT. Does growth hormone prevent or accelerate aging? *Exp Gerontol.* (1998) 33:675–87. doi: 10.1016/S0531-5565(98)00032-1
46. Laron Z. Do deficiencies in growth hormone and insulin-like growth factor-1 (IGF-1) shorten or prolong longevity? *Mechan Age Dev.* (2005) 126:305–7. doi: 10.1016/j.mad.2004.08.022
47. Parrella E, Longo VD. Insulin/IGF-I and related signaling pathways regulate aging in nondividing cells: from yeast to the mammalian brain. *Sci World J.* (2010) 10:161–77. doi: 10.1100/tsw.2010.8
48. Barbieri M, Bonafe M, Franceschi C, Paolisso G. Insulin/IGF-I-signaling pathway: an evolutionarily conserved mechanism of longevity from yeast to humans. *Am J Physiol Endocrinol Metabol.* (2003) 285:E1064–71. doi: 10.1152/ajpendo.00296.2003
49. Kenyon C. The plasticity of aging: insights from long-lived mutants. *Cell* (2005) 120:449–60. doi: 10.1016/j.cell.2005.02.002
50. Al-Regaiey KA, Masternak MM, Bonkowski M, Sun L, Bartke A. Long-lived growth hormone receptor knockout mice: interaction of reduced insulin-like growth factor i/insulin signaling and caloric restriction. *Endocrinology* (2005) 146:851–60. doi: 10.1210/en.2004-1120
51. Tissenbaum HA, Guarente L. Increased dosage of a sir-2 gene extends lifespan in Caenorhabditis elegans. *Nature* (2001) 410:227–30. doi: 10.1038/35065638
52. Lemieux ME, Yang X, Jardine K, He X, Jacobsen KX, Staines WA, et al. The Sirt1 deacetylase modulates the insulin-like growth factor signaling pathway in mammals. *Mech Age Dev.* (2005) 126:1097–105. doi: 10.1016/j.mad.2005.04.006
53. Kenyon C, Chang J, Gensch E, Rudner A, Tabtiang R. A *C. elegans* mutant that lives twice as long as wild type. *Nature* (1993) 366:461–4. doi: 10.1038/366461a0
54. Gan L, Han Y, Bastianetto S, Dumont Y, Unterman TG, Quirion R. FoxO-dependent and -independent mechanisms mediate SirT1 effects on IGFBP-1 gene expression. *Biochem Biophys Res Commun.* (2005) 337:1092–6. doi: 10.1016/j.bbrc.2005.09.169
55. Cohen DE, Supinski AM, Bonkowski MS, Donmez G, Guarente LP. Neuronal SIRT1 regulates endocrine and behavioral responses to calorie restriction. *Genes Dev.* (2009) 23:2812–7. doi: 10.1101/gad.1839209
56. Schwer B, Schumacher B, Lombard DB, Xiao C, Kurtev MV, Gao J, et al. Neural sirtuin 6 (Sirt6) ablation attenuates somatic growth and causes obesity. *Proc Natl Acad Sci USA.* (2010) 107:21790–4. doi: 10.1073/pnas.1016306107
57. Monteserin-Garcia J, Al-Massadi O, Seoane LM, Alvarez CV, Shan B, Stalla J, et al. Sirt1 inhibits the transcription factor CREB to regulate pituitary growth hormone synthesis. *FASEB J.* (2013) 27:1561–71. doi: 10.1096/fj.12-220129
58. Merimee TJ, Zapf J, Froesch ER. Insulin-like growth factors in the fed and fasted states. *J Clin Endocrinol Metabol.* (1982) 55:999–1002. doi: 10.1210/jcem-55-5-999
59. Fazeli PK, Klibanski A. Determinants of GH resistance in malnutrition. *J Endocrinol.* (2014) 220:R57–65. doi: 10.1530/JOE-13-0477
60. Yamamoto M, Iguchi G, Fukuoka H, Suda K, Bando H, Takahashi M, et al. SIRT1 regulates adaptive response of the growth hormone–insulin-like growth factor-I axis under fasting conditions in liver. *Proc Natl Acad Sci USA.* (2013) 110:14948–53. doi: 10.1073/pnas.1220606110

17

Anxiety and Cognition in Cre-Collagen Type II Sirt1 K/O Male Mice

Biana Shtaif[1,2], *Shay Henry Hornfeld*[2], *Michal Yackobovitch-Gavan*[1,3], *Moshe Phillip*[1,2,3] *and Galia Gat-Yablonski*[1,2,3*]

[1] *Sackler School of Medicine, Tel Aviv University, Tel Aviv, Israel,* [2] *Laboratory for Molecular Endocrinology and Diabetes, Felsenstein Medical Research Center, Petach Tikva, Israel,* [3] *The Jesse Z and Sara Lea Shafer Institute for Endocrinology and Diabetes, National Center for Childhood Diabetes, Schneider Children's Medical Center of Israel, Petach Tikva, Israel*

Correspondence:
Galia Gat-Yablonski
galiagy@tauex.tau.ac.il

Introduction: Using transgenic collagen type II-specific Sirt1 knockout (CKO) mice we studied the role of Sirt1 in nutritional induced catch up growth (CUG) and we found that these mice have a less organized growth plate and reduced efficiency of CUG. In addition, we noted that they weigh more than control (CTL) mice. Studying the reason for the increased weigh, we found differences in activity and brain function.

Methods: Several tests for behavior and activity were used: open field; elevated plus maze, Morris water maze, and home cage running wheels. The level of Glu- osteocalcin, known to connect bone and brain function, was measured by Elisa; brain Sirt1 was analyzed by western blot.

Results: We found that CKO mice had increased anxiety, with less spatial memory, learning capabilities and reduced activity in their home cages. No significant differences were found between CKO and CTL mice in Glu- osteocalcin levels; nor in the level of brain SIRT1.

Discussion/Conclusion: Using transgenic collagen type II-specific Sirt1 knockout (CKO) mice we found a close connection between linear growth and brain function. Using a collagen type II derived system we affected a central regulatory mechanism leading to hypo activity, increased anxiety, and slower learning, without affecting circadian period. As children with idiopathic short stature are more likely to have lower IQ, with substantial deficits in working memory than healthy controls, the results of the current study suggest that SIRT1 may be the underlying factor connecting growth and brain function.

Keywords: SIRT1, anxiety, cognition, collagen type II, osteocalcin

INTRODUCTION

In order to identify novel regulatory mechanisms in children's growth, we have been focusing on the epiphyseal growth plate (EGP) and the important role of SIRT1 in regulating the nutrition-growth connection was unraveled (1, 2). The sirtuin (SIRT) family of proteins consists of proteins that act predominately as nicotinamide adenine dinucleotide-dependent (NAD+) – deacetylases and convey diverse functions in a variety of physiological settings.

Abbreviations: CKO, collagen type II-specific Sirt1 knockout; CTL, control; Sirt1, sirtuin 1; OC, osteocalcin.

SIRT1, the most conserved enzyme of this family and the most extensively studied, is a central component of numerous basic pathways. The expression and activity of SIRT1 are tightly regulated. SIRT1 is usually localized to the nucleus but may also translocate to the cytosol (3). It interacts and deacetylates histones and non-histone proteins such as p53, E2F1, NF-kB, and FOXO (4, 5) and through them affects cell proliferation, senescence, autophagy, stress responses, and apoptosis. SIRT1 has been shown to have a substantial role in longevity (6), response to food restriction (1, 7), and linear growth (1, 2).

We studied nutritional-induced catch-up growth (CUG) using a model consisting of food restriction followed by refeeding. SIRT1 was among the few proteins that was increased in EGPs of food-restricted rats (2). Additionally, we showed that miR-140 and miR-22 were reduced at the EGP by food restriction, and their mutual target, SIRT1, showed a subsequent increase (1). Next, we knocked out Sirt1 expression using a collagen-type II-specific Cre-Lox system (2), and investigated its role in nutrition-induced CUG.

Depletion of SIRT1 by using the collagen-II-specific Cre-Lox system led to increased height of the proliferative zone with less organized EGP. The CKO mice were less responsive to the nutritional manipulation, and their CUG was less efficient. They remained shorter than the CTL mice who corrected the food restriction-induced growth deficit during the re-feeding period. In addition, we identified a crucial role of SIRT1 in the response of the cortical and trabecular bone fractions to nutritional manipulation. Furthermore, there was a significant effect on animal weight, with the knockout mice being heavier than their control littermates. The difference in weight was more pronounced with age. Others showed that Sirt1+/− mice presented with early onset, moderate osteoarthritis relative to their wild type littermates (8). Therefore, we hypothesized that, as our model is cartilage specific, it may also affects articular cartilage and thus mobility. This led us to monitor the locomotor activity of the knockout mice in the open field, and thereafter to perform additional tests to examine effects on anxiety and spatial memory.

MATERIALS AND METHODS

Animals

All the procedures and experiments were according to the Arrive guidelines (https://arriveguidelines.org) and approved by the Institutional Animal Care and Use Committee of Tel Aviv University, that follows the NIH guide for the care and use of laboratory animals (protocol approval number 01-16-052) prior to onset of the study. As most mice homozygous for the Sirt1-null allele do not survive for more than 1 month, we used the Cre-loxP system to knockout cartilage-specific Sirt1. Previous studies showed that crossing this floxed allele to a whole-body Cre-expressing mouse recapitulated the Sirt1-null phenotype (9). Sirt1-CKO (referred to throughout the manuscript as CKO) mice were generated as previously described (2); Col II-Cre-recombinase removes exon 4 of the floxed Sirt1 gene (encoding a catalytic domain of the protein) specifically in chondrocytes (2, 9). All mice were genotyped at the age of three weeks from tail snips (2). Male mice were chosen to eliminate the confounding factor of sex on linear growth. CKO mice were obtained at the expected Mendelian ratio, survived normally, and mated successfully. Sirt1 flox/flox littermate mice without the Cre transgene were used as controls (CTL). Mice were maintained under pathogen-free conditions (temperature controlled to 25 ± 1°C, humidity 50 ± 2%, 12h light/dark cycle (apart from the circadian rhythm study); lights off at 18:00h) and allowed free access to food (2018SC; Teklad Rodent Diet, Envigo, Madison, WI, USA) and tap water. The CKO and CTL mice showed no differences in size and weight at birth and no significant postnatal growth retardation. Mice were designated "young" when age was 4-8 months and "old" when age was >8-11 months.

The Open Field Test

In the open field test (OFT) mice were placed in a 47×47×51 cm arena for 30 min (CKO, n=37; CTL, n=32; **Table 1**). The total distance travelled and the duration of time exploring the periphery and the center of the arena were video-tracked under normal light conditions for 30 min using the EthoVision XT 11.5 software (EthoVision 3.1 Noldus Information Technology B.V., Wageningen, The Netherlands). Data was used to measure locomotor activity and to explore features indicative of greater anxiety-like behavior and decreased exploratory activity (10).

The Elevated Plus Maze Test

The elevated plus maze (EPM) test consists of two open arms (25 × 5 cm, with 3-mm-high ledges) and two closed arms (25 × 5 cm, with 15-cm-high transparent walls) of the same size. The arms of the same type were arranged at opposite sides; all the arms and central squares were made of white plastic plates and elevated above the floor. Each mouse was placed in the central square of the maze (5 × 5 cm), facing one of the closed arms, and was recorded for 6 min (CKO, n=15; CTL, n=15; **Table 2**). Time spent in the closed or open arms or in the center (seconds), the proportion of time spent in open or closed arms (% time), the distance traveled (cm), and the number of total entries into the arms were calculated automatically by the EthoVision software. EPM is a behavioral test widely employed to assess anxiety-like behaviors in mice, relying on the aversion of rodents to open spaces (11).

Morris Water Maze Test

Spatial learning and memory were measured using the Morris water maze test (MWM) in a circular water pool (diameter – 1.2 m) filled with water (22 ± 1oC). The water maze was divided into four quadrants according to the '+' shape; and a transparent platform was placed in the center of the 1st quadrant. The mice entered the water from the middle of the 1st, 2nd, 3rd and 4th quadrants, and the escape latency was recorded, namely the time from searching the platform to climbing the platform (CKO, n=15; CTL, n=15). If a platform was not found within 60 sec, the mouse was placed on the platform for 20 sec and then removed from the water maze, and the time was recorded as 60 sec. Each mouse was trained 4 times daily, and the mean time was

TABLE 1 | Comparison between CKO mice and CTL mice in the Open Field test (OFT) according to age group (data is presented as mean ± SD).

	All	Young (<9 months)	Old (≥9 months)	Within group (P1)
Table 1A (Open Field)				
N (number of measurements)				
CKO	37	22	15	
CTL	32	22	10	
Total distance (cm)				
CKO	8468.9±2530.3	9103.5±2437.6	7487.0±2531.3	0.064
CTL	3824.1±891.2	4002.7±928.8	3437.4±692.0	0.097
Between groups (P2)	<0.001	<0.001	<0.001	
Periphery (cm)				
CKO	5670.3±1655.3	5893.0±1612.7	5305.9±1776.8	0.313
CTL	2407.4±713.5	2633.6±717.7	1909.8±389.3	0.006
Between groups (P2)	<0.001	<0.001	<0.001	
Center (cm)				
CKO	2791.0±1257.4	3205.9±1307.7	2173.2±946.5	0.015
CTL	1406.4±608.1	1351.6±671.8	1527.0±444.2	0.459
Between groups (P2)	<0.001	<0.001	0.037	
Periphery (% of time)				
CKO	76.1±9.0	74.5±8.3	77.9±10.1	0.294
CTL	68.0±14.3	71.8±14.5	60.2±10.5	0.032
Between groups (P2)	0.010	0.455	<0.001	
Center (% of time)				
CKO	23.8±9.0	25.4±8.3	21.9±10.1	0.279
CTL	31.9±14.3	28.2±14.5	39.8±10.6	
Between groups (P2)	0.009	0.457	<0.001	0.032
Table 1B: (Open Field)				
N (number of measurements)				
CKO	37	22	15	
CTL	32	22	10	
Total distance (cm)				
CKO	19832.3±6407.2	22077.7±6370.5	16539.1±4998.0	0.008
CTL	8896.1±2022.3	9384.3±2040.7	7790.1±1558.5	0.036
Between groups (P2)	<0.001	<0.001	0.002	
Periphery (cm)				
CKO	13526.6±4215.1	14877.0±4152.0	11545.9±3571.9	0.016
CTL	5762.4±1579.2	6226.3±1563.9	4742.0±1095.8	0.011
Between groups (P2)	<0.001	<0.001	<0.001	
Center (cm)				
CKO	6286.4±2714.7	7176.2±2953.2	4981.4±1673.4	0.014
CTL	3100.1±1158.0	3124.9±1308.6	3045.5±786.6	0.861
Between groups (P2)	<0.001	<0.001	0.002	
Periphery (% of time)				
CKO	74.9±11.4	74.0±13.7	76.3±7.06	0.557
CTL	68.2±14.5	69.9±15.7	64.4±13.1	0.348
Between groups (P2)	0.041	0.354	0.007	
Center (% of time)				
CKO	24.9±11.4	26.0±13.7	23.5±7.07	0.531
CTL	31.8±14.9	30.1±15.7	35.5±13.0	0.351
Between groups (P2)	0.039	0.356	0.006	

(A)- at 10 minutes; (B)- at 30 minutes. P1- represents independent samples T Test analysis comparing young and old animals in each group. P2– represents T Test analysis comparing CKO vs CTL.

calculated. The experiment was conducted for 6 consecutive days. A place navigation test was performed in the first 3 days, a space exploration test on the 4th day, and a reversal phase test on the 5-6th day. Space exploration was performed when the platform in the 1st quadrant was removed, and the mice entered the water from the middle of the 2nd quadrant. The traversing times, within 60 sec, across the target quadrant (i.e., the 1st quadrant) and the swimming time were recorded. During the reversal phase, the platform was moved to another quarter of the maze and the time was recorded to reach the platform. Data were recorded using the automated EthoVision tracking system. The test assesses the ability of the animals to locate the underwater hidden platform, using surrounding visual cues; and is thus used to explore spatial memory and learning.

Voluntary Wheel Running

Mice were allowed to run freely on the open surface of a slanted plastic saucer-shaped wheel [Low-Profile Wireless Running Wheel (Med Associates, Fairfax, USA) for mouse (15.25 × 10.25 × 3.3 cm)] placed inside the mouse cage, within routine daily rhythmicity patterns in a non-stressed laboratory environment (CKO, n=15; CTL, n=14). Rotations were

TABLE 2 | Comparison between CKO and CTL animals in the Elevated Plus Maze (EPM) test according to age group (data is presented as mean±SD).

	All	Young (<9 months)	Old (≥9 months)	Within group (P1)
Table 2 (EPM test)				
N (number of mice)				
CKO	15	8	7	
CTL	15	8	7	
Total distance (cm)				
CKO	1555.5±333.4	1596.1±297.4	1509.1±389.1	0.632
CTL	1153.1±224.0	1253.4±64.2	1038.4±289.0	0.098
Between groups (P2)	0.001	0.014	0.025	
Open arms (cm)				
CKO	231.6±145.6	199.1±137.0	268.7±156.7	0.375
CTL	285.1±135.0	341.9±93.6	220.2±151.9	0.080
Between groups (P2)	0.306	0.029	0.567	
Open arms (% of time)				
CKO	15.8±8.4	14.3±7.5	17.6±9.5	0.463
CTL	24.6±10.2	29.6±7.9	18.9±9.8	0.035
Between groups (P2)	0.016	0.001	0.815	
Closed arms (cm)				
CKO	921.8±297.6	999.7±284.5	832.7±307.9	0.295
CTL	608.7±146.8	658.2±118.3	552.1±164.1	0.171
Between groups (P2)	0.002	0.007	0.055	
Closed arms (% of time)				
CKO	49.5±16.9	53.8±18.0	44.6±15.3	0.310
CTL	49.3±12.7	48.1±11.5	50.7±14.8	0.706
Between groups (P2)	0.974	0.463	0.462	
Center (cm)				
CKO	402.1±105.2	397.2±125.3	407.6±86.2	0.856
CTL	259.3±69.9	253.3±56.8	266.1±86.7	0.739
Between groups (P2)	<0.001	0.015	0.010	
Center (% of time)				
CKO	34.7±13.7	31.9±14.1	37.8±13.5	0.426
CTL	26.1±8.0	22.3±5.8	30.4±8.3	0.044
Between groups (P2)	0.048	0.096	0.243	
Entries –closed arms (n)				
CKO	34.9±12.3	37.8±9.8	31.7±14.8	0.362
CTL	20.6±3.2	20.9±3.5	20.3±3.1	0.736
Between groups (P2)	<0.001	0.001	0.088	
Entries –center (n)				
CKO	49.6±11.8	51.4±9.8	47.6±14.2	0.552
CTL	33.5±5.3	34.4±3.1	32.6±7.2	0.555
Between groups (P2)	<0.001	0.001	0.028	
Entries –open arms (n)				
CKO	19.6±8.0	20.6±9.5	18.4±6.3	0.614
CTL	14.7±4.6	14.9±1.6	14.4±6.7	0.869
Between groups (P2)	0.050	0.135	0.273	

P1- represents independent samples T Test analysis comparing young and old animals in each group. P2- represents T Test analysis comparing CKO vs CTL.

electronically transmitted to a USB hub (DIG-804 USB interface hub), such that the frequency and rate of running could be captured. Mice were individually housed so that accurate recordings could be made for each animal. The hourly sum of wheel revolutions (wheel spins) was collected by SOF-860-wheel manager software (Med Associates, Georgia, USA). Data were collected 6 days, 24 h a day (12, 13). The pattern of running during day (light time; L) and night (dark time; D) was analyzed and used to measure voluntary activity.

Serum Analysis of Uncarboxylated Osteocalcin (Glu- Osteocalcin)

Uncarboxylated osteocalcin (GluOC) was measured, since previous work showed that it may connect bone and brain function, especially anxiety (14). Serum samples (CKO, n=26; CTL, n=22) were analyzed using an Elisa kit (Cat # MK129; Takara, Japan) according to the manufacturers' instructions (detection limits=0.25ng/ml).

Western Blot Analysis of SIRT1

Brains of CKO and CTL mice were homogenized in a lysis buffer (200mM HEPES, 5mM EDTA, 150mM NaCl, 1% NP-40, 0.5% Na-deoxycholate), which was supplemented with a protease inhibitor cocktail (Roche, Basel, Switzerland) in a 1:12 ratio and phosphatase inhibitor cocktail (Roche, Basel, Switzerland) in a 1:12 ratio and phosphatase inhibitor cocktail (Roche, Basel, Switzerland) in a 1:10 ratio. Protein concentration was determined using the Pierce BCA Protein Assay Kit (Thermo Scientific, IL, USA), and 100μg proteins were analyzed per sample by sodium dodecyl sulfate (SDS)-polyacrylamide gel electrophoresis (PAGE), followed by western immunoblotting. Proteins were transferred to nitrocellulose membranes (GE Healthcare, NJ, USA) by the wet blotting system (Bio-Rad, Hercules, CA, USA). Nitrocellulose membranes were then incubated in TBS-T (10mM Tris-HCl, 150mM NaCl, 0.1% Tween 20) with 5% skim milk solution for one hour to block nonspecific binding, and then incubated with the primary antibody (anti Sirt1- Millipore Cat #07-131) overnight at 4°C. Membranes were washed with TBS-T, incubated with a secondary fluorescent antibody (LI-COR Biosciences, Lincoln, NE, USA) decorated with IRDye® for one hour and washed again. Alpha-Tubulin (Cat#2144 Cell Signaling) served as the reference. Quantification was performed using the Odyssey (2.1.) application Software (LI-COR Biosciences, Lincoln, NE, USA)

Statistical Analysis

2.8.1 A mixed-model repeated-measures analysis was conducted to compare the effect of group (CTL vs. CKO) on weight during the study period. This analysis enabled using all the available data from the full sample of randomized animals, without imputing missing values. The model was specified with a between-group factor (CTL vs. CKO), a within-group factor of time, and group x time interaction. For this analysis, data are expressed as estimated marginal means and standard error.

2.8.2 For the between group comparison of the behavioral test results (OFT, EPM, MWM), independent sample T-tests were conducted.

2.8.3 For the MWM test analyses, a Cox regression analysis was used to evaluate the effects of the group (CKO vs. CTL) and the animal age on the time until test success for each of the experiment days.

2.8.4 For the running wheels test, area under the curve (AUC) was calculated for each period of time and compared between the groups using Independent Samples Mann Whitney U tests (due to skewed distribution of the AUC).

2.8.5 Data were generated and analyzed with SPSS software, version 25.0 (IBM). Differences were considered statistically significant at $P<0.05$.

RESULTS

3.1. Effect on body weight: CKO mice were generally heavier (**Supplementary Figure 1**), with no significant differences in food consumption (average food consumption 3.68 ± 0.04 gr/day for the CTL mice and 3.56 ± 0.3 gr/day for the CKO mice; $p=0.27$). At the age of 21 days, no significant differences in weight were noted, however, there was a significant difference in the change over time between the CKO and CTL mice ($\beta=0.03$, $SE=0.01$, $P=0.006$), with a greater increase in weight gain in the CKO group [CTL group: y (weight) =14.92+0.16X (time); CKO group: y=14.08+0.19X] (2). We did not notice differences between the groups in behavior when they were in their home cages, either housed in small groups or in solitary cages (2).

3.2. Open field test (OFT) - using the OFT, no differences in gait were observed, however, there were significant differences in the number of steps (i.e. distance travelled). The results are presented in **Table 1** and **Figure 1** the first 10 minutes are

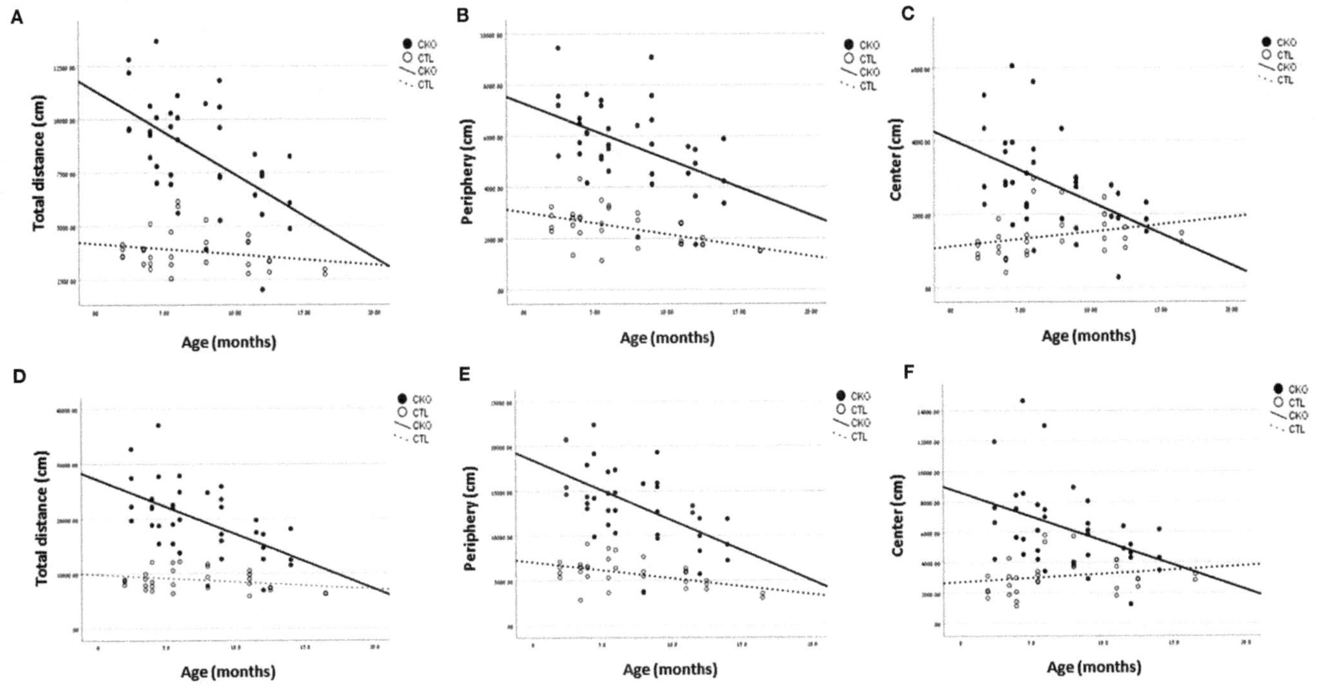

FIGURE 1 | Results of the open field test (OFT). Graphs showing, for each of the groups (CKO and CTL), correlations between the animal age and **(A, D)** The total distance covered, **(B, E)** distance travelled in peripheral zone, **(C, F)** distance travelled in central zone. **(A–C)**- 10 minutes; **(D–F)** 30 minutes.

presented in **Table 1A** and **Figures 1A–C**; results of the whole test (30 min.) are presented in **Table 1B** and **Figures 1D–F**. The distance covered by the CKO mice was substantially greater than that covered by the CTL mice, in both the first 10 minutes and when calculated for the whole duration of the test (in both P<0.001) (**Table 1**). While the effect of age was not significant in the first 10 minutes, the distance travelled during the whole period of the test (30 min.) decreased with age, in both CKO and CTL mice. Even though the distance was reduced with increased age of the CKO mice it was still significantly greater than in the CTL group (young CKO vs young CTL; Old CKO vs Old CTL, P<0.005 for both) (**Table 1**). CKO mice spent more time in the periphery and less in the center compared to CTL mice (p<0.05). To examine if greater anxiety might explain these differences, we performed a test that is more specific for anxiety assessment, the elevated plus maze test.

3.3. The elevated plus maze (EPM)- In the EPM test (**Table 2** and **Figure 2**), the CKO mice covered a significantly greater distance than did the CTL mice (P<0.001); the difference was significant for both younger (P=0.014) and older mice (P=0.025) (**Figure 2A**). The time spent in the open arms was significantly less in young CKO than in young CTL (P=0.001). However, the time was similar in the older age group (P=0.815). This was evident by less time spent in the open arms among older than younger CTL mice (P=0.035), yet no such difference by age was observed among the CKO mice (**Figure 2B**). The number of entries into all the sections of the maze were greater for CKO than CTL mice (P ≤ 0.05). This indicates that the CKO mice were moving about quickly, although differences from the CTL were statistically significant only in entries by younger CKO mice into the closed arms and the center (P=0.001), and in entries of older CKO mice into the center (P=0.028). Taken together, these results support the greater anxiety of CKO mice that was demonstrated in the OFT.

3.4. Morris water maze. We next compared spatial memory and learning abilities of CKO to CTL mice using the Morris water maze (**Figure 3** and **Table 3**). The study was conducted for six consecutive days. Both groups showed improved learning with time, and on the third day, all the animals (from both groups) reached the platform rapidly, with no significant differences between the groups. In the first three days an improvement was noted for both CKO and CTL mice, however, CKO mice were slower in finding the platform on the first (P=0.076) and second (P=0.014) days. Comprehensive Cox regression analysis for the first 3 days (**Table 3**) supported these results. No differences were observed between the CKO and CTL mice in the space exploration and the reversal phase tests (days 4-6; data not shown).

3.5. Free running wheels. Wheel running in the home cages was used to assess voluntary activity in contrast to other experimental platforms that we used. After mice were allowed to accustom to the free running wheels, their running activity was recorded. Both the CKO and CTL groups used the wheels mostly during the active dark period (**Figures 4A–C**). The young mice showed significantly greater activity than the older mice in both groups (P<0.001), both in the night and the day (**Figure 4C**). However, contrasting with the results of the OFT and the EPM, young CKO mice showed significantly reduced activity compared to the CTL mice (P=0.001) (**Figures 4A–D**). No differences in circadian period were observed (CTL 24.4 hours ± 0.88, CKO 24.0 ± 1.48; P=0.5).

3.6. Osteocalcin levels: Uncarboxylated osteocalcin (GluOC) was measured, since previous work showed that it may connect bone and brain function, especially anxiety (14). Levels of GluOC tended to be higher in the young CKO mice than in the young CTL mice, but the difference in magnitude was small (CKO 16.4 ± 1.3 ng/ml, CTL 15.0 ± 0.7 ng/ml; P=0.06). Levels were significantly reduced with age in both groups; differences between the CKO and CTL mice at age 3 months or older were not statistically significant.

3.7. Levels of* SIRT1 *in the brains of CKO and CTL mice were visualized using a western blot analysis, as several studies in mouse embryogenesis (9, 15–17), showed transient expression of Col type II mRNAs in the brain. No gross difference in the total amount of SIRT1 protein was observed. Three bands with apparent molecular weight of 100-130 kDa were observed per lane, a pattern that is commonly seen in samples taken from cytosols or whole cells, compared to a single band of 110 kDa

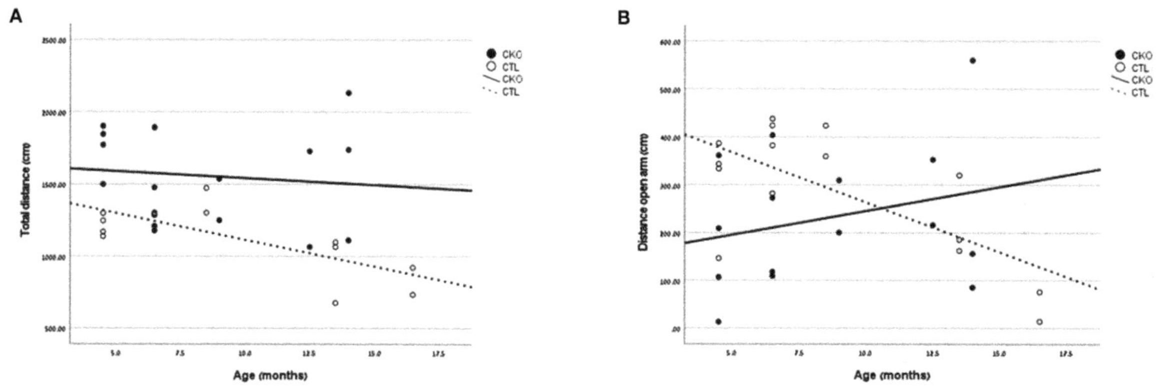

FIGURE 2 | Results of the elevated Plus Maze. Graphs showing, for each of the groups (CKO and CTL), correlations between the animal age and **(A)** total distance covered (cm) or **(B)** distance covered in the open arms (cm).

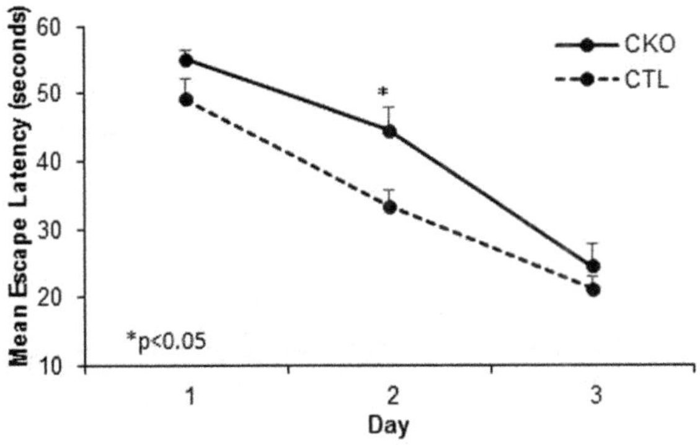

FIGURE 3 | Results of the Morris water maze (MWM). Cumulative escape latency in all 3 days comparing CKO and CTL mice. Data are presented as mean ± SD, *P < 0.05.

detected in nuclear extracts (18). In extracts derived from the CTL mice, the pattern was identical to that of a control mouse (C57Bl/6, which are the most widely used genetic background for genetically modified mice). In contrast, the relative distributions of the various bands differed substantially between the CKO and CTL mice; with the intermediate band more pronounced in extracts of CKO compared to CTL (**Figure 5**).

DISCUSSION

In this study, we found that Sirt1 knockout (CKO) mice have reduced activity, increased anxiety and decreased spatial learning and memory, compared to CTL mice. In a previous study (8), we found that the transgenic CKO mice had shorter bones with less organized EGP, had increased weight, reduced bone mineralization and were less responsive to the nutritional manipulation, with less efficient CUG.

While no gross effect was found in their gait, the CKO mice covered a significantly greater distance than the CTL mice in both the OF (19) and EPM tests (20, 21), and spent relatively more time in the sheltered areas of the arena or the maze, respectively. Increased levels of anxiety usually lead to less locomotion and decreased exploratory behavior with a

TABLE 3 | Multivariable Cox regression analysis for the MWM tests (time to platform) during the first three days.

Groups	Day	Point Estimate	95% Confidence Limits	Z Value	P
Table 3 (MWM test)					
CKO *vs* CTL	1	0.526	0.146-1.90	-0.98	0.327
CKO *vs* CTL	2	0.139	0.040-0.486	-3.09	<0.002
CKO *vs* CTL	3	0.577	0.177-1.884	-0.91	0.362
CKO	1 *vs* 2	0.223	0.085-0.584	-3.05	0.0023
CKO	2 *vs* 3	0.050	0.018-0.139	-5.74	<0.0001
CKO	1 *vs* 3	0.011	0.003-0.036	-7.51	<0.0001
CTL	1 *vs* 2	0.059	0.021-0.161	-5.50	<0.0001
CTL	2 *vs* 3	0.207	0.087-0.491	-3.57	0.0004
CTL	1 *vs* 3	0.012	0.004-0.040	-7.23	<0.0001
CKO young	1 *vs* 2	0.188	0.049-0.727	-2.42	0.015
CKO young	2 *vs* 3	0.019	0.005-0.077	-5.52	<0.0001
CKO young	1 *vs* 3	0.004	0.001-0.018	-6.8	<0.0001
CTL young	1 *vs* 2	0.06	0.017-0.218	-4.28	<0.0001
CTL young	2 *vs* 3	0.221	0.068-0.721	-2.5	0.0123
CTL young	1 *vs* 3	0.013	0.003-0.06	-5.6	<0.0001
CKO old	1 *vs* 2	0.174	0.042-0.714	-2.43	0.0152
CKO old	2 *vs* 3	0.086	0.022-0.333	-3.55	0.0004
CKO old	1 *vs* 3	0.015	0.003-0.066	-5.52	<0.0001
CTL old	1 *vs* 2	0.035	0.008-0.146	-4.60	<0.0001
CTL old	2 *vs* 3	0.161	0.049-0.534	-2.99	0.0028
CTL old	1 *vs* 3	0.006	0.001-0.028	-6.32	<0.0001
CKO young *vs* CKO old	1	1.61	0.225-11.497	0.47	0.635
CKO young *vs* CKO old	2	1.745	0.268-11.364	0.58	0.56
CKO young *vs* CKO old	3	0.378	0.062-2.309	-1.05	0.292
CTL young *vs* CTL old	1	0.644	0.092-4.483	-0.44	0.6566
CTL young *vs* CTL old	2	1.106	0.194-6.306	0.11	0.9093
CTL young *vs* CTL old	3	1.513	0.252-9.092	0.45	0.651
CKO young *vs* CTL young	1	0.303	0.044-2.079	-1.22	0.2242
CKO young *vs* CTL young	2	0.097	0.016-0.593	-2.53	0.0115
CKO young *vs* CTL young	3	1.15	0.20-6.614	0.16	0.875
CKO old *vs* CTL old	1	0.757	0.103-5.554	-0.27	0.7841
CKO old *vs* CTL old	2	0.153	0.022-1.045	-1.92	0.0555
CKO old *vs* CTL old	3	0.288	0.044-1.87	-1.3	0.192

CKO, collagen type II-specific Sirt1 knockout mice; CTL, Sirt1 flox/flox control mice without the Cre transgene.
These analyses clearly show that there is a significant difference between the groups on day 2 of the MWM, while no significant difference is found between young and old mice in both groups.

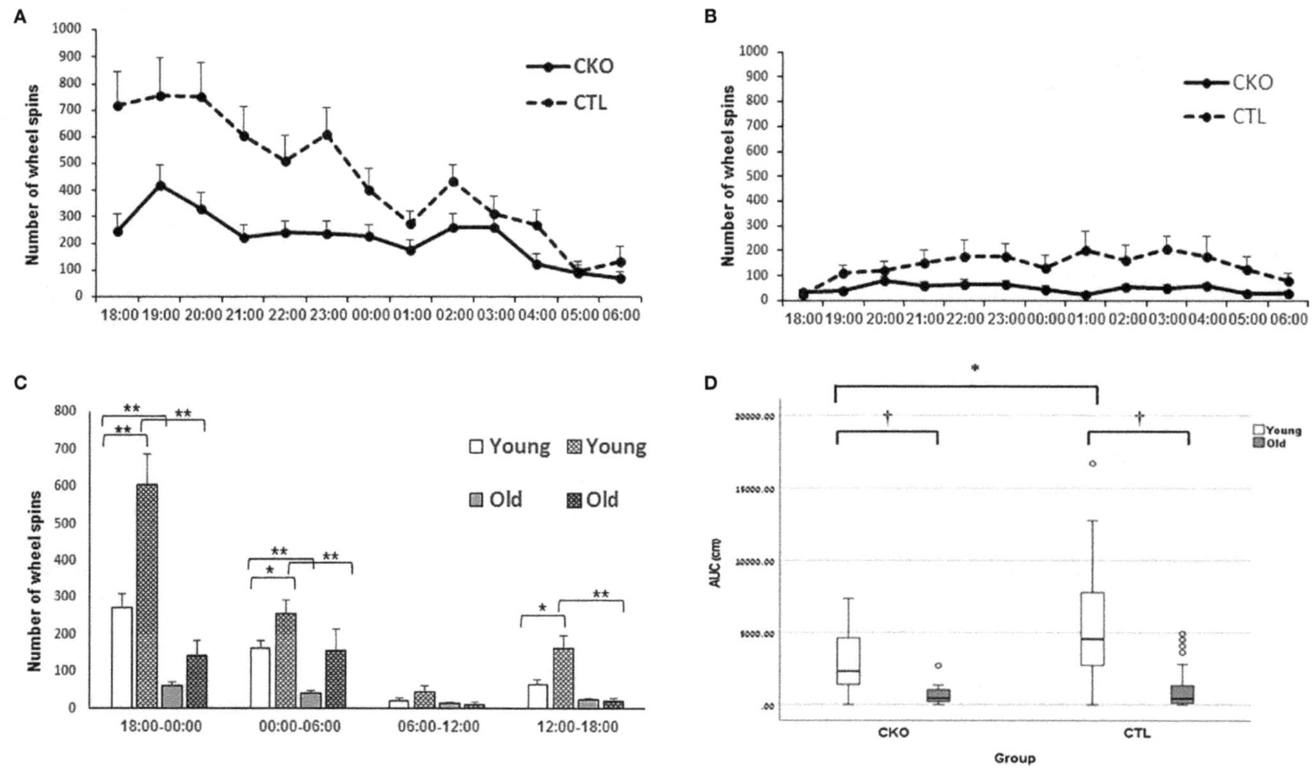

FIGURE 4 | Results of the free running wheels. The average sum of hourly wheel revolutions (wheel spins) of **(A)** young and **(B)** old mice old during the night cycle. **(C)** Hourly sum of wheel revolution according to 6 hours interval during the day and night (*$p < 0.05$; **$p = 0.001$). **(D)** AUC analysis of the hourly sum of wheel spins of the active period (night) presented in **A** and **B** (*$p < 0.05$; †< 0.01).

preference to stay close to the walls of the field; while in this case the animals showed increased activity with decreased exploratory behavior. In contrast to the increased activity in the above-mentioned tests, the use of home cage running wheels showed reduced activity. This indicates that the increased locomotion activity of the CKO mice in the OF and the EPM tests was due to increased anxiety, and the increased body weight we noted at the initiation of this research can be attributed to a lower level of activity in the home cage. Slower learning revealed by the MWM, was evident during the first two days of the tests (especially on the second day). Data from the home cage running wheels and from circadian rhythm analysis indicated that there was no significant difference between the groups in the circadian period, this is in contrast to the brain-specific SIRT1 knockout mice (BSKO) (22, 23) that showed elongated circadian period (24–26).

Compared to younger mice, older CTL tended to be less cautious in the OFT, exploring more willingly the center of the arena, consistent with previous reports of mice of a similar genetic background, C57BL/6J (27, 28); no such effect was observed for old CKO mice. On EPM, maybe due to the shorter duration of the test, there was no significant effect of

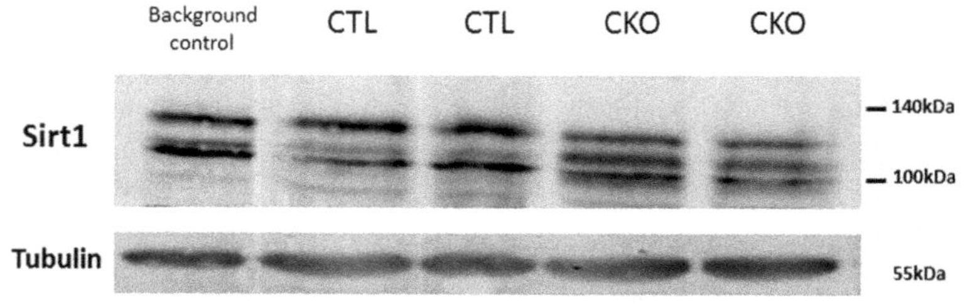

FIGURE 5 | Results of the western blot analysis of SIRT1. Significant differences in the pattern of SIRT1 in protein extracts derived from brains of C57BL mice (background control), CTL mice, CKO mice. The relative distribution of the different forms, in extracts derived from CTL mice is identical to that of other control mice (C57BL) and different from that of CKO mice.

age on the total distance traveled in both groups. However, old CTL spent more time in the center compared to young CTL ($P=0.044$), concomitant with a reduction in the % of time spent in the open arms ($p=0.035$), and similarly to the OFT, no such effect was noted in the CKO mice.

Taken together, our results indicate that the CKO mice entailed disruption in a central control mechanism that affects activity, anxiety and cognition. Since we used a common system of Cre/Col II, expected to be specific for cartilage, the explanation for the effect on cognitive function and behavior was elusive. An extensive review of the literature suggests several possible explanations.

One is that the knockout of SIRT1 from EGP cartilage, which affected bone mineralization and maturation (2), affected the level of osteocalcin (OC) and its un-carboxylated form (GluOC); the latter was shown to serve as a link between bone and brain function, especially anxiety (14). OC is expressed and secreted by osteoblasts, hypertrophic chondrocytes, and adipocytes (29), and is the most abundant non-collagenous protein in bone. OC was found to be involved in multiple physiological processes such as energy metabolism, adipogenesis, neuronal development, muscle growth, and male fertility (30). Despite the important role of OC in bone mineralization and calcium ion homeostasis, OC –/– mice showed only moderately increased bone mass (31). Interestingly, however, these mice showed unexpectedly increased anxiety (31). OC was later found to regulate proper brain development and function, and OC–/– mice had smaller and less developed brains. The mature OC is post-translationally modified on three glutamate residues; a process that increases the affinity of OC for hydroxyapatite crystal; thus, most secreted OC is embedded in the bone matrix. The acidic environment generated during bone resorption promotes decarboxylation of OC to GluOC, decreasing its affinity and promoting its release into the circulation. GluOC crosses the blood brain barrier, directly preventing anxiety and depressive behavior while also strengthening spatial learning and memory. Therefore, if GluOC activity would explain the findings of the current study, we would have expected to see lower levels of GluOC in the serum of CKO mice. Serum analysis showed that the levels of GluOC were significantly reduced with age in both groups as also reported by others (32), however, we found a small increase in GluOC levels in CKO mice, which tended to be significant only in young animals. This may be associated with the reduced bone mineralization in CKO mice (2). In addition, our mice mated and reproduced normally, with no difference between the groups, also supporting the finding that GluOC levels were comparable between the groups (30). Our findings contrast with a publication that reported an inverse association between GluOC and body weight (33). We therefore conclude that GluOC does not explain the increased anxiety and lower cognitive function in the CKO mice.

Another plausible explanation is that the Cre-Col II system affected brain SIRT1, as effects similar to those we see in learning, memory and anxiety were previously reported in brain-specific SIRT1 knockout mice (BSKO) (22, 23), this is in spite of the fact that the driver that we used for Cre was Col type II and not nestin (34). Indeed, a recent review summarized the off-target effect of many skeletal Cre lines, showing that most Cre lines show some level of unintended activity in other tissues (35), thus the notion that Cre lines are specific to a particular cell or tissue has been misleading. While collagen type II is usually considered a hallmark for chondrogenic differentiation, several publications on mouse embryogenesis (9, 15–17), as well as a study on the Cre Col II system (36) showed transient expression of Col type II mRNAs in a number of non-chondrogenic tissues such as notochord, sclerotome, pre-chondrogenic mesenchyme, heart, brain and eye. This transient expression (16), is suggested to have an important role in the proper development of all brain structures (17). The early expression of the collagen type II gene in the neuroepithelium at 9.5 days coincides with the period of extensive morphogenesis of the neural tube (15).

In BSKO it was shown that loss of function of SIRT1 impairs synaptic plasticity, memory formation and spatial learning, probably *via* a microRNA-mediated mechanism (22). SIRT1 has been suggested as a component of the molecular pathways that determine the fate of neuronal progenitor cells (37). Analysis of SIRT1 in the brain has shown that *Sirt1* mRNA is highly expressed in metabolically relevant sites, including, the hypothalamic arcuate, and some areas in the hindbrain (38). In addition, it was suggested that SIRT1 regulates anxiety by the de-acetylation of a transcription factor regulating the monoamine oxidase A gene in the brain, which is involved in oxidative deamination of dopamine, norepinephrine, and serotonin (39). Furthermore, in the same model, SIRT1 was shown to be involved in regulating the circadian rhythm (25).

There is a significant overlap between the expression of SIRT1 and sites of embryonic expression of collagen type II. However, western blot analysis of brain SIRT1 did not show the expected reduction in Sirt1 protein level, unlike the reduction shown in cartilage (2); in contrast, we found a significant difference in the pattern of SIRT1 forms. This may indicate changes in post-translational modifications, such as phosphorylation, as SIRT1 is known to be phosphorylated on numerous sites (40). Phosphorylation can increase its nuclear deacetylase activity (41, 42), and may also induce SIRT1 ubiquitination and proteasomal degradation (41).

It is important to note that there are several discrepancies between our findings and those of BSKO. For example, while it was reported that hypothalamic SIRT1 is crucially important for the central regulation of food intake (43), in our mice there was no difference in food consumption.

Furthermore, CKO mice showed hypo-activity when in their home cage, while brain POMC- SIRT1 k/o showed unaltered levels of activities (44). BSKO mice were reported to be dwarf (34), had reduced GH secretion, and reduced body weight and length at 10 weeks while in our study, CKO mice did not show gross growth inhibition; in contrast, their body weight was increased. In addition, BSKO mice were reported to have elongated circadian period, while the CKO and CTL show similar circadian period (26, 45–47)

Overall, it is still not clear what are the underlying causes for the differential behavior of the CKO mice. Some of the behavioral presentation of the CKO mice are reminiscent of Attention

Deficient Hyperactive Disorder (ADHD), in their reduced sensory regulation. Interestingly, a recent publication on children with ADHD showed significantly lower SIRT1 levels and significantly higher metalloproteinase-9 (MMP-9) levels in the serum (48). MMP-9, an endopeptidases involved in degradation of the extracellular matrix, is negatively regulated by SIRT1; MMP-9 and SIRT1 both act in the EGP and the brain and are important for brain development, synaptic plasticity, learning and memory (49). Their presence in the serum may suggest another link between EGP and brain.

Two thirds of the genetic syndromes with short stature as a feature listed in the genetics database, POSSUM (https://www.possum.net.au/) are associated with intellectual disability. Furthermore, more children with idiopathic short stature (ISS) were shown to have a lower IQ, lower fluid and quantitative reasoning, and substantial deficits in the visual-motor skills and working memory than healthy controls (50).

One possible explanation for lower test scores in intelligence and academic achievement tests in children with ISS might be an underlying condition that has caused both short stature and cognitive impairment, such as a genetic cause, malnutrition, improper psychosocial environment, the presence of general diseases and specific hormonal deficits. The influence of the environmental factors may be intertwined, making it difficult to ascertain the role of a specific factor in humans. Despite the significant progress in unraveling the complex mechanisms required for proper growth and development, the therapeutic options for both conditions are extremely limited. It has been proposed that pharmacological activation of SIRT1 with the SIRT1 activator, resveratrol, or with synthetic SIRT1-activating compounds (i.e.SRT2104) are used to treat neuropsychiatric disorders (51). Maybe these should be also considered for use in children with growth and development disorders, as we have previously shown that SIRT1 is required for efficient CUG (2). However, one should bear in mind that these studies were performed in a mice model and conclusions from this model to developmental process in children should be drawn with utmost caution.

Several publications show that SIRT1 plays an important role also in puberty, at least in females; over expression of SIRT1 in the hypothalamus was shown to cause delayed puberty in female mice (46, 47). Thus, in the current study, if the underlying cause for the behavioral changes had been due to reduction of SIRT1 in the brain, mice would have been expected to present with precocious puberty. No gross effect differences were noted in either male or females, although we did not check testosterone in males nor vaginal opening in the females, and this may be a limitation of the study (52). However, as most tests were performed on post pubertal mice, we do not consider it to be a significant confounding factor. Another limitation concerns the western blot, in which we have no explanation as to the different pattern of brain SIRT1 protein; it would have been best if we could have compared the brains to those of BSKO, however we could not obtain these mice.

The nature of the mechanism that enables the connection between growth and behavior is still elusive; we hope that in the future we will be able to decipher the underlying cause, and maybe find a common regulator that affects growth and cognition; this may open a new area for intervention and will enable development of novel therapeutic modalities.

ETHICS STATEMENT

The animal study was reviewed and approved by Institutional Animal Care and Use Committee of Tel Aviv University, that follows the NIH guide for the care and us of laboratory animals (protocol approval number 01-16-052) prior to onset of the study.

AUTHOR CONTRIBUTIONS

BS: conducted the study, analyzed the data and prepared the tables and figures. SHH helped performing and analyzing behavioral tests. MP: funding acquisition, MY-G performed the statistical analysis. GG-Y: conceived the idea, supervised the study, analyzed the data and wrote the paper. All authors contributed to the article and approved the submitted version.

ACKNOWLEDGMENTS

The authors are grateful to Prof. Mona Dvir-Ginzberg from the Hebrew University and Prof. Elazar Zelzer from The Weizmann Institute of Science, for the transgenic animals; to Prof. Noga Kronfeld- Schor and Dr. Rotem Cohen from the Tel Aviv University for their help with the circadian rhythm analysis; to Dr. Michal Taler from Felsenstein Medical Research Center and Dr. Lior Bikovski from the Myers Neuro-Behavioral Core Facility of Tel Aviv University for helpful discussion and to Ms. Cindy Cohen for editing this manuscript.

REFERENCES

1. Pando R, Even-Zohar N, Shtaif B, Edry L, Shomron N, Phillip M, et al. MicroRNAs in the Growth Plate Are Responsive to Nutritional Cues: Association Between miR-140 and SIRT1. *J Nutr Biochem* (2012) 23 (11):1474–81. doi: 10.1016/j.jnutbio.2011.09.010
2. Shtaif B, Bar-Maisels M, Gabet Y, Hiram-Bab S, Yackobovitch-Gavan M, Phillip M, et al. Cartilage -Specific Knockout of Sirt1 Significantly Reduces Bone Quality and Catch-Up Growth Efficiency. *Bone* (2020) 138:115468. doi: 10.1016/j.bone.2020.115468
3. Yanagisawa S, Baker JR, Vuppusetty C, Koga T, Colley T, Fenwick P, et al. The Dynamic Shuttling of SIRT1 Between Cytoplasm and Nuclei in Bronchial Epithelial Cells by Single and Repeated Cigarette Smoke Exposure. *PloS One* (2018) 13(3):e0193921. doi: 10.1371/journal.pone.0193921
4. Sin TK, Yung BY, Siu PM. Modulation of SIRT1-Foxo1 Signaling Axis by Resveratrol: Implications in Skeletal Muscle Aging and Insulin Resistance. *Cell Physiol Biochem* (2015) 35(2):541–52. doi: 10.1159/000369718
5. Blander G, Bhimavarapu A, Mammone T, Maes D, Elliston K, Reich C, et al. SIRT1 Promotes Differentiation of Normal Human Keratinocytes. *J Invest Dermatol* (2009) 129(1):41–9. doi: 10.1038/jid.2008.179
6. Herranz D, Serrano M. Impact of Sirt1 on Mammalian Aging. *Aging (Albany NY)* (2010) 2(6):315–6. doi: 10.18632/aging.100156
7. Kanfi Y, Peshti V, Gozlan YM, Rathaus M, Gil R, Cohen HY. Regulation of SIRT1 Protein Levels by Nutrient Availability. *FEBS Lett* (2008) 582 (16):2417–23. doi: 10.1016/j.febslet.2008.06.005
8. Gabay O, Oppenhiemer H, Meir H, Zaal K, Sanchez C, Dvir-Ginzberg M. Increased Apoptotic Chondrocytes in Articular Cartilage From Adult Heterozygous SirT1 Mice. *Ann Rheum Dis* (2012) 71(4):613–6. doi: 10.1136/ard.2011.200504
9. Cheng HL, Mostoslavsky R, Saito S, Manis JP, Gu Y, Patel P, et al. Developmental Defects and P53 Hyperacetylation in Sir2 Homolog (SIRT1)-Deficient Mice. *Proc Natl Acad Sci USA* (2003) 100(19):10794–9. doi: 10.1073/pnas.1934713100
10. David DJ, Samuels BA, Rainer Q, Wang JW, Marsteller D, Mendez I, et al. Neurogenesis-Dependent and -Independent Effects of Fluoxetine in an Animal Model of Anxiety/Depression. *Neuron* (2009) 62(4):479–93. doi: 10.1016/j.neuron.2009.04.017
11. Griebel G, Holmes A. 50 Years of Hurdles and Hope in Anxiolytic Drug Discovery. *Nat Rev Drug Discovery* (2013) 12(9):667–87. doi: 10.1038/nrd4075
12. Novak CM, Burghardt PR, Levine JA. The Use of a Running Wheel to Measure Activity in Rodents: Relationship to Energy Balance, General Activity, and Reward. *Neurosci Biobehav Rev* (2012) 36(3):1001–14. doi: 10.1016/j.neubiorev.2011.12.012
13. Sherwin CM. Voluntary Wheel Running: A Review and Novel Interpretation. *Anim Behav* (1998) 56(1):11–27. doi: 10.1006/anbe.1998.0836
14. Oury F, Khrimian L, Denny CA, Gardin A, Chamouni A, Goeden N, et al. Maternal and Offspring Pools of Osteocalcin Influence Brain Development and Functions. *Cell* (2013) 155(1):228–41. doi: 10.1016/j.cell.2013.08.042
15. Cheah KS, Lau ET, Au PK, Tam PP. Expression of the Mouse Alpha 1(II) Collagen Gene Is Not Restricted to Cartilage During Development. *Development* (1991) 111(4):945–53. doi: 10.1242/dev.111.4.945
16. Ng LJ, Tam PP, Cheah KS. Preferential Expression of Alternatively Spliced mRNAs Encoding Type II Procollagen With a Cysteine-Rich Amino-Propeptide in Differentiating Cartilage and Nonchondrogenic Tissues During Early Mouse Development. *Dev Biol* (1993) 159(2):403–17. doi: 10.1006/dbio.1993.1251
17. Leung AW, Wong SY, Chan D, Tam PP, Cheah KS. Loss of Procollagen IIA From the Anterior Mesendoderm Disrupts the Development of Mouse Embryonic Forebrain. *Dev Dyn* (2010) 239(9):2319–29. doi: 10.1002/dvdy.22366
18. Tulino R, Benjamin AC, Jolinon N, Smith DL, Chini EN, Carnemolla A, et al. SIRT1 Activity Is Linked to Its Brain Region-Specific Phosphorylation and Is Impaired in Huntington's Disease Mice. *PloS One* (2016) 11(1):e0145425. doi: 10.1371/journal.pone.0145425
19. Stead JD, Clinton S, Neal C, Schneider J, Jama A, Miller S, et al. Selective Breeding for Divergence in Novelty-Seeking Traits: Heritability and Enrichment in Spontaneous Anxiety-Related Behaviors. *Behav Genet* (2006) 36(5):697–712. doi: 10.1007/s10519-006-9058-7
20. Pellow S, Chopin P, File SE, Briley M. Validation of Open:Closed Arm Entries in an Elevated Plus-Maze as a Measure of Anxiety in the Rat. *J Neurosci Methods* (1985) 14(3):149–67. doi: 10.1016/0165-0270(85)90031-7
21. Lister RG. The Use of a Plus-Maze to Measure Anxiety in the Mouse. *Psychopharmacol (Berl)* (1987) 92(2):180–5. doi: 10.1007/BF00177912
22. Gao J, Wang WY, Mao YW, Graff J, Guan JS, Pan L, et al. A Novel Pathway Regulates Memory and Plasticity *via* SIRT1 and miR-134. *Nature* (2010) 466 (7310):1105–9. doi: 10.1038/nature09271
23. Michan S, Li Y, Chou MM, Parrella E, Ge H, Long JM, et al. SIRT1 Is Essential for Normal Cognitive Function and Synaptic Plasticity. *J Neurosci* (2010) 30 (29):9695–707. doi: 10.1523/JNEUROSCI.0027-10.2010
24. Belden WJ, Dunlap JC. SIRT1 Is a Circadian Deacetylase for Core Clock Components. *Cell* (2008) 134(2):212–4. doi: 10.1016/j.cell.2008.07.010
25. Asher G, Gatfield D, Stratmann M, Reinke H, Dibner C, Kreppel F, et al. SIRT1 Regulates Circadian Clock Gene Expression Through PER2 Deacetylation. *Cell* (2008) 134(2):317–28. doi: 10.1016/j.cell.2008.06.050
26. Chang HC, Guarente L. SIRT1 Mediates Central Circadian Control in the SCN by a Mechanism That Decays With Aging. *Cell* (2013) 153(7):1448–60. doi: 10.1016/j.cell.2013.05.027
27. Shoji H, Takao K, Hattori S, Miyakawa T. Age-Related Changes in Behavior in C57BL/6J Mice From Young Adulthood to Middle Age. *Mol Brain* (2016) 9:11. doi: 10.1186/s13041-016-0191-9
28. Tucker LB, McCabe JT. Behavior of Male and Female C57BL/6J Mice Is More Consistent With Repeated Trials in the Elevated Zero Maze Than in the Elevated Plus Maze. *Front Behav Neurosci* (2017) 11:13. doi: 10.3389/fnbeh.2017.00013
29. Lee NK, Sowa H, Hinoi E, Ferron M, Ahn JD, Confavreux C, et al. Endocrine Regulation of Energy Metabolism by the Skeleton. *Cell* (2007) 130(3):456–69. doi: 10.1016/j.cell.2007.05.047
30. Karsenty G, Oury F. Regulation of Male Fertility by the Bone-Derived Hormone Osteocalcin. *Mol Cell Endocrinol* (2014) 382(1):521–6. doi: 10.1016/j.mce.2013.10.008
31. Ducy P, Desbois C, Boyce B, Pinero G, Story B, Dunstan C, et al. Increased Bone Formation in Osteocalcin-Deficient Mice. *Nature* (1996) 382 (6590):448–52. doi: 10.1038/382448a0
32. Obri A, Khrimian L, Karsenty G, Oury F. Osteocalcin in the Brain: From Embryonic Development to Age-Related Decline in Cognition. *Nat Rev Endocrinol* (2018) 14(3):174–82. doi: 10.1038/nrendo.2017.181
33. Foresta C, Strapazzon G, De Toni L, Gianesello L, Calcagno A, Pilon C, et al. Evidence for Osteocalcin Production by Adipose Tissue and Its Role in Human Metabolism. *J Clin Endocrinol Metab* (2010) 95(7):3502–6. doi: 10.1210/jc.2009-2557
34. Cohen DE, Supinski AM, Bonkowski MS, Donmez G, Guarente LP. Neuronal SIRT1 Regulates Endocrine and Behavioral Responses to Calorie Restriction. *Genes Dev* (2009) 23(24):2812–7. doi: 10.1101/gad.1839209
35. Couasnay G, Madel MB, Lim J, Lee B, Elefteriou F. Sites of Cre-Recombinase Activity in Mouse Lines Targeting Skeletal Cells. *J Bone Miner Res* (2021) 36 (9):1661–79. doi: 10.1002/jbmr.4415
36. Sakai K, Hiripi L, Glumoff V, Brandau O, Eerola R, Vuorio E, et al. Stage-And Tissue-Specific Expression of a Col2a1-Cre Fusion Gene in Transgenic Mice. *Matrix Biol* (2001) 19(8):761–7. doi: 10.1016/s0945-053x(00)00122-0
37. Prozorovski T, Schulze-Topphoff U, Glumm R, Baumgart J, Schroter F, Ninnemann O, et al. Sirt1 Contributes Critically to the Redox-Dependent Fate of Neural Progenitors. *Nat Cell Biol* (2008) 10(4):385–94. doi: 10.1038/ncb1700
38. Ramadori G, Lee CE, Bookout AL, Lee S, Williams KW, Anderson J, et al. Brain SIRT1: Anatomical Distribution and Regulation by Energy Availability. *J Neurosci* (2008) 28(40):9989–96. doi: 10.1523/JNEUROSCI.3257-08.2008
39. Libert S, Pointer K, Bell EL, Das A, Cohen DE, Asara JM, et al. SIRT1 Activates MAO-A in the Brain to Mediate Anxiety and Exploratory Drive. *Cell* (2011) 147(7):1459–72. doi: 10.1016/j.cell.2011.10.054
40. Sasaki T, Maier B, Koclega KD, Chruszcz M, Gluba W, Stukenberg PT, et al. Phosphorylation Regulates SIRT1 Function. *PloS One* (2008) 3(12):e4020. doi: 10.1371/journal.pone.0004020
41. Nasrin N, Kaushik VK, Fortier E, Wall D, Pearson KJ, de Cabo R, et al. JNK1 Phosphorylates SIRT1 and Promotes Its Enzymatic Activity. *PloS One* (2009) 4(12):e8414. doi: 10.1371/journal.pone.0008414

42. Zschoernig B, Mahlknecht U. Carboxy-Terminal Phosphorylation of SIRT1 by Protein Kinase CK2. *Biochem Biophys Res Commun* (2009) 381(3):372–7. doi: 10.1016/j.bbrc.2009.02.085
43. Sasaki T, Kikuchi O, Shimpuku M, Susanti VY, Yokota-Hashimoto H, Taguchi R, et al. Hypothalamic SIRT1 Prevents Age-Associated Weight Gain by Improving Leptin Sensitivity in Mice. *Diabetologia* (2014) 57 (4):819–31. doi: 10.1007/s00125-013-3140-5
44. Ramadori G, Fujikawa T, Fukuda M, Anderson J, Morgan DA, Mostoslavsky R, et al. SIRT1 Deacetylase in POMC Neurons Is Required for Homeostatic Defenses Against Diet-Induced Obesity. *Cell Metab* (2010) 12(1):78–87. doi: 10.1016/j.cmet.2010.05.010
45. Bilu C, Einat H, Zimmet P, Vishnevskia-Dai V, Kronfeld-Schor N. Beneficial Effects of Daytime High-Intensity Light Exposure on Daily Rhythms, Metabolic State and Affect. *Sci Rep* (2020) 10(1):19782. doi: 10.1038/s41598-020-76636-8
46. Aylwin CF, Lomniczi A. Sirtuin (SIRT)-1: At the Crossroads of Puberty and Metabolism. *Curr Opin Endocr Metab Res* (2020) 14:65–72. doi: 10.1016/j.coemr.2020.06.001
47. Vazquez MJ, Toro CA, Castellano JM, Ruiz-Pino F, Roa J, Beiroa D, et al. SIRT1 Mediates Obesity- and Nutrient-Dependent Perturbation of Pubertal Timing by Epigenetically Controlling Kiss1 Expression. *Nat Commun* (2018) 9(1):4194. doi: 10.1038/s41467-018-06459-9
48. Uzun Cicek A, Mercan Isik C, Bakir S, Ulger D, Sari SA, Bakir D, et al. Evidence Supporting the Role of Telomerase, MMP-9, and SIRT1 in Attention-Deficit/Hyperactivity Disorder (ADHD). *J Neural Transm (Vienna)* (2020) 127(10):1409–18. doi: 10.1007/s00702-020-02231-w
49. Reinhard SM, Razak K, Ethell IM. A Delicate Balance: Role of MMP-9 in Brain Development and Pathophysiology of Neurodevelopmental Disorders. *Front Cell Neurosci* (2015) 9:280. doi: 10.3389/fncel.2015.00280
50. Wheeler PG, Bresnahan K, Shephard BA, Lau J, Balk EM. Short Stature and Functional Impairment: A Systematic Review. *Arch Pediatr Adolesc Med* (2004) 158(3):236–43. doi: 10.1001/archpedi.158.3.236
51. Xie J, Zhang X, Zhang L. Negative Regulation of Inflammation by SIRT1. *Pharmacol Res* (2013) 67(1):60–7. doi: 10.1016/j.phrs.2012.10.010
52. McCutcheon JE, Marinelli M. Age Matters. *Eur J Neurosci* (2009) 29(5):997–1014. doi: 10.1111/j.1460-9568.2009.06648.x

18

Activation of Sirtuin 1 Attenuates High Glucose-Induced Neuronal Apoptosis by Deacetylating p53

*Xiajie Shi[1,2], Linhua Pi[1], Shanlei Zhou[1], Xin Li[3], Fangyuan Min[3], Shan Wang[3], Zhenqi Liu[4] and Jing Wu[1]**

[1] Department of Endocrinology, Xiangya Hospital, Central South University, Changsha, China, [2] Department of Metabolism and Endocrinology, The Second Xiangya Hospital, Central South University, Changsha, China, [3] Department of Pharmaceutical Engineering, College of Chemistry and Chemical Engineering, Central South University, Changsha, China, [4] Division of Endocrinology and Metabolism, Department of Medicine, University of Virginia Health System, Charlottesville, VA, United States

***Correspondence:**
Jing Wu
wujing0731@163.com

Diabetes mellitus (DM) has been proven to be a key risk factor for cognitive impairment. Previous studies have implicated hippocampal neuronal apoptosis in diabetes-related cognitive impairment. However, the underlying mechanism remains unknown. Sirtuin 1 (SIRT1) is a protein deacetylase depended on nicotinamide adenine dinucleotide. Furthermore, it is indispensable in normal learning and memory. Whether SIRT1 is taken part in diabetes-induced neuronal apoptosis and thus involve in the development of diabetic cognitive impairment is still not clear. To address this issue, we examined the possible role of SIRT1 in hippocampal neuronal apoptosis in streptozotocin-induced diabetic mice. Furthermore, the possible mechanism was investigated in high glucose-induced SH-SY5Y cells. We found that downregulation of the activity and expression of SIRT1 was associated with increased hippocampal neuronal apoptosis in mice. *In vitro*, cell apoptosis induced by high glucose which was accompanied by a down-regulation of SIRT1 and an increased acetylation of p53. On the contrary, activation of SIRT1 using its agonist resveratrol ameliorated cell apoptosis *via* deacetylating p53. Our data suggest that high concentration of glucose can induce neuronal apoptosis through downregulation of SIRT1 and increased acetylation of p53, which likely contribute to the development of cognitive impairment in diabetes.

Keywords: diabetes, cognitive impairment, sirtuin 1, neuronal apoptosis, p53

INTRODUCTION

Diabetes has been characterized as a group of metabolic diseases caused by chronic hyperglycemia. Numerous epidemic studies have demonstrated that diabetes increases the risk of the development of cognitive impairment (1–3). With the fast growing number of diabetes and the ever-increasing aging people, diabetic-related diabetic cognitive impairment will challenge public health implication in the future. Therefore, a better insight into the molecular mechanism of the association between diabetes and dementia is of great importance for preventing and slowing the progression of cognitive dysfunction in people with diabetes. Interestingly, several previous studies have indicated that apoptosis in hippocampal neuron promoted the progression of diabetic cognitive dysfunction (4–7). However, the mechanism of neuronal apoptosis in diabetes is still unclear.

Sirtuin 1 (SIRT1), commonly known as a protein deacetylase depended on nicotinamide adenine dinucleotide (NAD^+), takes part in cell aging (8), differentiation (9), and apoptosis (10). Due to its deacetylating function, some data have indicated that SIRT1 may reduce cell apoptosis through deacetylating p53 (11, 12). p53 responds to various stress signals by modulating the expression of target genes which take part in DNA repair, metabolic pathways, and apoptosis (13, 14). Hyperacetylation of p53 has been shown to be positively associated with pro-apoptotic factors and can be reduced by the deacetylation activity of SIRT1 (15).

Thus, we hypothesized that SIRT1 may get involve in the neuronal apoptosis caused by hyperglycemia in diabetes *via* p53 signal pathway. To confirm the hypothesis, the expression of SIRT1 in streptozotocin (STZ)-induced diabetic mice and high glucose-treated neuroblastoma cells were measured. Then, we investigated whether activation of SIRT1 had a neuroprotective effect against high glucose-induced neuronal apoptosis *via* p53 signal pathway. These findings will offer new insights for diabetic cognitive impairment development and progression.

MATERIALS AND METHODS

Animals and Animal Experiment Procedure

After 1 week of acclimation, 17 C57BL/6 mice (Department of Laboratory Animals, Central South University) were randomly divided into two groups: the control group ($n = 8$) and the diabetes group ($n = 9$). The mice were raised in animal quarters with comfortable temperature and humidity. All procedures involving animal and their care were conducted in conformity with NIH Guidelines for Care and Use of Laboratory Animals. And the experiment was approved by the institutional animal care committee of Central South University.

After overnight fasting, the mice were modeled diabetes by a single intraperitoneal dose of STZ (Sigma, USA). At the same time, an equivalent volume of vehicle was infused into the control group. 0.1 M sodium citrate buffer (pH 4.4) was used to dissolve STZ. According to the previous study, the dose of 220 mg/kg was administered (16). To avoid hypoglycemic shock, 5% glucose was added into the water for 24 h after STZ injection. Three days after the administration of STZ, the blood from the tail vein was collected to measure the blood glucose for all mice. Mice with non-fasting blood glucose ≥16.7 mM in two consecutive tests were considered diabetic.

At the time of sacrifice, mice were anesthetized with pentobarbitol sodium. Then, we exposed the four mice' skulls from each group along the midline and placed the brain on a precooled cutting board for western blotting and SIRT1 activity test, and dissected hippocampus were snapped frozen in liquid nitrogen and preserved at −70°C. The remaining brains of mice were perfused with 4% paraformaldehyde and were then fixed in same solution for hematoxylin–eosin staining and immunohistochemistry staining.

Immunohistochemistry

Procedures were conducted according to instruction of the Vectastain ABC elite kit (ZSGB-BIO, China). Briefly, paraformaldehyde-fixed tissue sections were deparaffinized and rehydrated. Then, 10 mM sodium citrate (pH 6.0) was used to expose the antigen. To inactivate endogenous peroxidase, the slides were incubated with 0.3% hydrogen peroxide. Primary antibody was incubated overnight at 4°C after non-specific binding elimination. Then, the samples were treated with biotinylated secondary antibody for 60 min at room temperature, with streptavidin–biotin-horseradish peroxidase for another 60 min. 3,3′-Diaminobenzidine was used to visualize. Finally, the sections were counterstained with hematoxylin.

Cell Culture and Differentiation

SH-SY5Y cells obtained from the State Key Laboratory of Medical Genetics were used in the experiment. SH-SY5Y cells were cultured in DMEM/F12 (Gibco, USA), 10% fetal bovine serum (FBS; Gibco, USA), and 1% streptopenicillin (Gibco, USA) at 37°C in a humidified cell culture incubator with 5% carbon dioxide. The human neuroblastoma cells were incubated in the medium containing 1% FBS for 24 h and then treated with 10 μM all-*trans*-retinoic acid (RA; Sigma, USA) for 5 days before experiments.

Apoptosis Assay

According to the result of our previous study, SH-SY5Y cell was cultured in 75 mm glucose for 96 h to mimic the high glucose condition *in vitro*. Cell apoptosis was detected with DAPI nuclear staining. Briefly, after treatment, cells were gently washed with PBS and then stained using DAPI solution (Beyotime, China) for 5 min. The cells were subsequently visualized under a fluorescence microscope (Leica, Germany). To quantify apoptosis, two fields from five wells were blindly analyzed by an observer blinded to the photographers.

SIRT1 Agonist Treatment

Cells were cultured in 75 mM glucose for 96 h with or without SIRT1 agonist resveratrol (RV) (20 μM; Sigma, USA).

Western Blot

Proteins were extracted from the whole hippocampus of the mice or SH-SY5Y cells. The protein mass was detected by the bicinchoninic acid protein assay method (Beyotime, China). 50 μg of boiled proteins was separated by SDS-PAGE and blotted with anti-caspase-3 (cleaved form; Abacm, USA), anti-Bax antibody (Abcam, USA), anti-Bcl-2 antibody (Abcam, USA), anti-SIRT1 antibody (Abcam, USA), anti-p53 antibody (Abcam, USA), anti-Ace (K382)-p53 (Abcam, USA), and anti-β tubulin antibody (Abcam, USA).

SIRT1 Activity

Sirtuin 1 activity was measured by the SIRT1 colorimetric assay kit (Genmed, China) according to the instruction. Simply, synthesized substrate [Arg–His–Lys–Lys (Ac)] was incubated with hippocampus or SH-SY5Y cells. When SIRT1 is active, the acetylated substrate will be deacetylated, resulting in the change of colorimetric absorbance. The absorbance was detected by a M2 plate reader (Tecan, Austria).

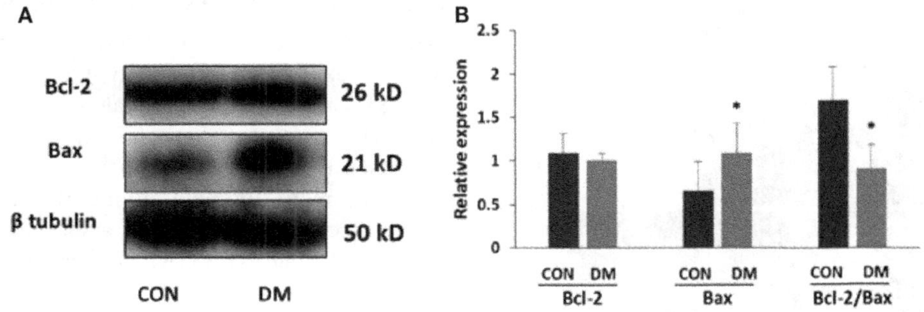

FIGURE 1 | Expression of apoptosis-related proteins in hippocampus of STZ-induced diabetic mice. **(A)** Representative Western blot gel images of Bcl-2 and Bax. **(B)** Summarized data of apoptosis-associated protein Bcl-2 and Bax in the hippocampus of STZ-induced diabetic mice and control. All values are expressed as the mean ± SD. Abbreviations: CON, control; DM, diabetes mellitus. *P < 0.05 versus control. N = 4.

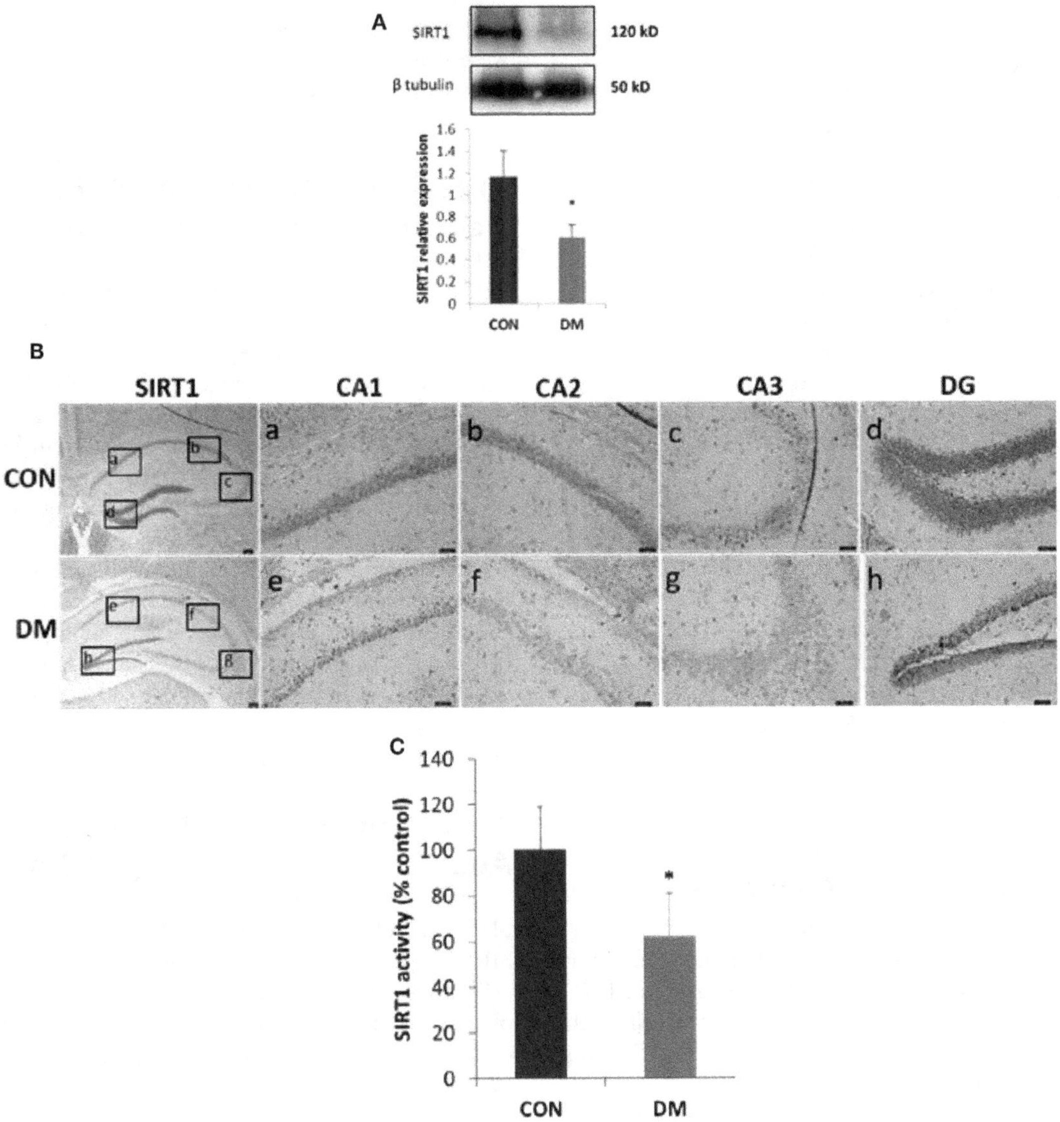

FIGURE 2 | Expression of sirtuin 1 (SIRT1) in hippocampus of STZ-induced diabetic mice. **(A)** Representative Western blot gel images and quantification data of SIRT1 (N = 4). **(B)** Immunohistochemical stainings of SIRT1. Represent the stainings of CA1, CA2, and CA3 sectors of the hippocampus and dentate gyrus (DG) in control group or diabetes group is shown in panel [**(B)**, a–d or e–h], respectively. Scale bars: 50 μm. **(C)** SIRT1 activity (N = 4). All values are expressed as the mean ± SD. Abbreviations: CON, control; DM, diabetes mellitus. *P < 0.05 versus control.

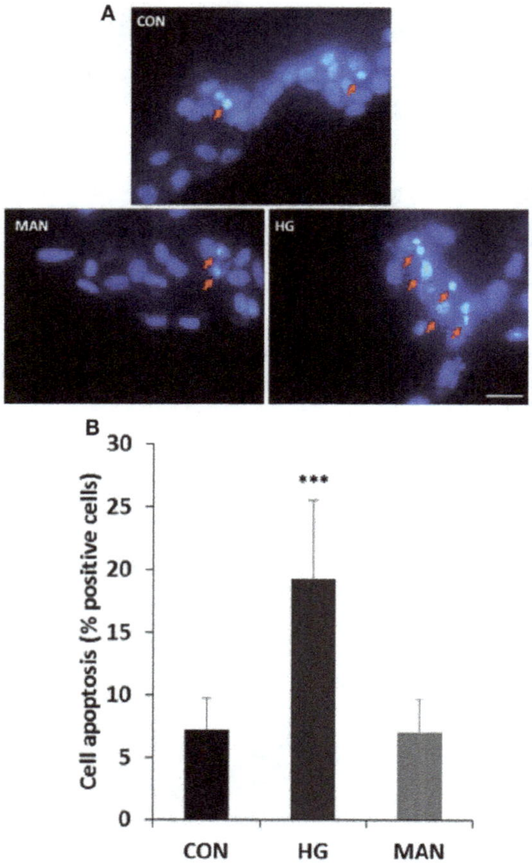

FIGURE 3 | Hyperglycemia induces apoptosis in cultured SH-SY5Y cells. **(A)** Representative fluorescence micrographs of DAPI staining of SH-SY5Y cells exposed to 5.5 mM (CON), 75 mM glucose (HG), or mannitol (MAN) for 96 h. The representative apoptotic cells were marked by arrows. Scale bar: 20 μm. **(B)** Percentage quantification of apoptotic cells. ***P<0.001 versus control.

Statistical Analysis

Independent t-test or Cochran and Cox t-test for continuous data was performed for comparison of two groups. Statistical analyses were performed with SPSS for windows (version 17.0). The significance level α is 0.05.

RESULTS

Hippocampus Neuronal Apoptosis in STZ-Induced Diabetic Mice

At the fourth week after STZ administration, changes in apoptosis-related proteins in hippocampus were examined. The protein levels of Bax (a protein facilitating apoptotic cell death) and Bcl-2 (a protein that is protective of apoptotic cell death) were measured by western blotting. In 4-week diabetic mice, the Bax expression was significantly increased. However, the level of Bcl-2 was not changed in diabetic mice. Nevertheless, our results showed that the ratio of Bcl-2 to Bax was significantly decreased (**Figure 1**, $P < 0.05$), indicating the enhanced neuronal apoptosis in hyperglycemia mice.

SIRT1 Is Decreased in Hippocampus Neuron of STZ-Induced Diabetic Mice

Sirtuin 1 expression and activity in hippocampus was detected after STZ administration of male C57BL/6J mice. Four weeks after STZ treatment, both SIRT1 levels and activities were decreased in hippocampus. To locate the alteration of SIRT1 in hippocampus, immunostaining was used. We found SIRT1 mainly decreased in cognition-associated areas such as CA1, CA3, and dentate gyrus (DG) (**Figure 2**).

Effect of High Glucose on SH-SY5Y Cells Apoptosis

Differentiated SH-SY5Y cells were cultured in 75 mM glucose or 69.5 mM mannitol (MAN) (plus 5.5 mM glucose in DMEM/F12 medium) for 96 h, and the cell apoptosis was measured with DAPI staining. A small number of apoptotic cells (7.2%) were measured in the control group. However, 19.3% apoptotic cells were detected by DAPI staining after high glucose treatment. Similar with the control group, the apoptotic rate in cells treated with MAN was 7.1% (**Figure 3**).

Alteration of SIRT1 and p53 in SH-SY5Y Cells Under High Glucose Condition

Differentiated neuroblastoma cells were cultured with 75 mM glucose for 96 h to explore whether high glucose could induce downregulation of SIRT1. Similar with the results in diabetic mice, both activity and expression of SIRT1 decreased significantly in high glucose-incubated SH-SY5Y cells. To investigate the possible mechanism between the downregulation of SIRT1 and cell apoptosis, we examined p53 protein by the Western blotting. The results showed an increase in acetylated p53 protein in cells treated with high glucose (**Figure 4**). To further characterize the trait of apoptotic mechanism, the status of Bax, Bcl-2, and caspase-3 was tested. SH-SY5Y cells showed a dramatic decrease in the ratio of Bcl-2 to Bax and an increase in the expression of caspase-3 under high glucose condition (**Figure 4**), suggesting that high glucose-induced apoptosis possibly be mediated by the mitochondrial pathway. Based on the above results, we guessed that SIRT1 may induce neuronal apoptosis through p53/Bax pathway.

Activation of SIRT1 Alleviated Cell Apoptosis *via* Decreasing p53 Acetylation

To explore the effects of SIRT1 activation on the differentiated SH-SY5Y cells, SIRT1 agonist RV was applied. Activation of SIRT1 significantly reduced the amount of apoptotic or necrotic cells induced by high glucose. As shown in **Figure 5**, the number of cells with positive DAPI staining was 12.3% in the presence of RV. However, without activator, the number reached up to 23.4%.

Then, we examined whether activation of SIRT1 could decrease the acetylated p53 level. Just as results shown in **Figure 5**, treatment with RV raised the SIRT1 expression and reduced the acetylated p53 level compared with cells incubated with high concentration of glucose.

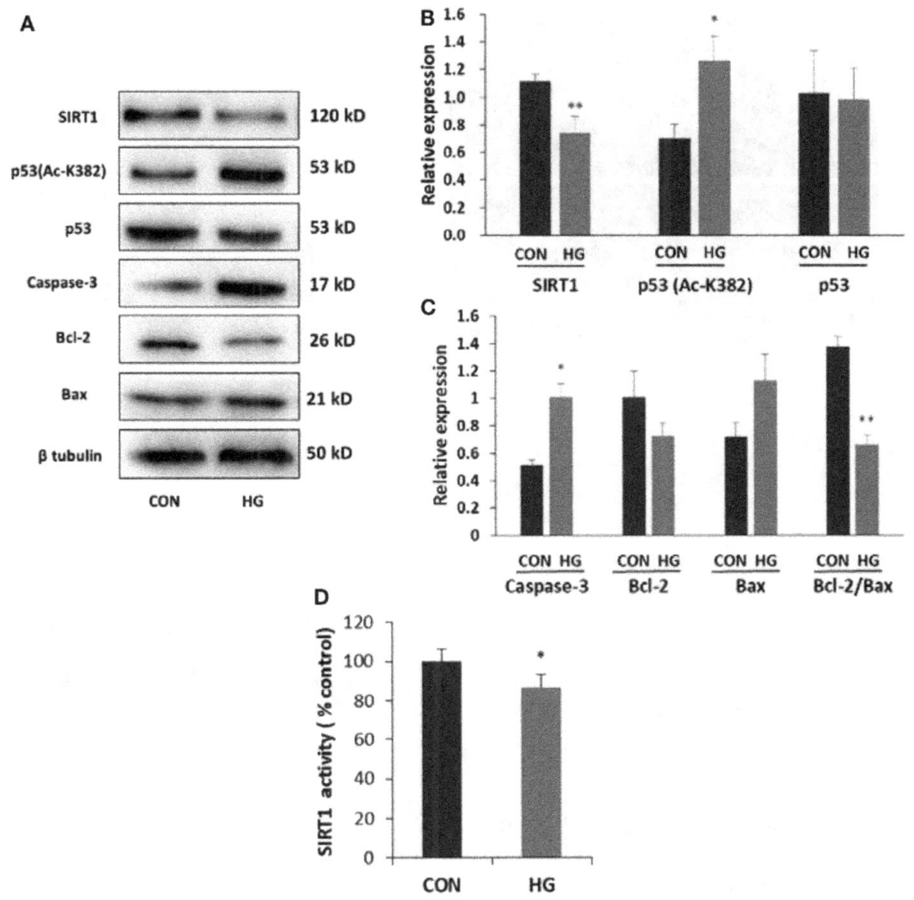

FIGURE 4 | Effects of high glucose on the expressions of sirtuin 1 (SIRT1), p53, Ac-p53, and apoptosis-associated proteins. SH-SY5Y cells were cultured in either 5.5 mM (CON) or 75 mM (HG) glucose-containing media for 96 h. **(A)** Representative Western blot images. **(B)** Quantifications of SIRT1, p53 (Ac-K382), and p53 expression. **(C)** Quantifications of caspase-3, Bcl-2, Bax, and Bcl-2/Bax expression. **(D)** SIRT1 activity. $^{*}P < 0.05$; $^{**}P < 0.01$ versus control. $N = 3$.

To further support these findings, several proteins associated with apoptotic cascade were assayed. The high glucose-induced increase of caspase-3 and the decline of the Bcl-2/Bax ratio were both partially reversed in the cells in the presence of SIRT1 activator.

DISCUSSION

The major aim of our work was to explore whether SIRT1 is involved in neuronal apoptosis induced by diabetes. Using STZ-induced diabetic mice and *in vitro* cultured differentiated SH-SY5Y cells, we found SIRT1 was obviously decreased. Activation of SIRT1 could alleviate high glucose-induced cell apoptosis by deacetylate p53. These findings revealed a novel molecular mechanism involving neuronal apoptosis in diabetes mellitus.

There has been a wide recognition that type 1 DM (T1DM) can cause cognitive impairment (17, 18). STZ is a commonly used reagent to model T1DM due to its preferentially toxic to beta cells in pancreas. Substantial evidence and our previous studies have demonstrated that single high dose of STZ can induced diabetic cognitive dysfunction at early stages of DM (19, 20). Hippocampus, an internal structure of the brain, plays a very important role in several key fields of cognitive function, such as spatial navigation, memory, and learning (21, 22). And previous studies have indicated that hippocampal neuronal apoptosis has close connection with diabetic cognitive impairment (23–26). Therefore, clarify of the mechanism in hippocampal neuronal apoptosis in diabetes will contribute a lot to the prevention and treatment for the diabetic cognitive impairment.

Sirtuin 1 is widely expressed and has been shown to be highly expressed in the developing mouse central nervous system (27), adult mouse and human brain (28). In the adult brain, SIRT1 is expressed in the most brain areas and is prominent in the hippocampal neuron (29), which is replicated in our results. Furthermore, SIRT1 was found highly decreased in the hippocampus with neuronal apoptosis, especially in the CA1, CA3, and DG subregions, which is closely related with memory and learning (30). And the activity of SIRT1 was also decreased. Bcl-2 family consists of a group of cytoplasmic proteins and is notable for its regulation of cell apoptosis. There

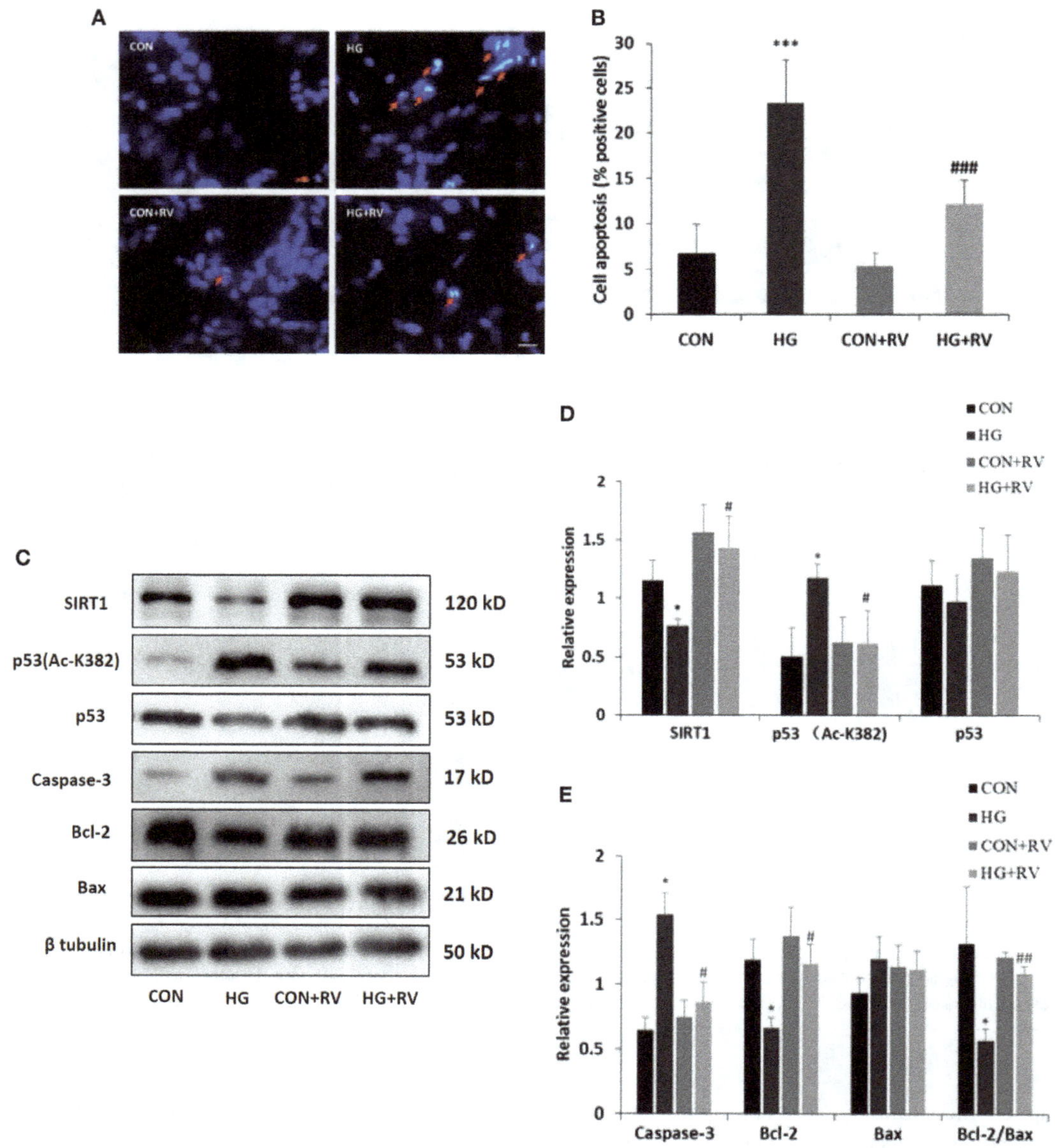

FIGURE 5 | Activation of sirtuin 1 (SIRT1) attenuates high glucose-induced cell apoptosis *via* deacetylating p53. SH-SY5Y cells were cultured in HG media for 96 h in the presence of 10 μM resveratrol (RV). **(A)** Representative fluorescence micrographs of DAPI staining of SH-SY5Y cells treated with or without RV. Arrow denotes cell apoptosis. **(B)** Quantification of cell apoptosis. **(C)** Representative Western blot images of protein expression. **(D)** Quantifications of SIRT1, p53 (Ac-K382), and p53 expression. **(E)** Quantifications of Caspase-3, Bcl-2, Bax, and Bcl-2/Bax expression. $^{*}P < 0.05$; $^{**}P < 0.01$; and $^{***}P < 0.001$ versus control. $^{\#}P < 0.05$; $^{\#\#}P < 0.01$; and $^{\#\#\#}P < 0.01$ versus HG. Scale bar: 20 μm. $N = 3$.

are two main proteins in this family, Bcl-2 and Bax. However, they are functionally opposite: Bax promotes apoptosis, whereas Bcl-2 counteracts this effect (31). And the ratio of Bcl-2 to Bax controls the cell life after an apoptotic stimulus. We found in this study, the ratio of Bcl-2 to Bax decreased in hippocampus of diabetic mice than that of the controls. These results indicated that hippocampal neuronal apoptosis in STZ-induced diabetic mice appeared to correlate with SIRT1. Thus, further study was conducted *in vitro*.

SH-SY5Y cell line, derived from SK-N-SH, is a widely used model for studying the neuronal mechanism. SH-SY5Y cells are able to differentiate into neuronal lineage by all-*trans*-RA treatment (32). Our previous study have proved that culturing differentiated SH-SY5Y cell in 75 mM glucose for 96 h is an appropriate choice to mimic high glucose condition *in vitro*. Another study also proved that SH-SY5Y cell cultured in high glucose (above 50 mM) occured hyperglycemic stress and cell injury (33). Our results indicated that the apoptotic cells were increased in the high glucose-cultured group. Besides, the ratio of Bcl-2 to Bax and the expression of caspase-3 were both changed in high glucose-cultured neuroblastoma cells. Similar with the findings *in vivo*, these results further indicated that glucose at high concentration could induce cell apoptosis through the mitochondria pathway.

Previous studies have proved that p53 can be deacetylated by SIRT1 by overexpression and dominant-negative strategies both *in vitro* and *in vivo* (11, 15). Multiple lysine residues of p53 can be acetylated in human, including K320, K373, and K382 (11). Acetylation at different residues induces diverse aspects of p53-mediated stress response. Acetylation of p53 on K382 residue facilitates p53 activation, which triggers the transcription of target genes associated with apoptosis (34). Our results showed that the increasing of acetylation of p53 K382 accompanied by decreasing of SIRT1. These findings strongly suggested that the decline of SIRT1 induced by high glucose resulted in acetylation of p53 at K382 lysine residues, which could mediate neuronal apoptosis.

Resveratrol is a well-known agonist of SIRT1 (35). So, we used RV in SH-SY5Y cells with neuron-like phenotypes to further prove the above view. This work indicated that the high glucose-induced decreasing of SIRT1 was reversed with RV. Then, we detected the effect of activation of SIRT1 on cell apoptosis and apoptosis-related protein. The most important finding of this work is that activation of SIRT1 can partially reverse the SH-SY5Y cell apoptosis mediated by high concentration of glucose. The reverse of the apoptosis-related protein, caspase-3 and the ratio of Bcl-2 to Bax, further confirmed it. Some previous studies also reported that RV had protective effect in the neuronal survival (36, 37). Although previous studies indicate that the activation of SIRT1 is a key aspect of RV action, the interaction between RV and other factors cannot be rule out.

Taken together, we demonstrate that decreasing of SIRT1 and neuronal apoptosis occures in the STZ-induced diabetic mice. In high glucose-incubated SH-SY5Y cells, decreasing of SIRT1, p53 acetylation, and cell apoptosis are confirmed, and activation of SIRT1 by RV attenuate the cell apoptosis *via* deacetylation of p53. It is therefore suggested that SIRT1 may be a therapeutic target for the treatment of diabetic cognitive impairment.

ETHICS STATEMENT

All procedures involving animal and their care were conducted in conformity with NIH Guidelines for Care and Use of Laboratory Animals, and the experiment was approved by the institutional animal care committee of Central South University.

AUTHOR CONTRIBUTIONS

JW and SW designed the experiments. The experimental procedures were performed by XS, LP, SZ, XL, and FM. XS and JW prepared the manuscript. ZL revised the manuscript.

ACKNOWLEDGMENTS

This study was mainly completed in the Institute of Medical Sciences, Xiangya Hospital of Central South University.

REFERENCES

1. Roberts RO, Knopman DS, Geda YE, Cha RH, Pankratz VS, Baertlein L, et al. Association of diabetes with amnestic and nonamnestic mild cognitive impairment. *Alzheimers Dement* (2014) 10(1):18–26. doi:10.1016/j.jalz.2013.01.001
2. Hilal S, Ikram MK, Saini M, Tan CS, Catindig JA, Dong YH, et al. Prevalence of cognitive impairment in Chinese: epidemiology of dementia in Singapore study. *J Neurol Neurosurg Psychiatry* (2013) 84(6):686–92. doi:10.1136/jnnp-2012-304080
3. Fu Z, Wu J, Nesil T, Li MD, Aylor KW, Liu Z. Long-term high-fat diet induces hippocampal microvascular insulin resistance and cognitive dysfunction. *Am J Physiol Endocrinol Metab* (2017) 312(2):E89–97. doi:10.1152/ajpendo.00297.2016
4. Liu J, Feng L, Ma D, Zhang M, Gu J, Wang S, et al. Neuroprotective effect of paeonol on cognition deficits of diabetic encephalopathy in streptozotocin-induced diabetic rat. *Neurosci Lett* (2013) 549:63–8. doi:10.1016/j.neulet.2013.06.002
5. Ye L, Wang F, Yang RH. Diabetes impairs learning performance and affects the mitochondrial function of hippocampal pyramidal neurons. *Brain Res* (2011) 1411:57–64. doi:10.1016/j.brainres.2011.07.011
6. Guo YJ, Wang SH, Yuan Y, Li FF, Ye KP, Huang Y, et al. Vulnerability for apoptosis in the hippocampal dentate gyrus of STZ-induced diabetic rats with cognitive impairment. *J Endocrinol Invest* (2014) 37(1):87–96. doi:10.1007/s40618-013-0030-0
7. Wang S, Zhou SL, Min FY, Ma JJ, Shi XJ, Bereczki E, et al. mTOR-mediated hyperphosphorylation of tau in the hippocampus is involved in cognitive deficits in streptozotocin-induced diabetic mice. *Metab Brain Dis* (2014) 29(3):729–36. doi:10.1007/s11011-014-9528-1
8. Satoh A, Brace CS, Rensing N, Cliften P, Wozniak DF, Herzog ED, et al. Sirt1 extends life span and delays aging in mice through the regulation of Nk2 homeobox 1 in the DMH and LH. *Cell Metab* (2013) 18(3):416–30. doi:10.1016/j.cmet.2013.07.013
9. Liu DJ, Hammer D, Komlos D, Chen KY, Firestein BL, Liu AY. SIRT1 knockdown promotes neural differentiation and attenuates the heat shock response. *J Cell Physiol* (2014) 229(9):1224–35. doi:10.1002/jcp.24556
10. Xiong H, Pang J, Yang H, Dai M, Liu Y, Ou Y, et al. Activation of miR-34a/SIRT1/p53 signaling contributes to cochlear hair cell apoptosis: implications for age-related hearing loss. *Neurobiol Aging* (2015) 36(4):1692–701. doi:10.1016/j.neurobiolaging.2014.12.034
11. Cheng HL, Mostoslavsky R, Saito S, Manis JP, Gu Y, Patel P, et al. Developmental defects and p53 hyperacetylation in Sir2 homolog (SIRT1)-deficient mice. *Proc Natl Acad Sci U S A* (2003) 100(19):10794–9. doi:10.1073/pnas.1934713100
12. Wang N, Zhang F, Yang L, Zou J, Wang H, Liu K, et al. Resveratrol protects against L-arginine-induced acute necrotizing pancreatitis in mice by enhancing SIRT1-mediated deacetylation of p53 and heat shock factor 1. *Int J Mol Med* (2017) 40(2):427–37. doi:10.3892/ijmm.2017.3012
13. Sen N, Kumari R, Singh MI, Das S. HDAC5, a key component in temporal regulation of p53-mediated transactivation in response to genotoxic stress. *Mol Cell* (2013) 52(3):406–20. doi:10.1016/j.molcel.2013.09.003
14. Yang W, Lu J, Weng J, Jia W, Ji L, Xiao J, et al. Prevalence of diabetes among men and women in China. *N Engl J Med* (2010) 362(12):1090–101. doi:10.1056/NEJMoa0908292
15. Li M, Lu Y, Hu Y, Zhai X, Xu W, Jing H, et al. Salvianolic acid B protects against acute ethanol-induced liver injury through SIRT1-mediated deacetylation of p53 in rats. *Toxicol Lett* (2014) 228(2):67–74. doi:10.1016/j.toxlet.2014.04.011
16. Ferber S, Halkin A, Cohen H, Ber I, Einav Y, Goldberg I, et al. Pancreatic and duodenal homeobox gene 1 induces expression of insulin genes in liver and ameliorates streptozotocin-induced hyperglycemia. *Nat Med* (2000) 6(5):568–72. doi:10.1038/75050

17. Nunley KA, Rosano C, Ryan CM, Jennings JR, Aizenstein HJ, Zgibor JC, et al. Clinically relevant cognitive impairment in middle-aged adults with childhood-onset type 1 diabetes. *Diabetes Care* (2015) 38(9):1768–76. doi:10.2337/dc15-0041
18. Kirchhoff BA, Jundt DK, Doty T, Hershey T. A longitudinal investigation of cognitive function in children and adolescents with type 1 diabetes mellitus. *Pediatr Diabetes* (2016). doi:10.1111/pedi.12414
19. Beauquis J, Roig P, De Nicola AF, Saravia F. Short-term environmental enrichment enhances adult neurogenesis, vascular network and dendritic complexity in the hippocampus of type 1 diabetic mice. *PLoS One* (2010) 5(11): e13993. doi:10.1371/journal.pone.0013993
20. Huang HJ, Chen YH, Liang KC, Jheng YS, Jhao JJ, Su MT, et al. Exendin-4 protected against cognitive dysfunction in hyperglycemic mice receiving an intrahippocampal lipopolysaccharide injection. *PLoS One* (2012) 7(7):e39656. doi:10.1371/journal.pone.0039656
21. Buzsaki G, Moser EI. Memory, navigation and theta rhythm in the hippocampal-entorhinal system. *Nat Neurosci* (2013) 16(2):130–8. doi:10.1038/nn.3304
22. Gruart A, Leal-Campanario R, Lopez-Ramos JC, Delgado-Garcia JM. Functional basis of associative learning and their relationships with long-term potentiation evoked in the involved neural circuits: lessons from studies in behaving mammals. *Neurobiol Learn Mem* (2015) 124:3–18. doi:10.1016/j.nlm.2015.04.006
23. Sun LJ, Hou XH, Xue SH, Yan F, Dai YJ, Zhao CH, et al. Fish oil modulates glycogen synthase kinase-3 signaling pathway in diabetes-induced hippocampal neurons apoptosis. *Brain Res* (2014) 1574:37–49. doi:10.1016/j.brainres.2014.05.050
24. Li ZG, Zhang W, Grunberger G, Sima AA. Hippocampal neuronal apoptosis in type 1 diabetes. *Brain Res* (2002) 946(2):221–31. doi:10.1016/S0006-8993(02)02887-1
25. Sima AA, Li ZG. The effect of C-peptide on cognitive dysfunction and hippocampal apoptosis in type 1 diabetic rats. *Diabetes* (2005) 54(5):1497–505. doi:10.2337/diabetes.54.5.1497
26. Wu J, Nie SD, Wang S. Tau pathology in diabetes mellitus. *Pharmazie* (2013) 68(8):649–52. doi:10.1691/ph.2013.2901
27. Ogawa T, Wakai C, Saito T, Murayama A, Mimura Y, Youfu S, et al. Distribution of the longevity gene product, SIRT1, in developing mouse organs. *Congenit Anom (Kyoto)* (2011) 51(2):70–9. doi:10.1111/j.1741-4520.2010.00304.x
28. Zakhary SM, Ayubcha D, Dileo JN, Jose R, Leheste JR, Horowitz JM, et al. Distribution analysis of deacetylase SIRT1 in rodent and human nervous systems. *Anat Rec (Hoboken)* (2010) 293(6):1024–32. doi:10.1002/ar.21116
29. Michan S, Li Y, Chou MM, Parrella E, Ge H, Long JM, et al. SIRT1 is essential for normal cognitive function and synaptic plasticity. *J Neurosci* (2010) 30(29):9695–707. doi:10.1523/JNEUROSCI.0027-10.2010
30. Kesner RP. Behavioral functions of the CA3 subregion of the hippocampus. *Learn Mem* (2007) 14(11):771–81. doi:10.1101/lm.688207
31. Siddiqui WA, Ahad A, Ahsan H. The mystery of BCL2 family: Bcl-2 proteins and apoptosis: an update. *Arch Toxicol* (2015) 89(3):289–317. doi:10.1007/s00204-014-1448-7
32. Lopes FM, Schroder R, Da FMJ, Zanotto-Filho A, Muller CB, Pires AS, et al. Comparison between proliferative and neuron-like SH-SY5Y cells as an in vitro model for Parkinson disease studies. *Brain Res* (2010) 1337:85–94. doi:10.1016/j.brainres.2010.03.102
33. Hsu YY, Tseng YT, Lo YC. Berberine, a natural antidiabetes drug, attenuates glucose neurotoxicity and promotes Nrf2-related neurite outgrowth. *Toxicol Appl Pharmacol* (2013) 272(3):787–96. doi:10.1016/j.taap.2013.08.008
34. Wang J, Qian J, Hu Y, Kong X, Chen H. ArhGAP30 promotes p53 acetylation and function in colorectal cancer. *Nat Commun* (2014) 5:4735. doi:10.1038/ncomms5735
35. Zhang W, Luo J, Yang F, Wang Y, Yin Y, Strom A, et al. BRCA1 inhibits AR-mediated proliferation of breast cancer cells through the activation of SIRT1. *Sci Rep* (2016) 6:22034. doi:10.1038/srep22034
36. Kim D, Nguyen MD, Dobbin MM, Fischer A, Sananbenesi F, Rodgers JT, et al. SIRT1 deacetylase protects against neurodegeneration in models for Alzheimer's disease and amyotrophic lateral sclerosis. *EMBO J* (2007) 26(13):3169–79. doi:10.1038/sj.emboj.7601758
37. Kairisalo M, Bonomo A, Hyrskyluoto A, Mudo G, Belluardo N, Korhonen L, et al. Resveratrol reduces oxidative stress and cell death and increases mitochondrial antioxidants and XIAP in PC6.3-cells. *Neurosci Lett* (2011) 488(3): 263–6. doi:10.1016/j.neulet.2010.11.042

19

The Versatility of Sirtuin-1 in Endocrinology and Immunology

*Fahmida Rasha[1], Brianyell McDaniel Mims[1], Isabel Castro-Piedras[1], Betsy J. Barnes[2,3], Matthew B. Grisham[1], Rakhshanda Layeequr Rahman[4] and Kevin Pruitt[1]**

[1] Department of Immunology and Molecular Microbiology, Texas Tech University Health Sciences Center, Lubbock, TX, United States, [2] Laboratory of Autoimmune and Cancer Research, Center for Autoimmune Musculoskeletal and Hematopoietic Disease, The Feinstein Institutes for Medical Research, Manhasset, NY, United States, [3] Department of Molecular Medicine and Department of Pediatrics, Zucker School of Medicine at Hofstra-Northwell, Hempstead, NY, United States, [4] Department of Surgery, Texas Tech University Health Sciences Center, Lubbock, TX, United States

***Correspondence:**
Kevin Pruitt
kevin.pruitt@ttuhsc.edu

Sirtuins belong to the class III family of NAD-dependent histone deacetylases (HDAC) and are involved in diverse physiological processes that range from regulation of metabolism and endocrine function to coordination of immunity and cellular responses to stress. Sirtuin-1 (SIRT1) is the most well-studied family member and has been shown to be critically involved in epigenetics, immunology, and endocrinology. The versatile roles of SIRT1 include regulation of energy sensing metabolic homeostasis, deacetylation of histone and non-histone proteins in numerous tissues, neuro-endocrine regulation via stimulation of hypothalamus-pituitary axes, synthesis and maintenance of reproductive hormones via steroidogenesis, maintenance of innate and adaptive immune system via regulation of T- and B-cell maturation, chronic inflammation and autoimmune diseases. Moreover, SIRT1 is an appealing target in various disease contexts due to the promise of pharmacological and/or natural modulators of SIRT1 activity within the context of endocrine and immune-related disease models. In this review we aim to provide a broad overview on the role of SIRT1 particularly within the context of endocrinology and immunology.

Keywords: SIRT1, SIRTUIN, endocrinology, immunology, autoimmune disease, cancer, development, therapy

INTRODUCTION

There are four classes of histone deacetylases (HDACs), namely, class I, II, III, and IV. HDAC1 – HDAC11 belong to class I, II, and IV while sirtuins belong to the class III HDAC family. Sirtuin-1 (SIRT1) is the most well-studied member of this family and its activity is NAD+-dependent, unlike the class I, II, and IV HDACs. Early on the yeast counterpart (Sir2) was shown to play a critical role in regulating DNA accessibility. However, over the last decade our understanding of the function and targets of sirtuins has increased. SIRT1 is an evolutionary conserved enzyme whose presence can be traced to archaea. The number of sirtuin family members, varies across species and varies from a single family member in bacteria to seven in mammals (Frye, 2000; Greiss and Gartner, 2009). Notably, human sirtuins are involved in a myriad of cellular processes that impact wide-ranging cellular processes from T cell differentiation to endocrine function. As key regulators of homeostasis, dysregulated sirtuin activity is associated with a wide spectrum of diseases. Even though our understanding of their role in aging, cancer, metabolic syndrome, neuropathologies, and autoimmune diseases (ADs) is increasing, the complexity of their contribution continues to make it difficult to draw firm conclusions about causation or mechanisms. However, regardless of this complexity, there is a consensus in recognizing that sirtuins may serve as potential therapeutic targets. This review will focus on SIRT1 and will discuss its role in the context of epigenetics, immunology, and endocrinology. It will provide a broad historical overview and will also highlight recent discoveries of the importance of post-translational acetylation particularly within the context of endocrinology and immunology. We point the reader to previous excellent reviews that focus more on the role of SIRT1 in aging (Longo and Kennedy, 2006), adaptive cellular responses (Anastasiou and Krek, 2006), and endocrine signaling (Yang et al., 2006).

Overview of Histone Deacetylases

Histone acetyltransferases (HATs), also referred to as lysine acetyltransferases (KATs), were the first enzymes shown to modify histones (Allfrey et al., 1964; Marmorstein, 2001; Allis et al., 2007; Pruitt, 2016) and have since been shown to modify numerous non-histone proteins (Saxena et al., 2013; Knyphausen et al., 2015; Pandey et al., 2015; Di et al., 2016; Tapias and Wang, 2017; Molehin et al., 2018). Protein acetylation involves acetyl-coenzyme A (acetyl-CoA) and therefore will be influenced by the cellular metabolic state (Peleg et al., 2016). While HATs/KATs are the writers of acetylation, the erasers are categorized as class I, II, III, and IV histone deacetylases. Additionally, the term lysine deacetylase (KDAC) will sometimes be used interchangeably with HDAC because this family deacetylates numerous non-histone proteins. The mechanism of deacetylation differentiates class I/II/IV HDACs from the sirtuins (class III). More than three decades ago histone deacetylase activity could be demonstrated; however, it was not until 1996 that the first HDAC was identified (Taunton et al., 1996). Subsequently, multiple HDAC family members were cloned and characterized (Ng and Bird, 2000). There are currently at least 18 distinct members of HDAC family. Class I HDACs (HDAC1, 2, 3, and 8) are largely nuclear proteins and are homologous to yeast RPD3 protein (Emiliani et al., 1998; Yang and Seto, 2008). Class II HDACs (HDAC4, 5, 6, 7, 9, and 10) shuttle between the nucleus and cytoplasm and are homologous to yeast Hda1 protein and are generally expressed in a tissue-specific manner (Fischle et al., 1999; Grozinger et al., 1999). HDAC 11 does not conform to the sequence similarity of class I or II, so it is considered a class IV HDAC (Gregoretti et al., 2004). In mammals, the sirtuin family (SIRT1-7) comprises the class III HDACs, and among them SIRT1 is the human homolog of yeast Sir2 (Blander and Guarente, 2004). While the class I, II, and IV, deacetylases are Zn^{2+}-dependent deacetylases, sirtuins catalyze the deacetylation reaction in a NAD^{+}-dependent manner. For the removal of every acetyl group from the substrate, one NAD^{+} is hydrolyzed resulting in a deacetylated protein and the reaction products, *O*-acetyl-ADP-ribose and nicotinamide. Nicotinamide is the amide derivative of vitamin B3 and can act as part of a negative feedback inhibitor of sirtuins. The role of the other reaction product, *O*-acetyl-ADP-ribose, is less clear, but some reports suggest that it influences cellular metabolic pathways (Pazienza et al., 2014), chromatin structure (Tung et al., 2017), and epigenetic gene silencing (Wang S. H. et al., 2019).

Role of SIRT1 in Histone Protein Deacetylation

It is remarkable that billions of cells with identical genomes show tissue-specificity. This is achieved by regulating transcription via a mechanism that links transcription potential with specific chromatin structures and epigenetic states. Chromatin can be defined as the sum of DNA, histones and associated RNA and it not only regulates transcription but also serves to compact and protect DNA. The general chromatin structure is influenced by epigenetic states. In general, "epigenetics" refers to a heritable pattern of gene expression that is not the result of alterations in the primary nucleotide sequence of a gene. The specific epigenetic state is the result of dynamic and reversible covalent modifications to DNA or post-translational modifications to histones. These so called "epigenetic marks" involve post-translational modifications to histone tails (such as acetylation, phosphorylation, ubiquitylation, methylation, and sumoylation) and methylation of DNA (Martin and Zhang, 2005; Nightingale et al., 2006; Ting et al., 2006). SIRT1 plays a role in deacetylating key lysines on histone H1, H3, and H4 which will directly impact chromatin structure and the accessibility of promoters to transcriptional activators (Pruitt et al., 2006; Alexander et al., 2007; Dawson and Kouzarides, 2012; Pruitt, 2016). SIRT1 has been shown to deacetylate a number of critical lysines such as histone H3 lysine 9 (H3K9) and histone H4 lysine 16 (H4K16) which collectively determine whether a gene is transcribed. CpG islands are typically associated with the promoter regions of genes where the methylation status correlates with transcription (Herman and Baylin, 2003). CpG methylation often works in concert with other epigenetic modifications such as histone hypoacetylation. The extent of histone acetylation impacts chromatin structure and gene transcription and the acetylation status of H3K9 and H4K16 influences recruitment of co-repressors and gene expression (Bannister et al., 2001; Nakayama et al., 2001). SIRT1 influences the epigenome in two distinct ways. First, as discussed above, it can directly deacetylate a number of key lysines on multiple histones. SIRT1 has been shown to regulate H3K9 and H4K16 at promoters wherein DNA methylation is enriched and contribute to epigenetic silencing of genes that modulate Wnt signaling (Pruitt et al., 2006). Second, SIRT1 can deacetylate other epigenetic enzymes that add (writers) or remove (erasers) epigenetic marks. In the case of an epigenetic writer that deposits DNA methylation on cytosine residues, DNA methyl transferase 1 (DNMT1) is a target of SIRT1 mediated deacetylation. However, the effect of DNMT1 deacetylation depends on the location of the lysine targeted and will dictate whether its DNA methyltransferase-dependent activity is augmented or whether its methyltransferase-independent transcription repression is limited (Peng et al., 2011). Regardless of whether SIRT1 is deacetylating histones or epigenetic writers, readers or erasers, the net effect will lead to important epigenomic changes. One particularly interesting example involves SIRT1 regulating the onset of puberty based on metabolic and nutritional cues. Kiss1 is a gene that controls the onset of female puberty based on its expression which is controlled by epigenetic mechanisms. Interestingly, SIRT1 is expressed in hypothalamic neurons and suppresses Kiss1 expression by partnering with polycomb group (PcG) proteins that mediate epigenetic silencing. With the onset of puberty, SIRT1 is evicted from the Kiss1 promoter, the gene is activated, and the brake on the hypothalamic-pituitary-gonad axis is released. Undernutrition has been shown to repress the onset of puberty whereas obesity has been shown to induce early onset (Vazquez et al., 2018). Moreover, beyond the effects in neurons, SIRT1 signaling in astrocytes also contributes to metabolic and reproductive regulation and deacetylase-deficient SIRT1 impairs the estrous cycles, decreases luteinizing hormone (LH) surges, and leads to fewer corpora lutea (Choi et al., 2019). While SIRT1 influences the epigenetic activation and repression of many critical genes, the recurring mechanism of its involvement will be to either directly regulate chromatin structure via histone-deacetylation or indirectly regulate it via deacetylation of chromatin modifying enzymes.

Role of SIRT1 in Non-histone Protein Deacetylation

Acetylation as a Regulator of Protein Function

Introduction of acetyl functional groups to histones was discovered more than five decades ago when it was associated with more accessible DNA (Allfrey et al., 1964). However, in recent years the study of acetylation is expanding outside its well-known histone context. Using high-resolution mass spectroscopy, Choudhary and his team were able to make an acetylome portrait by identifying 3600 lysine acetylation sites on 1750 proteins (Choudhary et al., 2009). Acetylation is recognized as one of the most common epigenetic modifications (Polevoda and Sherman, 2000) while also shaping the activity, location and stability of non-histone proteins. Acetylation regulates pathways in major cellular compartments including nucleus, plasma membrane, cytosol, and mitochondria and regulates metabolism, cell growth and insulin/insulin-like signaling (Pirola et al., 2012; Shi and Tu, 2014). Lysine acetylation of mitochondrial proteins was underappreciated until recently even though more than 20% of mitochondrial proteins are acetylated (Kim S. C. et al., 2006). Ghanta et al. (2013) propose that the mitochondrial acetylome acts as an energy consumption/storage switch. For instance, when a cell is exposed to constant energy excess or over-nutrition, malate dehydrogenase 2 (MDH2) is activated by hyperacetylation and inactivates energy consumption and promotes energy storage (e.g., gluconeogenesis) (Zhao et al., 2010). However, many other mitochondrial enzymes including superoxide dismutase 2 (Qiu et al., 2010), acetyl-CoA synthetases (Hallows et al., 2006), and glutamate dehydrogenase (Schlicker et al., 2008) are regulated by acetylation. Disturbance in lysine acetyl transferase activity causes cells to lose their ability to appropriately interpret the stress cues. Because of the reversibility of acetylation/deacetylation enzymatic reactions, there is increasing interest in exploiting this post-translational modification for therapeutic purposes. Currently, class I/II histone deacetylases are the targets of several molecule inhibitors in various phases of clinical trials, where some agents have yielded highly promising results (Johnstone, 2002; Rosato and Grant, 2004).

SIRT1 Deacetylates Many Non-histone Proteins

One of the challenges of sorting out the impact of pharmacologic inhibition of histone modifying enzymes is that non-histone proteins are also substrates. For example, SIRT1 knockdown in multiple colon cancer and breast cancer cells was shown to induce p53 activation by acetylation in the absence of conventional stress and induced either apoptosis or growth arrest, depending on the cell type (Ford et al., 2005). In a different study, SIRT1 was shown to bind and deacetylate estrogen related receptor α (ERRα) which resulted in enhancement of its DNA-binding potential (Wilson et al., 2010). Interestingly, ERRα is one of the transcription factors that regulates transcription of the CYP19A1 gene which encodes for the aromatase protein. Aromatase is the enzyme that converts testosterone to estrogen in the estrogen biosynthesis pathway and aromatase inhibitors are used for treatment of breast cancer. Another report demonstrated that inhibition of SIRT1 reduced aromatase mRNA and protein levels in estrogen receptor negative (ER−) breast cancer cells possibly due to loss of ERRα binding to the aromatase promoter and subsequent inhibition of aromatase transcription (Holloway et al., 2013). While SIRT1 is shown to promote many cancer phenotypes, a positive regulator of many cancer hallmarks (Hanahan and Weinberg, 2011), and is overexpressed in human cancer specimens compared to normal tissue, some reports from transgenic mouse models have identified tumor suppressor properties of SIRT1 (Firestein et al., 2008). Some of the controversy regarding whether SIRT1 acts in an oncogenic or tumor suppressive manner may be better reconciled as we consider the difference in multiple experimental designs. For example, two studies came to different conclusions regarding the *in vivo* influence of SIRT1 on tumor biology. Both studies used $APC^{min/+}$ mouse models (with germline mutation in the APC tumor suppressor gene) that enabled spontaneous adenomatous polyps and hyperplasia resulting in colon cancer. Both studies investigated the role of SIRT1 in colon tumorigenesis. Firestein et al. (2008) used conditional overexpression of SIRT1 in the intestine to show fewer polyps. However, Leko et al. (2013) used a conditional enterocyte-specific SIRT1 knockout and observed reduced tumor size and number of polyps, with no changes in proliferation but an increase in apoptosis of tumor cells in knockouts vs. wild type $APC^{min/+}$mice. Since the gain-of-function and loss-of function phenotypes were similar, Leko et al. (2013) argued that super-physiological levels of SIRT1 (as in the Firestein study) due to overexpression, might somehow be causing stoichiometry changes in protein complexes resulting in the inactivation of the overexpressed protein. These types of differences in experimental design need to be weighed as studies seeking to label chromatin regulators as tumor suppressers or oncogenes. More recent studies have identified several novel non-histone targets of SIRT1 including DNA methylation readers (MeCP2) and Dishevelled proteins which are critical regulators of Wnt signaling (Saxena et al., 2013; Knyphausen et al., 2015; Pandey et al., 2015; Di et al.,

2016; Tapias and Wang, 2017; Molehin et al., 2018). Both MeCP2 and DVL1 and 3 are deacetylated by SIRT1. MeCP2 deacetylation regulates its binding to co-repressors (Saxena et al., 2013; Knyphausen et al., 2015; Pandey et al., 2015; Di et al., 2016; Tapias and Wang, 2017; Molehin et al., 2018). SIRT1 activity regulates DVL1 binding to TIAM1, an activator of Rac that is important for cell migration. SIRT1-mediated DVL1 deacetylation on critical sites in the DIX and PDX domain regulates its sub-cellular localization and ability to activate CYP19A1 promoters (Sharma et al., 2018, 2019).

SIRT1 AND ENDOCRINE FUNCTION

The importance of SIRT1 in metabolism has been clearly established since its discovery and for a more in-depth review of the role of sirtuins in metabolism, we point the reader to other excellent reviews discussing sirtuins role in lipid metabolism (Simmons et al., 2015; Ye et al., 2017). In the following sections we will focus on the role of SIRT1 in the regulation of endocrine signaling and hormone production.

Connections With Hypothalamus-Pituitary Axes

Recent publications clearly demonstrate SIRT1 involvement in transcription and metabolic processes via hormonal production and homeostasis regulation in the neuroendocrine system (Yang et al., 2006; Cohen et al., 2009; Chang and Guarente, 2014). The hypothalamic pituitary axes play an integral role in mediating SIRT1 specific hormonal control in the neuroendocrine system. The hypothalamus regulates body temperature, hunger, thirst, energy expenses, emotion/behavior, circadian rhythm of organisms and thus maintains body homeostasis. In addition, hypothalamic cues such as synthesis or secretion of hypothalamic hormones induce or inhibit synthesis or secretion of pituitary hormones (Markakis, 2002; Xie and Dorsky, 2017). Pituitary hormones regulate hormone secretion by respective target organs via systemic blood circulation and hence a pathway is established from hypothalamus to target organs via the pituitary glands known as the 'hypothalamus-pituitary axis.' There are four major hypothalamus-pituitary axes found in the circulation based on specific target organ. These are: (i) hypothalamus-pituitary-adrenal (HPA) axis, (ii) hypothalamus-pituitary-thyroid (HPT) axis, (iii) hypothalamus-pituitary-gonadal (HPG) axis, and (iv) somatotropic axis (Yamamoto and Takahashi, 2018). Below we will briefly discuss the connection between SIRT1, hypothalamus and four different hypothalamus-pituitary axes in regulation of endocrine synthesis and signaling.

Hypothalamic SIRT1's Role in Maintenance of Body Homeostasis

Researchers reported SIRT1 expression in steroidogenic factor 1 (SF1), proopiomelanocortin (POMC) and agouti related peptide (AgRP) neurons of the ventromedial hypothalamic nucleus (VMH) and arcuate nucleus (ARH) respectively (Sasaki et al., 2014; Orozco-Solis et al., 2015). In addition, SF1 specific SIRT1 deletion induced insulin resistance while SIRT1 overexpression in SF1 resulted in insulin sensitivity and prevention of diet-induced obesity in skeletal muscles of transgenic type 2 diabetic mice (Ramadori et al., 2011). Moreover, targeted SIRT1 overexpression in POMC and/or AgRP neurons prevented weight gain and improved energy expenditure *in vivo* (Sasaki et al., 2014). Hypothalamic SIRT1 is also involved in regulation of feeding behavior, emotion, and physiological rhythms. For instance, SIRT1 regulates *in vitro* transcription of anorexigenic/orexigenic neuropeptides in HEK293 cells via Foxo1-induced AgRP promoter activity (Sasaki et al., 2010) while SIRT1 upregulation in the brain induced *in vivo* anxiety via increased transcription of genes encoding monoamine oxidase-A (Mo-A) enzyme (Mo-A inhibitors are involved in clinical depression and anxiety treatment) (Libert et al., 2011). Additionally, significant increase in food anticipatory activity was found among transgenic mice with brain-specific SIRT1 overexpression while SIRT1 knockdown reversed such activity in mice (Satoh et al., 2010). These results indicate crucial region-centric role of hypothalamic SIRT1 and its possible involvement in modulating hypothalamus-pituitary axes' metabolic functions in the neuroendocrine system.

The HPA axis is an important part of the neuroendocrine system that controls survival, metabolism, immunity, appetite, stress, emotion, and behavior of an organism. Stress response begins in the HPA axis with corticotrophin releasing hormone (CRH) secretion by the hypothalamic paraventricular nucleus (PVN) and via POMC production by the pituitary corticotroph. POMC respectively cleaved by prohormone convertase 1 and 2 (PC1 and PC2) in the pituitary corticotroph, thus results in synthesis of adrenocorticotropic hormone (ACTH) and α-melanocyte stimulating hormone (α-MSH). ACTH then triggers glucocorticoid production by the adrenal cortex responding to stress conditions (Yates et al., 2013; Yamamoto and Takahashi, 2018). Though researchers reported lack of connection between POMC specific SIRT1 induction/ablation with HPA axis activation during *in vivo* fasting conditions (Ramadori et al., 2010), SIRT1 increased PC2 levels in the PVN resulting in increased CRH production and HPA axis stimulation in high-fat diet fed mice (Toorie et al., 2016). Moreover, SIRT1 activator, resveratrol increased PC1 and PC2 levels while SIRT1 inhibitor, EX-527, decreased PC1 and PC2 levels in mouse corticotroph cell line (AtT20) suggesting indirect HPA axis modulating roles of SIRT1 via PC1 and PC2 (Toorie and Nillni, 2014; Toorie et al., 2016). Further, SIRT1 overexpression reduced corticosterone (CORT) mediated autophagy and induced apoptosis while SIRT1 knockdown reversed the results during chronic cellular stress *in vitro* indicating SIRT1 involvement in stress management via HPA axis (Jiang et al., 2019). Hence, these results clearly denote SIRT1 levels in hypothalamus, pituitary and adrenal glands regulate HPA axis functions in response to feeding/fasting and stress conditions.

Next, another major axis in hypothalamus and pituitary connection is the HPT axis which is activated when the hypothalamus senses reduced levels of thyroid hormone in the circulation. This is followed by release of thyrotropin-releasing hormone (TRH) from hypothalamus stimulating thyroid stimulating hormone (TSH) secretion by the pituitary and production of thyroid hormones (TH) by the thyroid organs. Thus normal TH level in the circulation is maintained (Sam and Frohman, 2008). SIRT1 is expressed in TSH producing thyrotroph cells and increases cellular endocytosis via deacetylation of enzyme involved in phosphatidylinositol-4,5-bisphosphate synthesis *in vitro*. On the other hand, *in vivo* SIRT1 knockout reduced TSH secretion via phosphatidylinositol-4-phosphate 5-kinase type 1γ (enzyme) acetylation indicating SIRT1 role in regulating hormone production possibly via HPT axis stimulation (Akieda-Asai et al., 2010). Similarly, serum thyroxin (T4) levels dropped in calorie-restricted SIRT1 knockout (KO) mice followed by reduced physical activity while non-calorie restricted SIRT1-KO mice were hypermetabolic, had inefficient hepatic mitochondria and increased lipid oxidation rates (Boily et al., 2008). In lieu, thyroxin treatment repressed hepatic SIRT1 expression and activity in 48 h fasted mice via TH receptor β indicating negative correlation between serum T4 and hepatic SIRT1 levels *in vivo* (Cordeiro et al., 2013). These data represent close connection between SIRT1 and HPT axis in hormonal regulation and energy metabolism.

The HPG axis plays major role in hypothalamus and pituitary connection via management of reproduction and life cycle. Gonadotropin-releasing hormone (GnRH) secreted from hypothalamic GnRH neurons forms a network which stimulates secretion of LH and follicle-stimulating hormone (FSH) by the pituitary gonadotroph cells followed by production of estrogen or testosterone by the gonads (Sam and Frohman, 2008). SIRT1 knockout mice showed diminished HPG endocrine signaling as identified by twofold reduction in hypothalamic GnRH expression, followed by reduced serum LH and FSH levels and arrested spermatogenesis as confirmed by histological analyses of animal testes (Kolthur-Seetharam et al., 2009). In addition, *in vitro* GnRH administration reduced post-transcriptional SIRT1 levels via induced action of miR-132/212 in the pituitary and downregulation of SIRT1 dependent Foxo1 deacetylation (Lannes et al., 2015). Besides recent investigations are also focused on SIRT1 role in puberty and infertility associated diseases during energy deficiency and abundance (Tatone et al., 2018; Vazquez et al., 2019), but their connections with HPG axis are yet to be explored.

In the somatotropic axis, the hypothalamus induces growth hormone (GH) secretion by pituitary somatotroph cells via releasing GH releasing hormone (GHRH). GH then binds to hepatic GH receptors leading to increased insulin like growth factor-1 (IGF-1) levels in the circulation. Additionally, local IGF-1 production by various tissues like bone, muscle and adipose tissue is also stimulated by GH (Sam and Frohman, 2008). Studies across different species reported progressive interaction between SIRT1 and the somatotropic pathways (Tissenbaum and Guarente, 2001; Al-Regaiey et al., 2005; Gan et al., 2005; Parrella and Longo, 2010) where reduced functionality in these pathways results in lifespan extension in both invertebrate and mammalian models (Bartke et al., 2013; Milman et al., 2016). SIRT1 brain-specific knockout (BS-KO) mice demonstrated dwarfism, smaller pituitary gland and diminished circulatory and hepatic levels of GH and IGF-1 though serum levels of other pituitary hormones remained unaltered in those animals (Cohen et al., 2009). This might be due to hypothalamic dysfunctions in absence of SIRT1 in those animals (Cohen et al., 2009), but how hypothalamic SIRT1 regulates somatotropic axis in hypothalamus-pituitary crosstalk is not known yet. Similarly, SIRT6 BS-KO mice exhibited postnatal growth retardation along with reduced serum GH and IGF-1 levels, however, hypothalamic GHRH and somatotropin release inhibiting factor (SRIF) levels were unchanged (Schwer et al., 2010). Such abnormalities might be due to impaired hypothalamic functions and dysregulated feedback mechanisms in absence of SIRT6 in those animals. Additionally, SIRT1 activation via resveratrol in rat somatotropic cells reduced GH secretory levels both *in vivo* and *in vitro*. Here, SIRT1 activation and overexpression suppressed cAMP response element binding protein (CREB) phosphorylation and glycogen synthase kinase 3 beta (GSK3β) deacetylation via protein phosphatase 1 which, in turn, transcriptionally deactivates CREB resulting in GHRH-mediated GH suppression (Monteserin-Garcia et al., 2013). From the above discussion, it is clear that SIRT1 is involved in regulating hormonal production and functions in the neuroendocrine system via modulating four major hypothalamic-pituitary axes. However, it is critical to understand that sirtuins can switch roles to adapt during low vs. high energy states by modulating hypothalamic-pituitary axes at various steps.

Connections to Steroidogenesis

Steroidogenesis involves conversion of cholesterol to sex hormones such as androgens, estrogens, and progesterone as well as to other steroid hormones such as glucocorticoids, mineralocorticoids to regulate cellular development and physiology via modulation of transcription and post-transcriptional modifications of various tissue-specific steroidogenic enzymes and co-factors (Bremer and Miller, 2014). SIRT1 can deacetylate histone and non-histone proteins in an energy-sensitive manner and regulate steroid hormone receptor activity. For example, SIRT1 can repress transcription of estrogen and androgen receptors via deacetylation while modulate progesterone receptors transcription via nucleo-cytosolic shuttling of the receptor and induction of slow vs. rapid progesterone response genes (Moore et al., 2012). Particularly, SIRT1 controls the activity of multiple steroid hormones via different mechanisms in cancer. Since SIRT1 overexpression is associated with poor survival and prognostic outcomes including higher lymph node metastases in cancer patients (Wu et al., 2012), post-translational modifications of SIRT1 such as deacetylation, phosphorylation, sumoylation determine hormonal dependence and -independence of multiple cancers through understanding the interactive association between SIRT1 and steroid hormone receptors. Moore et al. (2012) elaborately discussed different mechanisms involved in regulation of SIRT1 and steroid hormone receptors interaction. Below we will briefly discuss steroid hormone receptor modulatory roles of SIRT1 with respect to different diseased conditions.

(i) Regulation of androgen receptors (AR): SIRT1 is able to modulate AR activity via direct deacetylation, leading to inhibition of AR activation, translocation and transcription of AR-dependent genes, for instance in prostate cancer. SIRT1 inhibited AR-dependent prostate cancer cell growth and induced endogenous *AR* target genes repression while SIRT1 antagonists induced expression of AR-responsive target genes (*AR*) both *in vivo* and *in vitro* (Fu et al., 2006; Kojima et al., 2008). Similarly, shRNA mediated SIRT1 knockdown enhanced cell proliferation and reduced autophagy by inhibited phosphorylation of S6K and 4E-BP1 while SIRT1 activation by resveratrol reversed these effects in androgen-responsive prostate cancer cells (Fu et al., 2006; Li et al., 2013). On the other hand, androgen antagonists promote physical association of SIRT1 with transcriptional co-repressor, NCoR and AR, thus recruiting SIRT1 and NCoR to the AR target genes' promoter region followed by inducing local deacetylation of histone H3K9 in the promoter regions. This finding by Dai et al. (2007) demonstrated ligand-dependent recruitment of SIRT1 into a transcriptional co-repressor complex inducing AR-mediated transcriptional repression for the first time. Apart from this, researchers also reported AR-sensitive prostate cancer progression via (a) transcriptional association between NF-κB and SIRT1 (Jaganathan et al., 2014), (b) SIRT1 dependent transcriptional upregulation of VEGF-C and downregulation of the IGF-1R pathway (Li et al., 2005), and (c) via endogenous SIRT1 mediated induction of autophagy in cultured cells (Powell et al., 2011). Meanwhile, SIRT1 activation in BRCA1 overexpressed breast cancer cells inhibited AR expression and AR-stimulated cancer cell proliferation (Zhang et al., 2016). These results suggest critical role of SIRT1 in regulating cancer-specific AR signaling while loss of SIRT1 activity might result in loss of AR transcriptional control leading to ineffectual hormone-replacement therapy in multiple cancers.

(ii) Regulation of estrogen receptors (ER): SIRT1 leads to repressed ERα translocation from cytosol to nucleus resulting in reduced ERα binding and target gene transcription. SIRT1 expression is highly elevated by stimulated 17-β-estradiol (E2) levels in most ERα-positive breast cancer samples (Elangovan et al., 2011; Lee et al., 2011) while SIRT1 inhibition leads to ER signaling inhibition (Yao et al., 2010) implying SIRT1 role as ERα co-activator. SIRT1 dependent ERα inhibition resulted in E2-mediated suppression of cell growth in both healthy and malignant mammary epithelial cells (Yao et al., 2010). Moreover, SIRT1 has been found to interact with p300, PPARγ, PGC1α, and ERα transcriptomic co-activators thus regulating developmental processes such as chromatin remodeling (Picard et al., 2004; Rodgers et al., 2005). In addition, published work from our lab demonstrated that SIRT1 regulates estrogen production at two levels. First, SIRT1 binds multiple tissue-specific aromatase promoters and its inhibition decreases aromatase transcripts (Holloway et al., 2013; Molehin et al., 2018). Second, the aromatase protein itself is a target of SIRT1-mediated deacetylation (Holloway et al., 2013; Molehin et al., 2018). E2-mediated ERα activation also resulted in p300 mediated stabilization of the receptor via acetylation which can be reversed by SIRT1 (Kim M. Y. et al., 2006) implying SIRT1 inhibitory action on ER are mostly estrogen dependent. However, researchers also reported contradictory SIRT1 role as ERα repressor especially in breast cancer. Resveratrol inhibited breast cancer cell growth and upregulated SIRT1 mRNA and protein expression (Lin et al., 2010) while SIRT1 pharmacological inhibitor, sirtinol and splitomicin along with anti-SIRT1 siRNA demonstrated repressed SIRT1 activity, resulting in inhibited ERα-mediated cancer gene transcription in an estrogen-independent manner. Such SIRT1 inhibition (pharmacological/siRNA) leads to PI3K/Akt dependent ERα inhibition and repressed estrogen-dependent breast cancer cell growth (Moore et al., 2012). In addition, aberrant SIRT1 activity also leads to ER-dependent alterations in FOXO-family transcriptional deregulations (FOXOM1, FOXO3a) especially in triple negative breast cancer (Lee et al., 2016) while SIRT1 overexpression is observed in ER−/Her2+ breast cancer cells with E2 interactions with G-protein coupled ERs (GPER) via activation of EGFR/ERK/c-fos/AP-1 signal transduction pathways (Santolla et al., 2015). Intriguingly, induced cell proliferation via such interaction can be reversed by either SIRT1 inhibition or GPER silencing (Santolla et al., 2015). However, knowledge is still limited regarding the interplay between SIRT1 and GPER modulation in cancer progression. On a different note, SIRT1/ERα signaling has anti-oxidant function in different preclinical models of chronic disease and is involved in reducing oxidative stress, neuroinflammation and preventing arterial stiffness via ameliorating JNK/NF-κB signaling, and via upregulating endothelial nitric oxide synthase (eNOS) expression and reduced eNOS uncoupling, respectively (Khan et al., 2019; Li et al., 2019). Taken together, SIRT1 is integral in regulating ER-mediated transcriptional activity in different disease conditions, especially in cancers.

(iii) Inhibition of progesterone receptors (PR): SIRT1 via nucleo-cytoplasmic translocation of PR, leads to downstream activation of PR-regulated genes. The acetylated PR regulates the nuclear-cytosolic shuttling of the receptor and transcriptional activation of slow vs. rapid PR-responsive genes. For instance, acetylation-mimetics at the PR hinge region show delayed nuclear entry upon progesterone binding while acetylation-deficient mutants induced rapid *c-MYC* (a rapid PR-responsive gene) gene expression compared to wild type (Daniel et al., 2010). Additionally, SIRT1/c-MYC builds a negative feedback loop in such a way that c-MYC binds to SIRT1 promoter region upregulating its expression whereas SIRT1 deacetylates c-MYC reducing its transformative stability (Yuan et al., 2009). This further suppress cell proliferation and induce cell cycle arrest at G1/S phase suggesting PR-dependent SIRT1/c-MYC role in tumorigenesis (Mao et al., 2011). However, it is still not known whether SIRT1 is able to deacetylate PR itself in healthy vs. diseased condition. *In vitro* administration of SIRT1 agonists are also involved in induced progesterone secretion. Resveratrol enhanced serum progesterone levels by threefold after 48 h of culture while visfatin (an adipocytokine and SIRT1 inducer) treatment induced ~2-fold increase in progesterone secretion compared to basal state in rat and human granulosa cells, respectively (Morita et al., 2012; Reverchon et al., 2013). On the other hand, when T47D breast cancer cells were treated with nicotinamide (NAM), a SIRT1 inhibitor, PR-responsive gene transcription was decreased in a dose-dependent manner. Surprisingly, specific siRNA-mediated SIRT1 inhibition demonstrated SIRT1 independent PR-transcriptional repression. Hence, the authors reported a SIRT1 independent mechanism of NAM which inhibits the coordination of basal transcription machinery assembly of the progesterone-responsive promoter after chromatin remodeling and likelihood of off-target NAM effects apart from SIRT1 inhibitory effects (Aoyagi and Archer, 2008). Therefore, selecting a more specific SIRT1 inhibitor to investigate its role in PR regulation is warranted.

(iv) Regulation of glucocorticoid receptor (GR) signaling: SIRT1 and GR activity can be better described in light of myocyte metabolism. SIRT1 regulates deacetylation of the GR and its ability to interact with co-activator p300 through maintaining cellular NAD/NADH ratio. Induced GR ligand binding activates SIRT1 co-regulatory protein p300 leading to increased uncoupling protein-3 (UCP3) gene transcription (involved in mitochondrial stress response). SIRT1 then represses UCP3 transcription by preventing GR and p300 interaction at the promoter (Amat et al., 2007). Therefore, SIRT1 and GR interaction controls the metabolic state of cells, acting as an energy sensor via cellular NAD/NADH regulation and linking the transcriptional parameters of metabolic genes to the stress response. SIRT1 is involved in preventing glucocorticoid induced muscle wasting and mitochondrial dysfunction as reported by many researchers (Knobloch et al., 2014; Poulsen et al., 2014; Chiu et al., 2018; Ma et al., 2019). Resveratrol prevented dexamethasone-induced acetylation of FOXO1, expression of atrogin-1 and muscle ring finger protein-1 (MuRF1), and protein degradation in cultured myotubes in a SIRT1 dependent manner (Alamdari et al., 2012). Moreover, SIRT1-mediated enhancement of GR transcriptional activity independent of its deacetylation function was reported while SIRT1 knockdown reversed this phenomenon. At a molecular level, SIRT1 can physically interact with GR and glucocorticoid inducible proteins. SIRT1 further co-localizes with GR in the nucleus upon dexamethasone treatment and regulates GR transcriptional activity by cooperating with PGC1α in a deacetylase independent manner as shown in three different human cancer (cervical, colon, hepatic) cell lines (Suzuki et al., 2018). This suggests an important role of SIRT1 and GR interplay in various human diseases.

(v) Regulation of mineralocorticoid receptors (MR): SIRT1 regulates MR via enhanced binding to disruptor of telomeric silencing-1 (DOT1) and thus repression of MR-regulated genes, which is independent of SIRT1 deacetylase activity. The MR and its ligand, aldosterone, maintain electrolyte balance in the kidney via induced renal tubular sodium absorption and increased transcription of epithelial sodium channel α-subunit (α-ENaC) (Fan et al., 2011). SIRT1 modulates aldosterone signaling in a MR-dependent manner via its physical interaction with DOT1, which is a histone methyltransferase. This results in H3K79 global hypermethylation in chromatin and α-ENaC 5'-flanking region leading to transcriptional repression. Although this process requires SIRT1 to support DOT1 hypermethylation, it is independent of SIRT1 deacetylase activity indicating SIRT1 is a novel modulator of aldosterone pathway (Zhang D. et al., 2009). In lieu, SIRT1 overexpression prevented aldosterone-induced mitochondrial damage and podocyte injury via upregulating PGC-1α transcription and translation while resveratrol lessened aldosterone-induced mitochondrial malfunction *in vitro* and in aldosterone-infused mice (Yuan et al., 2012). Additionally, MR regulates obesity-associated cardiovascular complications through regulating adipose tissue mitochondrial functions. Hence, MR antagonists prevented adipocytes senescence *in vivo* via reducing SIRT1 levels and blocking p53/p21 pathway (Lefranc et al., 2019) indicating the possibility of MR and SIRT1 mediated stress response in obesity. Furthermore, SIRT1 regulates adipocyte renin-angiotensin-aldosterone system (RAAS) via targeting MR. When mouse preadipocytes were treated with angiotensin (Ang) II, they showed upregulated MR and reduced SIRT1 levels which was reversed by antioxidant heme oxygenase-1 (HO-1) administration. However, SIRT1 knockdown in preadipocytes by specific siRNA increased lipid accumulation and fatty acid synthase levels *in vitro* indicating SIRT1 mediated beneficial effects of HO-1 in rescuing Ang II-induced impaired MR upregulation in adipose tissue (Lakhani et al., 2019). Together, these data suggest novel MR regulatory roles of SIRT1 both dependent and independent of its deacetylase function in multiple disease conditions.

ROLE OF SIRT1 IN INNATE AND ADAPTIVE IMMUNITY

The body is continuously exposed to a variety of different bacteria, viruses and fungi which can produce potentially lethal infections. Defense against these unwanted invaders is mediated by a series of synchronized and highly regulated responses that are referred to as innate and adaptive immunity (**Figure 1**). These two arms of the immune system not only protect against pathogenic microbes, but they are also capable of recognizing and eliminating abnormal cells such as tumor cells. Innate immunity provides for the rapid response to invading pathogens whereas adaptive immunity requires more time to initiate its multifaceted, antigen specific responses. The innate immune system consists of myeloid cells that include polymorphonuclear neutrophils (neutrophils), monocytes, macrophages, eosinophils, basophils and dendritic cells (DCs) as well as innate lymphoid cells (iLCs), natural killer (NK) cells and natural killer T (NKT) cells. The adaptive immune system consists of T and B cells. Most innate immune cells begin their development within the bone marrow (BM) from self-renewing, multi-potent hematopoietic stem cells (HSCs) that will give rise to lineage-specific myeloid progenitor and lymphoid progenitor cells (**Figure 2**). Common myeloid progenitor cells give rise to all granulocytes (neutrophils, eosinophils, basophils), monocytes, erythrocytes, and platelets. The second major progenitor cell in the BM is the common lymphoid progenitor (CLP) cell that produces NK cells and B cells (**Figure 2**). Once produced, all myeloid cells, NK cells and B cells are released into the systemic circulation where they continuously patrol the body for evidence of microbial invasion. Circulating monocytes will ultimately leave the circulation and enter different tissues where they undergo maturation resulting in the formation of tissue macrophages (Macs) and DCs. Unlike innate immune cells, T cells undergo a different developmental pathway. Some of the BM-residing CLP cells that give rise to NK, iLC and B cells enter the systemic circulation and traffic to the thymus where they differentiate into MHC class I (MHC I)-restricted $CD8^+$ T cells, MHC class II (MHC II)-restricted

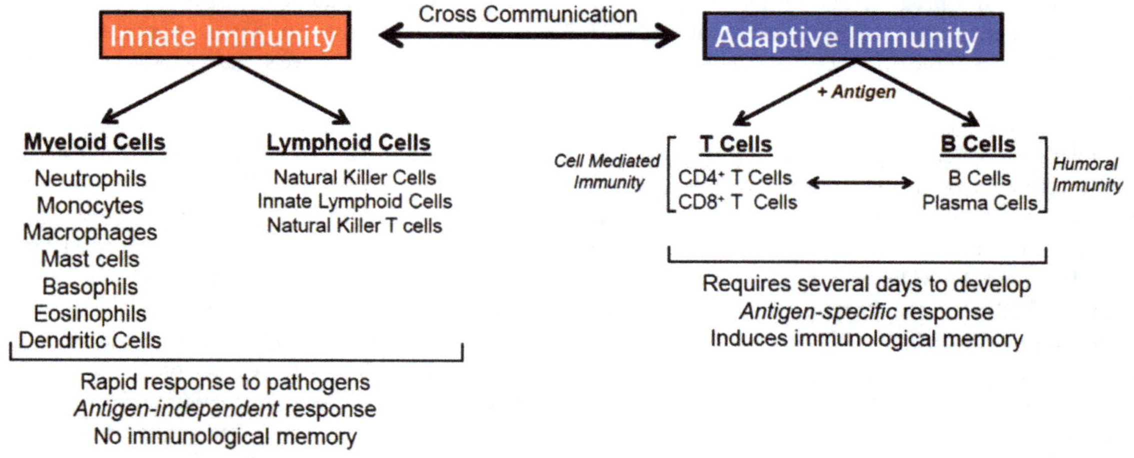

FIGURE 1 | Innate and adaptive immunity. Defense against invading microbes requires well-regulated interactions between innate and adaptive immune cells. Innate immune cells provide rapid responses (hours-days) to pathogens via the action of several different myeloid and lymphoid cells. Innate immune responses are antigen-independent and do not result in immunological memory. Adaptive immune cells (T and B cells) recognize a spectrum of microbial antigens that induce the activation and clonal expansion of thousands of antigen-specific lymphocytes. Highly specialized T and B cell responses to microbial antigens develop over the course of several days to weeks providing the host with long-lived memory T and B cells. T cells are required for cell-mediated immunity, a process by which activated T cells help kill pathogens that have been phagocytosed by macrophages and neutrophils. B cells and their tissue-associate counterparts (plasma cells) are required for humoral immunity via their ability to produce antigen specific antibodies that bind to and eliminate extracellular microorganisms. There are a number of interactions between and within innate and adaptive immune responses that enhance overall protection from pathogens.

$CD4^+$ T cells and NK T (NKT) cells (**Figure 2**). Mature $CD8^+$ T cells are referred to as cytotoxic T lymphocytes (CTLs) and are very effective at recognizing and killing host cells infected with intracellular pathogens (viruses, bacteria) or tumor cells. The thymus also produces a second lineage of $CD4^+$ T cells called thymus-derived regulatory T cells (tTregs) (Wing et al., 2019). These T cells express the transcription factor FOXP3 that is crucial for maintaining tolerance to self or autoantigens in the periphery. Although tTregs represent the majority of Tregs with in lymph nodes, BM and spleen, antigen activation of naïve $CD4^+$ T cells residing within the microenvironment of certain tissues such as the small and large bowel will induce the expression of Foxp3 thereby becoming peripheral Tregs (pTregs) (Wing et al., 2019; Campbell and Rudensky, 2020). Naïve $CD4^+$ T cells released by thymus will traffic to lymphoid tissue in search of their cognate antigens that are likely derived from invading microbes. Recognition of these antigens bound to MHC II on the surface of antigen presenting cells (e.g., DCs, Macs, B cells) will result in their activation, differentiation and clonal expansion of different subsets of antigen-specific T cells that produce a myriad of cytokines and chemokines. These mediators facilitate the recruitment and activation of other immune cells including macrophages, neutrophils, eosinophils, and basophils to sites of infection and inflammation where they help to destroy pathogenic micro-organisms. This section will discuss SIRT1 in immune cell development and how dysregulation may contribute to autoimmune and chronic inflammatory diseases.

Hematopoiesis

Numerous studies have suggested that SIRT1 plays an important role in HSC homeostasis, maturation, and lineage determination. Using global (i.e., germline) deletion of SIRT1, Leko et al. (2012) reported that *Sirt1*$^{-/-}$ mice contained frequencies and tissue distribution of hematopoietic progenitor populations as well as absolute numbers of differentiated blood cells similar to what was observed in wild type littermate controls. In addition, these investigators found that *Sirt1*$^{-/-}$ BM cells were capable of sustained reconstitution when transplanted into lethally irradiated recipients. Researchers concluded that SIRT1 signaling is dispensable in HSC homeostasis in mice. Because neonatal mortality in *Sirt1*$^{-/-}$ mice is relatively high with surviving littermates developing severe ADs (Zhang J. et al., 2009), investigators have generated mice with cell-specific deletion of Sirt1 to assess the role of this deacetylase in hematopoiesis. Singh et al. (2013) generated conditional Sirt1-deficient mice by interbreeding Sirt1-E4$^{floxed/floxed}$ mice to mice containing the 4-hydroxy-tamoxifen (4-OHT)–inducible ERT2-Cre transgene or by breeding Sirt1-E4$^{floxed/floxed}$ mice to mice containing the *vav-iCre* transgene which is predominantly expressed in BM progenitor cells. Both *Sirt1-E4*$^{fl/fl}$*/ERT2*^{Cre} and *Sirt1-E4*$^{fl/fl}$*/vav*^{iCre} were fed 4-OH for 11 weeks to ablate the *Sirt1* gene. These investigators demonstrated loss of Sirt1 in all tissues (*Sirt1-E4*$^{fl/fl}$*/ERT2*^{Cre} mice) or in BM-residing progenitor cells (*Sirt1-E4*$^{fl/fl}$*/vav*^{iCre}) promoted abnormal expansion of HSCs when mice were subjected to hematopoietic stress via administration of cytotoxic or genotoxic drugs (Singh et al., 2013). These atypical responses were associated with a high frequency of genomic mutations, DNA damage and loss of hematopoietic progenitor cells. In another study, Rimmele et al. (2014) reported that the conditional ablation of SIRT1 using a tamoxifen-inducible mouse model, resulted in defective self-renewal properties of HSCs, anemia and lymphocytopenia that was associated with an expansion of myeloid progenitor cells (i.e., granulocyte-monocyte progenitors).

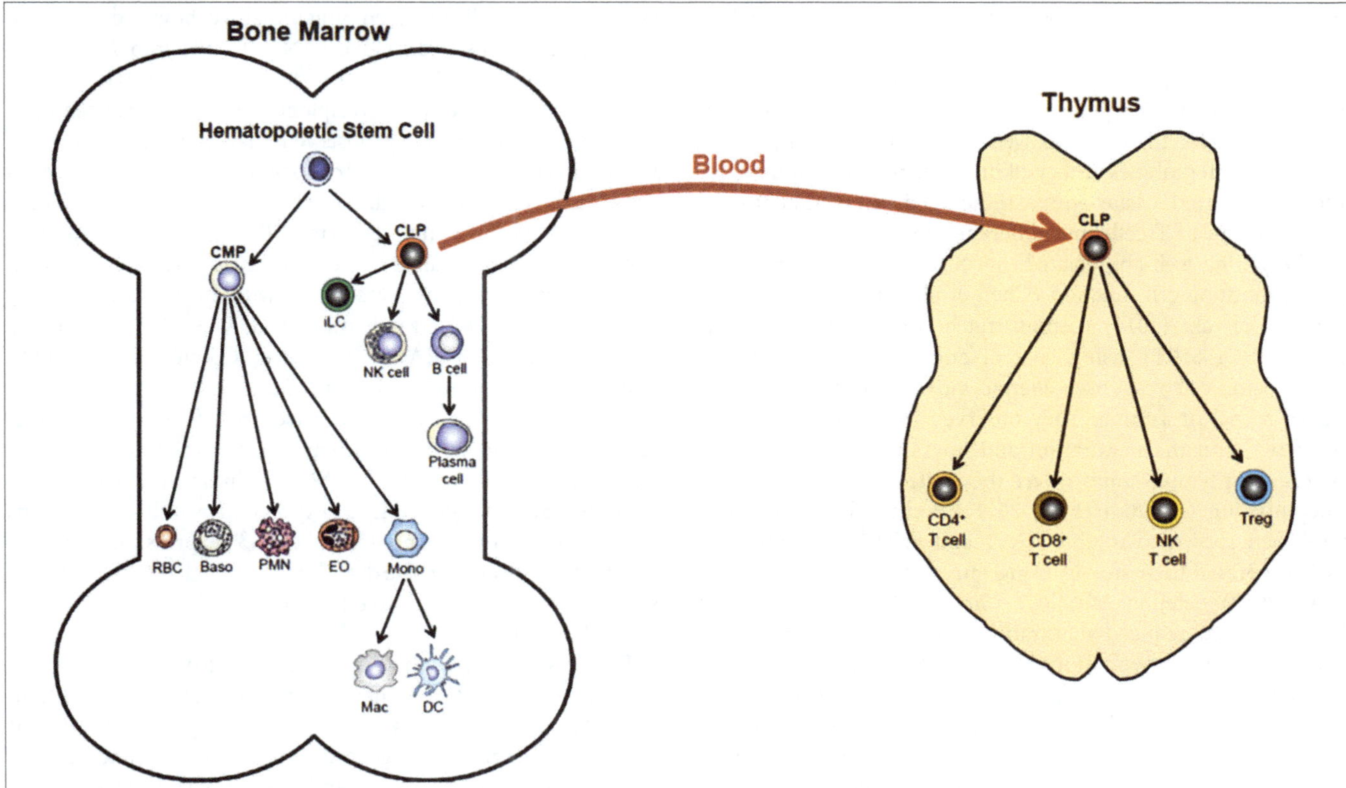

FIGURE 2 | Hematopoiesis. Differentiation of human multi-potent hematopoietic stem cells (HSCs) within the bone marrow (BM) is a complex and highly regulated process that produces most of all cellular elements of blood. The first step in differentiation of HSCs is the generation of lineage-specific progenitor cells called common myeloid progenitor cells (CMPs) and common lymphoid progenitor cells (CLPs). Differentiation of CMPs give rise to erythrocytes (RBC), basophils (Baso), polymorphonuclear neutrophils (PMN, neutrophils), eosinophils (EO) and monocytes (Mono). Monocytes may produce macrophages (Mac) and dendritic cells (DC) within the bone marrow. Monos also enter the blood and traffic to different tissue where they may give rise to Mac and DC. Differentiation of CLPs produce innate lymphoid cells (iLC), natural killer cells (NK cell), B cells and plasma cells. Some BM-residing CLPs will enter the blood and home to the thymus where they will differentiate into at least four additional immune cell populations including CD4+ T cells, CD8+ T cells, NK T cells and regulatory T cells (Treg). (This figure was modified from OpenStax Anatomy and Physiology, May18, 2016, with permission: Download for free at http://cnx.org/contents/14fb4ad7-39a1-4eee-ab6e-3ef2482e3e22@8.25).

It is well-known that HSCs in the BM reside and interact with a highly specialized microenvironment (called the BM niche) that actively regulates HSC homeostasis. The BM niche contains different stromal and progenitor cells, endothelial cells, extracellular matrix components and a number of secreted factors and surface receptors. Osteoblasts are stromal cells that underly the endosteal bone surface and are thus the major interface between calcified bone and the BM. This stromal niche has been shown to play a crucial role in regulating HSC renewal and expansion (Morrison and Scadden, 2014). Park et al. (2019) recently investigated the role that SIRT1 plays in the osteoblastic niche of BM. These investigators created mice with SIRT1 deficiency in the osteoblastic niche of BM by crossing $Sirt1^{flox/flox}$ mice with Ocn^{Cre} mice. Ocn^{Cre} mice are used to target osteoblasts in the BM niche. They observed that deletion of SIRT1 in BM osteoblasts did not alter circulating numbers of blood lymphocytes, neutrophils, monocytes, erythrocytes and platelets when compared to controls. In addition, Park et al. (2019) showed that $Sirt1^{\text{floxed/floxed}}/Ocn^{Cre}$ mice generated similar numbers of CD11b^{+} myeloid cells, T cells and B cells in the BM as did control mice. Furthermore, deletion of SIRT1 in the osteoblastic niche did not alter maturation of HSCs in mice subjected to hemopoietic stress induced by transplantation of HSCs into lethally irradiated or 5-fluorouracil- treated recipients. Park et al. (2019) concluded that in contrast to data reported by Rimmele et al. (2014) who showed that selective deletion of SIRT1 in HSCs caused anemia, lymphocytopenia and increased myeloid cell generation, deletion of SIRT1 in the osteoblastic niche had no effect on HSC maturation or lymphoid and myeloid lineage distribution in the BM.

Myeloid Cells

Neutrophils, monocytes, Macs, and DCs are the myeloid/innate immune cells that rapidly respond to and destroy invading pathogens. Much of what we have learned about the role of SIRT1 in the regulation of myeloid cell function has come from studies focused on DCs and Macs. Because DCs and Macs are required for robust T cell activation within lymphoid and non-lymphoid tissues, defects in their ability to endocytose (or phagocytose), process and present antigens would have dire consequences for host immunity. Thus, it is important to understand the different molecular and cellular mechanisms involved in DC and Mac function.

Dendritic cells play a crucial protective role following invasion of pathogenic microorganisms by promoting antigen-specific responses by T and B cells as well as by generating a plethora of different chemokines and cytokines that recruit immune cells into the infected tissue where these mediators influence the differentiation of T cells into different effector cell subsets. It is also becoming well-appreciated that SIRT1 plays an important role in immune cell function (Chen et al., 2015). For example, Legutko et al. (2011) demonstrated that pharmacological inhibition of SIRT1 using sirtinol and cambinol suppressed Th2 effector cell responses allergic airway inflammation in a mouse model of asthma. They observed that SIRT1 inhibition interfered with the maturation and migration of lung DCs to the draining lymph nodes where they failed to induce Th2 cell differentiation (Legutko et al., 2011). Because both inhibitors have been shown to inhibit SIRT1 and SIRT2, Legutko et al. (2011) repeated their studies using mice with DC-specific (Yang et al., 2013) deletion of SIRT1 ($Sirt1^{flox/flox}/CD11c^{Cre}$ mice). They observed reduced maturation and migration of DCs as well as an overall attenuation of Th2-mediated, antigen (OVA)-induced airway inflammation in these mice. Furthermore, these investigators reported that DC differentiation toward a pro-Th2 phenotype required SIRT1-mediated inhibition of peroxisome proliferator-activated receptor-γ (PPARγ). Using the same mice as Legutko and coworkers, Yang et al. (2013) have reported that DCs obtained from $Sirt1^{flox/flox}/CD11c^{Cre}$ mice exhibited increased production of IL-27 and IFN-β. They reported that co-culturing LPS-activated SIRT1-deficient DCs with $CD4^+$ T cells suppressed Th17 differentiation that was reversed by addition of anti-IL-27 and anti-IFN-β antibodies. These data suggested that SIRT1 acts as a negative regulator of IL-27 and IFN-β expression. Consistent with this hypothesis, these investigators demonstrated that DC-associated SIRT1 interacts with and deacetylates the transcription factor IRF-1 resulting in loss of transcriptional activity and suppression of IL-27 expression. Taken together, these data suggest that DC-associated SIRT1 plays an important role regulating Th17 differentiation during inflammation (Yang et al., 2013). Because both IL-27 and IFN-β function to suppress the generation of pro-inflammatory Th17 cells, Yang and coworkers reasoned that $Sirt1^{flox/flox}/CD11c^{Cre}$ mice may be less susceptible to induction of chronic inflammation. Indeed, they found that loss of SIRT1 function in DCs attenuated the development of chronic neuro-inflammation in a model of human multiple sclerosis called experimental autoimmune encephalomyelitis (EAE) (Yang W. B. et al., 2012). In addition, Liu et al. (2015) reported that DC-specific deletion of SIRT1 via the generation of $Sirt1^{flox/flox}/CD11c^{Cre}$ mice or SIRT1 inactivation of human DCs resulted in enhanced generation of IL-12 but suppressed production of TGF-β. Molecular studies revealed that DC-associated SIRT1 regulates IL-12 and TGF-β1 expression via HIF1α but not mTOR modulation. These data were consistent with their observation that targeted loss of SIRT1 in DCs induces the formation of Th1 cells while limiting the formation of Tregs (Liu et al., 2015). Similarly, Liu et al., 2015 tested their hypothesis *in vivo* using a well-established mouse model of Th1 cell-mediated inflammatory bowel disease. To do this, they transferred naïve $CD4^+$ T cells into *RAG-1*$^{-/-}$ mice devoid of DC SIRT1 ($Sirt1^{flox/flox}/CD11c^{Cre}/RAG\text{-}1^{-/-}$) or into DC-replete *RAG-1*$^{-/-}$ recipients and monitored the mice for signs of disease. They observed that adoptive transfer of T cells into $Sirt1^{flox/flox}/CD11c^{Cre}/RAG\text{-}1^{-/-}$ mice induced a marked acceleration in weight loss and an exacerbation of colonic inflammation when compared to their *RAG-1*$^{-/-}$ counterparts at 3 weeks post T cell transfer (Liu et al., 2015). The development of more severe colitis was associated with an increase in IFN-γ producing Th1 cells and reduction in $FOXP3^+$ Tregs compared to T cell-engrafted RAG-1$^{-/-}$ mice. Co-culturing of LPS-activated mouse or human DCs with their corresponding $CD4^+$ T cells in the presence of the selective SIRT1 inhibitor EX-527 recapitulated much of what was observed using mouse DCs with targeted deletion of SIRT1 including increases in the Th1/Treg ratio, IFN-γ and IL-12 expression as well as reductions in expression of mouse and human TGF-β1 expression (Liu et al., 2015). Taken together, these data demonstrate that DC-associated SIRT1 plays an important role in regulating the balance between Th1 cells and Tregs.

Extravasation of circulating monocytes from the blood and into the tissue initiates their maturation/differentiation into Macs. These phagocytes are well-known to play an important role in the immunopathogenesis of autoimmune and chronic inflammatory diseases. Importantly, Macs have been shown to proliferate in response to inflammatory cytokines and growth factors. Imperatore et al. (2017) recently reported that SIRT1 plays a crucial role in regulating self-renewal of Macs. They have shown that over- expressing SIRT1 in BM-derived Macs during differentiation enhanced their proliferative activity whereas pharmacologic inhibition or SIRT1 gene silencing (via shRNA) or deletion (via CRISPR/Cas9) diminished steady state and cytokine-induced proliferation of alveolar and peritoneal Macs *in vitro* and *in vivo* (Imperatore et al., 2017). Reduction in cell cycle progression and renewal induced by SIRT1 inhibition or gene silencing was associated with inhibition of transcription factors those promote cell cycle progression (e.g., E2F1 and Myc) as well as activation of a transcription factor that is known to induce cell cycle arrest (i.e., FoxO1). Another transcription factor that plays an important role in Mac-mediated immunity is NF-κB. Under steady state, this heterodimeric transcription factor (p50/p65) is localized to the cytoplasm via its binding to the inhibitor protein kB (IkB). Activation of Macs results in the degradation of IkB allowing NF-κB to translocate to the nucleus, where it binds and promotes inflammatory gene expression (Karin and Lin, 2002). It is also well-appreciated that SIRT1 inhibits NF-κB signaling by binding to and deacetylating the p65 subunit (Yeung et al., 2004). Schug et al. (2010) utilized $Sirt1^{flox/flox}/lysozyme^{Cre}$ to assess how the loss of SIRT1 in myeloid cells affects NF-κB signaling in these immune cells. They found that deletion of SIRT1 in myeloid cells caused hyperacetylation of the p65 subunit in NF-κB resulting in enhanced transcription of inflammatory cytokines including TNF-α and IL-1β in response to TNF-α or LPS stimulation *in vitro or in vivo* (Schug et al., 2010). In addition, these investigators showed that $Sirt1^{flox/flox}/lysozyme^{Cre}$ mice responded to a high fat diet with the infiltration of large numbers of activated Macs into the liver and adipose tissue that appeared to exacerbate insulin resistance and metabolic syndrome (Schug et al., 2010). Consistent with these observations, Yoshizaki et al. (2010) demonstrated that siRNA-mediated knockdown of SIRT1 in cultured RAW264.7 mouse macrophages enhanced LPS-induced phosphorylation of IkB kinase leading to an increase in IkB degradation, NF-κB activation, and enhanced expression of inflammatory genes. Taken together, these studies suggest that Mac-associated SIRT1 plays a crucial role in modulating NF-κB -mediated inflammation. Another transcription factor that is regulated by SIRT1 is activator protein-1 (AP-1) which is composed of the two submits c-Fos and c-Jun that together regulate inflammatory gene transcription. Zhang et al. (2010) found that SIRT1 directly interacts with the basic leucine zipper domains of c-Fos and c-Jun where it deacetylates c-Jun resulting in suppression of AP-1 transcriptional activity in peritoneal Macs. They also showed that SIRT1-mediated deacetylation of c-Jun reduced the AP-1 mediated expression of the two inflammatory mediators cyclooxygenase-2 and prostaglandin E2 resulting in diminished tumoricidal function (Zhang et al., 2010). Similarly, Yoshizaki et al. (2010) reported that SIRT1 actively suppresses inflammatory gene expression as siRNA knockdown of SIRT1 in cultured Macs enhanced LPS-induced phosphorylation of c-Jun N-terminal kinase (JNK) and c-JUN resulting in increased expression of several inflammatory genes including TNF-α, IL-1β, MMP-9, MCP-1 and IL-6 (Yoshizaki et al., 2010).

T and B Lymphocytes

The adaptive immune system is essential for mounting an effective and well-regulated immune response to invading microorganisms. This highly integrated immune response requires the participation of thymus-derived $CD4^+$ and $CD8^+$ T cells that is called cell-mediated immunity together with BM-derived B cells and plasma cells which mediate humoral immunity via their production of antibodies (**Figure 1**). Both cell-mediated and humoral immunity work in close association with the innate immune system to insure protection via long-term memory of infectious agents. As described above, interaction of $CD4^+$T cells with their cognate (i.e., microbial) antigen presented by antigen presenting cells in the context of MHC II results in the activation, differentiation and clonal expansion of a variety of different Th cell subsets including T helper 1 (Th1), Th2, Th17, pTreg, Th9 and T follicular (T_{FH}) cells (Russ et al., 2013) (**Figure 3**). The lineage-specific differentiation of the different Th effector cells depends upon the cytokines produced by the antigen presenting cells during their interaction with naive T cells. T_{FH} cells are a specialized subset of thymus-derived $CD4^+$ T cells that are produced and reside within lymph nodes, spleen and tonsils where they provide "help" to B cells to produce antibodies with high affinity that neutralize and remove pathogens (Ma et al., 2012). Differentiation of $CD4^+$ T cells is a complex process that is mediated by different cytokines, transcription factors and epigenetic alterations (Russ et al., 2013; Ellmeier and Seiser, 2018) (**Figure 3**). SIRT1 was originally reported to be a negative regulator of T cell function. Zhang J. et al. (2009) reported that $CD4^+$ T cells obtained from $Sirt1^{-/-}$mice responded to *in vitro* activation with greater proliferation and cytokine production than did wild type T cells. In addition, these investigators showed that $Sirt1^{-/-}$ mice developed more severe brain inflammation in the EAE model suggesting loss of tolerance to autoantigens (Zhang J. et al., 2009). However, subsequent studies have demonstrated that targeted deletion of SIRT1 in T cells actually promotes the generation of FOXP3-expressing Tregs with enhanced immunosuppressive activity (Chadha et al., 2019). For example, Beier et al. (2011) found that T cells obtained from mice with a T cell-specific deletion of SIRT1 (i.e., $Sirt1^{flox/flox}/CD4^{Cre}$ mice), were remarkably similar to wild type mice with respect to T cell numbers as well as their activation, proliferation and cytokine production *in vitro*. In addition, these investigators showed that targeted deletion of SIRT1 in conventional $CD4^+FOXP3^-$ T cells enhanced the expression of FOXP3 in these T cells resulting in the generation of Treg with immunosuppressive activity *in vitro* and *in vivo*. In fact, targeted deletion of SIRT1 in thymic-derived Tregs enhanced significantly their immunosuppressive properties (Beier et al., 2011). In addition, these investigators showed that major MHC mismatched heart allografts survived significantly longer when transplanted into $Sirt1^{flox/flox}/CD4^{Cre}$ mice or $Sirt1^{flox/flox}/Foxp3^{Cre}$ mice when compared to allograft transplantation into wild type mice or when transplanted into wild type mice and treated with selective SIRT1 inhibitors (Beier et al., 2011). More recent work by Levine et al. (2016) reported that MHC mismatched renal allografts survived significantly longer with better function when transplanted into $Sirt1^{flox/flox}/CD4^{Cre}$ vs. wild type mice or when transplanted into wild type recipients and treated with a selective SIRT1 inhibitor. These preclinical studies have prompted discussion to the use of selective targeting of T cell-associated SIRT1 as a possible therapeutic strategy to treat allograft transplantation rejection (Wang et al., 2018). One explanation for the differences in phenotypes and immune responses of T cells derived from $Sirt1^{-/-}$ mice vs. T cells obtained from $Sirt1^{flox/flox}/CD4^{Cre}$ mice is most likely due to alterations in thymic T cell selection in $Sirt1^{-/-}$ mice. It is well-known that SIRT1 plays an important role in regulating the expression of the transcription factor, autoimmune regulator (AIRE) that is required for robust thymic T cell selection (Chuprin et al., 2015). Indeed, this may be the reason why $Sirt1^{-/-}$ mice develop spontaneous and severe ADs that resembles Type 1 diabetes (Sequeira et al., 2008; Zhang J. et al., 2009).

Interaction of naïve $CD4^+$ T cells with DCs (or other antigen presenting cells) in the presence of IL-6, IL-23 and TGFβ induces the formation of Th17 cells (**Figure 3**). Although these IL-17 producing effector cells play a protective role against fungal and bacterial pathogens, Th17 cells have also been implicated in the immunopathogenesis of certain ADs (Omenetti et al., 2019). SIRT1 is highly expressed in Th17 and plays a major role in their generation. It has been well-described that SIRT1 binds to and deacetylates the transcription factor retinoid acid receptor related orphan receptor gamma (RORγt). The deacetylated form of RORγt induces differentiation of Th17 effector cells by activating the IL-17 promoter while repressing the IL-2 promoter (Lim et al., 2015). Lim et al. (2015) demonstrated that targeted

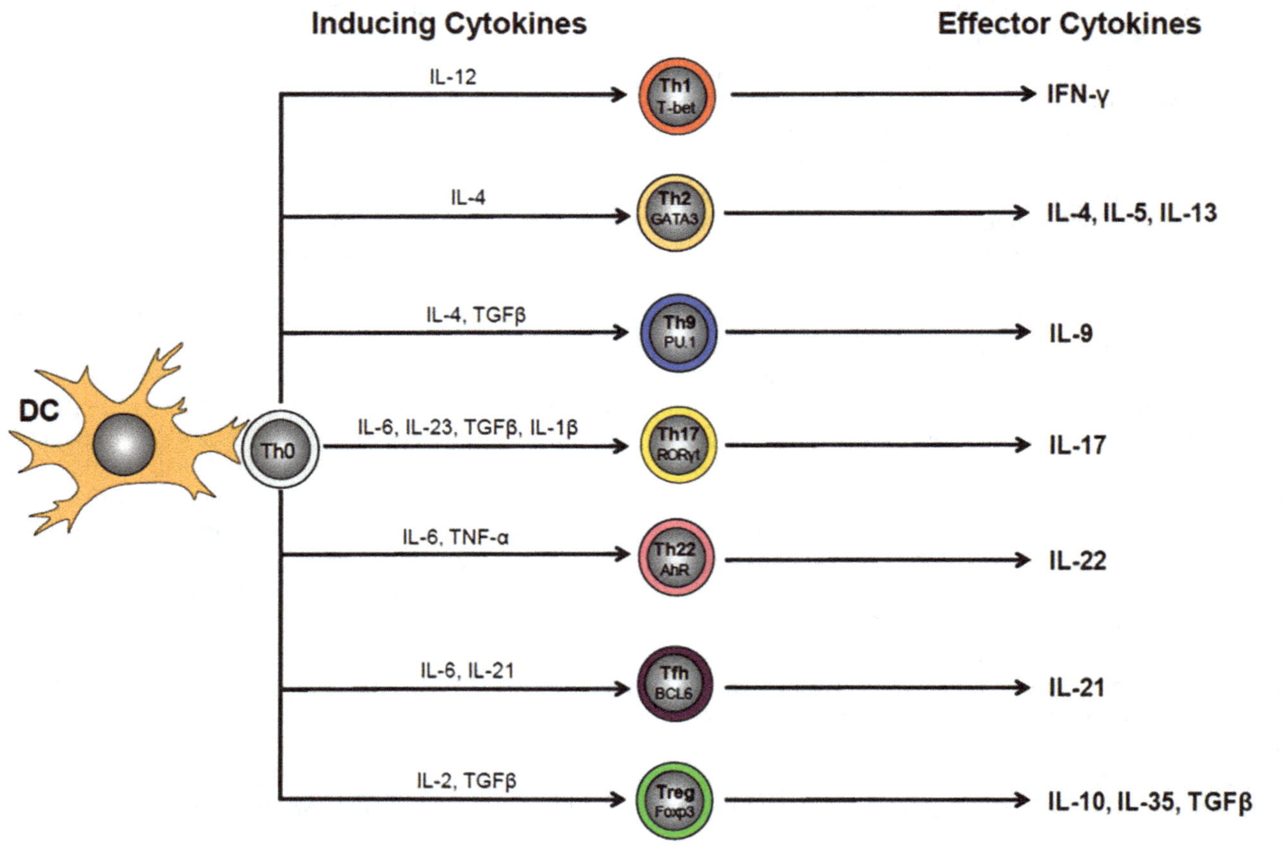

FIGURE 3 | Differentiation of CD4+ T helper (Th) cell subsets. Interaction of naïve (Th0) CD4+ T cells with its cognate antigen presented by dendritic cells (DCs) in the context of MHC II, induces their activation and differentiation into a variety of different Th cell subsets that is dependent upon the cytokine milieu of the microenvironment (e.g., IL-12 for Th1 cells). Th cell-inducing cytokines will upregulate lineage specific transcription factors that regulate and maintain Th cell-specific effector cell functions (e.g., Tbet for Th1 cells). The effector cytokines produced by the different Th subsets (e.g., Th1 cell-generated IFN-γ) act to eliminate the invading microbes that were responsible for the release of the inducing cytokines by DCs during Th0 cell activation.

deletion of T cell-associated SIRT1 in $Sirt1^{flox/flox}CD4^{cre}$ mice reduced Th17 differentiation by suppressing IL-17 expression while enhancing IL-2 generation. In addition to its ability to enhance the generation of Th17 cells, SIRT1 may also limit Th17 differentiation via its ability to deacetylate signal transducer and activator of transcription (STAT)-3 which is required for RORγt transcription (Limagne et al., 2017). In fact, a few studies have reported that enhancing rather than inhibiting SIRT1 may suppress Th17 development (Gardner et al., 2013, 2015). In order to directly assess the role of SIRT1 in Th17-mediated ADs, Lim et al. (2015) interbred $Sirt1^{flox/flox}$ mice with $ROR\gamma t^{Cre}$ mice producing offspring with selective deletion of Sirt1 in RORγt expressing T cells (i.e., $Sirt1^{flox/flox}/ROR\gamma t^{Cre}$ mice). Using these novel mice or a selective SIRT1 inhibitor (i.e., EX-527), these investigators observed marked suppression of Th17 differentiation, neuronal inflammation and demyelination in the EAE mouse model of multiple sclerosis (Lim et al., 2015). Taken together, these studies suggest that SIRT1 plays a pro-inflammatory role in Th17 effector cells and that selective inhibition of this deacetylase may be useful in treating certain ADs. A third group of Th cells that appear to be regulated by SIRT1 are Th9 effector cells (**Figure 3**). These IL-9 secreting effector cells have been shown to possess anti-parasitic and antitumor activities; however, other studies have suggested that Th9 cells may be important mediators of allergic diseases (Kaplan et al., 2015). Work by Wang et al. (2016) has demonstrated that SIRT1 serves to negatively regulate the Th9 cell differentiation. They found that targeted deletion of SIRT1 in mouse $CD4^{+}$T cells *(*$Sirt1^{flox/flox}CD4^{cre}$) or SIRT1 silencing in mouse or human T cells (via siRNA inactivation) enhanced Th9 cell differentiation and production of IL-9 (Wang et al., 2016). Conversely, they showed that ectopic expression of SIRT1 reduced IL-9 production and Th9 effector cell numbers. In addition, Wang et al. (2016) found that IL-9 produced by SIRT1 deficient T cells delayed melanoma growth and enhanced development of allergic airway inflammation *in vivo*. In the following sections of this review, we will elaborately discuss T cell mediated SIRT1 roles in multiple ADs (section "The Role of SIRT1 in Autoimmune Disease").

A second group of T cells that are critically important in cell-mediated immunity against viral infections and tumor cells are the $CD8^{+}$ T cells. Interaction of naïve $CD8^{+}$ T cells with their cognate antigen expressed on the surface of most cells in the context of MHC I, induces antigen-specific activation, differentiation and clonal expansion of cytotoxic lymphocytes

(CTLs). Although the role of epigenetic regulation is recognized as an important determinant for CD8$^+$ T cell differentiation (Henning et al., 2018), relatively little is known about the role that SIRT1 plays in the generation and activity of CTLs. Kuroda et al. (2011) have shown that suppressing the expression of basic leucine zipper transcription factor, ATF-like (BATF) in CD8$^+$ T cells via insertion of GFP cDNA into the *Batf* locus reduced CD8 differentiation *in vivo*. They observed that in the presence of IL-12, co-stimulation of CD8$^+$ T cells enhanced expression of BATF, a transcription factor that is required for IL-12 mediated acetylation of histone proteins as well as survival and differentiation of CD8$^+$ T cells. In addition, Kuroda et al. (2011) demonstrated that both BATF and c-Jun were responsible for negatively regulating transcription of SIRT1 thereby promoting histone acetylation and expression of the critical transcription factor T-bet. In the absence of BATF, Kuroda et al. (2011) showed that SIRT1 expression was greatly increased in activated CD8$^+$ T cells and was associated with deacetylation of T-bet and limited T cell differentiation. Taken together, these data demonstrate that BATF and c-Jun promote CD8$^+$ T cell differentiation by negatively regulating SIRT1 expression. Another group of lymphocytes whose function is required for mediating humoral immunity are B cells and their terminally differentiated progeny, plasma cells. These lymphocytes are responsible for generating antibodies that bind, neutralize, and eliminate extracellular microbes and their toxins. Gan et al. (2020) recently reported that SIRT1 plays an important role in regulating antibody maturation in B cells. They found that activation of B cells leads to the down regulation of SIRT1 with concurrent upregulation of activation-induced cytidine deaminase (AICDA), the master regulator of secondary antibody diversification (Gan et al., 2020). Using B cells obtained from mice with B cell-specific ablation of SIRT1 ($Sirt1^{flox/flox}/Aicda^{Cre}$ mice), Gan et al. (2020) found reduced deacetylation of histone proteins associated with the *AICDA* promoter and non-histone proteins (e.g., Dnmt1 and p65/NF-κB) in activated B cells resulting in increased expression of AICDA and induction of CSR/SHM antibody maturation. Conversely, transgenic overexpression of SIRT1 in B cells was found to reduce expression of AICDA and CSR/SHM confirming its role in silencing AICDA expression. Interestingly, Gan et al. (2020) observed that loss of SIRT1 in activated B cells resulted in the production of several systemic lupus erythematosus (SLE)-associated autoantibodies including antibodies to nuclear antigens, double-stranded DNA, histones, ribonucleoprotein, and RNA IgG. In addition, these investigators reported that B cells obtained from mice that develop spontaneous SLE (e.g., MRL/Faslpr/lpr and BXD2 mice) or from patients with SLE, exhibited increased expression of AICDA that was associated with decreased SIRT1 expression when compared to healthy control mice or humans. Taken together, these data suggest that loss of SIRT1 expression in B cells may promote SLE by driving the generation of SLE-associated autoantibodies.

The Role of SIRT1 in Infection

Upon invasion of the body by an infectious organism, cells of the immune system undergo proliferation and differentiation, and specify specific lineages that combat the infection by triggering a transition in immune cells from quiescent to an activated state. A key change in this activation involves a metabolic switch within the immune cells that equip them to meet the energetic requirements. For example, myeloid cells undergo a metabolic switch from oxidative phosphorylation during quiescence to glycolysis during activation. This switch to glycolysis is often triggered by Toll-like receptor (TLR) activation which promotes the robust expression and production of inflammatory cytokines. Metabolic reprogramming is important and during immune cell activation can favor specific immune responses. While the shift from oxidative phosphorylation to glycolysis may favor myeloid cell activation, the energy derived may be used to generate more reactive oxygen species in the case of Macs (O'Neill and Pearce, 2016) or synthesize more fatty acids in the case of DCs (Everts et al., 2012). Regardless of the specifics of these metabolic shifts, SIRT1 has been shown to regulate key metabolic pathways including glycolysis, gluconeogenesis, fatty acid synthesis and oxidative phosphorylation. SIRT1 exerts its influence on metabolic pathways by regulating chromatin structure through histone deacetylation as well as through deacetylation of non-histone proteins including transcription factors such as SREBP, a master regulator of fatty acid synthesis (Simmons et al., 2015) or mTOR/HIF1α signaling that regulate genes controlling glycolysis (Wang et al., 2016). NF-κB activity is also regulated by SIRT1 deacetylation, where in Macs SIRT1 deficiency drives an increase in pro-inflammatory cytokines in response to LPS (Schug et al., 2010). Myeloid cells can also be targeted by parasitic infections. One type of parasitic infection spread by insects that can directly impact myeloid cells and modulate metabolic reprogramming involves trypanosomes, which are unicellular protozoa belonging to the *trypanosoma* genus. For example, infection of host cells by *Trypanosoma cruzi* (Tc) can lead to Chagas disease (CD) and a range of mild to severe pathologies. Tc infection can lead to enlargement of the liver, spleen and lymph node and in the case of severe disease can lead to inflammation of the brain and heart and fatal accumulation of fluid around the heart. *In vivo* models of CD show that administration of a SIRT1 activator (SRT1720) suppresses oxidative stress and inflammation associated with chronic Tc infection (Wan et al., 2016, 2019). Wan et al. (2019) demonstrated that SRT1720 had no significant effect on the total population of splenic cells but caused a significant decrease in subpopulations of monocytes and Macs in the spleen of chronically infected mice and a decrease in the CD80$^+$/CD64$^+$ M1 phenotype Chagas mice. Interestingly, investigators demonstrated that SRT1720 administration had no effect on parasite survival and persistence as measured by parasite DNA in splenic monocytes/macrophages, while there was a significant reduction in the mono/mac ratio in the spleen and heart and an improvement of left ventricular function in Chagas mice. Further investigation of links with SIRT1 and other parasitic infections by other groups found an association with Leishmania, another genus of trypanosomes, which is responsible for the disease leishmaniasis. *Leishmania infantum* (*L. infantum*) which can infect Macs were also shown to trigger metabolic switches in host cells infected with intracellular *L. infantum*. Moreira et al. (2015) demonstrated that infection of Macs with

L. infantum induces a switch from early glycolytic metabolism to oxidative phosphorylation in a manner that is dependent on SIRT1, liver kinase B1, and AMPK (Roy et al., 2019). Liver kinase B1 plays a key role in HSC maintenance while AMPK critically regulates autophagy in monocytes and Macs based on cellular energy levels. More investigation of other parasites including *Leishmania donovani* (*L. donovani*) further revealed the importance of the competition for metabolic resources between the normal host cell and the parasite-infected host cell. Therefore, the SIRT1 signaling axes linked with AMPK activity has proven to be critical for metabolic programs that influence the pathology associated with parasitic infections (Moreira et al., 2015; Roy et al., 2019).

THE ROLE OF SIRT1 IN AUTOIMMUNE DISEASE

Autoimmune diseases are a heterogeneous group of diseases affecting 8–10% of the Western population, characterized by the loss of ability of the immune system to differentiate self from non-self. Nowadays, AD patients are subjected to comorbidities, short life expectancy and progressive disability as the current therapeutic strategies are based on systemic immunosuppression (IS) (Alexander et al., 2019). Even though this is a diverse group of diseases, recent research using genome-wide association studies show that the immune pathogenesis shared by the major ADs is dictated by distinct pathways (Cho and Gregersen, 2011), in which SIRT1 plays an integral role (**Table 1**).

Role of SIRT1 in Inflammatory Bowel Disease (IBD)

A group of inflammatory diseases that are driven by certain Th effector cells are the inflammatory bowel diseases (IBD; Crohn's disease ulcerative colitis). These diseases are characterized by chronic and unrelenting inflammation of the small and/or large intestine (Uhlig and Powrie, 2018). There is good evidence suggesting that chronic gut inflammation may arise from a complex interaction among genetics, the immune system and the intestinal microbiota (Uhlig and Powrie, 2018). Akimova et al. (2014) utilized two different models of IBD to ascertain the role of T cell associated SIRT1 in the induction and/or perpetuation of chronic colitis in mice. In their first series of studies using the well-established T cell transfer model, they found that adoptive transfer of syngeneic $CD4^{+}CD25^{-}FOXP3^{-}$ T cells obtained from wild type C57BL/6 (Bl6) into immunodeficient Bl6 RAG-$1^{-/-}$ recipients induced Th1 effector cell-mediated chronic and unrelenting colitis that was characterized by expansion of disease producing Th1 effector cells that is associated with weight loss, splenomegaly and the infiltration of large numbers of T cells into the colon (Akimova et al., 2014). In contrast, adoptive transfer of Bl6 T cells devoid of SIRT1 (obtained from $Sirt1^{flox/flox}/CD4^{Cre}$ mice) into Bl6 RAG-$1^{-/-}$ recipients, induced less weight loss and splenomegaly as well as much milder disease when compared to mice that received wild type T cells. The protective effect of eliminating SIRT1 in $CD4^{+}$ T cells corresponded with a 2.8-fold increase in the generation of iTregs when compared to WT T cell engrafted recipients (Akimova et al., 2014). These data suggest that in the absence of SIRT1, differentiation of naïve T cells is skewed toward the generation of iTregs. Using a second model of colitis, Akimova et al. (2014) induced chronic colitis via multiple cycles of drinking water containing the colitogenic polymer dextran sodium sulfate (DSS) that were alternated with drinking water alone. They found that daily administration of the selective SIRT1 inhibitor EX-527 markedly attenuated weight loss and chronic colitis as well as increased the production of iTregs (Akimova et al., 2014). Similarly, Caruso et al. (2014) examined the expression, regulation, and function of SIRT1 in IBD. They found that relative to normal controls, SIRT1 RNA and protein expression was less pronounced in whole biopsies and lamina propria mononuclear cells (LPMCs) of IBD patients. They also reported that SIRT1 expression was downregulated in control LPMC and upregulated in IBD LPMC by neutralizing TNF-α and IL-21 antibodies. Moreover, they found that infliximab-treated IBD patients showed increased SIRT1 expression in mucosal samples and IBD LPMC treated with a specific SIRT1 activator showed reduced NF-κB activation and inhibited inflammatory cytokine synthesis while a SIRT1 inhibitor increased IFN-γ in control LPMC. Overall, assessing patient samples and mouse models of experimental colitis, using a combination of SIRT1 activators and inhibitors, they conclude that SIRT1 is downregulated in IBD patients and colitic mice, and suggest that SIRT1 activation can help attenuate inflammatory signals in the gut (Caruso et al., 2014). Together, these data suggest that T cell associated SIRT1 may represent a potential therapeutic target for treating patients with IBD.

Role of SIRT1 in Type 1 Diabetes (T1D)

Aside from intestinal/GI-linked autoimmune pathologies, SIRT1 has also been linked with type I diabetes (T1D) and mutations in the SIRT1 gene have been identified in a family with T1D (Biason-Lauber et al., 2013). SIRT1 has been shown to be prominently expressed in beta cells and regulates insulin secretion. In mice, targeted overexpression of SIRT1 in beta cells enhances insulin secretion. In view of this, a mutation in the SIRT1 gene could lead to autoimmune disease. Biason-Lauber and investigators studied a SIRT1 mutation (L107P) that was found in a family harboring this mutation. Four of the five family members developed T1D while 1 in 5 developed colitis. To understand how the mutation might be linked with autoimmune defects, the investigators tested the known functions of SIRT1 and observed whether these functions were altered because of the mutation. Analysis of SIRT1-L107P influence on cytokine production showed increased cytokine-induced nitric oxide synthase expression and TNF-α relative to the wildtype SIRT1 gene. Moreover, in a mouse model of pancreatic insulitis induced by streptozotocin, $Sirt1^{-/-}$ mice showed increased islet destruction and hyperglycemia. They also reported that myoblasts from patients harboring this mutation generated insulin resistance in the mice (Biason-Lauber et al., 2013).

Role of SIRT1 in Rheumatoid Arthritis (RA)

One of the most prevalent ADs in the US is rheumatoid arthritis (RA). This chronic inflammatory disorder is characterized by

TABLE 1 | Summary of immune regulatory pathways and their interaction with SIRT1 in modulating autoimmune diseases (ADs).

Pathway	Gene	SIRT1	References
Lymphocyte activation	Cytotoxic T-lymphocyte antigen 4 (CTLA4)	• In Tregs lymphocytes, depletion of SIRT1-increases mRNA levels of CTLA4.	Beier et al., 2011
	Tumor necrosis factor α-induced protein 3 (TNFAIP3)	• In macrophages, SIRT1 binds to TNFAIP3 loci and participates in its downregulation.	Li et al., 2020
	Tumor Necrosis Factor Receptor Superfamily Member 5, CD40 Antigen (CD40)	• In HUVEC endothelial cells, SIRT1 inhibits TNF-α-induced CD40 expression by deacetylating the RelA/p65 subunit of NF-κB. • In LPS-stimulated renal inner medullary collecting duct (IMCD) cells, SIRT1 overexpression or activation by SRT1720 diminished the expression of CD40, which was reversed by SIRT1 siRNA or inhibitors EX-527 and sirtinol. • In 3T3-L1 adipocytes, SIRT1 regulates TNF-α-induced expression of CD40 via NF-κB pathway.	Lin et al., 2012, 2017; Yang L. et al., 2012
Cytokines and cytokines receptors	Interleukin 23 Receptor (IL23R)	• In T cells, the treatment with a low dose of metformin (SIRT1 agonist) decreases the expression of IL23R.	Limagne et al., 2017
	Interleukin 2 Receptor Subunit Alpha (IL2RA)	• In macrophages, SIRT1 participates in downregulation of IL2RA. • In Treg lymphocytes, the transfection of miR-124a and miR-155 (miRNAs repressing SIRT1) induce the expression of IL2RA.	Heyn et al., 2016; Li et al., 2020
	Interleukin 10 (IL10)	• In microglia (CNS), resveratrol (SIRT1 activator) induces IL10 mRNA expression.	Song et al., 2014
Transcription factors	Signal transducer and activator of transcription 3 (STAT3)	• SIRT1 induces STAT3 deacetylation • SIRT1-null MEF cells display increase of STAT3 levels in mitochondria through constitutive activation of NF-κB	Nie et al., 2009; Bernier et al., 2011

progressive and unrelenting immune cell-mediated destruction of cartilage and bone in the joints. It has been well-described that myeloid cells such as monocytes and Macs play important roles in the development and perpetuation of chronic joint inflammation (McInnes and Schett, 2011). In an attempt to better understand the role that myeloid cell derived SIRT1 plays in the pathogenesis of experimental arthritis, Hah et al. (2014) used the well-characterized mouse model of arthritis in which serum from arthritic K/BxN mice was injected into control or *Sirt1*$^{flox/flox}$/*lysozyme*^{Cre} mice. Joint inflammation in recipients is promoted by the presence of autoantibodies directed against the self-antigen, glucose-6-phosphate isomerase that leads to the formation of immune complexes within joints. These immune complexes will activate complement as well as a number of innate immune cells such as Macs, neutrophils and possibly DCs (Christensen et al., 2016). Hah et al. (2014) demonstrated that transfer of serum from arthritic K/BxN donors induced more severe arthritis in *Sirt1*$^{flox/flox}$/*lysozyme*^{Cre} mice that correlated with significant increases in protein levels of IL-1β and TNF-α as well as increases in TRAP-positive osteoclasts and F4/80+ macrophages in the ankles. BM-derived monocytes and Macs obtained from these mice with selective deletion of SIRT1 exhibited hyperacetylation of p65 and activation of NF-κB that correlated with enhanced polarization, migration and inflammatory cytokine production in these phagocytes when compared to control cells. These data suggest that SIRT1 may act to limit the activation of innate immune cells resulting in less joint inflammation. Although this model induces robust arthritis in 100% of most mouse strains, it is more of an acute form of arthritis that does not involve interactions among T cells, B cells and innate immune cells that are required for the development of chronic disease. Mouse models of chronic arthritis require a priming step in which mice are immunized with self-antigens (e.g., collagen II) to induce T and B cell-dependent production autoantibodies. The second (i.e., effector) phase for the development of chronic arthritis is essentially the same as that involved in the serum transfer model. That is, autoantibodies generated during the priming step enter the synovial space where they bind to collagen II and initiate immune complex deposition and joint inflammation. The priming and effector phases in this model of collagen induced arthritis (CIA), are thought occur in human RA (Christensen et al., 2016). Thus, Woo et al. (2016) undertook a follow up study to assess the role of myeloid cell derived SIRT1 in the CIA model. Interestingly, in contrast to their previous study, Woo et al. (2016) observed less joint inflammation and bone loss in *Sirt1*$^{flox/flox}$/*lysozyme*^{Cre} mice when compared to their wild type controls. Attenuation of disease correlated with reductions in inflammatory cytokines, MMPs and ROR-γT as well as decreases in the numbers of Th1, Th17 and DCs. Indeed, maturation of DCs obtained from *Sirt1*$^{flox/flox}$/*lysozyme*^{Cre} mice was impaired as was their ability to induce differentiation and proliferation of disease producing Th1 and Th17 effector cells. SIRT1 has also been shown to be increased in patients with RA (Woo et al., 2016). Another study used resveratrol to assess the role of SIRT1 in CIA. Resveratrol has been shown to be protective against cardiovascular disease and has been connected to increased life spans. Resveratrol affects immune response by inhibiting proliferation of spleen cells, production of TNF-α, IL-12 and T and B cell activity by upregulating CTLA4 and down-regulating CD28 and CD80 (Zou et al., 2013). Zou et al. (2013) reported that SIRT1 inhibition in T cells diminished the resveratrol-induced inhibition of T cell activation and also coincided with changes in c-Jun acetylation and the incidence and severity of collagen-induced arthritis.

Role od SIRT1 in Acute and Chronic Graft Versus Host Disease (GVHD)

In addition to solid organ transplantation (i.e., host vs. graft reaction), preclinical studies have shown that selective deletion of T cell associated SIRT1 provides protection to mice that receive allogeneic hematopoietic stem cell transplantation (HSCT). This protocol is a potential cure for severe and/or relapsing hematological malignancies, ADs or blood disorders (Niederwieser et al., 2016). Unfortunately, the beneficial effects of HSCT are limited by the development of a multi-organ inflammatory condition called acute graft versus host disease (aGVHD) (Zeiser and Blazar, 2017; Toubai et al., 2018). Typically, inflammatory tissue damage involves the gastrointestinal tract, skin, liver and lungs (Zeiser and Blazar, 2017; Toubai et al., 2018).Though the immuno-pathogenesis of aGVHD has not been completely defined, experimental and clinical studies demonstrate that T cells within the donor BM are the major effector cells responsible for mediating inflammatory tissue injury in the different target tissues (Zeiser and Blazar, 2017). A recent study by Daenthanasanmak et al. (2019) demonstrated that engraftment of allogeneic BM supplemented with allogeneic T cells obtained from mice with targeted deletion of SIRT1 in their T cells produced significantly less aGVHD and chronic GVHD (cGVHD) when compared to wild type recipients that received that same allogeneic BM and T cell suspension. They also observed increased generation of Tregs that were derived from the donor T cells. These induced Tregs exhibited greater FOXP3 stability and immunosuppressive activity *in vitro and in vivo.* In addition, Daenthanasanmak et al. (2019) found that administration of the selective SIRT1 inhibitor EX-527 to mice that received wild type allogeneic BM and T cells significantly increased survival of the recipients that was associated with reduced production of IL-17 and IFN-γ by donor T cells. These results suggest that T cell associated SIRT1 may be a possible target for the treatment of acute and chronic GVHD. Together these findings demonstrate an increasing interest between the crosstalk of endocrine, nervous and immune systems and reveal the interaction between gene expression, cytokine release and hormone action in ADs with SIRT1 (Tanriverdi et al., 2003; Silverman and Sternberg, 2008).

PROSPECTS FOR TARGETING SIRTUINS PHARMACOLOGICALLY

Recognition of the epigenetic defects in tumorigenesis and decades of research led to the clinical use of several FDA-approved therapies that target some of the epigenetic "erasers" (Kelly et al., 2010; Cheng et al., 2019). Several class I/II HDAC inhibitors have either been approved (Suraweera et al., 2018) or are currently advancing in various phases of clinical trials (Ramalingam et al., 2010; O'Connor et al., 2013; Foss et al., 2016; Sborov et al., 2017) for the treatment of multiple types of cancer. However, there are no approved therapies that target SIRT1 by increasing or decreasing its activity, but several studies hint of future promise. For example, SIRT1 may be an important therapeutic target in patients whose complications involve chronic inflammatory responses (Dai et al., 2018; Zhou et al., 2018; Wang Y. et al., 2019). **Table 2** lists some of the sirtuin inhibitors potentially effective in diseases with dysfunctional endocrine and immune regulation. One of the promising areas where modulating SIRT1 activity therapeutically may be important involves managing cellular dysfunction associated with protozoa infection involving models of CD where SIRT1 regulates myeloid responses to infection (Wan et al., 2016, 2019). Additionally, other parasites including *Leishmania infantum* and *L. donovani* are capable of subverting key SIRT1 signaling axes linked with AMPK activity. Ultimately, this aberrant engagement of SIRT1 leads to a switch in metabolic programs that favor the pathology associated with infection. Consequently, as we learn more about how SIRT1 mediates metabolic reprogramming of infected cells, this could yield potential new therapeutic targets for treatment of leshmaniasis (Moreira et al., 2015; Roy et al., 2019). Studies have also suggested that targeting SIRT1 may also be effective in decreasing neurodegeneration associated with multiple sclerosis (MS), which is linked with progressive disease despite success in reducing inflammation. Application of SIRT1 activators have been reported to both reduce the degeneration associated with decreased ATP synthesis and increased inflammation in MS models (Fonseca-Kelly et al., 2012; Nimmagadda et al., 2017). While these studies are important, it should be noted that the use of some resveratrol-based inhibitors may elicit effects on uncharacterized targets that are modulated independent of SIRT1. Other inflammation-linked diseases in which modulating SIRT1 activity may show benefit include non-alcoholic fatty liver disease (NAFLD) and diet-induced non-alcoholic steatohepatitis (NASH) (Simmons et al., 2015). SIRT1 has been repeatedly shown to be expressed at high levels in tissues that play a dominant role in the regulation of metabolism and in models of NAFLD, targeting SIRT1 ameliorates inflammation associated with these pathologies (Kume et al., 2010).

Apart from the inhibitors listed in **Table 2**, natural SIRT1 inhibitors are currently under investigation due to their anticancer roles. For instance, Subramaniyan et al. (2017) reported Wnt-mediated inhibition of SIRT1 signaling in SW480 colorectal cancer cells by sodium salt 'Burtin' extracted from *Butea monosperma* flowers. Similarly, betulinic acid derivative (B10) increased FOXO3a transcription and reduced SIRT1 expression leading to induced apoptosis *in vitro* and reduced *in vivo* tumor growth and hence B10 is a novel therapeutic candidate for glioma treatment (Huo et al., 2017). It is intriguing that the SIRT1 inhibitor, nicotinamide, is the amide derivative of vitamin B3. This begs the question as to what role does diet or the supplementation of specific vitamins have on disease progression and the regulation of protein/histone acetylation? Along these lines, the cancer-preventative soy peptide, lunasin, is also known to regulate the dynamics of acetylation-deacetylation

TABLE 2 | List of existing potent SIRT inhibitors and their possible therapeutic implications.

Name	Study objective	Treatment group	Study type	Mechanism of action	References
Clinical research					
Nicotinamide	Anticancer Activity of Nicotinamide on Lung Cancer	EGFR Mutated Lung Cancer Terminal Stage Patients	Phase II/Phase III clinical trial (active, not recruiting)	Results not published yet	NCT02416739, https://clinicaltrials.gov
EX-527 (Selisistat)	SIRT1 Antagonist Therapy Before Embryo Transfer to Improve Endometrial Receptivity and Life Pregnancy Rates	Endometriosis, Uterine Diseases, Endometrial Diseases, Infertility, Unexplained Infertility; Female Non-implantation	Double blind, placebo-controlled Phase II clinical trial	Protective SIRT1 inhibitor functions of EX-527 in Huntington's disease treatment (Süssmuth et al., 2015)	NCT04184323, https://clinicaltrials.gov
Preclinical research					
Nicotinamide	Anticancer effects of SIRT1 inhibitor	Human leukemia and prostate cancer cells	*In vitro*	(i) Blocked cancer cell proliferation and promoted apoptosis via p53 dependent caspase-3 and miR-34a induction (ii) Inhibited cancer cell growth and viability through SIRT1 mediated inhibition of Foxo1 acetylation	Jung-Hynes et al., 2009; Audrito et al., 2011
AK-7	Neuroprotective action via SIRT2 inhibition	Huntington's disease naïve neuronal cell model	*In vitro*	Brain permeability with limited metabolic stability via induced SREBP-2 cytosolic retention and downregulated transcription of cholesterol biosynthesizing enzymes	Taylor et al., 2011
EX-527	Antinociceptive and anticancer effects of SIRT1 inhibitor	BALB/c Mice injected with bone cancer cells; Human leukemia cells; PABPN1 transgenic nematodes; Primary human mammary epithelial cells	*In vitro*, *In vivo*	(i) induced cellular apoptosis in cancers (ii) protected against muscular dystrophy (iii) Increased P53 acetylation in breast epithelial cells after DNA damage	Solomon et al., 2006; Pasco et al., 2010; Cea et al., 2011; Lux et al., 2019
AC-93253	Anticancer effects via SIRT1-3 inhibition	Prostate DU145, Pancreas MiaPaCa, Lung A549 and NCI-H460 cancer cells	*In vitro*	Cytotoxic effects against a panel of cancer cell lines	Zhang Y. et al., 2009
Inauhzin	Anticancer effects of SIRT1 inhibitor	Human lung cancer, H460 and colon cancer, HCT116 cells; Wildtype and lung/colon tumor bearing SCID mice	*In vitro*; *In vivo*	Reactivated p53 via SIRT1 inhibition thus: (i) Repressed cancer cell proliferation, (ii) Stimulated cancer cell senescence and apoptosis without genotoxicity, and (iii) Repressed the xenograft tumor growth	Zhang et al., 2012
Sirtinol	Anticancer effects of SIRT1/2 inhibitor	Human Breast cancer MCF7, Lung cancer H1299, Prostate cancer PC3 and Du145 cell lines	*In vitro*	(i) Induced senescence-like growth arrest with impaired activation of RAS-MAPK pathway (ii) P53 dependent cell apoptosis (iii) Increased sensitivity to chemotherapeutic agents along with inhibited cell proliferation	Ota et al., 2006; Kojima et al., 2008; Jin et al., 2010; Wang et al., 2012
Salermide	Anticancer effects of SIRT1/2 inhibitor	Human cancer cell lines: Leukemia (MOLT4 and KG1A); Breast cancer (MCF7 and MDA-MB-231); Colon cancer (SW480); and non-small-cell lung cancer lines	*In vitro*	Induces apoptosis, growth arrest and reduces cancer cell proliferation in a panel of cancer cell lines via p53-independent and dependent inhibition of SIRT1/2; have potent cytotoxic and anti-proliferative effects against cancer	Lara et al., 2009; Peck et al., 2010; Liu et al., 2012; Rotili et al., 2012a

(Continued)

TABLE 2 | Continued

Name	Study objective	Treatment group	Study type	Mechanism of action	References
Cambinol	Anticancer, inflammatory and immune response effects of SIRT1/2 inhibitor	Human lymphoma and breast cancer cell line; Mouse Burkitt lymphoma model; Bone marrow cells from BALB/c mice housed in pathogen free conditions	*In vitro*; *In vivo*	Promotes cell cycle arrest via hyperacetylation of tubulin, p53, Foxo3a, and KU70; reduced xenograft tumor growth in a mouse Burkitt lymphoma model; reduced neuroblastoma formation in N-Myc transgenic mice; and Repressed aromatase transcription via ERα deacetylation in breast cancer Decreased proinflammatory cytokines expression and macrophage response upon microbial stimulation (TLR) *in vivo*	Heltweg et al., 2006; Marshall et al., 2011; Holloway et al., 2013; Lugrin et al., 2013
Splitomicin and its analogues	Anticancer effects of SIRT1/2 inhibitor	Human colon (DLD-1), cervical (HeLa), breast (MCF7) cancer, and colorectal, glioblastoma cancer stem cells	*In vitro*	Weak or anti-proliferative effects against a panel of human cancer cell lines and cancer stem cells	Neugebauer et al., 2008; Rotili et al., 2010, 2012b
Tenovin-1/-6	Anticancer effects of SIRT1/2 inhibitor	Human breast (MCF7, MDA-MB-231), gastric cancer (MKN-45, NUGC-4, STKM-2, SNU-1), lymphoma (BL2 Burkitt's), and melanoma (ARN8) cell lines; ARN8 mouse xenograft model	*In vitro*; *In vivo*	Cytotoxic to a panel of cancer cell lines (breast, gastric, lymphoma, melanoma); delayed xenograft tumor growth and disease progression partly via p53 activation and death receptor-5 (DR-5) upregulation	Lain et al., 2008; Hirai et al., 2014; Jin et al., 2015

(de Lumen, 2005). Studies have demonstrated that consumption of soy milk more than once a day is associated with a 70% reduction in prostate cancer risk compared with no soy milk intake (Hebert et al., 1998). Although we are still early in our exploration of the impact of acetylation on protein function, there are several landmarks indicating that the journey is still worth the effort. Taken together, given the potential therapeutic implication of sirtuin inhibitors in cancer and other immune modulatory diseases, good selectivity and optimization practices should be employed for future clinical and preclinical studies.

Finally, examples are increasingly emerging that hint the promise of targeting SIRT1 and its downstream effectors therapeutically that may involve an intersection of endocrinology and immunology. For example, the accumulation of excess lipids and cholesterol esters in arterial walls is characteristic of atherosclerosis, and macrophage-derived foam cells play a critical role in this process. Macrophage-derived foam cells localize to blood vessel walls wherein fat accumulation is enriched, and within this vascular microenvironment, they uptake low-density lipoproteins, thereby promoting atherosclerosis. Retinoid signaling regulates cholesterol deposition and removal in macrophages, in part, by regulating the steroidogenic acute regulatory (StAR) protein (Manna et al., 2016). StAR activity and other pathways linked with retinoid and hormone signaling have been shown to regulate this process. For example, we demonstrated that the activation of cAMP/PKA signaling promotes retinoid-induced macrophage cholesterol efflux and increased LXR activity, a process that may reduce the formation of atherosclerotic lesions. Moreover, we found that treatment of mouse macrophages with retinoids increased cholesterol efflux to apolipoprotein AI (Apo-A1) and elevated StAR promoter activity while macrophages overexpressing hormone-sensitive lipase increased the hydrolysis of cholesterol esters (Manna et al., 2015a). Not only can retinoids modulate StAR activity in macrophages, but they also regulate StAR at multiple levels across a wide spectrum of cell types (Manna et al., 2015b). StAR is well recognized for its ability to mediate intra-mitochondrial transport of cholesterol in target tissues, however, only recently has it been shown to be a target of SIRT1 as well as other lysine deacetylases (Manna et al., 2019). While much remains to be discovered about how endocrine linked signaling modulates key regulators of immune responses, it is clear that the intersection of these fields of study will likely find SIRT1 at the crossroads.

CONCLUDING REMARKS

From these examples and others not discussed at length here (Hu et al., 2014; Dai et al., 2018; Zhou et al., 2018; Wang S. H. et al., 2019), it is apparent that epigenetic drugs that regulate acetylation/deacetylation will likely prove beneficial in the treatment of several diseases. Combination therapies involving deacetylase inhibitors and immunotherapy may provide yet another means for treating numerous disorders. Finally, these agents might also be effective for chemopreventive approaches for individuals who have not yet acquired neoplastic lesions or advanced stage disorders. Likewise, our understanding of the role that SIRT1 plays in cellular transformation and tumorigenesis is still murky; however, there is enough evidence that warrants further investigation of the link. Moreover, it is becoming increasingly appreciated that SIRT1 plays an important role in innate and adaptive immunity as well as in the pathogenesis of certain autoimmune or chronic inflammatory diseases. Studies presented in this review reveal that the role of this histone deacetylase is context specific, as SIRT1 acts as a positive or negative regulator of gene expression depending upon the specific immune cell and its environment. For example, T cell associated SIRT1 appears to play an important role in promoting the generation of Th1, Th9 and Th17 effector cells as well as inducing certain autoimmune or chronic inflammatory diseases. In contrast, B cell associated SIRT1, in the steady state, appears to act as a negative regulator for the production and maturation of protective antibodies. Many of the studies described in this review discuss the therapeutic potential of cell specific SIRT1 targeting in the treatment of different autoimmune and chronic inflammatory disease. Additionally, evidence demonstrates that chronic inflammation and autoimmunity are associated with the development of malignancy (Franks and Slansky, 2012; Yu et al., 2016) and patients with a primary malignancy may develop autoimmune-like disease (Valencia et al., 2019). These relationships imply a need for deeper understanding of the role of up- or down-regulation of SIRT1 and surveillance of patients on immunomodulatory therapies for potential secondary disease processes.

AUTHOR CONTRIBUTIONS

All the authors were involved in manuscript writing and revision. FR and KP finalized the draft. FR submitted the manuscript with consent from all authors.

REFERENCES

1. Akieda-Asai, S., Zaima, N., Ikegami, K., Kahyo, T., Yao, I., Hatanaka, T., et al. (2010). SIRT1 regulates thyroid-stimulating hormone release by enhancing PIP5Kγ activity through deacetylation of specific lysine residues in mammals. *PLoS One* 5:e11755. doi: 10.1371/journal.pone.0011755
2. Akimova, T., Xiao, H., Liu, Y., Bhatti, T. R., Jiao, J., Eruslanov, E., et al. (2014). Targeting sirtuin-1 alleviates experimental autoimmune colitis by induction of Foxp3+ T-regulatory cells. *Mucosal Immunol.* 7, 1209–1220. doi: 10.1038/mi. 2014.10
3. Alamdari, N., Aversa, Z., Castillero, E., Gurav, A., Petkova, V., Tizio, S., et al. (2012). Resveratrol prevents dexamethasone-induced expression of the muscle atrophy-related ubiquitin ligases atrogin-1 and MuRF1 in cultured myotubes through a SIRT1-dependent mechanism. *Biochem. Biophys. Res. Commun.* 417, 528–533. doi: 10.1016/j.bbrc.2011.11.154
4. Alexander, J. S., Mathis, J. M., and Pruitt, K. (2007). Interaction of microsatellite instability and loss of heterozygosity in adenocarcinoma: multiple markers in adenocarcinoma: an introduction to 'Genetic changes in Slovenian patients with gastric adenocarcinoma evaluated in terms of microsatellite DNA.' *Eur. J. Gastroenterol. Hepatol.* 19, 1038–1040. doi: 10.1097/meg.0b013e3282f 1a295
5. Alexander, T., Sharrack, B., Rovira, M., Farge, D., and Snowden, J. A. (2019). "Autoimmune disease," in *The EBMT Handbook: Hematopoietic Stem Cell Transplantation and Cellular Therapies*, eds E. Carreras, C. Dufour, M. Mohty, and N. Kroger (Cham: Springer), 677–683.
6. Allfrey, V. G., Faulkner, R., and Mirsky, A. E. (1964). Acetylation and methylation of histones and their possible role in the regulation of RNA synthesis. *Proc. Natl. Acad. Sci. U.S.A.* 51, 786–794. doi: 10.1073/pnas.51.5.786
7. Allis, C. D., Berger, S. L., Cote, J., Dent, S., Jenuwien, T., Kouzarides, T., et al. (2007). New nomenclature for chromatin-modifying enzymes. *Cell* 131, 633–636. doi: 10.1016/j.cell.2007.10.039
8. Al-Regaiey, K. A., Masternak, M. M., Bonkowski, M., Sun, L., and Bartke, A. (2005). Long-lived growth hormone receptor knockout mice: interaction of reduced insulin-like growth factor i/insulin signaling and caloric restriction. *Endocrinology* 146, 851–860. doi: 10.1210/en.2004-1120
9. Amat, R., Solanes, G., Giralt, M., and Villarroya, F. (2007). SIRT1 is involved in glucocorticoid-mediated control of uncoupling protein-3 gene transcription. *J. Biol. Chem.* 282, 34066–34076. doi: 10.1074/jbc.m707114200
10. Anastasiou, D., and Krek, W. (2006). SIRT1: linking adaptive cellular responses to aging-associated changes in organismal physiology. *Physiology* 21, 404–410. doi: 10.1152/physiol.00031.2006
11. Aoyagi, S., and Archer, T. K. (2008). Nicotinamide uncouples hormone-dependent chromatin remodeling from transcription complex assembly. *Mol. Cell. Biol.* 28, 30–39. doi: 10.1128/mcb.01158-07
12. Audrito, V., Vaisitti, T., Rossi, D., Gottardi, D., D'Arena, G., Laurenti, L., et al. (2011). Nicotinamide blocks proliferation and induces apoptosis of chronic lymphocytic leukemia cells through activation of the p53/miR-34a/SIRT1 tumor suppressor network. *Cancer Res.* 71, 4473–4483. doi: 10.1158/0008- 5472.can-10-4452
13. Bannister, A. J., Zegerman, P., Partridge, J. F., Miska, E. A., Thomas, J. O., Allshire, R. C., et al. (2001). Selective recognition of methylated lysine 9 on histone H3 by the HP1 chromo domain. *Nature* 410, 120–124. doi: 10.1038/35065138
14. Bartke, A., Sun, L. Y., and Longo, V. (2013). Somatotropic signaling: trade-offs between growth, reproductive development, and longevity. *Physiol. Rev.* 93, 571–598. doi: 10.1152/physrev.00006.2012
15. Beier, U. H., Wang, L., Bhatti, T. R., Liu, Y., Han, R., Ge, G., et al. (2011). Sirtuin- 1 targeting promotes Foxp3+ T-regulatory cell function and prolongs allograft survival. *Mol. Cell. Biol.* 31, 1022–1029. doi: 10.1128/mcb.01206-10
16. Bernier, M., Paul, R. K., Martin-Montalvo, A., Scheibye-Knudsen, M., Song, S., He, H. J., et al. (2011). Negative regulation of STAT3 protein-mediated cellular respiration by SIRT1 protein. *J. Biol. Chem.* 286, 19270–19279. doi: 10.1074/jbc. M110.200311
17. Biason-Lauber, A., Boni-Schnetzler, M., Hubbard, B. P., Bouzakri, K., Brunner, A., Cavelti-Weder, C., et al. (2013). Identification of a SIRT1 mutation in a family with type 1 diabetes. *Cell Metab.* 17, 448–455. doi: 10.1016/j.cmet.2013.02.001
18. Blander, G., and Guarente, L. (2004). The Sir2 family of protein deacetylases. *Annu. Rev. Biochem.* 73, 417–435. doi: 10.1146/annurev.biochem.73.011303.073651 Boily, G., Seifert, E. L., Bevilacqua, L., He, X. H., Sabourin, G., Estey, C., et al. (2008).
19. SirT1 regulates energy metabolism and response to caloric restriction in mice. *PLoS One* 3:e1759. doi: 10.1371/journal.pone.0001759
20. Bremer, A. A., and Miller, W. L. (2014). "Regulation of steroidogenesis," in *Cellular Endocrinology in Health and Disease*, eds A. Aguirre and P. M. Conn (Amsterdam: Elsevier), 207–227. doi: 10.1016/b978-0-12-408134-5.00013-5
21. Campbell, C., and Rudensky, A. (2020). Roles of regulatory T cells in tissue pathophysiology and metabolism. *Cell Metab.* 31, 18–25. doi: 10.1016/j.cmet.2019.09.010
22. Caruso, R., Marafini, I., Franze, E., Stolfi, C., Zorzi, F., Monteleone, I., et al. (2014). Defective expression of SIRT1 contributes to sustain inflammatory pathways in the gut. *Mucosal Immunol.* 7, 1467–1479. doi: 10.1038/mi.2014.35

23. Cea, M., Soncini, D., Fruscione, F., Raffaghello, L., Garuti, A., Emionite, L., et al. (2011). Synergistic interactions between HDAC and sirtuin inhibitors in human leukemia cells. *PLoS One* 6:e22739. doi: 10.1371/journal.pone.0022739
24. Chadha, S., Wang, L., Hancock, W. W., and Beier, U. H. (2019). Sirtuin-1 in immunotherapy: a Janus-headed target. *J. Leukoc. Biol.* 106, 337–343. doi: 10. 1002/JLB.2RU1118-422R
25. Chang, H.-C., and Guarente, L. (2014). SIRT1 and other sirtuins in metabolism. *Trends Endocrinol. Metab.* 25, 138–145. doi: 10.1016/j.tem.2013.12.001
26. Chen, X., Lu, Y., Zhang, Z., Wang, J., Yang, H., and Liu, G. (2015). Intercellular interplay between Sirt1 signalling and Cell Metabolism in immune cell biology. *Immunology* 145, 455–467. doi: 10.1111/imm.12473
27. Cheng, Y., He, C., Wang, M., Ma, X., Mo, F., Yang, S., et al. (2019). Targeting epigenetic regulators for cancer therapy: mechanisms and advances in clinical trials. *Signal Transduct. Target. Ther.* 4, 1–39.
28. Chiu, H. C., Chiu, C. Y., Yang, R. S., Chan, D. C., Liu, S. H., and Chiang, C. K. (2018). Preventing muscle wasting by osteoporosis drug alendronate in vitro and in myopathy models via sirtuin-3 down-regulation. *J. Cachexia Sarcopenia Muscle* 9, 585–602. doi: 10.1002/jcsm.12289
29. Cho, J. H., and Gregersen, P. K. (2011). Genomics and the multifactorial nature of human autoimmune disease. *N. Engl. J. Med.* 365, 1612–1623. doi: 10.1056/ NEJMra1100030
30. Choi, I., Rickert, E., Fernandez, M., and Webster, N. J. G. (2019). SIRT1 in astrocytes regulates glucose metabolism and reproductive function. *Endocrinology* 160, 1547–1560. doi: 10.1210/en.2019-00223
31. Choudhary, C., Kumar, C., Gnad, F., Nielsen, M. L., Rehman, M., Walther, T. C., et al. (2009). Lysine acetylation targets protein complexes and co-regulates major cellular functions. *Science* 325, 834–840. doi: 10.1126/ science.1175371
32. Christensen, A. D., Haase, C., Cook, A. D., and Hamilton, J. A. (2016). K/ BxN serum-transfer arthritis as a model for human inflammatory arthritis. *Front. Immunol.* 7:213. doi: 10.3389/fimmu.2016.00213
33. Chuprin, A., Avin, A., Goldfarb, Y., Herzig, Y., Levi, B., Jacob, A., et al. (2015). The deacetylase Sirt1 is an essential regulator of Aire-mediated induction of central immunological tolerance. *Nat. Immunol.* 16, 737–745. doi: 10.1038/ni. 3194
34. Cohen, D. E., Supinski, A. M., Bonkowski, M. S., Donmez, G., and Guarente, L. P. (2009). Neuronal SIRT1 regulates endocrine and behavioral responses to calorie restriction. *Genes Dev.* 23, 2812–2817. doi: 10.1101/gad.1839209
35. Cordeiro, A., de Souza, L. L., Oliveira, L. S., Faustino, L. C., Santiago, L. A., Bloise, F. F., et al. (2013). Thyroid hormone regulation of Sirtuin 1 expression and implications to integrated responses in fasted mice. *J. Endocrinol.* 216, 181–193. doi: 10.1530/joe-12-0420
36. Daenthanasanmak, A., Iamsawat, S., Chakraborty, P., Nguyen, H. D., Bastian, D., Liu, C., et al. (2019). Targeting Sirt-1 controls GVHD by inhibiting T-cell allo-response and promoting Treg stability in mice. *Blood* 133, 266–279. doi: 10.1182/blood-2018-07-863233
37. Dai, H., Sinclair, D. A., Ellis, J. L., and Steegborn, C. (2018). Sirtuin activators and inhibitors: promises, achievements, and challenges. *Pharmacol. Ther.* 188, 140–154. doi: 10.1016/j.pharmthera.2018.03.004
38. Dai, Y., Ngo, D., Forman, L. W., Qin, D. C., Jacob, J., and Faller, D. V. (2007). Sirtuin 1 is required for antagonist-induced transcriptional repression of androgen- responsive genes by the androgen receptor. *Mol. Endocrinol.* 21, 1807–1821. doi: 10.1210/me.2006-0467
39. Daniel, A. R., Gaviglio, A. L., Czaplicki, L. M., Hillard, C. J., Housa, D., and Lange, C. A. (2010). The progesterone receptor hinge region regulates the kinetics of transcriptional responses through acetylation, phosphorylation, and nuclear retention. *Mol. Endocrinol.* 24, 2126–2138. doi: 10.1210/me.2010-0170
40. Dawson, M. A., and Kouzarides, T. (2012). Cancer epigenetics: from mechanism to therapy. *Cell* 150, 12–27. doi: 10.1016/j.cell.2012.06.013
41. de Lumen, B. O. (2005). Lunasin: a cancer-preventive soy peptide. *Nutr. Rev.* 63, 16–21. doi: 10.1301/nr.2004.janr.16-21
42. Di, M. M., Del, B. D., and Trisciuoglio, D. (2016). The multifaceted role of lysine acetylation in cancer: prognostic biomarker and therapeutic target. *Oncotarget* 7, 55789–55810. doi: 10.18632/oncotarget.10048
43. Elangovan, S., Ramachandran, S., Venkatesan, N., Ananth, S., Gnana-Prakasam, P., Martin, P. M., et al. (2011). SIRT1 is essential for oncogenic signaling by estrogen/estrogen receptor α in breast cancer. *Cancer Res.* 71, 6654–6664. doi: 10.1158/0008-5472.can-11-1446
44. Ellmeier, W., and Seiser, C. (2018). Histone deacetylase function in CD4(+) T cells. *Nat. Rev. Immunol.* 18, 617–634. doi: 10.1038/s41577-018-0037-z
45. Emiliani, S., Fischle, W., Van, L. C., Al-Abed, Y., and Verdin, E. (1998). Characterization of a human RPD3 ortholog, HDAC3. *Proc. Natl. Acad. Sci. U.S.A.* 95, 2795–2800. doi: 10.1073/pnas.95.6.2795
46. Everts, B., Amiel, E., van der Windt, G. J., Freitas, T. C., Chott, R., Yarasheski, K. E., et al. (2012). Commitment to glycolysis sustains survival of NO-producing inflammatory dendritic cells. *Blood* 120, 1422–1431. doi: 10.1182/ blood-2012- 03-419747
47. Fan, Y.-Y., Kohno, M., Hitomi, H., Kitada, K., Fujisawa, Y., Yatabe, J., et al. (2011). Aldosterone/mineralocorticoid receptor stimulation induces cellular senescence in the kidney. *Endocrinology* 152, 680–688. doi: 10.1210/en.2010-0829
48. Firestein, R., Blander, G., Michan, S., Oberdoerffer, P., Ogino, S., Campbell, J., et al. (2008). The SIRT1 deacetylase suppresses intestinal tumorigenesis and colon cancer growth. *PLoS One* 3:e2020. doi: 10.1371/journal.pone.0002020
49. Fischle, W., Emiliani, S., Hendzel, M. J., Nagase, T., Nomura, N., Voelter, W., et al. (1999). A new family of human histone deacetylases related to Saccharomyces cerevisiae HDA1p. *J. Biol. Chem.* 274, 11713–11720.
50. Fonseca-Kelly, Z., Nassrallah, M., Uribe, J., Khan, R. S., Dine, K., Dutt, M., et al. (2012). Resveratrol neuroprotection in a chronic mouse model of multiple sclerosis. *Front. Neurol.* 3:84. doi: 10.3389/fneur.2012.00084
51. Ford, J., Jiang, M., and Milner, J. (2005). Cancer-specific functions of SIRT1 enable human epithelial cancer cell growth and survival. *Cancer Res.* 65, 10457–10463. doi: 10.1158/0008-5472.can-05-1923
52. Foss, F., Horwitz, S., Pro, B., Prince, H. M., Sokol, L., Balser, B., et al. (2016). Romidepsin for the treatment of relapsed/refractory peripheral T cell lymphoma: prolonged stable disease provides clinical benefits for patients in the pivotal trial. *J. Hematol. Oncol.* 9:22. doi: 10.1186/s13045-016-0243-8
53. Franks, A. L., and Slansky, J. E. (2012). Multiple associations between a broad spectrum of autoimmune diseases, chronic inflammatory diseases and cancer. *Anticancer Res.* 32, 1119–1136.
54. Frye, R. A. (2000). Phylogenetic classification of prokaryotic and eukaryotic Sir2- like proteins. *Biochem. Biophys. Res. Commun.* 273, 793–798. doi: 10.1006/bbrc. 2000.3000
55. Fu, M., Liu, M., Sauve, A. A., Jiao, X., Zhang, X., Wu, X., et al. (2006). Hormonal control of androgen receptor function through SIRT1. *Mol. Cell. Biol.* 26, 8122–8135. doi: 10.1128/mcb.00289-06
56. Gan, H., Shen, T., Chupp, D. P., Taylor, J. R., Sanchez, H. N., Li, X., et al. (2020). B cell Sirt1 deacetylates histone and non-histone proteins for epigenetic modulation of AID expression and the antibody response. *Sci. Adv.* 6:eaay2793. doi: 10.1126/sciadv.aay2793
57. Gan, L., Han, Y., Bastianetto, S., Dumont, Y., Unterman, T. G., and Quirion, R. (2005). FoxO-dependent and-independent mechanisms mediate SirT1 effects on IGFBP-1 gene expression. *Biochem. Biophys. Res. Commun.* 337, 1092–1096. doi: 10.1016/j.bbrc.2005.09.169
58. Gardner, P. J., Joshi, L., Lee, R. W., Dick, A. D., Adamson, P., and Calder, V. L. (2013). SIRT1 activation protects against autoimmune T cell-driven retinal disease in mice via inhibition of IL-2/Stat5 signaling. *J. Autoimmun.* 42, 117–129. doi: 10.1016/j.jaut.2013.01.011
59. Gardner, P. J., Yazid, S., Chu, C. J., Copland, D. A., Adamson, P., Dick, A. D., et al. (2015). TNFalpha Regulates SIRT1 cleavage during ocular autoimmune disease. *Am. J. Pathol.* 185, 1324–1333. doi: 10.1016/j.ajpath.2015.01.017
60. Ghanta, S., Grossmann, R. E., and Brenner, C. (2013). Mitochondrial protein acetylation as a cell-intrinsic, evolutionary driver of fat storage: chemical and metabolic logic of acetyl-lysine modifications. *Crit. Rev. Biochem. Mol. Biol.* 48, 561–574. doi: 10.3109/10409238.2013.838204
61. Gregoretti, I. V., Lee, Y. M., and Goodson, H. V. (2004). Molecular evolution of the histone deacetylase family: functional implications of phylogenetic analysis. *J. Mol. Biol.* 338, 17–31. doi: 10.1016/j.jmb.2004.02.006
62. Greiss, S., and Gartner, A. (2009). Sirtuin/Sir2 phylogeny, evolutionary considerations and structural conservation. *Mol. Cells* 28, 407–415. doi: 10. 1007/s10059-009-0169-x
63. Grozinger, C. M., Hassig, C. A., and Schreiber, S. L. (1999). Three proteins define a class of human histone deacetylases related to yeast Hda1p. *Proc. Natl. Acad. Sci. U.S.A.* 96, 4868–4873. doi: 10.1073/pnas.96.9.4868
64. Hah, Y. S., Cheon, Y. H., Lim, H. S., Cho, H. Y., Park, B. H., Ka, S. O., et al. (2014). Myeloid deletion of SIRT1 aggravates serum transfer arthritis in mice via nuclear factor-kappaB activation. *PLoS One* 9:e87733. doi: 10.1371/ journal. pone.0087733
65. Hallows, W. C., Lee, S., and Denu, J. M. (2006). Sirtuins deacetylate and activate mammalian acetyl-CoA synthetases. *Proc. Natl. Acad. Sci. U.S.A.* 103, 10230– 10235. doi: 10.1073/pnas.0604392103

66. Hanahan, D., and Weinberg, R. A. (2011). Hallmarks of cancer: the next generation. *Cell* 144, 646–674. doi: 10.1016/j.cell.2011.02.013
67. Hebert, J. R., Hurley, T. G., Olendzki, B. C., Teas, J., Ma, Y., and Hampl, J. S. (1998). Nutritional and socioeconomic factors in relation to prostate cancer mortality: a cross-national study. *J. Natl. Cancer Inst.* 90, 1637–1647. doi: 10.1093/jnci/90.21.1637
68. Heltweg, B., Gatbonton, T., Schuler, A. D., Posakony, J., Li, H., Goehle, S., et al. (2006). Antitumor activity of a small-molecule inhibitor of human silent information regulator 2 enzymes. *Cancer Res.* 66, 4368–4377. doi: 10.1158/0008-5472.can-05-3617
69. Henning, A. N., Roychoudhuri, R., and Restifo, N. P. (2018). Epigenetic control of CD8(+) T cell differentiation. *Nat. Rev. Immunol.* 18, 340–356. doi: 10.1038/nri. 2017.146
70. Herman, J. G., and Baylin, S. B. (2003). Gene silencing in cancer in association with promoter hypermethylation. *N. Engl. J. Med.* 349, 2042–2054. doi: 10.1056/ nejmra023075
71. Heyn, J., Luchting, B., Hinske, L. C., Hubner, M., Azad, S. C., and Kreth, S. (2016). miR-124a and miR-155 enhance differentiation of regulatory T cells in patients with neuropathic pain. *J. Neuroinflammation* 13:248. doi: 10.1186/s12974-016- 0712-6
72. Hirai, S., Endo, S., Saito, R., Hirose, M., Ueno, T., Suzuki, H., et al. (2014). Antitumor effects of a sirtuin inhibitor, tenovin-6, against gastric cancer cells via death receptor 5 up-regulation. *PLoS One* 9:e102831. doi: 10.1371/journal.pone.0102831
73. Holloway, K. R., Barbieri, A., Malyarchuk, S., Saxena, M., Nedeljkovic-Kurepa, A., Cameron Mehl, M., et al. (2013). SIRT1 positively regulates breast cancer associated human aromatase (CYP19A1) expression. *Mol. Endocrinol.* 27, 480– 490. doi: 10.1210/me.2012-1347
74. Hu, J., Jing, H., and Lin, H. (2014). Sirtuin inhibitors as anticancer agents. *Future Med. Chem.* 6, 945–966. doi: 10.4155/fmc.14.44
75. Huo, L., Bai, X., Wang, Y., and Wang, M. (2017). Betulinic acid derivative B10 inhibits glioma cell proliferation through suppression of SIRT1, acetylation of FOXO3a and upregulation of Bim/PUMA. *Biomed. Pharmacother.* 92, 347–355. doi: 10.1016/j.biopha.2017.05.074
76. Imperatore, F., Maurizio, J., Vargas Aguilar, S., Busch, C. J., Favret, J., Kowenz-Leutz, E., et al. (2017). SIRT1 regulates macrophage self-renewal. *EMBO J.* 36, 2353–2372. doi: 10.15252/embj.201695737
77. Jaganathan, A., Chaurasia, P., Xiao, G.-Q., Philizaire, M., Lv, X., Yao, S., et al. (2014). Coactivator MYST1 regulates nuclear factor-κB and androgen receptor functions during proliferation of prostate cancer cells. *Mol. Endocrinol.* 28, 872–885. doi: 10.1210/me.2014-1055
78. Jiang, Y., Botchway, B. O., Hu, Z., and Fang, M. (2019). Overexpression of SIRT1 Inhibits Corticosterone-Induced Autophagy. *Neuroscience* 411, 11–22. doi: 10.1016/j.neuroscience.2019.05.035
79. Jin, K. L., Park, J.-Y., Noh, E. J., Hoe, K. L., Lee, J. H., Kim, J.-H., et al. (2010). The effect of combined treatment with cisplatin and histone deacetylase inhibitors on HeLa cells. *J. Gynecol. Oncol.* 21, 262–268. doi: 10.3802/jgo.2010.21. 4.262
80. Jin, Y., Cao, Q., Chen, C., Du, X., Jin, B., and Pan, J. (2015). Tenovin-6-mediated inhibition of SIRT1/2 induces apoptosis in acute lymphoblastic leukemia (ALL) cells and eliminates ALL stem/progenitor cells. *BMC Cancer* 15:226. doi: 10. 1186/s12885-015-1282-1
81. Johnstone, R. W. (2002). Histone-deacetylase inhibitors: novel drugs for the treatment of cancer. *Nat. Rev. Drug Discov.* 1, 287–299. doi: 10.1038/nrd772 Jung-Hynes, B., Nihal, M., Zhong, W., and Ahmad, N. (2009). Role of sirtuin histone deacetylase SIRT1 in prostate cancer a target for prostate cancer management via its inhibition? *J. Biol. Chem.* 284, 3823–3832. doi: 10.1074/ jbc.m807869200
82. Kaplan, M. H., Hufford, M. M., and Olson, M. R. (2015). The development and in vivo function of T helper 9 cells. *Nat. Rev. Immunol.* 15, 295–307. doi: 10.1038/nri3824
83. Karin, M., and Lin, A. (2002). NF-kappaB at the crossroads of life and death. *Nat. Immunol.* 3, 221–227. doi: 10.1038/ni0302-221
84. Kelly, T. K., De Carvalho, D. D., and Jones, P. A. (2010). Epigenetic modifications as therapeutic targets. *Nat. Biotechnol.* 28, 1069–1078.
85. Khan, M., Ullah, R., Rehman, S. U., Shah, S. A., Saeed, K., Muhammad, T., et al. (2019). 17β-Estradiol Modulates SIRT1 and halts oxidative stress-mediated cognitive impairment in a male aging mouse model. *Cells* 8:928. doi: 10.3390/ cells8080928
86. Kim, M. Y., Woo, E. M., Chong, Y. T. E., Homenko, D. R., and Kraus, W. L. (2006). Acetylation of estrogen receptor α by p300 at lysines 266 and 268 enhances the deoxyribonucleic acid binding and transactivation activities of the receptor. *Mol. Endocrinol.* 20, 1479–1493. doi: 10.1210/me.2005-0531
87. Kim, S. C., Sprung, R., Chen, Y., Xu, Y., Ball, H., Pei, J., et al. (2006). Substrate and functional diversity of lysine acetylation revealed by a proteomics survey. *Mol. Cell* 23, 607–618. doi: 10.1016/j.molcel.2006.06.026
88. Knobloch, J., Wahl, C., Feldmann, M., Jungck, D., Strauch, J., Stoelben, E., et al. (2014). Resveratrol attenuates the release of inflammatory cytokines from human bronchial smooth muscle cells exposed to lipoteichoic acid in chronic obstructive pulmonary disease. *Basic Clin. Pharmacol. Toxicol.* 114, 202–209. doi: 10.1111/bcpt.12129
89. Knyphausen, P., Kuhlmann, N., de, B. S., and Lammers, M. (2015). Lysine-acetylation as a fundamental regulator of Ran function: implications for signaling of proteins of the Ras-superfamily. *Small GTPases* 6, 189–195. doi: 10.1080/21541248.2015.1103399
90. Kojima, K., Ohhashi, R., Fujita, Y., Hamada, N., Akao, Y., Nozawa, Y., et al. (2008). A role for SIRT1 in cell growth and chemoresistance in prostate cancer PC3 and DU145 cells. *Biochem. Biophys. Res. Commun.* 373, 423–428. doi: 10.1016/j.bbrc.2008.06.045
91. Kolthur-Seetharam, U., Teerds, K., de Rooij, D. G., Wendling, O., McBurney, M., Sassone-Corsi, P., et al. (2009). The histone deacetylase SIRT1 controls male fertility in mice through regulation of hypothalamic-pituitary gonadotropin signaling. *Biol. Reprod.* 80, 384–391. doi: 10.1095/biolreprod.108.070193
92. Kume, S., Uzu, T., Kashiwagi, A., and Koya, D. (2010). SIRT1, a calorie restriction mimetic, in a new therapeutic approach for type 2 diabetes mellitus and diabetic vascular complications. *Endocr. Metab. Immune Disord. Drug Targets* 10, 16–24. doi: 10.2174/187153010790827957
93. Kuroda, S., Yamazaki, M., Abe, M., Sakimura, K., Takayanagi, H., and Iwai, Y. (2011). Basic leucine zipper transcription factor, ATF-like (BATF) regulates epigenetically and energetically effector CD8 T-cell differentiation via Sirt1 expression. *Proc. Natl. Acad. Sci. U.S.A.* 108, 14885–14889. doi: 10.1073/pnas. 1105133108
94. Lain, S., Hollick, J. J., Campbell, J., Staples, O. D., Higgins, M., Aoubala, M., et al. (2008). Discovery, in vivo activity, and mechanism of action of a small-molecule p53 activator. *Cancer Cell* 13, 454–463. doi: 10.1016/j.ccr.2008.03.004
95. Lakhani, H. V., Zehra, M., Pillai, S. S., Puri, N., Shapiro, J. I., Abraham, N. G., et al. (2019). Beneficial Role of HO-1-SIRT1 Axis in Attenuating Angiotensin II-Induced Adipocyte Dysfunction. *Int. J. Mol. Sci.* 20:3205. doi: 10.3390/ ijms20133205
96. Lannes, J., L'Hôte, D., Garrel, G., Laverrière, J.-N., Cohen-Tannoudji, J., and Quérat, B. (2015). Rapid communication: a microRNA-132/212 pathway mediates GnRH activation of FSH expression. *Mol. Endocrinol.* 29, 364–372. doi: 10.1210/me.2014-1390
97. Lara, E., Mai, A., Calvanese, V., Altucci, L., Lopez-Nieva, P., Martinez-Chantar, M., et al. (2009). Salermide, a Sirtuin inhibitor with a strong cancer-specific proapoptotic effect. *Oncogene* 28, 781–791. doi: 10.1038/onc.2008.436
98. Lee, H., Kim, K. R., Noh, S. J., Park, H. S., Kwon, K. S., Park, B.-H., et al. (2011). Expression of DBC1 and SIRT1 is associated with poor prognosis for breast carcinoma. *Hum. Pathol.* 42, 204–213. doi: 10.1016/j.humpath.2010.05.023
99. Lee, J. J., Lee, H. J., Son, B. H., Kim, S. B., Ahn, J. H., Ahn, S. D., et al. (2016). Expression of FOXM 1 and related proteins in breast cancer molecular subtypes. *Int. J. Exp. Pathol.* 97, 170–177.
100. Lefranc, C., Friederich-Persson, M., Braud, L., Palacios-Ramirez, R., Karlsson, S., Boujardine, N., et al. (2019). MR (mineralocorticoid receptor) induces adipose tissue senescence and mitochondrial dysfunction leading to vascular dysfunction in obesity. *Hypertension* 73, 458–468. doi: 10.1161/hypertensionaha.118.11873
101. Legutko, A., Marichal, T., Fievez, L., Bedoret, D., Mayer, A., de Vries, H., et al. (2011). Sirtuin 1 promotes Th2 responses and airway allergy by repressing peroxisome proliferator-activated receptor-gamma activity in dendritic cells. *J. Immunol.* 187, 4517–4529. doi: 10.4049/jimmunol.1101493
102. Leko, V., Park, G. J., Lao, U., Simon, J. A., and Bedalov, A. (2013). Enterocyte-specific inactivation of SIRT1 reduces tumor load in the APC(+/min) mouse model. *PLoS. One* 8:e66283. doi: 10.1371/journal.pone.0066283
103. Leko, V., Varnum-Finney, B., Li, H., Gu, Y., Flowers, D., Nourigat, C., et al. (2012). SIRT1 is dispensable for function of hematopoietic stem cells in adult mice. *Blood* 119, 1856–1860. doi: 10.1182/blood-2011-09-377077
104. Levine, M. H., Wang, Z., Xiao, H., Jiao, J., Wang, L., Bhatti, T. R., et al. (2016). Targeting Sirtuin-1 prolongs murine renal allograft survival and function. *Kidney Int.* 89, 1016–1026. doi: 10.1016/j.kint.2015.12.051
105. Li, G., Rivas, P., Bedolla, R., Thapa, D., Reddick, R. L., Ghosh, R., et al. (2013). Dietary resveratrol prevents development of high-grade prostatic intraepithelial neoplastic lesions: involvement of SIRT1/S6K axis. *Cancer Prev. Res.* 6, 27–39. doi: 10.1158/1940-6207.capr-12-0349

106. Li, H., Xia, N., Hasselwander, S., and Daiber, A. (2019). Resveratrol and vascular function. *Int. J. Mol. Sci.* 20:2155. doi: 10.3390/ijms20092155
107. Li, J., Wang, E., Rinaldo, F., and Datta, K. (2005). Upregulation of VEGF-C by androgen depletion: the involvement of IGF-IR-FOXO pathway. *Oncogene* 24, 5510–5520. doi: 10.1038/sj.onc.1208693
108. Li, T., Garcia-Gomez, A., Morante-Palacios, O., Ciudad, L., Ozkaramehmet, S., Van Dijck, E., et al. (2020). SIRT1/2 orchestrate acquisition of DNA methylation and loss of histone H3 activating marks to prevent premature activation of inflammatory genes in macrophages. *Nucleic Acids Res.* 48, 665–681. doi: 10. 1093/nar/gkz1127
109. Libert, S., Pointer, K., Bell, E. L., Das, A., Cohen, D. E., Asara, J. M., et al. (2011). SIRT1 activates MAO-A in the brain to mediate anxiety and exploratory drive. *Cell* 147, 1459–1472. doi: 10.1016/j.cell.2011.10.054
110. Lim, H. W., Kang, S. G., Ryu, J. K., Schilling, B., Fei, M., Lee, I. S., et al. (2015). SIRT1 deacetylates RORgammat and enhances Th17 cell generation. *J. Exp. Med.* 212, 607–617. doi: 10.1084/jem.20132378
111. Limagne, E., Thibaudin, M., Euvrard, R., Berger, H., Chalons, P., Vegan, F., et al. (2017). Sirtuin-1 activation controls tumor growth by impeding Th17 differentiation via STAT3 Deacetylation. *Cell Rep.* 19, 746–759. doi: 10.1016/j.celrep.2017.04.004
112. Lin, J.-N., Lin, V. C.-H., Rau, K.-M., Shieh, P.-C., Kuo, D.-H., Shieh, J.-C., et al. (2010). Resveratrol modulates tumor cell proliferation and protein translation via SIRT1-dependent AMPK activation. *J. Agric. Food Chem.* 58, 1584–1592. doi: 10.1021/jf9035782
113. Lin, Q. Q., Geng, Y. W., Jiang, Z. W., and Tian, Z. J. (2017). SIRT1 regulates lipopolysaccharide-induced CD40 expression in renal medullary collecting duct cells by suppressing the TLR4-NF-kappaB signaling pathway. *Life Sci.* 170, 100–107. doi: 10.1016/j.lfs.2016.11.026
114. Lin, Q. Q., Yan, C. F., Lin, R., Zhang, J. Y., Wang, W. R., Yang, L. N., et al. (2012). SIRT1 regulates TNF-alpha-induced expression of CD40 in 3T3-L1 adipocytes via NF-kappaB pathway. *Cytokine* 60, 447–455. doi: 10.1016/j.cyto.2012.05.025 Liu, G., Bi, Y., Xue, L., Zhang, Y., Yang, H., Chen, X., et al. (2015). Dendritic cell SIRT1-HIF1alpha axis programs the differentiation of CD4+ T cells through IL- 12 and TGF-beta1. *Proc. Natl. Acad. Sci. U.S.A.* 112, E957–E965. doi: 10.1073/ pnas.1420419112
115. Liu, G., Su, L., Hao, X., Zhong, N., Zhong, D., Singhal, S., et al. (2012). Salermide up-regulates death receptor 5 expression through the ATF4-ATF3-CHOP axis and leads to apoptosis in human cancer cells. *J. Cell. Mol. Med.* 16, 1618–1628. doi: 10.1111/j.1582-4934.2011.01401.x
116. Longo, V. D., and Kennedy, B. K. (2006). Sirtuins in aging and age-related disease. *Cell* 126, 257–268. doi: 10.1016/j.cell.2006.07.002
117. Lugrin, J., Ciarlo, E., Santos, A., Grandmaison, G., Dos Santos, I., Le Roy, D., et al. (2013). The sirtuin inhibitor cambinol impairs MAPK signaling, inhibits inflammatory and innate immune responses and protects from septic shock. *Biochim. Biophys. Acta* 1833, 1498–1510. doi: 10.1016/j.bbamcr.2013.03.004
118. Lux, S., Lobos, N., Lespay-Rebolledo, C., Salas-Huenuleo, E., Kogan, M. J., Flores, C., et al. (2019). The antinociceptive effect of resveratrol in bone cancer pain is inhibited by the Silent Information Regulator 1 inhibitor selisistat. *J. Pharm. Pharmacol.* 71, 816–825. doi: 10.1111/jphp.13064
119. Ma, J., Fu, Q., Wang, Z., Zhou, P., Qiao, S., Wang, B., et al. (2019). Sodium hydrosulfide mitigates dexamethasone-induced osteoblast dysfunction by interfering with mitochondrial function. *Biotechnol. Appl. Biochem.* 66, 690–697. doi: 10.1002/bab.1786
120. Ma, Z., Faulkner, M. J., and Helmann, J. D. (2012). Origins of specificity and cross- talk in metal ion sensing by *Bacillus subtilis* Fur. *Mol. Microbiol.* 86, 1144–1155. doi: 10.1111/mmi.12049
121. Manna, P. R., Ahmed, A. U., Vartak, D., Molehin, D., and Pruitt, K. (2019). Overexpression of the steroidogenic acute regulatory protein in breast cancer: regulation by histone deacetylase inhibition. *Biochem. Biophys. Res. Commun.* 509, 476–482. doi: 10.1016/j.bbrc.2018.12.145
122. Manna, P. R., Sennoune, S. R., Martinez-Zaguilan, R., Slominski, A. T., and Pruitt, (2015a). Regulation of retinoid mediated cholesterol efflux involves liver X receptor activation in mouse macrophages. *Biochem. Biophys. Res. Commun.* 464, 312–317. doi: 10.1016/j.bbrc.2015.06.150
123. Manna, P. R., Stetson, C. L., Daugherty, C., Shimizu, I., Syapin, P. J., Garrel, G., et al. (2015b). Up-regulation of steroid biosynthesis by retinoid signaling: implications for aging. *Mech. Ageing Dev.* 150, 74–82. doi: 10.1016/j.mad.2015. 08.007
124. Manna, P. R., Stetson, C. L., Slominski, A. T., and Pruitt, K. (2016). Role of the steroidogenic acute regulatory protein in health and disease. *Endocrine* 51, 7–21. doi: 10.1007/s12020-015-0715-6
125. Mao, B., Zhao, G., Lv, X., Chen, H.-Z., Xue, Z., Yang, B., et al. (2011). Sirt1 deacetylates c-Myc and promotes c-Myc/Max association. *Int. J. Biochem. Cell Biol.* 43, 1573–1581. doi: 10.1016/j.biocel.2011.07.006
126. Markakis, E. A. (2002). Development of the neuroendocrine hypothalamus. *Front. Neuroendocrinol.* 23, 257–291. doi: 10.1016/s0091-3022(02)00003-1
127. Marmorstein, R. (2001). Structure and function of histone acetyltransferases. *Cell. Mol. Life Sci.* 58, 693–703. doi: 10.1007/pl00000893
128. Marshall, G. M., Liu, P. Y., Gherardi, S., Scarlett, C. J., Bedalov, A., Xu, N., et al. (2011). SIRT1 promotes N-Myc oncogenesis through a positive feedback loop involving the effects of MKP3 and ERK on N-Myc protein stability. *PLoS Genet.* 7:e1002135. doi: 10.1371/journal.pgen.1002135
129. Martin, C., and Zhang, Y. (2005). The diverse functions of histone lysine methylation. *Nat. Rev. Mol. Cell Biol.* 6, 838–849. doi: 10.1038/nrm1761
130. McInnes, I. B., and Schett, G. (2011). The pathogenesis of rheumatoid arthritis. *N. Engl. J. Med.* 365, 2205–2219. doi: 10.1056/NEJMra1004965
131. Milman, S., Huffman, D. M., and Barzilai, N. (2016). The somatotropic axis in human aging: framework for the current state of knowledge and future research. *Cell Metab.* 23, 980–989. doi: 10.1016/j.cmet.2016.05.014
132. Molehin, D., Castro-Piedras, I., Sharma, M., Sennoune, S. R., Arena, D., Manna, P. R., et al. (2018). Aromatase acetylation patterns and altered activity in response to sirtuin inhibition. *Mol. Cancer Res.* 16, 1530–1542. doi: 10.1158/ 1541-7786.MCR-18-0047
133. Monteserin-Garcia, J., Al-Massadi, O., Seoane, L. M., Alvarez, C. V., Shan, B., Stalla, J., et al. (2013). Sirt1 inhibits the transcription factor CREB to regulate pituitary growth hormone synthesis. *FASEB J.* 27, 1561–1571. doi: 10.1096/fj.12-22 0129
134. Moore, R., Dai, Y., and Faller, D. (2012). Sirtuin 1 (SIRT1) and steroid hormone receptor activity in cancer. *J. Endocrinol.* 213, 37–48. doi: 10.1530/joe-11-0217 Moreira, D., Rodrigues, V., Abengozar, M., Rivas, L., Rial, E., Laforge, M., et al. (2015). Leishmania infantum modulates host macrophage mitochondrial metabolism by hijacking the SIRT1-AMPK axis. *PLoS Pathog.* 11:e1004684. doi: 10.1371/journal.ppat.1004684
135. Morita, Y., Wada-Hiraike, O., Yano, T., Shirane, A., Hirano, M., Hiraike, H., et al. (2012). Resveratrol promotes expression of SIRT1 and StAR in rat ovarian granulosa cells: an implicative role of SIRT1 in the ovary. *Reproduct. Biol. Endocrinol.* 10:14. doi: 10.1186/1477-7827-10-14
136. Morrison, S. J., and Scadden, D. T. (2014). The bone marrow niche for haematopoietic stem cells. *Nature* 505, 327–334. doi: 10.1038/nature12984 Nakayama, J., Rice, J. C., Strahl, B. D., Allis, C. D., and Grewal, S. I. (2001). Role of histone H3 lysine 9 methylation in epigenetic control of heterochromatin assembly. *Science* 292, 110–113. doi: 10.1126/science.1060118
137. Neugebauer, R. C., Uchiechowska, U., Meier, R., Hruby, H., Valkov, V., Verdin, E., et al. (2008). Structure–activity studies on splitomicin derivatives as sirtuin inhibitors and computational prediction of binding mode. *J. Med. Chem.* 51, 1203–1213. doi: 10.1021/jm700972e
138. Ng, H. H., and Bird, A. (2000). Histone deacetylases: silencers for hire. *Trends Biochem. Sci.* 25, 121–126. doi: 10.1016/s0968-0004(00)01551-6
139. Nie, Y., Erion, D. M., Yuan, Z., Dietrich, M., Shulman, G. I., Horvath, T. L., et al. (2009). STAT3 inhibition of gluconeogenesis is downregulated by SirT1. *Nat. Cell Biol.* 11, 492–500. doi: 10.1038/ncb1857
140. Niederwieser, D., Baldomero, H., Szer, J., Gratwohl, M., Aljurf, M., Atsuta, Y., et al. (2016). Hematopoietic stem cell transplantation activity worldwide in 2012 and a SWOT analysis of the Worldwide Network for Blood and Marrow Transplantation Group including the global survey. *Bone Marrow Transplant.* 51, 778–785. doi: 10.1038/bmt.2016.18
141. Nightingale, K. P., O'Neill, L. P., and Turner, B. M. (2006). Histone modifications: signalling receptors and potential elements of a heritable epigenetic code. *Curr. Opin. Genet. Dev.* 16, 125–136. doi: 10.1016/j.gde.2006.02.015
142. Nimmagadda, V. K., Makar, T. K., Chandrasekaran, K., Sagi, A. R., Ray, J., Russell, J. W., et al. (2017). SIRT1 and NAD+ precursors: therapeutic targets in multiple sclerosis a review. *J. Neuroimmunol.* 304, 29–34. doi: 10.1016/j.jneuroim.2016. 07.007
143. O'Connor, O. A., Masszi, T., Savage, K. J., Pinter-Brown, L. C., Foss, F. M., Popplewell, L., et al. (2013). *Belinostat, a Novel Pan-Histone Deacetylase Inhibitor (HDACi), in Relapsed or Refractory Peripheral T-Cell Lymphoma (R/R PTCL): Results from the BELIEF Trial.* Alexandria, VA: American Society of Clinical Oncology.
144. Omenetti, S., Bussi, C., Metidji, A., Iseppon, A., Lee, S., Tolaini, M., et al. (2019). The intestine harbors functionally distinct homeostatic tissue-resident and inflammatory Th17 cells. *Immunity* 51, 77–89.e6. doi: 10.1016/j.immuni.2019. 05.004

145. O'Neill, L. A., and Pearce, E. J. (2016). Immunometabolism governs dendritic cell and macrophage function. *J. Exp. Med.* 213, 15–23. doi: 10.1084/jem.20151570 Orozco-Solis, R., Ramadori, G., Coppari, R., and Sassone-Corsi, P. (2015). SIRT1 relays nutritional inputs to the circadian clock through the sf1 neurons of the ventromedial hypothalamus. *Endocrinology* 156, 2174–2184. doi: 10.1210/en. 2014-1805

146. Ota, H., Tokunaga, E., Chang, K., Hikasa, M., Iijima, K., Eto, M., et al. (2006). Sirt1 inhibitor, Sirtinol, induces senescence-like growth arrest with attenuated Ras- MAPK signaling in human cancer cells. *Oncogene* 25, 176–185. doi: 10.1038/sj. onc.1209049

147. Pandey, S., Simmons, G. E. Jr., Malyarchuk, S., Calhoun, T. N., and Pruitt, K. (2015). A novel MeCP2 acetylation site regulates interaction with ATRX and HDAC1. *Genes Cancer* 6, 408–421. doi: 10.18632/genesandcancer.84

148. Park, S. M., Kim, J., Hong, C. M., Shin, D. H., Kim, J. Y., Park, D. Y., et al. (2019). SIRT1 is dispensable for maturation of hematopoietic stem cell in the bone marrow niche. *Exp. Ther. Med.* 18, 2341–2345. doi: 10.3892/etm.2019.7813

149. Parrella, E., and Longo, V. D. (2010). Insulin/IGF-I and related signaling pathways regulate aging in nondividing cells: from yeast to the mammalian brain. *Sci. World J.* 10, 161–177. doi: 10.1100/tsw.2010.8

150. Pasco, M. Y., Rotili, D., Altucci, L., Farina, F., Rouleau, G. A., Mai, A., et al. (2010). Characterization of sirtuin inhibitors in nematodes expressing a muscular dystrophy protein reveals muscle cell and behavioral protection by specific sirtinol analogues. *J. Med. Chem.* 53, 1407–1411. doi: 10.1021/jm9013345

151. Pazienza, V., Borghesan, M., Mazza, T., Sheedfar, F., Panebianco, C., Williams, R., et al. (2014). SIRT1-metabolite binding histone macroH2A1.1 protects hepatocytes against lipid accumulation. *Aging* 6, 35–47. doi: 10.18632/aging.100632

152. Peck, B., Chen, C.-Y., Ho, K.-K., Di Fruscia, P., Myatt, S. S., Coombes, R. C., et al. (2010). SIRT inhibitors induce cell death and p53 acetylation through targeting both SIRT1 and SIRT2. *Mol. Cancer Ther.* 9, 844–855. doi: 10.1158/1535-7163. mct-09-0971

153. Peleg, S., Feller, C., Ladurner, A. G., and Imhof, A. (2016). The metabolic impact on histone acetylation and transcription in ageing. *Trends Biochem. Sci.* 41, 700–711. doi: 10.1016/j.tibs.2016.05.008

154. Peng, L., Yuan, Z., Ling, H., Fukasawa, K., Robertson, K., Olashaw, N., et al. (2011). SIRT1 deacetylates the DNA methyltransferase 1 (DNMT1) protein and alters its activities. *Mol. Cell. Biol.* 31, 4720–4734. doi: 10.1128/mcb.06147-11

155. Picard, F., Kurtev, M., Chung, N., Topark-Ngarm, A., Senawong, T., de Oliveira, R. M., et al. (2004). Sirt1 promotes fat mobilization in white adipocytes by repressing PPAR-γ. *Nature* 429, 771–776. doi: 10.1038/nature02583

156. Pirola, L., Zerzaihi, O., Vidal, H., and Solari, F. (2012). Protein acetylation mechanisms in the regulation of insulin and insulin-like growth factor 1 signalling. *Mol. Cell. Endocrinol.* 362, 1–10. doi: 10.1016/j.mce.2012.05.011

157. Polevoda, B., and Sherman, F. (2000). Nalpha -terminal acetylation of eukaryotic proteins. *J. Biol. Chem.* 275, 36479–36482. doi: 10.1074/jbc.R000023200

158. Poulsen, R. C., Watts, A. C., Murphy, R. J., Snelling, S. J., Carr, A. J., and Hulley, P. A. (2014). Glucocorticoids induce senescence in primary human tenocytes by inhibition of sirtuin 1 and activation of the p53/p21 pathway: *in vivo* and *in vitro* evidence. *Ann. Rheum. Dis.* 73, 1405–1413. doi: 10.1136/annrheumdis- 2012-203146

159. Powell, M. J., Casimiro, M. C., Cordon-Cardo, C., He, X., Yeow, W.-S., Wang, C., et al. (2011). Disruption of a Sirt1-dependent autophagy checkpoint in the prostate results in prostatic intraepithelial neoplasia lesion formation. *Cancer Res.* 71, 964–975. doi: 10.1158/0008-5472.can-10-3172

160. Pruitt, K. (2016). Molecular and cellular changes during cancer progression resulting from genetic and epigenetic alterations. *Prog. Mol. Biol. Transl. Sci.* 144, 3–47. doi: 10.1016/bs.pmbts.2016.09.001

161. Pruitt, K., Zinn, R. L., Ohm, J. E., McGarvey, K. M., Kang, S. H., Watkins, D. N., et al. (2006). Inhibition of SIRT1 reactivates silenced cancer genes without loss of promoter DNA hypermethylation. *PLoS Genet.* 2:e40. doi: 10.1371/journal. pgen.0020040

162. Qiu, X., Brown, K., Hirschey, M. D., Verdin, E., and Chen, D. (2010). Calorie restriction reduces oxidative stress by SIRT3-mediated SOD2 activation. *Cell Metab.* 12, 662–667. doi: 10.1016/j.cmet.2010.11.015

163. Ramadori, G., Fujikawa, T., Anderson, J., Berglund, E. D., Frazao, R., Michán, S., et al. (2011). SIRT1 deacetylase in SF1 neurons protects against metabolic imbalance. *Cell Metab.* 14, 301–312. doi: 10.1016/j.cmet.2011.06.014

164. Ramadori, G., Fujikawa, T., Fukuda, M., Anderson, J., Morgan, D. A., Mostoslavsky, R., et al. (2010). SIRT1 deacetylase in POMC neurons is required for homeostatic defenses against diet-induced obesity. *Cell Metab.* 12, 78–87. doi: 10.1016/j.cmet.2010.05.010

165. Ramalingam, S. S., Kummar, S., Sarantopoulos, J., Shibata, S., LoRusso, P., Yerk, M., et al. (2010). Phase I study of vorinostat in patients with advanced solid tumors and hepatic dysfunction: a National Cancer Institute Organ Dysfunction Working Group study. *J. Clin. Oncol.* 28, 4507–4512. doi: 10.1200/jco.2010. 30.2307

166. Reverchon, M., Cornuau, M., Cloix, L., Rame, C., Guerif, F., Royère, D., et al. (2013). Visfatin is expressed in human granulosa cells: regulation by metformin through AMPK/SIRT1 pathways and its role in steroidogenesis. *Mol. Hum. Reprod.* 19, 313–326. doi: 10.1093/molehr/gat002

167. Rimmele, P., Bigarella, C. L., Liang, R., Izac, B., Dieguez-Gonzalez, R., Barbet, G., et al. (2014). Aging-like phenotype and defective lineage specification in SIRT1-deleted hematopoietic stem and progenitor cells. *Stem Cell Rep.* 3, 44–59. doi: 10.1016/j.stemcr.2014.04.015

168. Rodgers, J. T., Lerin, C., Haas, W., Gygi, S. P., Spiegelman, B. M., and Puigserver, P. (2005). Nutrient control of glucose homeostasis through a complex of PGC-1α and SIRT1. *Nature* 434, 113–118. doi: 10.1038/nature03354

169. Rosato, R. R., and Grant, S. (2004). Histone deacetylase inhibitors in clinical development. *Expert. Opin. Investig. Drugs* 13, 21–38.

170. Rotili, D., Tarantino, D., Carafa, V., Lara, E., Meade, S., Botta, G., et al. (2010). Identification of tri-and tetracyclic pyrimidinediones as sirtuin inhibitors. *ChemMedChem* 5, 674–677. doi: 10.1002/cmdc.201000030

171. Rotili, D., Tarantino, D., Carafa, V., Paolini, C., Schemies, J., Jung, M., et al. (2012a). Benzodeazaoxaflavins as sirtuin inhibitors with antiproliferative properties in cancer stem cells. *J. Med. Chem.* 55, 8193–8197. doi: 10.1021/jm301115r

172. Rotili, D., Tarantino, D., Nebbioso, A., Paolini, C., Huidobro, C., Lara, E., et al. (2012b). Discovery of salermide-related sirtuin inhibitors: binding mode studies and antiproliferative effects in cancer cells including cancer stem cells. *J. Med. Chem.* 55, 10937–10947. doi: 10.1021/jm3011614

173. Roy, S., Saha, S., Gupta, P., Ukil, A., and Das, P. K. (2019). Crosstalk of PD- 1 signaling with the SIRT1/FOXO-1 axis during the progression of visceral leishmaniasis. *J. Cell Sci.* 132:jcs226274. doi: 10.1242/jcs.226274

174. Russ, B. E., Prier, J. E., Rao, S., and Turner, S. J. (2013). T cell immunity as a tool for studying epigenetic regulation of cellular differentiation. *Front. Genet.* 4:218. doi: 10.3389/fgene.2013.00218

175. Sam, S., and Frohman, L. A. (2008). Normal physiology of hypothalamic pituitary regulation. *Endocrinol. Metab. Clin. North Am.* 37, 1–22. doi: 10.1016/j.ecl. 2007.10.007

176. Santolla, M. F., Avino, S., Pellegrino, M., De Francesco, E., De Marco, P., Lappano, R., et al. (2015). SIRT1 is involved in oncogenic signaling mediated by GPER in breast cancer. *Cell Death Dis.* 6:e1834. doi: 10.1038/cddis.2015.201

177. Sasaki, T., Kikuchi, O., Shimpuku, M., Susanti, V. Y., Yokota-Hashimoto, H., Taguchi, R., et al. (2014). Hypothalamic SIRT1 prevents age-associated weight gain by improving leptin sensitivity in mice. *Diabetologia* 57, 819–831. doi: 10.1007/s00125-013-3140-5

178. Sasaki, T., Kim, H.-J., Kobayashi, M., Kitamura, Y.-I., Yokota-Hashimoto, H., Shiuchi, T., et al. (2010). Induction of hypothalamic Sirt1 leads to cessation of feeding via agouti-related peptide. *Endocrinology* 151, 2556–2566. doi: 10.1210/ en.2009-1319

179. Satoh, A., Brace, C. S., Ben-Josef, G., West, T., Wozniak, D. F., Holtzman, D. M., et al. (2010). SIRT1 promotes the central adaptive response to diet restriction through activation of the dorsomedial and lateral nuclei of the hypothalamus. *J. Neurosci.* 30, 10220–10232. doi: 10.1523/jneurosci.1385-10.2010

180. Saxena, M., Dykes, S. S., Malyarchuk, S., Wang, A. E., Cardelli, J. A., and Pruitt, K. (2013). The sirtuins promote Dishevelled-1 scaffolding of TIAM1, Rac activation and cell migration. *Oncogene* 34, 188–198. doi: 10.1038/onc.2013.549 Sborov, D. W., Canella, A., Hade, E. M., Mo, X., Khountham, S., Wang, J., et al. (2017). A phase 1 trial of the HDAC inhibitor AR-42 in patients with multiple myeloma and T- and B-cell lymphomas. *Leuk. Lymphoma* 58, 2310–2318. doi: 10.1080/10428194.2017.1298751

181. Schlicker, C., Gertz, M., Papatheodorou, P., Kachholz, B., Becker, C. F., and Steegborn, C. (2008). Substrates and regulation mechanisms for the human mitochondrial sirtuins Sirt3 and Sirt5. *J. Mol. Biol.* 382, 790–801. doi: 10.1016/j.jmb.2008.07.048

182. Schug, T. T., Xu, Q., Gao, H., Peres-da-Silva, A., Draper, D. W., Fessler, M. B., et al. (2010). Myeloid deletion of SIRT1 induces inflammatory signaling in response to environmental stress. *Mol. Cell. Biol.* 30, 4712–4721. doi: 10.1128/MCB.00657-10
183. Schwer, B., Schumacher, B., Lombard, D. B., Xiao, C., Kurtev, M. V., Gao, J., et al. (2010). Neural sirtuin 6 (Sirt6) ablation attenuates somatic growth and causes obesity. *Proc. Natl. Acad. Sci. U.S.A.* 107, 21790–21794. doi: 10.1073/pnas. 1016306107
184. Sequeira, J., Boily, G., Bazinet, S., Saliba, S., He, X., Jardine, K., et al. (2008). sirt1-null mice develop an autoimmune-like condition. *Exp. Cell Res.* 314, 3069–3074. doi: 10.1016/j.yexcr.2008.07.011
185. Sharma, M., Castro-Piedras, I., Simmons, G. E. Jr., and Pruitt, K. (2018). Dishevelled: a masterful conductor of complex Wnt signals. *Cell Signal.* 47, 52–64. doi: 10.1016/j.cellsig.2018.03.004
186. Sharma, M., Molehin, D., Castro-Piedras, I., Martinez, E. G., and Pruitt, K. (2019). Acetylation of conserved DVL-1 lysines regulates its nuclear translocation and binding to gene promoters in triple-negative breast cancer. *Sci. Rep.* 9:16257. doi: 10.1038/s41598-019-52723-3
187. Shi, L., and Tu, B. P. (2014). Protein acetylation as a means to regulate protein function in tune with metabolic state. *Biochem. Soc. Trans.* 42, 1037–1042. doi: 10.1042/bst20140135
188. Silverman, M. N., and Sternberg, E. M. (2008). Neuroendocrine-immune interactions in rheumatoid arthritis: mechanisms of glucocorticoid resistance. *Neuroimmunomodulation* 15, 19–28. doi: 10.1159/000135620
189. Simmons, G. E. Jr., Pruitt, W. M., and Pruitt, K. (2015). Diverse roles of SIRT1 in cancer biology and lipid metabolism. *Int. J. Mol. Sci.* 16, 950–965. doi: 10.3390/ijms16010950
190. Singh, S. K., Williams, C. A., Klarmann, K., Burkett, S. S., Keller, J. R., and Oberdoerffer, P. (2013). Sirt1 ablation promotes stress-induced loss of epigenetic and genomic hematopoietic stem and progenitor cell maintenance. *J. Exp. Med.* 210, 987–1001. doi: 10.1084/jem.20121608
191. Solomon, J. M., Pasupuleti, R., Xu, L., McDonagh, T., Curtis, R., DiStefano, P. S., et al. (2006). Inhibition of SIRT1 catalytic activity increases p53 acetylation but does not alter cell survival following DNA damage. *Mol. Cell. Biol.* 26, 28–38. doi: 10.1128/mcb.26.1.28-38.2006
192. Song, J., Cheon, S. Y., Jung, W., Lee, W. T., and Lee, J. E. (2014). Resveratrol induces the expression of interleukin-10 and brain-derived neurotrophic factor in BV2 microglia under hypoxia. *Int. J. Mol. Sci.* 15, 15512–15529. doi: 10.3390/ijms150915512
193. Subramaniyan, B., Kumar, V., and Mathan, G. (2017). Effect of sodium salt of Butrin, a novel compound isolated from *Butea monosperma* flowers on suppressing the expression of SIRT1 and Aurora B kinase-mediated apoptosis in colorectal cancer cells. *Biomed. Pharmacother.* 90, 402–413. doi: 10.1016/j.biopha.2017.03.086
194. Suraweera, A., O'Byrne, K. J., and Richard, D. J. (2018). Combination therapy with histone deacetylase inhibitors (HDACi) for the treatment of cancer: achieving the full therapeutic potential of HDACi. *Front. Oncol.* 8:92. doi: 10.3389/fonc. 2018.00092
195. Süssmuth, S. D., Haider, S., Landwehrmeyer, G. B., Farmer, R., Frost, C., Tripepi, G., et al. (2015). An exploratory double-blind, randomized clinical trial with selisistat, a SirT1 inhibitor, in patients with Huntington's disease. *Br. J. Clin. Pharmacol.* 79, 465–476. doi: 10.1111/bcp.12512
196. Suzuki, S., Iben, J. R., Coon, S. L., and Kino, T. (2018). SIRT1 is a transcriptional enhancer of the glucocorticoid receptor acting independently to its deacetylase activity. *Mol. Cell. Endocrinol.* 461, 178–187. doi: 10.1016/j.mce.2017.09.012
197. Tanriverdi, F., Silveira, L. F., MacColl, G. S., and Bouloux, P. M. (2003). The hypothalamic-pituitary-gonadal axis: immune function and autoimmunity. *J. Endocrinol.* 176, 293–304. doi: 10.1677/joe.0.1760293
198. Tapias, A., and Wang, Z. Q. (2017). Lysine acetylation and deacetylation in brain development and neuropathies. *Genomics Proteomics Bioinformatics* 15, 19–36. doi: 10.1016/j.gpb.2016.09.002
199. Tatone, C., Di Emidio, G., Barbonetti, A., Carta, G., Luciano, A. M., Falone, S., et al. (2018). Sirtuins in gamete biology and reproductive physiology: emerging roles and therapeutic potential in female and male infertility. *Hum. Reprod. Update* 24, 267–289. doi: 10.1093/humupd/dmy003
200. Taunton, J., Hassig, C. A., and Schreiber, S. L. (1996). A mammalian histone deacetylase related to the yeast transcriptional regulator Rpd3p. *Science* 272, 408–411. doi: 10.1126/science.272.5260.408
201. Taylor, D. M., Balabadra, U., Xiang, Z., Woodman, B., Meade, S., Amore, A., et al. (2011). A brain-permeable small molecule reduces neuronal cholesterol by inhibiting activity of sirtuin 2 deacetylase. *ACS Chem. Biol.* 6, 540–546. doi: 10.1021/cb100376q
202. Ting, A. H., McGarvey, K. M., and Baylin, S. B. (2006). The cancer epigenome- components and functional correlates. *Genes Dev.* 20, 3215–3231. doi: 10.1101/ gad.1464906
203. Tissenbaum, H. A., and Guarente, L. (2001). Increased dosage of a sir-2 gene extends lifespan in Caenorhabditis elegans. *Nature* 410, 227–230. doi: 10.1038/ 35065638
204. Toorie, A. M., Cyr, N. E., Steger, J. S., Beckman, R., Farah, G., and Nillni, E. A. (2016). The nutrient and energy sensor sirt1 regulates the hypothalamic-pituitary-adrenal (HPA) axis by altering the production of the prohormone convertase 2 (PC2) essential in the maturation of Corticotropin-releasing Hormone (CRH) from its prohormone in male rats. *J. Biol. Chem.* 291, 5844–5859. doi: 10.1074/jbc.m115.675264
205. Toorie, A. M., and Nillni, E. A. (2014). Minireview: Central Sirt1 regulates energy balance via the melanocortin system and alternate pathways. *Mol. Endocrinol.* 28, 1423–1434. doi: 10.1210/me.2014-1115
206. Toubai, T., Rossi, C., Tawara, I., Liu, C., Zajac, C., Oravecz-Wilson, K., et al. (2018). Murine models of steroid refractory graft-versus-host disease. *Sci. Rep.* 8:12475. doi: 10.1038/s41598-018-30814-x
207. Tung, S. Y., Wang, S. H., Lee, S. P., Tsai, S. P., Shen, H. H., Chen, F. J., et al. (2017). Modulations of SIR-nucleosome interactions of reconstructed yeast silent pre- heterochromatin by O-acetyl-ADP-ribose and magnesium. *Mol. Biol. Cell* 28, 381–386. doi: 10.1091/mbc.e16-06-0359
208. Uhlig, H. H., and Powrie, F. (2018). Translating immunology into therapeutic concepts for inflammatory bowel disease. *Annu. Rev. Immunol.* 36, 755–781. doi: 10.1146/annurev-immunol-042617-053055
209. Valencia, J. C., Egbukichi, N., and Erwin-Cohen, R. A. (2019). Autoimmunity and cancer, the paradox comorbidities challenging therapy in the context of preexisting autoimmunity. *J. Interferon Cytokine Res.* 39, 72–84. doi: 10.1089/jir.2018.0060
210. Vazquez, M. J., Toro, C. A., Castellano, J. M., Ruiz-Pino, F., Roa, J., Beiroa, D., et al. (2018). SIRT1 mediates obesity- and nutrient-dependent perturbation of pubertal timing by epigenetically controlling Kiss1 expression. *Nat. Commun.* 9:4194. doi: 10.1038/s41467-018-06459-9
211. Vazquez, M. J., Velasco, I., and Tena-Sempere, M. (2019). Novel mechanisms for the metabolic control of puberty: implications for pubertal alterations in early-onset obesity and malnutrition. *J. Endocrinol.* 242, R51–R65.
212. Wan, X., Chowdhury, I. H., Jie, Z., Choudhuri, S., and Garg, N. J. (2019). Origin of Monocytes/Macrophages Contributing to Chronic Inflammation in Chagas Disease: SIRT1 Inhibition of FAK-NFκB-Dependent Proliferation and Proinflammatory Activation of Macrophages. *Cells* 9:80. doi: 10.3390/ cells9010080
213. Wan, X., Wen, J. J., Koo, S. J., Liang, L. Y., and Garg, N. J. (2016). SIRT1-PGC1α- NFκB Pathway of Oxidative and Inflammatory Stress during Trypanosoma cruzi Infection: Benefits of SIRT1-Targeted Therapy in Improving Heart Function in Chagas Disease. *PLoS Pathog.* 12:e1005954. doi: 10.1371/journal. ppat.1005954
214. Wang, J., Kim, T. H., Ahn, M. Y., Lee, J., Jung, J. H., Choi, W. S., et al. (2012). Sirtinol, a class III HDAC inhibitor, induces apoptotic and autophagic cell death in MCF-7 human breast cancer cells. *Int. J. Oncol.* 41, 1101–1109. doi: 10.3892/ijo.2012.1534
215. Wang, L., Beier, U. H., Akimova, T., Dahiya, S., Han, R., Samanta, A., et al. (2018). Histone/protein deacetylase inhibitor therapy for enhancement of Foxp3+ T-regulatory cell function posttransplantation. *Am. J. Transplant.* 18, 1596–1603. doi: 10.1111/ajt.14749
216. Wang, S. H., Tung, S. Y., Su, K. C., Shen, H. H., Hong, J. Y., Tsai, M. S., et al. (2019). Enhancer role of a native metabolite, O-acetyl-ADP-ribose, on the Saccharomyces cerevisiae chromatin epigenetic gene silencing. *Genes Cells* 24, 449–457. doi: 10.1111/gtc.12685
217. Wang, Y., Bi, Y., Chen, X., Li, C., Li, Y., Zhang, Z., et al. (2016). Histone Deacetylase SIRT1 Negatively Regulates the Differentiation of Interleukin-9-Producing CD4(+) T Cells. *Immunity* 44, 1337–1349. doi: 10.1016/j.immuni.2016.05.009
218. Wang, Y., He, J., Liao, M., Hu, M., Li, W., Ouyang, H., et al. (2019). An overview of Sirtuins as potential therapeutic target: structure, function and modulators. *Eur. J. Med. Chem.* 161, 48–77. doi: 10.1016/j.ejmech.2018.10.028
219. Wilson, B. J., Tremblay, A. M., Deblois, G., Sylvain-Drolet, G., and Giguere, V. (2010). An acetylation switch modulates the transcriptional activity of estrogen-related receptor alpha. *Mol. Endocrinol.* 24, 1349–1358. doi: 10.1210/me.2009-0441
220. Wing, J. B., Tanaka, A., and Sakaguchi, S. (2019). Human FOXP3(+) regulatory T cell heterogeneity and function in autoimmunity and cancer. *Immunity* 50, 302–316. doi: 10.1016/j.immuni.2019.01.020

221. Woo, S. J., Lee, S. M., Lim, H. S., Hah, Y. S., Jung, I. D., Park, Y. M., et al. (2016). Myeloid deletion of SIRT1 suppresses collagen-induced arthritis in mice by modulating dendritic cell maturation. *Exp. Mol. Med.* 48:e221. doi: 10.1038/ emm.2015.124

222. Wu, M., Wei, W., Xiao, X., Guo, J., Xie, X., Li, L., et al. (2012). Expression of SIRT1 is associated with lymph node metastasis and poor prognosis in both operable triple-negative and non-triple-negative breast cancer. *Med. Oncol.* 29, 3240–3249. doi: 10.1007/s12032-012-0260-6

223. Xie, Y., and Dorsky, R. I. (2017). Development of the hypothalamus: conservation, modification and innovation. *Development* 144, 1588–1599. doi: 10.1242/dev. 139055

224. Yamamoto, M., and Takahashi, Y. (2018). The essential role of SIRT1 in hypothalamic-pituitary axis. *Front. Endocrinol.* 9:605. doi: 10.3389/fendo.2018. 00605

225. Yang, H., Lee, S. M., Gao, B., Zhang, J., and Fang, D. (2013). Histone deacetylase sirtuin 1 deacetylates IRF1 protein and programs dendritic cells to control Th17 protein differentiation during autoimmune inflammation. *J. Biol. Chem.* 288, 37256–37266. doi: 10.1074/jbc.M113.527531

226. Yang, L., Zhang, J., Yan, C., Zhou, J., Lin, R., Lin, Q., et al. (2012). SIRT1 regulates CD40 expression induced by TNF-alpha via NF-kB pathway in endothelial cells. *Cell. Physiol. Biochem.* 30, 1287–1298. doi: 10.1159/000343318

227. Yang, T., Fu, M., Pestell, R., and Sauve, A. A. (2006). SIRT1 and endocrine signaling. *Trends Endocrinol. Metab.* 17, 186–191. doi: 10.1016/j.tem.2006.04.002

228. Yang, W. B., Liang, Q. L., Ye, Z. J., Niu, C. M., Ma, W. L., Xiong, X. Z., et al. (2012). Cell origins and diagnostic accuracy of interleukin 27 in pleural effusions. *PLoS One* 7:e40450. doi: 10.1371/journal.pone.0040450

229. Yang, X. J., and Seto, E. (2008). The Rpd3/Hda1 family of lysine deacetylases: from bacteria and yeast to mice and men. *Nat. Rev. Mol. Cell Biol.* 9, 206–218. doi: 10.1038/nrm2346

230. Yao, Y., Li, H., Gu, Y., Davidson, N. E., and Zhou, Q. (2010). Inhibition of SIRT1 deacetylase suppresses estrogen receptor signaling. *Carcinogenesis* 31, 382–387. doi: 10.1093/carcin/bgp308

231. Yates, R., Katugampola, H., Cavlan, D., Cogger, K., Meimaridou, E., Hughes, C., et al. (2013). Adrenocortical development, maintenance, and disease. *Curr. Top. Dev. Biol.* 106, 239–312. doi: 10.1016/b978-0-12-416021-7.00007-9

232. Ye, X., Li, M., Hou, T., Gao, T., Zhu, W. G., and Yang, Y. (2017). Sirtuins in glucose and lipid metabolism. *Oncotarget* 8, 1845–1859. doi: 10.18632/ oncotarget. 12157

233. Yeung, F., Hoberg, J. E., Ramsey, C. S., Keller, M. D., Jones, D. R., Frye, R. A., et al. (2004). Modulation of NF-kappaB-dependent transcription and cell survival by the SIRT1 deacetylase. *EMBO J.* 23, 2369–2380. doi: 10.1038/ sj.emboj.760 0244

234. Yoshizaki, T., Schenk, S., Imamura, T., Babendure, J. L., Sonoda, N., Bae, E. J., et al. (2010). SIRT1 inhibits inflammatory pathways in macrophages and modulates insulin sensitivity. *Am. J. Physiol. Endocrinol. Metab.* 298, E419–E428. doi: 10.1152/ajpendo.00417.2009

235. Yu, K.-H., Kuo, C.-F., Huang, L. H., Huang, W.-K., and See, L.-C. (2016). Cancer risk in patients with inflammatory systemic autoimmune rheumatic diseases: a nationwide population-based dynamic cohort study in Taiwan. *Medicine* 95:e3540. doi: 10.1097/md.0000000000003540

236. Yuan, J., Minter-Dykhouse, K., and Lou, Z. (2009). A c-Myc–SIRT1 feedback loop regulates cell growth and transformation. *J. Cell Biol.* 185, 203–211. doi: 10.1083/jcb.200809167

237. Yuan, Y., Huang, S., Wang, W., Wang, Y., Zhang, P., Zhu, C., et al. (2012). Activation of peroxisome proliferator-activated receptor-γ coactivator 1α ameliorates mitochondrial dysfunction and protects podocytes from aldosterone-induced injury. *Kidney Int.* 82, 771–789. doi: 10.1038/ki.2012.188 Zeiser, R., and Blazar, B. R. (2017). Acute graft-versus-host disease - biologic process, prevention, and therapy. *N. Engl. J. Med.* 377, 2167–2179. doi: 10.1056/ NEJMra1609337

238. Zhang, D., Li, S., Cruz, P., and Kone, B. C. (2009). Sirtuin 1 functionally and physically interacts with disruptor of telomeric silencing-1 to regulate α-ENaC transcription in collecting duct. *J. Biol. Chem.* 284, 20917–20926. doi: 10.1074/ jbc.m109.020073

239. Zhang, J., Lee, S. M., Shannon, S., Gao, B., Chen, W., Chen, A., et al. (2009). The type III histone deacetylase Sirt1 is essential for maintenance of T cell tolerance in mice. *J. Clin. Invest.* 119, 3048–3058. doi: 10.1172/JCI38902

240. Zhang, Q., Zeng, S. X., Zhang, Y., Zhang, Y., Ding, D., Ye, Q., et al. (2012). A small molecule Inauhzin inhibits SIRT1 activity and suppresses tumour growth through activation of p53. *EMBO Mol. Med.* 4, 298–312. doi: 10.1002/emmm. 201100211

241. Zhang, R., Chen, H. Z., Liu, J. J., Jia, Y. Y., Zhang, Z. Q., Yang, R. F., et al. (2010). SIRT1 suppresses activator protein-1 transcriptional activity and cyclooxygenase-2 expression in macrophages. *J. Biol. Chem.* 285, 7097–7110. doi: 10.1074/jbc.M109.038604

242. Zhang, W., Luo, J., Yang, F., Wang, Y., Yin, Y., Strom, A., et al. (2016). BRCA1 inhibits AR-mediated proliferation of breast cancer cells through the activation of SIRT1. *Sci. Rep.* 6:22034.

243. Zhang, Y., Au, Q., Zhang, M., Barber, J. R., Ng, S. C., and Zhang, B. (2009). Identification of a small molecule SIRT2 inhibitor with selective tumor cytotoxicity. *Biochem. Biophys. Res. Commun.* 386, 729–733. doi: 10.1016/j. bbrc.2009.06.113

244. Zhao, S., Xu, W., Jiang, W., Yu, W., Lin, Y., Zhang, T., et al. (2010). Regulation of cellular metabolism by protein lysine acetylation. *Science* 327, 1000–1004. doi: 10.1126/science.1179689

245. Zhou, Z., Ma, T., Zhu, Q., Xu, Y., and Zha, X. (2018). Recent advances in inhibitors of sirtuin1/2: an update and perspective. *Future Med. Chem.* 10, 907–934. doi: 10.4155/fmc-2017-0207

246. Zou, T., Yang, Y., Xia, F., Huang, A., Gao, X., Fang, D., et al. (2013). Resveratrol Inhibits CD4+ T cell activation by enhancing the expression and activity of Sirt1. *PLoS One* 8:e75139. doi: 10.1371/journal.pone.0075139

20

SIRT1 Antagonizes Oxidative Stress in Diabetic Vascular Complication

Teng Meng [1,2,3], *Weifeng Qin* [1,2] *and Baohua Liu* [1,2*]

[1] *Shenzhen Key Laboratory for Systemic Aging and Intervention, National Engineering Research Center for Biotechnology (Shenzhen), Medical Research Center, Shenzhen University Health Science Center, Shenzhen, China,* [2] *Key Laboratory of Optoelectronic Devices and Systems of Ministry of Education and Guangdong Province, College of Optoelectronic Engineering, Shenzhen University, Shenzhen, China,* [3] *Guangdong Key Laboratory of Genome Stability and Human Disease Prevention, Department of Biochemistry & Molecular Biology, School of Basic Medical Sciences, Shenzhen University, Shenzhen, China*

Correspondence:
Baohua Liu
ppliew@szu.edu.cn

Diabetic mellitus (DM) is a significant public health concern worldwide with an increased incidence of morbidity and mortality, which is particularly due to the diabetic vascular complications. Several pivotal underlying mechanisms are associated with vascular complications, including hyperglycemia, mitochondrial dysfunction, inflammation, and most importantly, oxidative stress. Oxidative stress triggers defective angiogenesis, activates pro-inflammatory pathways and causes long-lasting epigenetic changes to facilitate the development of vascular complications. Therefore, therapeutic interventions targeting oxidative stress are promising to manage diabetic vascular complications. Sirtuin1 (SIRT1), a class III histone deacetylase belonging to the sirtuin family, plays critical roles in regulating metabolism and ageing-related pathological conditions, such as vascular diseases. Growing evidence has indicated that SIRT1 acts as a sensing regulator in response to oxidative stress and attenuates vascular dysfunction via cooperating with adenosine-monophosphate-activated protein kinase (AMPK) to activate antioxidant signals through various downstream effectors, including peroxisome proliferator-activated receptor-gamma co-activator 1 (PGC-1α), forkhead transcription factors (FOXOs), and peroxisome proliferative-activated receptor α (PPARα). In addition, SIRT1 interacts with hydrogen sulfide (H2S), regulates NADPH oxidase, endothelial NO synthase, and mechanistic target of rapamycin (mTOR) to suppress oxidative stress. Furthermore, mRNA expression of sirt1 is affected by microRNAs in DM. In the current review, we summarize recent advances illustrating the importance of SIRT1 in antagonizing oxidative stress. We also discuss whether modulation of SIRT1 can serve as a therapeutic strategy to treat diabetic vascular complications.

Keywords: SIRT1, oxidative stress, diabetic vascular complications, adenosine-monophosphate-activated protein kinase, mechanistic target of rapamycin, microRNAs

INTRODUCTION

Diabetes mellitus (DM) is a complicated age-related diseases worldwide (1) and the main characteristics of DM are hyperglycemia and insulin resistance caused by β-cell dysfunction, resulting in increased risk for vascular disease (2–4). Notably, DM patients always accompany with various diseases associated with diabetic vascular complications, such as acquired blindness, atherosclerosis, end-stage renal failure, and neuropathies. Generally, diabetic vascular complications are classified into microvascular and macrovascular complications, the latter of which occur more frequently in patients with diabetes. The central pathological symptoms in macrovascular disease include hypertension, atherosclerosis, diabetic heart diseases, peripheral arterial disease, and stroke. Actually, diabetic patients have two times higher risk of developing stroke and hypertension than those who are healthy adults (5). On the contrary, microvascular complications involve diabetic nephropathy, neurophathy, and retinopathy (6–9). Considering the increased prevalence and the emergent requirement of therapeutic interventions to prevent these complications, it is important to explore the underlying connections between vascular disease and diabetes (10).

Advances in understanding of diabetes have made it clear that abnormal angiogenesis and endothelial dysfunction are two well-documented pathological characteristics of diabetic vascular complications (11–13). In particular, endothelial dysfunction plays central roles in the development of vascular complications, which is characterized by diminished bioavailability of nitric oxide, increased endothelium-derived contracting factors, and the impaired vasodilation. In addition, endothelial dysfunction is accompanied by the accumulation of cytokines and chemokines within the vascular microenvironment (14, 15). Therefore, elucidating the etiology and mechanisms of endothelial dysfunction will facilitate the development of diagnosis, prevention, and treatment even during suboptimal metabolic control of DM.

OXIDATIVE STRESS IN DIABETIC VASCULAR COMPLICATIONS

Oxidative stress is manifested as an overload of free radical accumulations, such as reactive oxygen species (ROS), and decreased antioxidants in the microvasculature, which always result in endothelial dysfunction. Importantly, amount of works have demonstrated that oxidative stress is one of the greatest contributors to the pathogenesis of vascular disorders and DM (16–18). For one hand, oxidative stress alters the endothelial signaling transduction and regulates the activation of transcriptional factors in response to redox, and thereby enhances vascular endothelial permeability and leukocyte adhesion. For another hand, oxidative stress contributes to insulin resistance, β-cell dysfunction, and hyperglycemia-mediated cellular injury, leading to the development of DM (16–18).

Specifically, metabolic abnormalities of DM, especially hyperglycemia and hyperlipidemia, can activate NADPH oxidases (NOXs) and endothelial Nitric Oxide Synthase (eNOS), increase advanced glycation end-products (AGE), and interrupt the polyol pathway as well as the mitochondrial respiratory chain, to impinge on oxidative stress (19). Consequently, oxidative stress may impair β-cell function *via* reducing insulin synthesis, hindering proinsulin inclusion, and inducing the apoptotic cell death of pancreatic cells (20). Mitochondrial collapse induced by oxidative stress is another important contributor to insulin resistance. Many high glucose levels associated biochemical pathways, such as glucose autoxidation, prostanoid synthesis, and protein glycation, crumble mitochondrial and promote mitochondria-mediated overproduction of ROS (predominantly superoxide anion) (21). As a result, excess ROS triggers several cellular mechanisms, including polyol pathway, mitogen-activated protein kinase (MAPK), adenosine-monophosphate-activated protein kinase (AMPK), NF-κB signaling pathways, and transcription factors such as forkhead transcription factors (FOXO), Nrf2 and AP-1, to initiate inflammation and deregulate insulin signaling pathways (22, 23). Taken together, therapeutic interventions aiming to reduce oxidative stress, such as anti-oxidative agents, are promising strategies reversing insulin resistance, ameliorating endothelial function and preventing cardiovascular morbidity in patients with diabetes.

STRUCTURE AND REGULATION OF SIRT1

The mammalian sirtuins are nicotinamide adenine dinucleotide (NAD^+)-dependent histone deacetylases, which regulate numerous cellular processes involved in DNA repair, cell survival and senescence, stress-stimulated metabolism alternations (24, 25). They require NAD^+ as a cofactor for deacetylation of histone or non-histone substrates and are generally not inhibited by compounds that inhibit zinc-dependent deacetylases. Importantly, increasing reports have demonstrated that the sirtuin family participates in the development of vascular physiology and pathology (26, 27), suggesting the sirtuins as therapeutic targets in DM.

In mammals, the sirtuin family is comprised of seven members (SIRT1-SIRT7). Among these mammalian Sirts, SIRT1 has been investigated most extensively (28). SIRT1 has 747 amino acids and three independent domains, the central deacetylase domain conservative in species, the N-terminal region containing nuclear localization/export signals, and the C-terminal region containing the essential for SIRT1 activity (ESA) domain (**Figure 1**). Structurally, a substrate and a NAD+ binding pocket exists in the catalytic domain, whereas the regulatory element and binding domain of SIRT1 co-activator/co-repressor distribute in the N- and C-terminus. SIRT1 removes the acetyl groups from multiple cytoplasmic substrates rather than histones, such as peroxisome proliferator-activated receptor-gamma co-activator 1 (PGC-1α), farnesoid X receptor (FXR), liver X receptor (LXR), sterol-regulatory element binding protein 1 (SREBP1), peroxisome proliferative-activated receptor (PPAR) to exert various functions in cellular metabolism (gluconeogenesis, insulin sensitivity, fat mobilization, and lipid metabolism) (29, 30). In addition, SIRT1 also regulate mechanistic target of rapamycin (mTOR), p53, KU70, E2F, and FOXO to affect cell survival and senescence (**Figure 1**).

Multiple studies on the regulation of SIRT1 activity have shown that post-translational modifications (PTMs), such as

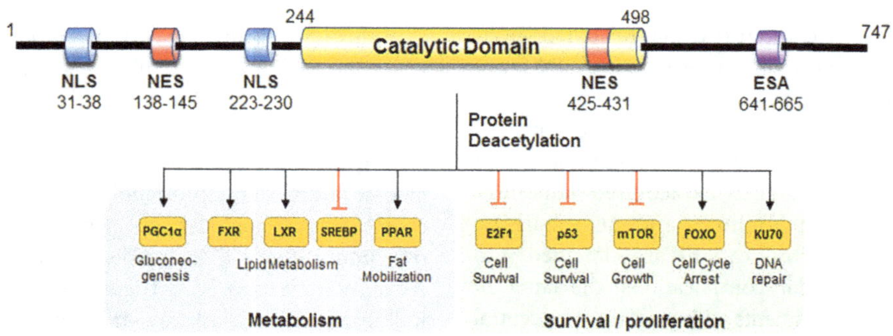

FIGURE 1 | Structure and function of human SIRT1. Important domains and substrates of human SIRT1 are shown, and their corresponding functions are presented. NLS, nuclear localization signal; NES, nuclear export signal; ESA, essential for Sirt1 activity; FXR, farnesoid X receptor; LXR, liver X receptor; SREBP1, sterol-regulatory element binding protein 1.

phosphorylation, S-nitrosylation, and SUMOylation, modulate SIRT1 protein level and its deacetylase activity (31). For instance, SIRT1 contains several sites for phosphorylation (e.g., N-terminus with seven residues and C-terminus with eight residues). In most cases, phosphorylation of SIRT1 mediated by different kinases, such as C-Jun N-terminal kinase 1, casein kinase 2, and cyclin-dependent kinase 1, enhances SIRT1 deacetylase activity and regulates its function in a substrate-dependent manner (31). In addition, SUMO is an ubiquitin like-modifier that exerts opposite effect of ubiquitin and covalently addition of SUMO protein to lysine residues (the so-called SUMOylation) can stabilize proteins. SUMOylation of SIRT1 at Lys 734 also increase its deacetylase activity and protein stability. Conversely, deSUMOylation of SIRT1 by specific deSUMOylating enzyme, sentrin-specific protease 1 (SENP1), reduces its deacetylase activity (32). Unlike SUMOylation, the covalently incorporating a nitric oxide moiety into Cys 387 and 390 of SIRT1 (S-nitrosylation) significantly reduces the deacetylase activity of SIRT1 toward to a widely reported substrate PGC-1α (33). Furthermore, SIRT1 activity is also regulated by protein-protein interaction. For instance, and deleted in breast cancer 1 (DBC1) and active regulator of SIRT1 (AROS) are negative and positive regulator of SIRT1, respectively. AROS binds to the N-terminus of SIRT1 to increase the SIRT1 activity (34), whereas DBC1 binds to the "essential for SIRT1 activity" (ESA) domain or the SIRT1 deacetylase core domain to inactivate SIRT1 (35). Finally, there are several small chemicals able to modify the activity of SIRT1, such as polyphenol resveratrol, sirtinol, and splitomicin (36). Resveratrol is a stilbenoid and is well-known for its ability to activating SIRT1 to exert its anti-aging, anti-diabetic, and anti-cardiovascular functions. Further works are inspired to discover more SIRT1 PTMs and protein regulators and to explore the possible crosstalk among different SIRT1 PTMs.

SIRT1 ANTAGONIZES OXIDATIVE STRESS IN DIABETIC MELLITUS

Recently published studies have clearly revealed that SIRT1 antagonizes oxidative stress in the pathogenesis of diabetic vasculopathy (37–39). For instance, the downregulation of SIRT1 by hyperglycemia caused vascular dysfunction in DM (40). On the contrary, upregulation of SIRT1 attenuated oxidative stress-induced endothelial senescence in diabetic mice (41). Notably, SIRT1 attenuates oxidative stress to regulate diabetic vascular complications through several important signal mediators, such as AMPK, NADPH oxidase, endothelial NO synthase, mTOR, and miRNAs (**Figure 2**). It seems that SIRT1 relies on the availability of different substrates to regulate cellular oxidative stress.

SIRT1 Cooperates With AMPK to Antagonize Oxidative Stress in Diabetic Mellitus

AMPK is the main cellular mediator of metabolic stress and is activated by glucose deprivation (42). Importantly, AMPK and SIRT1 both regulate each other and have similar effects on various cellular processes such as cell metabolism, DNA repair, mitochondrial function, and cell growth (43). For instance, AMPK manipulates energy expenditure by increasing the intercellular NAD+ concentration to enhance SIRT1 activity (44). Alternatively, SIRT1 deacetylates and activates LKB1, the upstream kinase of AMPK, to activate AMPK and to suppress ROS production (45, 46). Furthermore, SIRT1 and AMPK share many common targets, such as forkhead transcription factors (FOXOs), peroxisome proliferative-activated receptor α (PPARα), and PGC-1α (43). The joint activation of AMPK and SIRT1 can individually or combinatory activates these downstream effectors to exert antioxidant protective response and to ameliorate oxidative stress in DM (47, 48).

Inhibition of Oxidative Stress by SIRT1-AMPK-PGC-1α

PGC-1α is recognized as a key metabolic sensor and regulator in response to malnutrition and hypoxia (49, 50). Upon activation, PGC-1α regulates mitochondrial biogenesis and thus ROS production by controlling many transcription factors to initiate the expression of mitochondrial genes, resulting in reduced oxidative stress (51). PGC-1α is activated either by

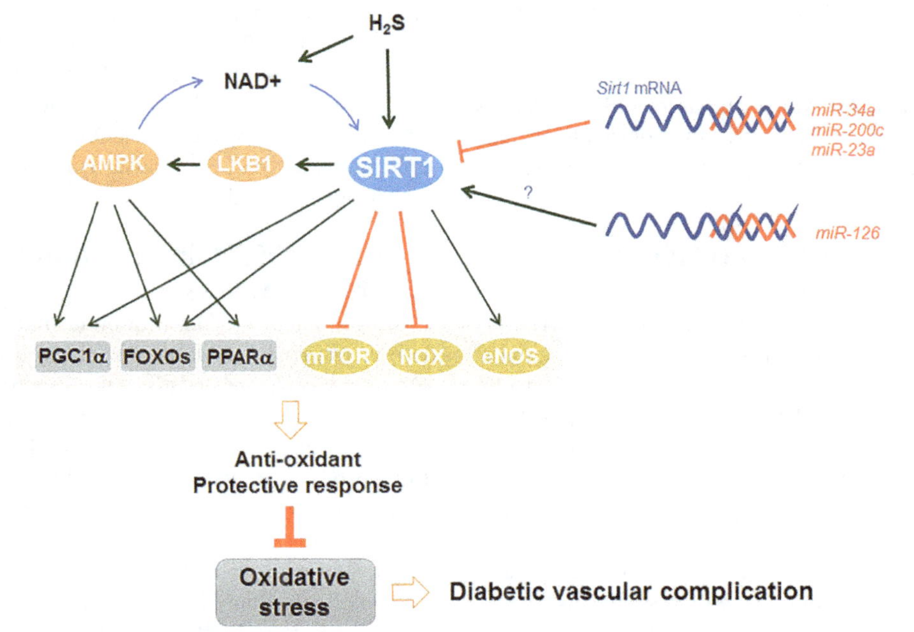

FIGURE 2 | SIRT1 antagonizes oxidative stress in diabetic vascular complications. SIRT1 directly or cooperatively with AMPK to activate various downstream effectors, including PGC1α, FOXOs, and PPARα. SIRT1 also stimulate eNOS and inhibit NOX and mTOR to trigger anti-oxidant protective response. In addition, H_2S can either activate SIRT1 directly *via* sulfydration, or indirectly *via* increasing NAD+ level. Furthermore, several miRNAs, such as miR-34a, miR-200c, and miR-23a, directly inhibit the mRNA expression of *sirt1* in DM, while other miRNAs including miR-126 promote *sirt1* expression indirectly with unclear mechanism.

AMPK-mediated phosphorylation or SIRT1-mediated deacetylation in an NAD^+-dependent manner (43, 52). Notably, amount of evidence has proved that SIRT1 cooperates with AMPK to enhance the ability of PGC-1α to attenuate endothelial dysfunction *via* stimulating mitochondrial biogenesis (53) and activating gluconeogenic fatty acid oxidation genes (54, 55). In addition, SIRT1-AMPK-PGC-1α pathway exerts its anti-oxidative activity in other diabetic vascular complications including brain complications (56), diabetic cardiomyopathy, and diabetic nephropathy (57, 58). Furthermore, PGC-1α can be directly activated by SIRT1 without AMPK to ease metabolic disorders in high glucose-induced endothelial oxidative damage (59) and Drp-mediated mitochondrial fission in diabetic hearts (60). Therefore, whether SIRT1 regulates the PGC-1α-mediated mitochondrial respiration and ROS production, with or without the help of AMPK activation, rests on a context-dependent way.

Inhibition of Oxidative Stress by SIRT1-AMPK-FOXOs

The significance of FOXOs in regulating the metabolic activity of vascular endothelium has been gradually addressed (61). There are four FOXO members in mammals, FOXO1, FOXO3, FOXO4, and FOXO6. SIRT1 deacetylates FOXO1, FOXO3 and FOXO4, and stimulates FOXO-dependent expression of antioxidants to scavenge ROS, such as catalase, manganese superoxide dismutase (MnSOD), and thioredoxin, either positively or negatively (62, 63). For instance, SIRT1 deacetylated FOXO1 to combat oxidative stress in diabetic vascular complications, diabetic nephropathy, and particularly in diabetic cardiomyopathy under the treatment of resveratrol (64–66). Besides, SIRT1 directly deacetylated FOXO3a and promoted the expression of MnSOD and catalase that are involved in stress resistance, which in turn attenuated oxidative stress in diabetic cardiomyopathy and nephropathy (67, 68). Moreover, SIRT1 bound to FOXO4 and increased its transactivation capacity to inhibit NF-κB signaling and inflammation (63). Interestingly, AMPK has also been shown to phosphorylate and activate FOXOs, yet the precise mechanism of AMPK in SIRT1-FOXO pathway remains unclear (44, 64). It seems that AMPK can regulate the function of FOXOs either by direct phosphorylation or indirectly *via* the SIRT1-induced activation.

Inhibition of Oxidative Stress by SIRT1-AMPK-PPARα

As a transcriptional factor, PPARα is mainly expressed in many oxidative tissues that require high capacity of fatty acid oxidation and is essential for the regulation of glucose metabolism (69). Additionally, PPARα is able to attenuate oxidative stress and inflammation through repressing NF-κB-mediated gene transcription, as well as increasing NO expression and release (70–72). It has been proved that expression of PPARα was reduced by hyperglycemia, and SIRT1 activated PPARα pathway to reduce ROS in diabetic vascular diseases (73, 74). In addition, AMPK-SIRT1-PPARα was activated by resveratrol to alleviate oxidative stress and endothelial dysfunction in type 2 diabetic nephropathy (58). However, unlike FOXOs, PPARα is not a directly target deacetylated by SIRT1, but its activity can be enhanced by SIRT1 indirectly through the coactivators, such as AMPK and PGC-1α (75, 76). Moreover, various PPAR agonists have been proved to prevent diabetes in the non-obese diabetic mouse model, suggesting the therapeutic function of SIRT1-PPARα axis in DM.

SIRT1 Regulates eNOS and NOX to Suppress Oxidative Stress

Nicotinamide adenine dinucleotide phosphate (NADPH) oxidase (NOX) family protein are primary sources of regulated production of ROS and play critical functions in the pathogenesis of the macro and micro-vascular complications of diabetes (77). Several important mediators of DM, such as hyperglycemia, oxidized or glycated low-density lipoproteins (LDL) and AGEs, can activate NOX to generate ROS, resulting in cell and tissue injury characteristic of diabetic complications (19). Importantly, the closely connection between NOX and SIRT1 has been gradually recognized, which shows that SIRT1 inhibits NOX to diminish ROS. For instance, resveratrol-mediated activation of SIRT1 inhibited the expression of NOX4 and the NADPH oxidative activity to reduce vascular superoxide production and to ameliorate endothelial dysfunction (78). Besides, dulaglutide, a glucagon-like peptide-1 receptor agonist used to treat type 2 DM, activated SIRT1 to suppress high glucose-induced activation of NLRP3 inflammasome and to downregulate NOX4 expression and the generation of ROS in human umbilical vein endothelial cells (79). In addition, SIRT1 was activated by quercetin to antagonize oxidized LDL-induced endothelial oxidative damage through activating AMPK and inhibiting NOX2 and NOX4 activity (80). Although the detailed mechanisms about how SIRT1 inhibits NOX directly or indirectly though AMPK have not been eliminated, SIRT1 has an antergic action on NOX-mediated ROS production.

Endothelial NO synthase (eNOS) is the primary enzyme producing NO, which participate in mitochondrial biogenesis and has various anti-atherosclerotic functions. Patients with DM demonstrate uncoupled eNOS in blood vessels, resulting in excessive superoxide anion ($O2^-$) production and diminished NO availability (81). Up to now, there are extensive connections between SIRT1 and eNOS in counteracting oxidative stress. For instance, in response to calorie restriction, SIRT1 promoted eNOS activity and NO bioavailability *via* the deacetylation of eNOS at lysine 496 and 506 (82, 83). In addition to deacetylation, SIRT1 also positively regulated the phosphorylation of eNOS to affect its ability in reducing oxidative stress and premature senescence (84). Except for SIRT1, AMPK has also been demonstrated to promote NO secretion by increasing eNOS phosphorylation as serine 633, which was another effective way for SIRT1 to overcome caloric restriction and facilitate vascular reconditioning after ischemia *via* activating the AMPK/eNOS axis (85, 86). In addition, SIRT1 enhances eNOS expression as evidenced by that resveratrol induced SIRT1-dependent upregulation of eNOS in endothelial cells, and endothelial-specific overexpression of *Sirt1* led to elevation of eNOS expression (87–89). Furthermore, under resveratrol-stimulated conditions, knockdown of FOXO1 or FOXO3a by siRNAs led to a downregulation of eNOS transcription, implying that SIRT1 activates FOXOs to elevate eNOS (90). Taken together, SIRT1 either enhances eNOS expression or eNOS enzymatic activity to protect against oxidative stress and endothelial dysfunction.

H_2S and SIRT1 Interaction Suppress Oxidative Stress

Hydrogen sulfide (H_2S) is a gasotransmitter playing an important role in physiological conditions, dysregulation of which always occurs in vascular-related diseases. Amount of evidence has clearly demonstrated that interaction between H_2S and SIRT1 is critical modulator of oxidative stress (91, 92). For one hand, H_2S limits ROS production *via* directly enhancing SIRT1 activity or expression (93–96). H_2S promotes the S-sulfydration of two CXXC motifs in the catalytic domain of SIRT1, resulting in elevated protein stability and deacetylase activity (96). H_2S is also able to activate SIRT1 indirectly by increasing intracellular NAD^+ levels (97). Furthermore, H_2S exerts its anti-inflammatory and anti-oxidant effects against diabetic complications *via* stimulating AMPK (92). One possible mechanism is that H_2S mediates the S-sulfydration of calcium/calmodulin-dependent protein kinase kinase β (CaMKKβ), one important upstream regulator of AMPK, to phosphorylate AMPK and to activate its downstream effector, the SIRT1/PGC-1α axis (98, 99). Taken together, H_2S and SIRT1 interaction represents a protective mechanism against oxidative stress in DM.

SIRT1 Regulates mTOR Pathway to Repress Oxidative Stress

The mechanistic target of rapamycin (mTOR) is a nutrient sensor and initiator of cell growth, forming structurally and functionally distinct mTOR complex 1 (mTORC1) and complex 2 (mTORC2) (100). Importantly, mTOR is an important regulator of oxidative stress through regulating mitochondrial biogenesis and enhancing oxidative metabolism *via* PGC-1α pathway (101). Besides, insulin-mediated PI3K/Akt/mTOR signaling axis is one of the most well-known mechanisms in regulating cell cycle, glucose metabolism and endothelial dysfunction in DM (102, 103). Interestingly, under calorie restriction, mTOR was inhibited whereas SIRT1 activity was upregulated (104, 105), suggesting the feedback action between mTOR and SIRT1. Indeed, numerous studies have revealed their possible reciprocal connections. For instance, hepatic SIRT1 deficiency disrupted mTORC2/Akt signaling to cause hyperglycemia and oxidative stress in mice model (106). One possible mechanism is that SIRT1 directly regulated mTOR *via* erythropoietin to protect vascular cells in DM (107, 108). Another example is that SIRT1 activated the mTORC2 signaling *via* activating a cascade of Akt and FOXO phosphorylation, which in turn ameliorated myocardial ischemia or reperfusion injury in DM (103). Together, all the observations imply that SIRT1-mTOR pathway could be potentially therapeutic targets for diabetic vascular complications.

Regulation of *Sirt1* by MicroRNAs in Diabetic Mellitus

MicroRNAs (miRNAs) are cluster of non-coding RNAs that trigger mRNA degradation and repress translation function mainly by targeting messenger RNAs (mRNAs) (109). Recently, the importance of miRNAs-mediated *sirt1* regulation in diabetic vascular complications has gradually emerged (110). One extensively investigated miRNA was miR-34a (111, 112). Hyperglycemia-mediated oxidative stress recruited p66SHc, which then upregulated miR-34a to impair angiogenesis in endothelial cells *via* directly suppressing the stability of *sirt1* mRNA, leading to the reduced protein level of SIRT1 (112–114). Besides, regulation of miR-34a, SIRT1, and eNOS synthesis promoted kallistatin to inhibit antioxidant gene expression in endothelial progenitor cells (115). In addition to miR-34a, miR-200c and miR-23a were also related to oxidative stress-induced diabetic vascular complications. Hyperglycemia triggered ROS production and upregulated miR-200c expression, which subsequently inhibited the mRNA expression of *sirt1* to facilitate endothelial dysfunction in DM (116, 117). However, unlike miR-34a and miR-200c, increased level of miR-126 could facilitate the expressions of *sirt1* and *sod-2* to enhance oxidative stress and aggravate diabetic vascular complications, with unclear mechanism (118). Aside from miRNAs discussed above, many other miRNAs, such as miR-195, miR-9, and miR-132, have also been reported to target the mRNA of *sirt1* (119–121). Whether they play a role in DM remains to be determined.

SIRT1 AS A THERAPEUTIC TARGET FOR DIABETIC MELLITUS

As discussed above, SIRT1 antagonises oxidative stress *via* different substrates in DM, implying activating SIRT1 as potent therapeutic strategy. Importantly, SIRT1 can be activated directly or indirectly by some naturally polyphenols *in vitro* and *in vivo*, such as resveratrol, quercetin, and catechins (122, 123). For instance, resveratrol is one of the well-studied SIRT1 activators that binds to SIRT1 to promote its substrate binding activity. Resveratrol exhibits various biological functions *via* activating SIRT1 and numerous clinical trials have been performed to test its protective effect against several diseases, such as neurodegeneration, type 2 diabetes, and insulin resistance (123). In addition, some completed phase 1/2 clinical trials have clearly showed that resveratrol is able to improve metabolic and vascular health of diabetes subjects (123). Notably, those natural SIRT1-activating compounds are mostly used as nutraceuticals in management of diabetic vascular complications. Whether their therapeutic effects rely on SIRT1 activation in DM remains to be examined. Considering that most natural compounds possess pleiotropic effects, more selective and specific SIRT1 activators are required, which may facilitate to establish a direct link between SIRT1 activation and human diseases. There are several other SIRT1 activators, such as SRT1720 (an analogue of resveratrol), that have been shown to enhance SIRT1 activity in mammals (36, 124). Whether these activators can exhibit higher specificity and activity than naturally polyphenols, as well as their potentially clinical application, remain to be determined.

CONCLUSION

SIRT1 plays a key role in many signaling pathways and regulates various important biological phenomena, especially in metabolism, inflammation, aging, and stress resistance through deacetylating transcription factors and histones. The involvement of SIRT1 in diabetic vascular complications has increased, and the diverse mechanisms of SIRT1 against oxidative stress gradually emerges, suggesting that modulation of SIRT1 activity may be an available therapeutic intervention against diabetes-induced vascular diseases (125). However, many detailed molecular interactions remain unsolved. For instance, a comprehensive understanding of how SIRT1 and AMPK are intertwined in mediating vascular diseases is still needed. It is difficult to parse how specific interactions between SIRT1 and AMPK contribute to cross-regulation in each vascular complication. Besides, except for SIRT1, there are still other members of the sirtuin family (e.g., SIRT3, SIRT6, and SIRT7) that are active in modulating vascular function (126, 127), which inspires further works to investigate their associations with oxidative stress and diabetic vascular complications. Finally, substantial efforts aiming to develop novel specifically pharmacological SIRT1 activators under active clinical investigation is needed.

AUTHOR CONTRIBUTIONS

TM and WQ synthesized and generally organized the manuscript, **Figures 1** and **2**. BL supervised and edited the manuscript. All authors contributed to the article and approved the submitted version.

REFERENCES

1. Disease GBD, Injury I, Prevalence C. Global, regional, and national incidence, prevalence, and years lived with disability for 328 diseases and injuries for 195 countries, 1990-2016: a systematic analysis for the Global Burden of Disease Study 2016. *Lancet* (2017) 390:1211–59. doi: 10.1016/S0140-6736(17)32154-2
2. van den Born JC, Hammes HP, Greffrath W, van Goor H, Hillebrands JL. Complications DGIRTGDM. Gasotransmitters in Vascular Complications of Diabetes. *Diabetes* (2016) 65:331–45. doi: 10.2337/db15-1003
3. Koulis C, Watson AM, Gray SP, Jandeleit-Dahm KA. Linking RAGE and Nox in diabetic micro- and macrovascular complications. *Diabetes Metab* (2015) 41:272–81. doi: 10.1016/j.diabet.2015.01.006
4. Gregg EW, Williams DE, Geiss L. Changes in diabetes-related complications in the United States. *N Engl J Med* (2014) 371:286–7. doi: 10.1056/NEJMc1406009
5. Shaikh A. A Practical Approach to Hypertension Management in Diabetes. *Diabetes Ther* (2017) 8:981–9. doi: 10.1007/s13300-017-0310-3
6. Leung A, Amaram V, Natarajan R. Linking diabetic vascular complications with LncRNAs. *Vascul Pharmacol* (2019) 114:139–44. doi: 10.1016/j.vph.2018.01.007
7. Yamazaki D, Hitomi H, Nishiyama A. Hypertension with diabetes mellitus complications. *Hypertens Res* (2018) 41:147–56. doi: 10.1038/s41440-017-0008-y
8. Choby B. Diabetes Update: Prevention and Management of Diabetes Complications. *FP Essent* (2017) 456:36–40.
9. Maric-Bilkan C. Sex differences in micro- and macro-vascular complications of diabetes mellitus. *Clin Sci (Lond)* (2017) 131:833–46. doi: 10.1042/CS20160998
10. Paneni F, Beckman JA, Creager MA, Cosentino F. Diabetes and vascular disease: pathophysiology, clinical consequences, and medical therapy: part I. *Eur Heart J* (2013) 34:2436–43. doi: 10.1093/eurheartj/eht149
11. Sorrentino FS, Matteini S, Bonifazzi C, Sebastiani A, Parmeggiani F. Diabetic retinopathy and endothelin system: microangiopathy versus endothelial dysfunction. *Eye (Lond)* (2018) 32:1157–63. doi: 10.1038/s41433-018-0032-4
12. Sena CM, Pereira AM, Seica R. Endothelial dysfunction - a major mediator of diabetic vascular disease. *Biochim Biophys Acta* (2013) 1832:2216–31. doi: 10.1016/j.bbadis.2013.08.006
13. Shi Y, Vanhoutte PM. Macro- and microvascular endothelial dysfunction in diabetes. *J Diabetes* (2017) 9:434–49. doi: 10.1111/1753-0407.12521
14. Capitão M, Soares R. Angiogenesis and Inflammation Crosstalk in Diabetic Retinopathy. *J Cell Biochem* (2016) 117:2443–53. doi: 10.1002/jcb.25575
15. Dinh QN, Drummond GR, Sobey CG, Chrissobolis S. Roles of inflammation, oxidative stress, and vascular dysfunction in hypertension. *BioMed Res Int* (2014) 2014:406960. doi: 10.1155/2014/406960
16. Odegaard AO, Jacobs DRJr, Sanchez OA, Goff DCJr, Reiner AP, Gross MD. Oxidative stress, inflammation, endothelial dysfunction and incidence of type 2 diabetes. *Cardiovasc Diabetol* (2016) 15:51. doi: 10.1186/s12933-016-0369-6
17. Pitocco D, Tesauro M, Alessandro R, Ghirlanda G, Cardillo C. Oxidative stress in diabetes: implications for vascular and other complications. *Int J Mol Sci* (2013) 14:21525–50. doi: 10.3390/ijms141121525
18. Ceriello A, Testa R, Genovese S. Clinical implications of oxidative stress and potential role of natural antioxidants in diabetic vascular complications. *Nutr Metab Cardiovasc Dis* (2016) 26:285–92. doi: 10.1016/j.numecd.2016.01.006
19. Rochette L, Zeller M, Cottin Y, Vergely C. Diabetes, oxidative stress and therapeutic strategies. *Biochim Biophys Acta* (2014) 1840(9):2709–29. doi: 10.1016/j.bbagen.2014.05.017
20. Yaribeygi H, Sathyapalan T, Atkin SL, Sahebkar A. Molecular Mechanisms Linking Oxidative Stress and Diabetes Mellitus. *Oxid Med Cell Longev* (2020) 2020:8609213. doi: 10.1155/2020/8609213
21. Kaludercic N, Di Lisa F. Mitochondrial ROS Formation in the Pathogenesis of Diabetic Cardiomyopathy. *Front Cardiovasc Med* (2020) 7:12. doi: 10.3389/fcvm.2020.00012
22. Keane KN, Cruzat VF, Carlessi R, de Bittencourt PIJr, Newsholme P. Molecular Events Linking Oxidative Stress and Inflammation to Insulin Resistance and β-Cell Dysfunction. *Oxid Med Cell Longev* (2015) 2015:181643. doi: 10.1155/2015/181643
23. Volpe CMO, Villar-Delfino PH, Dos Anjos PMF, Nogueira-Machado JA. Cellular death, reactive oxygen species (ROS) and diabetic complications. *Cell Death Dis* (2018) 9(2):119. doi: 10.1038/s41419-017-0135-z
24. Chalkiadaki A, Guarente L. Sirtuins mediate mammalian metabolic responses to nutrient availability. *Nat Rev Endocrinol* (2012) 8:287–96. doi: 10.1038/nrendo.2011.225
25. Haigis MC, Sinclair DA. Mammalian sirtuins: biological insights and disease relevance. *Annu Rev Pathol* (2010) 5:253–95. doi: 10.1146/annurev.pathol.4.110807.092250
26. D'Onofrio N, Servillo L, Balestrieri ML. SIRT1 and SIRT6 Signaling Pathways in Cardiovascular Disease Protection. *Antioxid Redox Signal* (2018) 28:711–32. doi: 10.1089/ars.2017.7178
27. Sosnowska B, Mazidi M, Penson P, Gluba-Brzozka A, Rysz J, Banach M. The sirtuin family members SIRT1, SIRT3 and SIRT6: Their role in vascular biology and atherogenesis. *Atherosclerosis* (2017) 265:275–82. doi: 10.1016/j.atherosclerosis.2017.08.027
28. Zhang HN, Dai Y, Zhang CH, Omondi AM, Ghosh A, Khanra I, et al. Sirtuins family as a target in endothelial cell dysfunction: implications for vascular ageing. *Biogerontology* (2020) 21(5):495–516. doi: 10.1007/s10522-020-09873-z
29. Brooks CL, Gu W. How does SIRT1 affect metabolism, senescence and cancer? *Nat Rev Cancer* (2009) 9:123–8. doi: 10.1038/nrc2562
30. Hwang JW, Yao H, Caito S, Sundar IK, Rahman I. Redox regulation of SIRT1 in inflammation and cellular senescence. *Free Radic Biol Med* (2013) 61:95–110. doi: 10.1016/j.freeradbiomed.2013.03.015
31. Revollo JR, Li X. The ways and means that fine tune Sirtl activity. *Trends Biochem Sci* (2013) 38:160–7. doi: 10.1016/j.tibs.2012.12.004
32. Yang Y, Fu W, Chen J, Olashaw N, Zhang X, Nicosia SV, et al. SIRT1 sumoylation regulates its deacetylase activity and cellular response to genotoxic stress. *Nat Cell Biol* (2007) 9:1253–62. doi: 10.1038/ncb1645
33. Kornberg MD, Sen N, Hara MR, Juluri KR, Nguyen JV, Snowman AM, et al. GAPDH mediates nitrosylation of nuclear proteins. *Nat Cell Biol* (2010) 12:1094–100. doi: 10.1038/ncb2114
34. Kim EJ, Kho JH, Kang MR, Um SJ. Active regulator of SIRT1 cooperates with SIRT1 and facilitates suppression of p53 activity. *Mol Cell* (2007) 28:277–90. doi: 10.1016/j.molcel.2007.08.030
35. Kim JE, Chen J, Lou Z. DBC1 is a negative regulator of SIRT1. *Nature* (2008) 451:583–6. doi: 10.1038/nature06500
36. Dai H, Sinclair DA, Ellis JL, Steegborn C. Sirtuin activators and inhibitors: Promises, achievements, and challenges. *Pharmacol Ther* (2018) 188:140–54. doi: 10.1016/j.pharmthera.2018.03.004
37. Mishra M, Duraisamy AJ, Kowluru RA. Sirtl: A Guardian of the Development of Diabetic Retinopathy. *Diabetes* (2018) 67:745–54. doi: 10.2337/db17-0996
38. Karbasforooshan H, Karimi G. The role of SIRT1 in diabetic retinopathy. *BioMed Pharmacother* (2018) 97:190–4. doi: 10.1016/j.biopha.2017.10.075
39. Kume S, Uzu T, Kashiwagi A, Koya D. SIRT1, a calorie restriction mimetic, in a new therapeutic approach for type 2 diabetes mellitus and diabetic vascular complications. *Endocr Metab Immune Disord Drug Targets* (2010) 10(1):16–24. doi: 10.2174/187153010790827957
40. Orimo M, Minamino T, Miyauchi H, Tateno K, Okada S, Moriya J, et al. Protective role of SIRT1 in diabetic vascular dysfunction. *Arterioscler Thromb Vasc Biol* (2009) 29:889–94. doi: 10.1161/ATVBAHA.109.185694
41. Ota H, Eto M, Kano MR, Kahyo T, Setou M, Ogawa S, et al. Induction of Endothelial Nitric Oxide Synthase, SIRT1, and Catalase by Statins Inhibits Endothelial Senescence Through the Akt Pathway. *Arterioscl Throm Vas* (2010) 30:2205–U2411. doi: 10.1161/ATVBAHA.110.210500
42. Herzig S, Shaw RJ. AMPK: guardian of metabolism and mitochondrial homeostasis. *Nat Rev Mol Cell Biol* (2018) 19:121–35. doi: 10.1038/nrm.2017.95
43. Ruderman NB, Xu XJ, Nelson L, Cacicedo JM, Saha AK, Lan F, et al. AMPK and SIRT1: a long-standing partnership? *Am J Physiol Endocrinol Metab* (2010) 298:E751–60. doi: 10.1152/ajpendo.00745.2009
44. Canto C, Gerhart-Hines Z, Feige JN, Lagouge M, Noriega L, Milne JC, et al. AMPK regulates energy expenditure by modulating NAD+ metabolism and SIRT1 activity. *Nature* (2009) 458:1056–60. doi: 10.1038/nature07813

45. Zheng Z, Chen H, Li J, Li T, Zheng B, Zheng Y, et al. Sirtuin 1-mediated cellular metabolic memory of high glucose *via the* LKB1/AMPK/ROS pathway and therapeutic effects of metformin. *Diabetes* (2012) 61:217–28. doi: 10.2337/db11-0416
46. Chen S, Xiao X, Feng X, Li W, Zhou N, Zheng L, et al. Resveratrol induces Sirt1-dependent apoptosis in 3T3-L1 preadipocytes by activating AMPK and suppressing AKT activity and survivin expression. *J Nutr Biochem* (2012) 23:1100–12. doi: 10.1016/j.jnutbio.2011.06.003
47. Manna P, Achari AE, Jain SK. Vitamin D supplementation inhibits oxidative stress and upregulate SIRT1/AMPK/GLUT4 cascade in high glucose-treated 3T3L1 adipocytes and in adipose tissue of high fat diet-fed diabetic mice. *Arch Biochem Biophys* (2017) 615:22–34. doi: 10.1016/j.abb.2017.01.002
48. Tikoo K, Lodea S, Karpe PA, Kumar S. Calorie restriction mimicking effects of roflumilast prevents diabetic nephropathy. *Biochem Biophys Res Commun* (2014) 450:1581–6. doi: 10.1016/j.bbrc.2014.07.039
49. Cheng CF, Ku HC, Lin H. PGC-1α as a Pivotal Factor in Lipid and Metabolic Regulation. *Int J Mol Sci* (2018) 19(11):3447. doi: 10.3390/ijms19113447
50. Arany Z, Foo SY, Ma Y, Ruas JL, Bommi-Reddy A, Girnun G, et al. HIF-independent regulation of VEGF and angiogenesis by the transcriptional coactivator PGC-1alpha. *Nature* (2008) 451:1008–12. doi: 10.1038/nature06613
51. Rius-Pérez S, Torres-Cuevas I, Millán I, Ortega ÁL, Pérez S. PGC-1α, Inflammation, and Oxidative Stress: An Integrative View in Metabolism. *Oxid Med Cell Longev* (2020) 2020:1452696. doi: 10.1155/2020/1452696
52. Iwabu M, Yamauchi T, Okada-Iwabu M, Sato K, Nakagawa T, Funata M, et al. Adiponectin and AdipoR1 regulate PGC-1alpha and mitochondria by Ca(2+) and AMPK/SIRT1. *Nature* (2010) 464:1313–9. doi: 10.1038/nature08991
53. Yuan Y, Shi M, Li L, Liu J, Chen B, Chen Y, et al. Mesenchymal stem cell-conditioned media ameliorate diabetic endothelial dysfunction by improving mitochondrial bioenergetics *via the* Sirt1/AMPK/PGC-1alpha pathway. *Clin Sci (Lond)* (2016) 130:2181–98. doi: 10.1042/CS20160235
54. Rodgers JT, Lerin C, Haas W, Gygi SP, Spiegelman BM, Puigserver P. Nutrient control of glucose homeostasis through a complex of PGC-1alpha and SIRT1. *Nature* (2005) 434:113–8. doi: 10.1038/nature03354
55. Rodgers JT, Lerin C, Gerhart-Hines Z, Puigserver P. Metabolic adaptations through the PGC-1 alpha and SIRT1 pathways. *FEBS Lett* (2008) 582:46–53. doi: 10.1016/j.febslet.2007.11.034
56. Zheng A, Li H, Xu J, Cao K, Li H, Pu W, et al. Hydroxytyrosol improves mitochondrial function and reduces oxidative stress in the brain of db/db mice: role of AMP-activated protein kinase activation. *Br J Nutr* (2015) 113:1667–76. doi: 10.1017/S0007114515000884
57. Gallardo-Montejano VI, Saxena G, Kusminski CM, Yang C, McAfee JL, Hahner L, et al. Nuclear Perilipin 5 integrates lipid droplet lipolysis with PGC-1alpha/SIRT1-dependent transcriptional regulation of mitochondrial function. *Nat Commun* (2016) 7:12723. doi: 10.1038/ncomms12723
58. Park HS, Lim JH, Kim MY, Kim Y, Hong YA, Choi SR, et al. Resveratrol increases AdipoR1 and AdipoR2 expression in type 2 diabetic nephropathy. *J Transl Med* (2016) 14:176. doi: 10.1186/s12967-016-0967-9
59. Cheng L, Li B, Chen X, Su J, Wang H, Yu S, et al. CTRP9 induces mitochondrial biogenesis and protects high glucose-induced endothelial oxidative damage *via* AdipoR1 -SIRT1- PGC-1alpha activation. *Biochem Biophys Res Commun* (2016) 477:685–91. doi: 10.1016/j.bbrc.2016.06.120
60. Ding M, Feng N, Tang D, Feng J, Li Z, Jia M, et al. Melatonin prevents Drp1-mediated mitochondrial fission in diabetic hearts through SIRT1-PGC1alpha pathway. *J Pineal Res* (2018) 65(2):e12491. doi: 10.1111/jpi.12491
61. Wilhelm K, Happel K, Eelen G, Schoors S, Oellerich MF, Lim R, et al. FOXO1 couples metabolic activity and growth state in the vascular endothelium. *Nature* (2016) 529:216–20. doi: 10.1038/nature16498
62. Giannakou ME, Partridge L. The interaction between FOXO and SIRT1: tipping the balance towards survival. *Trends Cell Biol* (2004) 14(8):408–12. doi: 10.1016/j.tcb.2004.07.006
63. Kobayashi Y, Furukawa-Hibi Y, Chen C, Horio Y, Isobe K, Ikeda K, et al. SIRT1 is critical regulator of FOXO-mediated transcription in response to oxidative stress. *Int J Mol Med* (2005) 16(2):237–43. doi: 10.3892/ijmm.16.2.237
64. Brunet A, Sweeney LB, Sturgill JF, Chua KF, Greer PL, Lin Y, et al. Stress-dependent regulation of FOXO transcription factors by the SIRT1 deacetylase. *Science* (2004) 303:2011–5. doi: 10.1126/science.1094637
65. Wang B, Yang Q, Sun YY, Xing YF, Wang YB, Lu XT, et al. Resveratrol-enhanced autophagic flux ameliorates myocardial oxidative stress injury in diabetic mice. *J Cell Mol Med* (2014) 18:1599–611. doi: 10.1111/jcmm.12312
66. Mori J, Patel VB, Ramprasath T, Alrob OA, DesAulniers J, Scholey JW, et al. Angiotensin 1-7 mediates renoprotection against diabetic nephropathy by reducing oxidative stress, inflammation, and lipotoxicity. *Am J Physiol Renal Physiol* (2014) 306:F812–821. doi: 10.1152/ajprenal.00655.2013
67. Wang X, Meng L, Zhao L, Wang Z, Liu H, Liu G, et al. Resveratrol ameliorates hyperglycemia-induced renal tubular oxidative stress damage *via* modulating the SIRT1/FOXO3a pathway. *Diabetes Res Clin Pract* (2017) 126:172–81. doi: 10.1016/j.diabres.2016.12.005
68. Yerra VG, Kalvala AK, Kumar A. Isoliquiritigenin reduces oxidative damage and alleviates mitochondrial impairment by SIRT1 activation in experimental diabetic neuropathy. *J Nutr Biochem* (2017) 47:41–52. doi: 10.1016/j.jnutbio.2017.05.001
69. Kersten S P, Desvergne B, Wahli W. Roles of PPARs in health and disease. *Nature* (2000) 405:421–4. doi: 10.1038/35013000
70. Poynter ME, Daynes RA. Peroxisome proliferator-activated receptor alpha activation modulates cellular redox status, represses nuclear factor-kappaB signaling, and reduces inflammatory cytokine production in aging. *J Biol Chem* (1998) 273:32833–41. doi: 10.1074/jbc.273.49.32833
71. Guellich A, Damy T, Lecarpentier Y, Conti M, Claes V, Samuel JL, et al. Role of oxidative stress in cardiac dysfunction of PPARalpha-/- mice. *Am J Physiol Heart Circ Physiol* (2007) 293(1):H93–H102. doi: 10.1152/ajpheart.00037.2007
72. Goya K, Sumitani S, Xu X, Kitamura T, Yamamoto H, Kurebayashi S, et al. Peroxisome proliferator-activated receptor alpha agonists increase nitric oxide synthase expression in vascular endothelial cells. *Arterioscler Thromb Vasc Biol* (2004) 24:658–63. doi: 10.1161/01.ATV.0000118682.58708.78
73. Kim MY, Kang ES, Ham SA, Hwang JS, Yoo TS, Lee H, et al. The PPARdelta-mediated inhibition of angiotensin II-induced premature senescence in human endothelial cells is SIRT1-dependent. *Biochem Pharmacol* (2012) 84:1627–34. doi: 10.1016/j.bcp.2012.09.008
74. Zhao S, Li J, Wang N, Zheng B, Li T, Gu Q, et al. Fenofibrate suppresses cellular metabolic memory of high glucose in diabetic retinopathy *via a* sirtuin 1-dependent signalling pathway. *Mol Med Rep* (2015) 12:6112–8. doi: 10.3892/mmr.2015.4164
75. Purushotham A, Schug TT, Xu Q, Surapureddi S, Guo X, Li X. Hepatocyte-specific deletion of SIRT1 alters fatty acid metabolism and results in hepatic steatosis and inflammation. *Cell Metab* (2009) 9(4):327–38. doi: 10.1016/j.cmet.2009.02.006
76. Hayashida S, Arimoto A, Kuramoto Y, Kozako T, Honda S, Shimeno H, et al. Fasting promotes the expression of SIRT1, an NAD+ -dependent protein deacetylase, *via* activation of PPARalpha in mice. *Mol Cell Biochem* (2010) 339(1-2):285–92. doi: 10.1007/s11010-010-0391-z
77. Zarzuelo MJ, López-Sepúlveda R, Sánchez M, Romero M, Gómez-Guzmán M, Ungvary Z, et al. SIRT1 inhibits NADPH oxidase activation and protects endothelial function in the rat aorta: implications for vascular aging. *Biochem Pharmacol* (2013) 85(9):1288–96. doi: 10.1016/j.bcp.2013.02.015
78. Gano LB, Donato AJ, Pasha HM, Hearon CMJr, Sindler AL, Seals DR. The SIRT1 activator SRT1720 reverses vascular endothelial dysfunction, excessive superoxide production, and inflammation with aging in mice. *Am J Physiol Heart Circ Physiol* (2014) 307(12):H1754–63. doi: 10.1152/ajpheart.00377.2014
79. Luo X, Hu Y, He S, Ye Q, Lv Z, Liu J, et al. Dulaglutide inhibits high glucose-induced endothelial dysfunction and NLRP3 inflammasome activation. *Arch Biochem Biophys* (2019) 671:203–9. doi: 10.1016/j.abb.2019.07.008
80. Hung CH, Chan SH, Chu PM, Tsai KL. Quercetin is a potent anti-atherosclerotic compound by activation of SIRT1 signaling under oxLDL stimulation. *Mol Nutr Food Res* (2015) 59(10):1905–17. doi: 10.1002/mnfr.201500144
81. Triggle CR, Ding H. A review of endothelial dysfunction in diabetes: a focus on the contribution of a dysfunctional eNOS. *J Am Soc Hypertens* (2010) 4 (3):102–15. doi: 10.1016/j.jash.2010.02.004

82. Nisoli E, Tonello C, Cardile A, Cozzi V, Bracale R, Tedesco L, et al. Calorie restriction promotes mitochondrial biogenesis by inducing the expression of eNOS. *Science* (2005) 310(5746):314–7. doi: 10.1126/science.1117728
83. Mattagajasingh I, Kim CS, Naqvi A, Yamamori T, Hoffman TA, Jung SB, et al. SIRT1 promotes endothelium-dependent vascular relaxation by activating endothelial nitric oxide synthase. *Proc Natl Acad Sci U S A* (2007) 104(37):14855–60. doi: 10.1073/pnas.0704329104
84. Sun Y, Hu X, Hu G, Xu C, Jiang H. Curcumin Attenuates Hydrogen Peroxide-Induced Premature Senescence *via the* Activation of SIRT1 in Human Umbilical Vein Endothelial Cells. *Biol Pharm Bull* (2015) 38 (8):1134–41. doi: 10.1248/bpb.b15-00012
85. Morrow VA, Foufelle F, Connell JM, Petrie JR, Gould GW, Salt IP. Direct activation of AMP-activated protein kinase stimulates nitric-oxide synthesis in human aortic endothelial cells. *J Biol Chem* (2003) 278(34):31629–39. doi: 10.1074/jbc.M212831200
86. Chen Z, Peng IC, Sun W, Su MI, Hsu PH, Fu Y, et al. AMP-activated protein kinase functionally phosphorylates endothelial nitric oxide synthase Ser633. *Circ Res* (2009) 104(4):496–505. doi: 10.1161/CIRCRESAHA.108.187567
87. Kondo M, Shibata R, Miura R, Shimano M, Kondo K, Li P, et al. Caloric restriction stimulates revascularization in response to ischemia *via* adiponectin-mediated activation of endothelial nitric-oxide synthase. *J Biol Chem* (2009) 284(3):1718–24. doi: 10.1074/jbc.M805301200
88. Csiszar A, Labinskyy N, Pinto JT, Ballabh P, Zhang H, Losonczy G, et al. Resveratrol induces mitochondrial biogenesis in endothelial cells. *Am J Physiol Heart Circ Physiol* (2009) 297(1):H13–20. doi: 10.1152/ajpheart.00368.2009
89. Zhang QJ, Wang Z, Chen HZ, Zhou S, Zheng W, Liu G, et al. Endothelium-specific overexpression of class III deacetylase SIRT1 decreases atherosclerosis in apolipoprotein E-deficient mice. *Cardiovasc Res* (2008) 80(2):191–9. doi: 10.1093/cvr/cvn224
90. Xia N, Strand S, Schlufter F, Siuda D, Reifenberg G, Kleinert H, et al. Role of SIRT1 and FOXO factors in eNOS transcriptional activation by resveratrol. *Nitric Oxide* (2013) 32:29–35. doi: 10.1016/j.niox.2013.04.001
91. Arumugam TV, Kennedy BK. H(2)S to Mitigate Vascular Aging: A SIRT1 Connection. *Cell* (2018) 173(1):8–10. doi: 10.1016/j.cell.2018.03.011
92. Testai L, Citi V, Martelli A, Brogi S, Calderone V. Role of hydrogen sulfide in cardiovascular ageing. *Pharmacol Res* (2020) 160:105125. doi: 10.1016/j.phrs.2020.105125
93. Jiang T, Yang W, Zhang H, Song Z, Liu T, Lv X. Hydrogen Sulfide Ameliorates Lung Ischemia-Reperfusion Injury Through SIRT1 Signaling Pathway in Type 2 Diabetic Rats. *Front Physiol* (2020) 11:596. doi: 10.3389/fphys.2020.00596
94. Ahmed HH, Taha FM, Omar HS, Elwi HM, Abdelnasser M. Hydrogen sulfide modulates SIRT1 and suppresses oxidative stress in diabetic nephropathy. *Mol Cell Biochem* (2019) 57(1-2):1–9. doi: 10.1007/s11010-019-03506-x
95. Wang CY, Zou W, Liang XY, Jiang ZS, Li X, Wei HJ, et al. Hydrogen sulfide prevents homocysteine–induced endoplasmic reticulum stress in PC12 cells by upregulating SIRT-1. *Mol Med Rep* (2017) 16(3):3587–93. doi: 10.3892/mmr.2017.7004
96. Du C, Lin X, Xu W, Zheng F, Cai J, Yang J, et al. Sulfhydrated Sirtuin-1 Increasing Its Deacetylation Activity Is an Essential Epigenetics Mechanism of Anti-Atherogenesis by Hydrogen Sulfide. *Antioxid Redox Signal* (2019) 30 (2):184–97. doi: 10.1089/ars.2017.7195
97. Das A, Huang GX, Bonkowski MS, Longchamp A, Li C, Schultz MB, et al. Impairment of an Endothelial NAD(+)-H(2)S Signaling Network Is a Reversible Cause of Vascular Aging. *Cell* (2018) 173(1):74–89. doi: 10.1016/j.cell.2018.02.008
98. Zhou X, Cao Y, Ao G, Hu L, Liu H, Wu J, et al. CaMKKβ-dependent activation of AMP-activated protein kinase is critical to suppressive effects of hydrogen sulfide on neuroinflammation. *Antioxid Redox Signal* (2014) 21 (12):1741–58. doi: 10.1089/ars.2013.5587
99. Shimizu Y, Polavarapu R, Eskla KL, Nicholson CK, Koczor CA, Wang R, et al. Hydrogen sulfide regulates cardiac mitochondrial biogenesis *via the* activation of AMPK. *J Mol Cell Cardiol* (2018) 116:29–40. doi: 10.1016/j.yjmcc.2018.01.011
100. Tee AR. The Target of Rapamycin and Mechanisms of Cell Growth. *Int J Mol Sci* (2018) 19:E880. doi: 10.3390/ijms19030880
101. Cunningham JT, Rodgers JT, Arlow DH, Vazquez F, Mootha VK, Puigserver P. mTOR controls mitochondrial oxidative function through a YY1-PGC-1alpha transcriptional complex. *Nature* (2007) 450(7170):736–40. doi: 10.1038/nature06322
102. Vergès B, Cariou B. mTOR inhibitors and diabetes. *Diabetes Res Clin Pract* (2015) 110(2):101–8. doi: 10.1016/j.diabres.2015.09.014
103. Zhao D, Yang J, Yang L. Insights for Oxidative Stress and mTOR Signaling in Myocardial Ischemia/Reperfusion Injury under Diabetes. *Oxid Med Cell Longev* (2017) 2017:6437467. doi: 10.1155/2017/6437467
104. Igarashi M, Guarente L. mTORC1 and SIRT1 Cooperate to Foster Expansion of Gut Adult Stem Cells during Calorie Restriction. *Cell* (2016) 166:436–50. doi: 10.1016/j.cell.2016.05.044
105. Ma L, Dong W, Wang R, Li Y, Xu B, Zhang J, et al. Effect of caloric restriction on the SIRT1/mTOR signaling pathways in senile mice. *Brain Res Bull* (2015) 116:67–72. doi: 10.1016/j.brainresbull.2015.06.004
106. Wang RH, Kim HS, Xiao C, Xu X, Gavrilova O, Deng CX. Hepatic Sirt1 deficiency in mice impairs mTorc2/Akt signaling and results in hyperglycemia, oxidative damage, and insulin resistance. *J Clin Invest* (2011) 121:4477–90. doi: 10.1172/JCI46243
107. Maiese K. Programming apoptosis and autophagy with novel approaches for diabetes mellitus. *Curr Neurovasc Res* (2015) 12:173–88. doi: 10.2174/1567202612666150305110929
108. Maiese K. Erythropoietin and mTOR: A "One-Two Punch" for Aging-Related Disorders Accompanied by Enhanced Life Expectancy. *Curr Neurovasc Res* (2016) 13:329–40. doi: 10.2174/1567202613666160729164900
109. Ruiz MA, Chakrabarti S. MicroRNAs: the underlying mediators of pathogenetic processes in vascular complications of diabetes. *Can J Diabetes* (2013) 37:339–44. doi: 10.1016/j.jcjd.2013.07.003
110. Maiese K. Harnessing the Power of SIRT1 and Non-coding RNAs in Vascular Disease. *Curr Neurovasc Res* (2017) 14:82–8. doi: 10.2174/1567202613666161129112822
111. Li Q, Kim YR, Vikram A, Kumar S, Kassan M, Gabani M, et al. P66Shc-Induced MicroRNA-34a Causes Diabetic Endothelial Dysfunction by Downregulating Sirtuin1. *Arterioscler Thromb Vasc Biol* (2016) 36:2394–403. doi: 10.1161/ATVBAHA.116.308321
112. Arunachalam G, Lakshmanan AP, Samuel SM, Triggle CR, Ding H. Molecular Interplay between microRNA-34a and Sirtuin1 in Hyperglycemia-Mediated Impaired Angiogenesis in Endothelial Cells: Effects of Metformin. *J Pharmacol Exp Ther* (2016) 356:314–23. doi: 10.1124/jpet.115.226894
113. Zhou S, Chen HZ, Wan YZ, Zhang QJ, Wei YS, Huang S, et al. Repression of P66Shc expression by SIRT1 contributes to the prevention of hyperglycemia-induced endothelial dysfunction. *Circ Res* (2011) 109:639–48. doi: 10.1161/CIRCRESAHA.111.243592
114. Paneni F, Volpe M, Luscher TF, Cosentino F. SIRT1, p66(Shc), and Set7/9 in vascular hyperglycemic memory: bringing all the strands together. *Diabetes* (2013) 62:1800–7. doi: 10.2337/db12-1648
115. Guo Y, Li P, Gao L, Zhang J, Yang Z, Bledsoe G, et al. Kallistatin reduces vascular senescence and aging by regulating microRNA-34a-SIRT1 pathway. *Aging Cell* (2017) 16:837–46. doi: 10.1111/acel.12615
116. Carlomosti F, D'Agostino M, Beji S, Torcinaro A, Rizzi R, Zaccagnini G, et al. Oxidative Stress-Induced miR-200c Disrupts the Regulatory Loop Among SIRT1, FOXO1, and eNOS. *Antioxid Redox Signal* (2017) 27:328–44. doi: 10.1089/ars.2016.6643
117. Zhao S, Li T, Li J, Lu Q, Han C, Wang N, et al. miR-23b-3p induces the cellular metabolic memory of high glucose in diabetic retinopathy through a SIRT1-dependent signalling pathway. *Diabetologia* (2016) 59:644–54. doi: 10.1007/s00125-015-3832-0
118. Togliatto G, Trombetta A, Dentelli P, Gallo S, Rosso A, Cotogni P, et al. Unacylated ghrelin induces oxidative stress resistance in a glucose intolerance and peripheral artery disease mouse model by restoring endothelial cell miR-126 expression. *Diabetes* (2015) 64:1370–82. doi: 10.2337/db14-0991
119. Rane S, He M, Sayed D, Vashistha H, Malhotra A, Sadoshima J, et al. Downregulation of miR-199a derepresses hypoxia-inducible factor-1alpha and Sirtuin 1 and recapitulates hypoxia preconditioning in cardiac myocytes. *Circ Res* (2009) 104:879–86. doi: 10.1161/CIRCRESAHA.108.193102
120. Ramachandran D, Roy U, Garg S, Ghosh S, Pathak S, Kolthur-Seetharam U. Sirt1 and mir-9 expression is regulated during glucose-stimulated insulin

secretion in pancreatic β-islets. *FEBS J* (2011) 278:1167–74. doi: 10.1111/j.1742-4658.2011.08042.x

121. Strum JC, Johnson JH, Ward J, Xie H, Feild J, Hester A, et al. MicroRNA 132 regulates nutritional stress-induced chemokine production through repression of SirT1. *Mol Endocrinol* (2009) 23:1876–84. doi: 10.1210/me.2009-0117
122. Chung S, Yao H, Caito S, Hwang JW, Arunachalam G, Rahman I. Regulation of SIRT1 in cellular functions: role of polyphenols. *Arch Biochem Biophys* (2010) 501:79–90. doi: 10.1016/j.abb.2010.05.003
123. Iside C, Scafuro M, Nebbioso A, Altucci L. SIRT1 Activation by Natural Phytochemicals: An Overview. *Front Pharmacol* (2020) 11:1225. doi: 10.3389/fphar.2020.01225
124. Milne JC, Lambert PD, Schenk S, Carney DP, Smith JJ, Gagne DJ, et al. Small molecule activators of SIRT1 as therapeutics for the treatment of type 2 diabetes. *Nature* (2007) 450:712–6. doi: 10.1038/nature06261
125. Kitada M, Ogura Y, Koya D. The protective role of Sirt1 in vascular tissue: its relationship to vascular aging and atherosclerosis. *Aging (Albany NY)* (2016) 8:2290–307. doi: 10.18632/aging.101068
126. Aditya R, Kiran AR, Varma DS, Vemuri R1, Gundamaraju R. A Review on SIRtuins in Diabetes. *Curr Pharm Des* (2017) 23:2299–307. doi: 10.2174/1381612823666170125153334
127. Song J, Yang B, Jia X, Li M, Tan W, Ma S, et al. Distinctive Roles of Sirtuins on Diabetes, Protective or Detrimental? *Front Endocrinol (Lausanne)* (2018) 9:724. doi: 10.3389/fendo.2018.00724

Permissions

All chapters in this book were first published by Frontiers; hereby published with permission under the Creative Commons Attribution License or equivalent. Every chapter published in this book has been scrutinized by our experts. Their significance has been extensively debated. The topics covered herein carry significant findings which will fuel the growth of the discipline. They may even be implemented as practical applications or may be referred to as a beginning point for another development.

The contributors of this book come from diverse backgrounds, making this book a truly international effort. This book will bring forth new frontiers with its revolutionizing research information and detailed analysis of the nascent developments around the world.

We would like to thank all the contributing authors for lending their expertise to make the book truly unique. They have played a crucial role in the development of this book. Without their invaluable contributions this book wouldn't have been possible. They have made vital efforts to compile up to date information on the varied aspects of this subject to make this book a valuable addition to the collection of many professionals and students.

This book was conceptualized with the vision of imparting up-to-date information and advanced data in this field. To ensure the same, a matchless editorial board was set up. Every individual on the board went through rigorous rounds of assessment to prove their worth. After which they invested a large part of their time researching and compiling the most relevant data for our readers.

The editorial board has been involved in producing this book since its inception. They have spent rigorous hours researching and exploring the diverse topics which have resulted in the successful publishing of this book. They have passed on their knowledge of decades through this book. To expedite this challenging task, the publisher supported the team at every step. A small team of assistant editors was also appointed to further simplify the editing procedure and attain best results for the readers.

Apart from the editorial board, the designing team has also invested a significant amount of their time in understanding the subject and creating the most relevant covers. They scrutinized every image to scout for the most suitable representation of the subject and create an appropriate cover for the book.

The publishing team has been an ardent support to the editorial, designing and production team. Their endless efforts to recruit the best for this project, has resulted in the accomplishment of this book. They are a veteran in the field of academics and their pool of knowledge is as vast as their experience in printing. Their expertise and guidance has proved useful at every step. Their uncompromising quality standards have made this book an exceptional effort. Their encouragement from time to time has been an inspiration for everyone.

The publisher and the editorial board hope that this book will prove to be a valuable piece of knowledge for researchers, students, practitioners and scholars across the globe.

List of Contributors

Yu Liu, Weilu Huang, Ke-Yu Deng, Yisong Qian and Hong-Bo Xin
Cardiovascular Research Center, Institute of Translational Medicine, Nanchang University, Nanchang, China

Yinfang Guo
Department of Medical Records, The First Affiliated Hospital of Nanchang University, Nanchang, China

Birsen Elibol
Department of Medical Biology, Faculty of Medicine, Bezmialem Vakif University, Istanbul, Turkey

Ulkan Kilic
Department of Medical Biology, Faculty of Medicine, University of Health Sciences, Istanbul, Turkey

Xihong Zhou and Xin Wu
Key Laboratory of Agro-Ecological Processes in Subtropical Region, Institute of Subtropical Agriculture, Chinese Academy of Sciences, Changsha, China

Haiwen Zhang
Key Laboratory of Tropical Animal Breeding and Epidemic Disease Research of Hainan Province, Hainan University, Haikou, China

Liuqin He
Laboratory of Animal Nutrition and Human Health, College of Life Sciences, Hunan Normal University, Changsha, China

Yulong Yin
Key Laboratory of Agro-Ecological Processes in Subtropical Region, Institute of Subtropical Agriculture, Chinese Academy of Sciences, Changsha, China
Laboratory of Animal Nutrition and Human Health, College of Life Sciences, Hunan Normal University, Changsha, China

Jie Song
School of Traditional Chinese Pharmacy, China Pharmaceutical University, Nanjing, China
Affiliated Hospital on Integration of Chinese and Western Medicine, Nanjing University of Chinese Medicine, Nanjing, China

Xiaobin Jia, Xinhong Shi and Liang Feng
School of Traditional Chinese Pharmacy, China Pharmaceutical University, Nanjing, China

Bing Yang
School of Traditional Chinese Pharmacy, China Pharmaceutical University, Nanjing, China
Nanjing University of Chinese Medicine, Nanjing, China

Mingyu Li
Nanjing University of Chinese Medicine, Nanjing, China

Wei Tan
Affiliated Hospital on Integration of Chinese and Western Medicine, Nanjing University of Chinese Medicine, Nanjing, China

Shitang Ma
Life and Health college, Anhui Science and Technology University, Fengyang, China

Raffaele Frazzi
Laboratory of Translational Research, Azienda Unità Sanitaria Locale - IRCCS di Reggio Emilia, Reggio Emilia, Italy

Di Wu
Key Laboratory of Carcinogenesis and Translational Research (Ministry of Education), Beijing Key Laboratory of Protein Posttranslational Modifications and Cell Function, Peking University Health Science Center, School of Basic Medical Sciences, Beijing, China
School of Basic Medical Sciences, Institute of Systems Biomedicine, Peking University Health Science Center, Beijing, China

Yinglu Li and Wei-Guo Zhu
Department of Biochemistry and Molecular Biology, Shenzhen University Health Science Center, Shenzhen, China

Kathy S. Zhu
Peking University Health Science Center, School of Public Health, Beijing, China

Haiying Wang
Key Laboratory of Carcinogenesis and Translational Research (Ministry of Education), Beijing Key Laboratory of Protein Posttranslational Modifications and Cell Function, Peking University Health Science Center, School of Basic Medical Sciences, Beijing, China
Department of Biochemistry and Molecular Biology, Peking University Health Science Center, School of Basic Medical Sciences, Beijing, China

Hanna Artsi, Irina Gurt, Gal Ben Shalom, Einav Cohen-Kfir, Eva Abramowitz and Rivka Dresner-Pollak
Division of Medicine, Department of Endocrinology and Metabolism, Faculty of Medicine, The Hadassah Medical Center, Hebrew University of Jerusalem, Jerusalem, Israel

Madi El-Haj, Leonid Kandel and Ori Safran
Department of Orthopedics, Faculty of Medicine, The Hadassah Medical Center, Hebrew University of Jerusalem, Jerusalem, Israel

Ralph Müller and Gisela A. Kuhn
Department of Health Sciences and Technology, Institute for Biomechanics, ETH Zurich, Zurich, Switzerland

Yifei Zhong
Division of Nephrology, Longhua Hospital, Shanghai University of Traditional Chinese Medicine, Shanghai, China

Kyung Lee
Division of Nephrology, Department of Medicine, Icahn School of Medicine at Mount Sinai, New York City, NY, United States

John Cijiang He
Division of Nephrology, Department of Medicine, Icahn School of Medicine at Mount Sinai, New York City, NY, United States
Renal Section, James J. Peters VA Medical Center, Bronx, NY, United States

Munehiro Kitada and Daisuke Koya
Department of Diabetology and Endocrinology, Kanazawa Medical University, Uchinada, Japan
Division of Anticipatory Molecular Food Science and Technology, Medical Research Institute, Kanazawa Medical University, Uchinada, Japan

Yoshio Ogura and Itaru Monno
Department of Diabetology and Endocrinology, Kanazawa Medical University, Uchinada, Japan

Zheying Min
Beijing Key Laboratory of Reproductive Endocrinology and Assisted Reproductive Technology and Key Laboratory of Assisted Reproduction, Ministry of Education, Department of Obstetrics and Gynecology, Center for Reproductive Medicine, Peking University Third Hospital, Beijing, China
Peking-Tsinghua Center for Life Sciences, Academy for Advanced Interdisciplinary Studies, Peking University, Beijing, China

Jiangman Gao and Yang Yu
Beijing Key Laboratory of Reproductive Endocrinology and Assisted Reproductive Technology and Key Laboratory of Assisted Reproduction, Ministry of Education, Department of Obstetrics and Gynecology, Center for Reproductive Medicine, Peking University Third Hospital, Beijing, China

Jing Xu, Charlie W. Jackson, Nathalie Khoury, Iris Escobar and Miguel A. Perez-Pinzon
Cerebral Vascular Disease Research Laboratories, Department of Neurology, Leonard M. Miller School of Medicine, University of Miami, Miami, FL, United States
Department of Neurology, Leonard M. Miller School of Medicine, University of Miami, Miami, FL, United States

Min Sun
Department of General Surgery, Taihe Hospital, Hubei University of Medicine, Shiyan, China
Department of Anesthesiology, Institute of Anesthesiology, Taihe Hospital, Hubei University of Medicine, Shiyan, China

Mengyu Du, Xingrui Gong, Jin Zha and Hongrui Zhu
Department of Anesthesiology, Institute of Anesthesiology, Taihe Hospital, Hubei University of Medicine, Shiyan, China

Wenhua Zhang
Department of Pharmaceutical Sciences, College of Pharmacy, Hubei University of Medicine, Shiyan, China

Sisi Xiong
School of Nursing, Hubei University of Medicine, Shiyan, China

Peijie Lei
The First Clinical School, Hubei University of Medicine, Shiyan, China

Heng Li and Dong Huang
Department of General Surgery, Taihe Hospital, Hubei University of Medicine, Shiyan, China

Xinsheng Gu
Department of Pharmacology, College of Basic Medical Sciences, Hubei University of Medicine, Shiyan, China

Sergio Liarte and Francisco José Nicolás
Laboratorio de Oncología Molecular y TGFβ, Instituto Murciano de Investigaciones Biosanitarias Arrixaca, Murcia, Spain

José Luis Alonso-Romero
Servicio de Oncología, Hospital Clínico Universitario Virgen de la Arrixaca, Murcia, Spain

Consolato Sergi
Department of Orthopedics, Tianyou Hospital, Wuhan University of Science and Technology, Wuhan, China
Department of Laboratory Medicine and Pathology, University of Alberta, Edmonton, AB, Canada
Department of Pediatrics, Stollery Children's Hospital, Edmonton, AB, Canada

Fan Shen
Department of Laboratory Medicine and Pathology, University of Alberta, Edmonton, AB, Canada

Song-Mei Liu
Center for Gene Diagnosis, Zhongnan Hospital of Wuhan University, Wuhan, China

Shuang Zhou
Internal Medicine, Peking Union Medical College Hospital, Beijing, China

Xiaoqiang Tang
Key Laboratory of Birth Defects and Related Diseases of Women and Children of MOE, State Key Laboratory of Biotherapy, West China Second University Hospital, Sichuan University, Chengdu, China

Hou-Zao Chen
State Key Laboratory of Medical Molecular Biology, Department of Biochemistry and Molecular Biology, Institute of Basic Medical Sciences, Chinese Academy of Medical Sciences & Peking Union Medical College, Beijing, China

Masaaki Yamamoto
Pituitary Center, Department of Medicine, Cedars-Sinai Medical Center, Los Angeles, CA, United States

Yutaka Takahashi
Division of Diabetes and Endocrinology, Department of Internal Medicine, Kobe University Graduate School of Medicine, Kobe, Japan

Biana Shtaif
Sackler School of Medicine, Tel Aviv University, Tel Aviv, Israel
Laboratory for Molecular Endocrinology and Diabetes, Felsenstein Medical Research Center, Petach Tikva, Israel

Shay Henry Hornfeld
Laboratory for Molecular Endocrinology and Diabetes, Felsenstein Medical Research Center, Petach Tikva, Israel

Michal Yackobovitch-Gavan
Sackler School of Medicine, Tel Aviv University, Tel Aviv, Israel
The Jesse Z and Sara Lea Shafer Institute for Endocrinology and Diabetes, National Center for Childhood Diabetes, Schneider Children's Medical Center of Israel, Petach Tikva, Israel

Moshe Phillip and Galia Gat-Yablonski
Sackler School of Medicine, Tel Aviv University, Tel Aviv, Israel
Laboratory for Molecular Endocrinology and Diabetes, Felsenstein Medical Research Center, Petach Tikva, Israel
The Jesse Z and Sara Lea Shafer Institute for Endocrinology and Diabetes, National Center for Childhood Diabetes, Schneider Children's Medical Center of Israel, Petach Tikva, Israel

Xiajie Shi
Department of Endocrinology, Xiangya Hospital, Central South University, Changsha, China
Department of Metabolism and Endocrinology, The Second Xiangya Hospital, Central South University, Changsha, China

Linhua Pi, Shanlei Zhou and Jing Wu
Department of Endocrinology, Xiangya Hospital, Central South University, Changsha, China

Xin Li, Fangyuan Min and Shan Wang
Department of Pharmaceutical Engineering, College of Chemistry and Chemical Engineering, Central South University, Changsha, China,

Zhenqi Liu
Division of Endocrinology and Metabolism, Department of Medicine, University of Virginia Health System, Charlottesville, VA, United States

Fahmida Rasha, Brianyell McDaniel Mims, Isabel Castro-Piedras, Matthew B. Grisham and Kevin Pruitt
Department of Immunology and Molecular Microbiology, Texas Tech University Health Sciences Center, Lubbock, TX, United States

Betsy J. Barnes
Laboratory of Autoimmune and Cancer Research, Center for Autoimmune Musculoskeletal and Hematopoietic Disease, The Feinstein Institutes for Medical Research, Manhasset, NY, United States
Department of Molecular Medicine and Department of Pediatrics, Zucker School of Medicine at Hofstra-Northwell, Hempstead, NY, United States

Rakhshanda Layeequr Rahman
Department of Surgery, Texas Tech University Health Sciences Center, Lubbock, TX, United States

Teng Meng
Shenzhen Key Laboratory for Systemic Aging and Intervention, National Engineering Research Center for Biotechnology (Shenzhen), Medical Research Center, Shenzhen University Health Science Center, Shenzhen, China
Key Laboratory of Optoelectronic Devices and Systems of Ministry of Education and Guangdong Province, College of Optoelectronic Engineering, Shenzhen University, Shenzhen, China
Guangdong Key Laboratory of Genome Stability and Human Disease Prevention, Department of Biochemistry & Molecular Biology, School of Basic Medical Sciences, Shenzhen University, Shenzhen, China

Weifeng Qin and Baohua Liu
Shenzhen Key Laboratory for Systemic Aging and Intervention, National Engineering Research Center for Biotechnology (Shenzhen), Medical Research Center, Shenzhen University Health Science Center, Shenzhen, China
Key Laboratory of Optoelectronic Devices and Systems of Ministry of Education and Guangdong Province, College of Optoelectronic Engineering, Shenzhen University, Shenzhen, China

Index

P

R

S

T

U